11/06

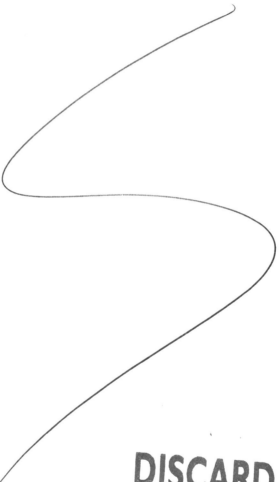

DISCARD

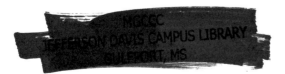

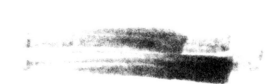

VOLUME

8

Personality Disorders

WPA Series
Evidence and Experience in Psychiatry

Other Titles in the *WPA Series* Evidence and Experience in Psychiatry

VOLUME

8

Personality Disorders

Edited by

Mario Maj
University of Naples, Italy

Hagop S. Akiskal
University of California, San Diego, USA

Juan E. Mezzich
Mount Sinai School of Medicine, New York, USA

Ahmed Okasha
Ain Shams University, Cairo, Egypt

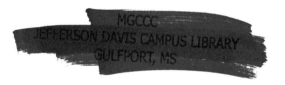

WPA Series
Evidence and Experience in Psychiatry

John Wiley & Sons, Ltd

Other Wiley Editorial Offices

John Wiley & Sons Inc., 111 River Street, Hoboken, NJ 07030, USA

Jossey-Bass, 989 Market Street, San Francisco, CA 94103-1741, USA

Wiley-VCH Verlag GmbH, Boschstr. 12, D-69469 Weinheim, Germany

John Wiley & Sons Australia Ltd, 33 Park Road, Milton, Queensland 4064, Australia

John Wiley & Sons (Asia) Pte Ltd, 2 Clementi Loop #02-01, Jin Xing Distripark, Singapore
129809

John Wiley & Sons Canada Ltd, 22 Worcester Road, Etobicoke, Ontario, Canada M9W 1L1

Wiley also publishes its books in a variety of electronic formats. Some content that appears in
print may not be available in electronic books.

Library of Congress Cataloguing-in-Publication Data

Personality disorders / edited by Mario Maj ... [et al.].
    p. ; cm. - - (WPA series, evidence and experience in psychiatry ; v. 8)
    Includes bibliographical references and index.
    ISBN 0-470-09036-7 (alk. paper)
    1. Personality disorders. I. Maj, Mario, 1953–   II. Series.
    [DNLM: 1. Personality Disorders. WM 190 P4667 2005]
    RC554.P468 2005
    616.85′81--dc22

British Library Cataloguing in Publication Data

A catalogue record for this book is available from the British Library

ISBN 0-470-09036-7 (HB)

Typeset in 10/12 Palatino by Dobbie Typesetting Ltd, Tavistock, Devon
Printed and bound in Great Britain by T.J. International Ltd, Padstow, Cornwall
This book is printed on acid-free paper responsibly manufactured from sustainable forestry
in which at least two trees are planted for each one used for paper production.

In Memory of Paul E. Meehl

Contents

List of Review Contributors

Hagop S. Akiskal   University of California at San Diego, La Jolla, and Veterans Administration Hospital, 3350 La Jolla Village Drive, San Diego, CA 92161, USA

Kareen Akiskal   International Mood Center, University of California at San Diego, La Jolla 92093-0603, USA

Michael Bagby   Laboratory of Personality and Cognition, Intramural Research Program, National Institute on Aging, National Institutes of Health, Gerontology Research Center, 5600 Nathan Shock Drive, Baltimore, MD 21224, USA

Pierre Bovet   Département Universitaire de Psychiatrie Adulte, Université de Lausanne, Hôpital de Cery, 1008 Prilly, Switzerland

C. Robert Cloninger   Washington University School of Medicine, Department of Psychiatry and Sansone Center for Well-Being, Campus Box 8134, 660 S. Euclid, St. Louis, MO 63110, USA

Paul T. Costa   Laboratory of Personality and Cognition, Intramural Research Program, National Institute on Aging, National Institutes of Health, Gerontology Research Center, 5600 Nathan Shock Drive, Baltimore, MD 21224, USA

Lee Daffin   Laboratory of Personality and Cognition, Intramural Research Program, National Institute on Aging, National Institutes of Health, Gerontology Research Center, 5600 Nathan Shock Drive, Baltimore, MD 21224, USA

Deborah Licht   Danish National Research Foundation, Center for Subjectivity Research, University of Copenhagen, Købmagergade 46, 1150 Copenhagen K, Denmark

Hillary Norton   Laboratory of Personality and Cognition, Intramural Research Program, National Institute on Aging, National Institutes of Health, Gerontology Research Center, 5600 Nathan Shock Drive, Baltimore, MD 21224, USA

Josef Parnas   Cognitive Research Unit, University Department of Psychiatry, Hvidovre Hospital and Danish National Research

Foundation, Center for Subjectivity Research, University of Copenhagen, Købmagergade 46, 1150 Copenhagen K, Denmark

Elsa Ronningstam   McLean Hospital, Harvard Medical School, Belmont, MA 02478, USA

Jack Samuels   Laboratory of Personality and Cognition, Intramural Research Program, National Institute on Aging, National Institutes of Health, Gerontology Research Center, 5600 Nathan Shock Drive, Baltimore, MD 21224, USA

Michael H. Stone   Columbia College of Physicians and Surgeons, 225 Central Park West, New York, NY 10024, USA

Peter Tyrer   Department of Psychological Medicine, Imperial College London, Charing Cross Campus, Claybrook Centre, St. Dunstan's Road, London W6 8RP, UK

Preface

This eighth volume of the WPA series "Evidence and Experience in Psychiatry"—the most extensive of the series and the one which took the longest time to complete—reflects the complexity of the ongoing debate on the diagnosis and management of personality disorders.

Many aspects of the current conceptualization and classification of these disorders emerge as problematic from the six reviews, the eighty commentaries and the epilogue composing the book.

The present general definition of a personality disorder is the first of these aspects. On the one hand, it appears debatable whether the "dysfunction-distress" criterion is really fulfilled by all the conditions currently classified as personality disorders (see, for instance, the reviews on the obsessive-compulsive, narcissistic and schizoid disorders), which has obvious consequences for help seeking and adherence to treatment. On the other hand, it seems questionable whether all the above conditions really represent "enduring patterns of experience and behavior", since more than a half of people with a DSM-IV diagnosis of a personality disorder do not show diagnostic stability even over a one-year period.

The issue of the relationship and the boundary between "normal" personality traits and personality disorders is certainly another critical one, recurring in almost all the chapters, and expanding into the debate about the advantages and limitations of a dimensional approach to the classification of these disorders, and on the pros and cons of the dimensional models which have been recently proposed (in particular, Widiger et al.'s five-factor model and Cloninger's tridimensional approach).

Another recurring theme is the mixture of traits, behaviors and symptoms in the current definition of several personality disorders, so that some of them (notably, schizotypal and borderline disorders) appear like "syndromes", which would be better accommodated in the DSM-IV Axis I (analogously to what the ICD-10 has done for schizotypal disorder). This is related to the critical question of the boundary between DSM-IV Axis I and II disorders, which emerges as particularly relevant in the case of Cluster A disorders (with respect to schizophrenia) and Cluster C disorders (with respect to major depression and anxiety disorders).

Finally, the issue of the extremely high frequency of probably spurious comorbidity between the various personality disorders (and in particular between some of them, even belonging to different DSM-IV clusters) emerges repeatedly as an indicator of the questionable validity of current classification systems in this area.

Additional concerns which are expressed more sporadically throughout the book, but appear not less significant, are those about the validity of personality assessments carried out by questionnaires in the absence of any external source of information (will people with obsessive-compulsive or narcissistic personality traits admit these traits when requested directly?); the dramatic cross-cultural variability in the expression of personality traits, in the meaning of these traits and in the "threshold" for pathology; and the impact of experts' opinions and fashions, in the absence of solid empirical evidence, on the history of several personality disorders.

The last chapter of the book deals with the contemporary renaissance of the ancient temperament approach to personology. This approach emphasizes not only what makes an individual vulnerable to emotional excesses or breakdowns, but also the positive adaptive potential in each temperament type. The conceptual model of temperament is vital for clinical work, because it balances countertransference with what makes therapeutic alliance possible.

The overall impression is that of an area in which a significant change in the approach to classification is now overdue. The hope is that this volume will be of some usefulness in this respect, by providing an overview of the research evidence and the possible solutions to the current problems, and allowing a direct comparison of the state of the art for the various groups of disorders.

The other critical area covered in the volume is that of the management of personality disorders. This is a problem which is emerging as extremely important throughout the world: the more widespread becomes the awareness—not only among psychiatrists and other mental health professionals, but also in the general public—of the broad range and high prevalence of personality disorders, the more the current shortage of empirical evidence concerning the treatment of these conditions becomes a matter of concern. This volume emphasizes the need for well-designed studies in this area, but also reviews what has been done up to now, which appears promising even in areas traditionally dominated by pessimism and disenchantment (like that of antisocial personality disorder). The importance of the context where the treatment is carried out and of the therapeutic alliance which is established, when dealing with people with personality disorders, is a recurring theme in this respect.

It has taken more than two years to put this volume together and to amalgamate the various contributions. We hope that this effort will be

regarded as worthwhile by the readers, and that this book will be useful both to researchers, in their current work aimed to re-shape the classification of personality disorders, and to clinicians, in their daily struggle with these complex and demanding conditions.

Mario Maj
Hagop S. Akiskal
Juan E. Mezzich
Ahmed Okasha

Cluster A Personality Disorders: A Review

Josef Parnas[1,2], Deborah Licht[2] and Pierre Bovet[2,3]

[1]*Cognitive Research Unit, University Department of Psychiatry, Hvidovre Hospital, Copenhagen, Denmark*
[2]*Danish National Research Foundation, Center for Subjectivity Research, University of Copenhagen, Denmark*
[3]*Département Universitaire de Psychiatrie Adulte, Lausanne, Switzerland*

INTRODUCTION

Schizoid (SdPD), paranoid (PPD), and schizotypal (SPD) personality disorders together form the so-called Cluster A personality disorders of the DSM-IV classification [1], a cluster that is believed to bear a symptomatic and genetic relationship to schizophrenia. SPD is character-ized by an "odd" pattern of affectivity and cognition, interpersonal isolation, and transient psychotic experiences. Introversion and lack of enjoyment from social relations, but an absence of the affective-cognitive peculiarities and sub-psychotic symptoms found in SPD, dominate the schizoid pattern. The criteria of PPD emphasize a distrustful, guarded attitude and suspiciousness-related interpersonal problems, and a lack of SPD-type peculiarities (for details see the section on clinical aspects). Individuals can be diagnosed with more than one of these disorders (because of the overlapping criteria) and, in clinical samples, SPD and PPD exhibit moderate to high levels of Axis I co-morbidity (especially with depression, anxiety, and substance abuse) [2,3].

The DSM's general definition of personality disorders emphasizes an "enduring pattern of inner experience and behavior that (...) leads to distress or impairment" [1]. As such, a schizoid person defined according to the DSM SdPD criteria (as well as a proportion of individuals with symptom patterns of SPD and PPD) would typically not fulfill such a dysfunction-distress criterion (e.g. one would not seek help from a doctor

Personality Disorders. Edited by Mario Maj, Hagop S. Akiskal, Juan E. Mezzich and Ahmed Okasha.
©2005 John Wiley & Sons Ltd: ISBN 0-470-09036-7

for disliking a talkative environment or because of harbouring a magical conviction).

It is important to realize that, in the ICD-10 [4], schizotypy is *not* a personality disorder, but is rather a *syndrome*, listed just after schizophrenia. This difference between the DSM and the ICD has important implications for clinical diagnosis, which are addressed at the end of this chapter. In an examination of cross-system concordance, diagnostic agreement between the DSM-IV and ICD-10 categories showed good agreement for PPD and schizotypy (PPD: Cohen's $\kappa = 0.74$; schizotypy: $\kappa = 0.66$) and poor agreement for SdPD ($\kappa = 0.37$). The dimensional correlations (Pearson's r) between pairs of the diagnostic criteria sets were much higher (PPD: $r = 0.88$; SdPD: $r = 0.88$; schizotypy: $r = 0.89$) [5].

Although the current literature demonstrates massive research on the construct of schizotypy (including, but not limited to, SPD), SdPD and PPD have not stimulated a corresponding interest, perhaps because of their rarity, and, in the case of SdPD, because of its apparent lack of genetic affinity to schizophrenia. In the following, we shall therefore concentrate on SPD, occasionally (when appropriate) referring to PPD and SdPD, as well as including a summary at the end of this chapter of some of the information pertinent to PPD and SdPD.

Another important issue to note is that modern SPD literature, especially the one dealing with the neurobiological and cognitive correlates of the construct, concerns at least three variants of SPD subjects: patients identified in clinical settings, persons diagnosed in genetic family studies, and "psychometric" samples (usually college students or people recruited through newspapers) recruited on the basis of high scores on self-report questionnaires targeting presumed schizotypal dimensions.

EPIDEMIOLOGY

Descriptive Epidemiology in Non-Psychiatric Populations

In a recent study of a community sample comprising 2053 subjects aged 18 to 65 years in Oslo, Torgersen *et al.* [6] found an overall prevalence of 13.4% for any personality disorder (assessed using the Semistructured Interview for DSM-III-R Personality Disorders, SIDP-R). The figure for the Cluster A personality disorders was 4.1% (PPD: 2.4%; SdPD: 1.7%; SPD: 0.6%; some subjects met criteria for more than one Cluster A personality disorder). SdPD was found to be twice as frequent in men than it was in women (not statistically significantly different). Several personality disorders, particularly those of Cluster A, were diagnosed most frequently in subjects aged 50 and above (a highly problematic finding, considering the general definition of a personality disorder), and were more frequent among less educated subjects, those living without a partner, and those living in the centre of the city.

In a review of previous community studies, Torgersen *et al.* [6] noted considerable variation in the estimated prevalence of Cluster A personality disorders, ranging from 0% to 4.5% for PPD, 0% to 4.1% for SdPD, and 0% to 5.1% for SPD. These figures can be compared with those provided in genetic-epidemiological studies (see Table 1.3), which evaluated the frequency of Cluster A personality disorders in control probands or their first-degree relatives (FDR). However, these control samples are relatively small, and further they are biased, because they often contain multiple members from families. Frangos *et al.* [7] found a rate of 1.68% for Cluster A personality disorders; rates for PPD have ranged from 0.4% [8] to 2.7% [9]; for SdPD, from 0% [9] to 0.5% [10]; and for SPD, from 0.3% [10] to 6.5% [9]. Battaglia *et al.* [11], studying the factorial structure of SPD, using direct diagnostic interviews, found a rate of 0.8% for SPD among non-patients. And finally, Koenigsberg *et al.* [12] examined 2462 patients with general medical conditions; 11 of these patients had PPD (0.4%), none had SdPD, and 48 (1.9%) had SPD, of a total of 885 (35.9%) patients with at least one personality disorder.

As a point of reference, we would like to note here that Meehl [13], drawing on theoretical considerations, suggested a base rate of 0.10 for schizotaxia and predicted that approximately 10% of schizotypes would decompensate into schizophrenia. Moreover, he suggested that close to 2/3 of all psychiatric patients suffered from schizophrenia spectrum disorders.

The Search for Aetiological Factors

Most of the epidemiological studies devoted to aetiological factors of Cluster A personality disorders are concerned with genetics or gene–environment interactions; these are addressed in a separate section, where several aetiological models are also presented.

M. Bleuler [14] suggested that environmental factors, mainly pertaining to family structure, functioning and emotional climate, should not be overlooked as potentially implicated in pathogenetic processes, a position shared by Meehl [15]. Few inquiries found significant correlations between type of familial environment and the development of Cluster A personality disorders or features [16–18]. Other environmental factors have been proposed: Susser *et al.* [19] found prenatal exposure to famine to be a risk factor for SdPD; Venables [20] suggested that maternal exposure to influenza might be related to positive schizotypy scores, whereas cold temperatures might be related to anhedonic traits. The results from the

Copenhagen High Risk study (see below) indicate that high-risk adult offspring with SdPD diagnoses suffered less early environmental stress than did the high-risk subjects who developed schizophrenia [21].

"Co-morbidity"

Epidemiological studies addressing both general and clinical populations find high rates of psychiatric (and somatic) co-morbidities in subjects with personality disorders. In Torgersen et al.'s [6] sample, 29% of those with at least one personality disorder met criteria for at least another one (5.2% met criteria for more than three personality disorders). Similar findings were reported by Stuart et al. [22]. In a clinical sample, Fossati et al. [23] found that over 70% of the patients diagnosed with SPD received one or more additional personality disorder diagnoses; significant positive associations were observed between SPD and both SdPD and PPD. The frequency of Axis I disorders is also elevated (notably for dysthymic and anxious disorders) [24,25]. Moreover, an association between SPD and obsessive–compulsive disorder (OCD) has been observed: in one study approximately 50% of the OCD subjects fulfilled the DSM-IV SPD criteria [26].

Clinical and Operational Diagnosis and Diagnostic Frequency

The pre-operational diagnostic systems offered several unclearly defined possibilities for diagnosing conditions corresponding to SPD (e.g. ICD-8 included latent, pseudoneurotic schizophrenia, schizoid personality, border-line cases), which were used differently at different sites. The introduction of an explicit SPD category into the operational classification systems (such as DSM-III/IV and ICD-10), in principle, should entail a modifying influence on the definitions of all other non-psychotic and non-organic disorders. It is an intrinsic feature of a closed conceptual system (a classificatory system is one typical example) that adding a new concept to it (such as SPD) entails widespread repercussions on the conceptual validity (diagnostic status) of all remaining (non-psychotic) categories. Since no systematic studies were conducted to examine the potential effect of the SPD category on the diagnostic validity of other entities (e.g. anxiety disorders, certain depressions, dysthymic states, dissociative and somatoform disorders, social phobias, and OCD), a clinician using contemporary diagnostic schemes is confronted by many dilemmas and ambiguities. For example, numerous patients with such non-psychotic diagnoses would fulfill the SPD criteria, if these were rigorously applied, and if, as it seems to be the case in the ICD-10, the schizotypy diagnosis hierarchically overrides these other categories.

Recent empirical data from Denmark illustrate that such problems are quite real in the daily clinical use of the schizotypy diagnosis (as a *syndrome* diagnosis). In one study, operational research diagnoses (ICD-10) were assigned to 100 consecutive first admission patients (younger than 40 years of age) at the Department of Psychiatry of Hvidovre Hospital in Copenhagen [27]: 37% were diagnosed with schizophrenia or another non-affective psychosis, 25% were schizotypes, 36% suffered from disorders outside the schizophrenia spectrum, and 2% suffered from organic disorders. Yet, according to the statistics from the Danish Institute of Psychiatric Demography, the frequencies of ICD-10 schizophrenia and schizotypy as the principal *clinical* diagnoses in patients discharged in 2001 and 2002 from seven, mutually independent, psychiatric departments (jointly serving Greater Copenhagen) ranged from a low of 17% (schizophrenia) and 0.4% (schizotypy) to a high of 36% (schizophrenia) and 10% (schizotypy; mean $= 2.7\%$). Thus, the frequency of the schizotypy diagnosis as made by clinicians was incommensurably lower than its strictly operational prevalence. The observed inter-departmental differences cannot be accounted for by socio-economic differences in the catchment area populations, nor was a low frequency of schizotypy diagnosis at a given site reflective of a more frequent use of schizophrenia diagnosis (in the sense that schizotypy simply becomes absorbed by the schizophrenia diagnosis). On the contrary, there was a positive and significant association between the tendencies (high or low) to use both diagnostic categories within each department ($n = 7$; Spearman's rho $= 0.818$; $p = 0.024$). In other words, the less frequent schizophrenia diagnosis was at a given site, the lower the frequency of the schizotypy diagnosis was as well. These findings question a widely held assumption that criteria-based diagnostic systems have improved everyday clinical reliability.

The frequency of the operational DSM SPD diagnosis (in this case, Axis II diagnosis) in patient populations varies across the studies, but generally is lower than 25%. Fossati *et al.* [23] reported that 66% of mixed in/out patients (yet with unclear representativeness) had a personality disorder; the rate for SPD was approximately 5%, and close to 10% among inpatients. In other clinically based studies, prevalence rates of DSM-III-R PPD ranged from 1% to 30% [3], whereas the rates for SdPD ranged from 1% to 16% [28].

EVOLUTION OF THE SCHIZOPHRENIA SPECTRUM AND SCHIZOTYPY CONCEPTS

Although historically several theorists have approached this topic from a truly diachronic perspective [29,30], we attempt here to portray the

evolution of the schizophrenia spectrum concept as a layering or inter-
penetration of different conceptual perspectives, with each perspective
having its own theoretical background and specific focus. The first four
perspectives rely on purported prototypical clinical descriptions, mainly
from third person perspectives, and with the notion of autism at the core of
the described features. The next three approaches address the investigated
phenomena from the patient's (subjective) first person perspective, and
each claims some basic distortion of selfhood and intersubjectivity as
specifying or defining the nature of schizophrenia and its related disorders
(thus addressing the issue of the conceptual [31] or "non-empirical"
validity of schizophrenia spectrum disorders [32]). Finally, the last and
most recent approach addresses the construction of the DSM-III Cluster A
diagnostic categories.

The first thing to be noted is that the very idea of a spectrum of illness is
as old as psychiatry itself. In his "Traité des maladies mentales" from 1860,
Morel [33] pointed to the difficulties encountered in recognizing "the
demarcation line dividing sanity from madness". He observed "temperamental" predispositions to mental illness and acknowledged that if certain
"neuropathic states" were manifestations of the "incubation period of
madness", many people appeared to spend their whole lives in such states,

TABLE 1.1 Outline of the evolution of the schizophrenia spectrum and schizotypy
concepts

Authors	Focus
Earliest descriptions: e.g. Kahlbaum	*Intersubjective* peculiarities of behaviour
Eugen Bleuler	*Autism* as a trait phenomenon: radical intersubjective displacement, clinically manifest in several modalities
Kretschmer	*Autism* and coexisting hyper- and hypo-sensitivity
Zilboorg, Hoch, Polatin, Kety *et al.*	Pseudo-neurotic/borderline schizophrenia: polymorphic features, *disintegration*
Minkowski	*Autism* as a "generative disorder": altered structure of experience
Gadelius, Berze, Gruhle, Blankenburg	*Altered structure* of subjective experience (altered structure of consciousness)
Rado, Meehl	*Schizotypal organization:* anhedonia and proprioceptive diathesis
DSM-III	Operational criteria for *schizoid, paranoid and schizotypal personality disorders*

without ever succumbing to psychosis. This idea was then further elaborated during the next 100 years by numerous authors.

Kraepelin [34], Berze [35], Hoch [36] and many others described some of the relatives of dementia praecox patients as people with eccentric personalities, and used a variety of designations to name these states. "Heboidophrenia" was a term proposed by Kahlbaum [37] in 1890 and "praekatatonia" was another, proposed by Gadelius [38] in 1909. The terms "schizoid personality" and "schizoidia" were informally coined at staff conferences at Eugen Bleuler's clinic around 1910 [14] to denote peculiarities observable in some relatives of schizophrenic patients, as well as the features that seemed to characterize schizophrenic patients premorbidly (i.e. prior to their illness onset).

The concept of schizoidia gave rise to detailed clinical descriptions and very vibrant scientific controversies during the first half of the 20th century. Diem's [39] "simple" schizophrenia, Bleuler's [40] "latent" schizophrenia, and later proposals of "ambulatory schizophrenias" [41], "pseudoneurotic schizophrenia" [42], "schizotypal organization" [15,43,44], "psychotic character" [45], and "borderline schizophrenia" [46] together have formed the conceptual basis for the elaboration of the "schizotypal personality disorder" as it was defined in the DSM-III and its successive revisions.

Prototypical Approaches Linked to the Concept of Autism

Earliest Clinical Descriptions: Intersubjective Peculiarities

The very first and rather loose descriptions, from 1890 to 1920, stressed the schizoids' eccentricity, lack of attunement, seclusiveness, and the difficulties that these people encountered in their relationships with the "outer world" and mainly so in the interpersonal domains.

(...) heboidophrenia (is) characterized (by) deviations of (...) this complex of mental qualities which chiefly constitute the psychic individuality of human beings in social relationships, (...) deviations and unusualness of life's drives, which have to be conceived of as defects (...) of habits (...) [37].

Among the *praekatatonic,* there are a great many who definitively shut their ears to arguments, and are entirely preoccupied with some craze or other (Gadelius, 1910, quoted in [38]).

To this diagnostic group [schizoid psychopathy] belong autistic people, who may appear as curt, cold, often hurting, but (...) who may achieve great success in some specific professions; (...) or odd and eccentric people with strange ideas, which they are unable to justify; (...) and people who fail in all domains, but who do not learn anything neither from what one might tell them, nor from what they encounter in their life [47].

Kretschmer: The "Psychaesthetic Proportion"

In 1921, Kretschmer published a book on bodily and psychological types, written in a particularly brilliant style, which ensured a widespread dissemination of the concept of schizoidia among psychiatrists and psychologists, as well as among the general public. Kretschmer [48] described two fundamental "temperament types" ("schizothymia" and "cyclothymia"), which intrinsically corresponded to the two "endoge-neous" psychoses, schizophrenia and manic-depressive. The transition happened through morbid characterological accentuations, schizoidia and cycloidia respectively. Personality deviation was seen here as a sub-syndromic component on a continuum from normality to psychosis. A fundamental concept introduced by Kretschmer was "psychaesthetic proportion". Schizothymia and schizoidia are not marked by dullness and hyposensitivity or hypersensitivity; rather, they are a mixture of both hypo- and hypersensitivity. Whereas the apparent coldness of schizoids strikes every superficial observer, it is essential, warned Kretschmer, not to overlook a "deeper" level of extreme sensitivity, the constantly wounded, "mimosa-like" nature of the schizoid, whom Kretschmer called "of the Hölderlin type".

> He alone, however, has the key to the schizoid temperament who has clearly recognized that the majority of schizoids are not *either* over-sensitive *or* cold, but that they are over-sensitive *and* cold at the same time, and, indeed, in quite different relational mixtures.

Kretschmer described various "subtypes" of schizoid temperament, determined by varying proportions of hyperaesthetic and anaesthetic dimensions, and other character features such as a liability to outward emotional expression (e.g. a shut-in dreamy type and an acting out type). In schizoids, the psychaesthetic proportion does not fluctuate smoothly, but in a jerking way. Kretschmer noted that, with aging, this proportion is progressively dominated by the anaesthetic pole. Bleuler [49] shared most of Kretschmer's views. But rather than "schizothymia" and "cyclothymia", he proposed the terms "schizoidia" and "syntonia", because, he argued, these modes of reaction do not solely concern affectivity, but cognition as well and, among normal individuals, "cyclothymia" is not cyclic at all. In summary, the important aspects of Kretschmer's contribution are (a) the linking of major psychosis with a corresponding personality disorder; and (b) the conceptualization of schizoidia as intrinsically marked by inconsistent, or even apparently contradictory, hyper- and hypo-sensitivity, a kind of inner discordance that was then pointed out by numerous other authors.

E. Bleuler: The Concept of Autism

Bleuler's elaboration of autism had a major influence on the conceptualization of schizoidia (including Kretschmer's views). Autism was defined as a detachment from outer reality accompanied by the predominance of inner fantasy life, an unfortunate definition that did not account for apparently extraverted schizophrenics or schizophrenics with obvious paucity of mental life [50]. Autism was considered to be diagnostically pathognomonic for schizophrenia (schizoidia and latent schizophrenia as well), although it was seen as secondary from a pathogenetic point of view. Despite its debatable abstract definition, autism was a central clinical concept of pre-World War II psychiatry. It was not a symptom or sign (Bleuler designated it as a "complex fundamental symptom"), but rather a generic term indicating a peculiar intersubjective displacement of a patient with schizophrenia, a displacement that could manifest itself in many domains of behaviour, expression, and experience. This notion of "displacement" points to the fact that the intersubjective functioning or skill is not simply reduced but also qualitatively altered. The patient's world and the shared or intersubjective world are not superposable, but only overlapping by varying degree. Thus, under the heading of autism, Bleuler, Kretschmer and others described a variety of manifestations of this intersubjective deficit: poor ability to enter into contact with others; withdrawal and inaccessibility (in the extreme cases, negativism); indifference; rigid attitudes, opinions and behaviours (the patient was typically unyielding to external influences); overvalued and strongly held strange ideas; existential patterns with an altered hierarchy of values and goals; inappropriate behaviour; idiosyncratic logic and odd ways of thinking; and even a propensity to delusional thinking. Although Bleuler referred to the patient's "inner life" in his definition of autism, all the clinical features were basically described as "third-person" phenomena (i.e. as observable "external" behaviours or "signs"), without systematic attempts to describe the patient's subjectivity and world-view from his/her own perspective.

It is also important to note that the concept of "latent schizophrenia" was not introduced by Bleuler [40] in order to designate yet another clinical subtype within his "group of schizophrenias", but rather in order to capture the constitutional ground, the potentiality of an individual to develop the disease. Such individuals may exhibit any of the autistic features described above, usually in attenuated form: they are often irritable, bizarre, "lunatic", lonely, and may present subtle catatonic or paranoid symptoms in a diluted, masked way. Latent and simple schizophrenia, according to Bleuler, were rarely diagnosed, although they were not infrequent among relatives of schizophrenics and among "reformers of the world, philosophers, writers, and artists" [40].

The diagnostic importance of autism pervades the subsequent clinical descriptions of schizoidia. For a person to be diagnosed as having a schizoid personality (in the assessment of premorbid personality in schizophrenia), Kasanin and Rosen [51] required that all five of the following traits be present: few friends; preference for solitary amusements; shy and a follower in groups; close-mouthed; and extremely sensitive. Kallmann [52], in a study of 2000 offspring of schizophrenic patients, subdivided schizoidia into "eccentric borderline cases" (a precursor of borderline schizophrenia) and "schizoid psychopaths", who were characterized by secretiveness, social withdrawal, and impulsive delinquency of an illogical or senseless nature (subsequently designated as "pseudo-psychopathic" schizophrenia).

Further Descriptions of Autism: Shifting Focus Towards Disintegration

Gradually the focus shifted from strictly behavioural descriptions towards the issues of personality disintegration and disturbed sense of identity, i.e. underlying subtle characteristics of the autistic existence. Several authors [36,53] stressed the peculiarities of schizoid sexuality, ranging from abstinence to chaotic experiences. Psychoanalytic literature also focused on disintegrative aspects of personality. Deutsch [54] described the so-called "as-if" personalities, emphasizing the dissociation between "inner" and "outer" aspects of psychic life, whereas Fairbairn [55] stressed the schizoids' "overvaluation of the internal at the expense of the external world". Zilboorg [41] emphasized chaotic sexuality, hypochondriac complaints, and conflicts with the law. He stressed that the outward appearance of shallowness of affect should not be mistaken for its absence or for some disturbance of the "emotional sphere"; rather, "the emotion appears lacking in the schizophrenic only because that part of his personality which deals with external realities of life (...) acts more as a perceptive registering apparatus (...) and does not seem integrated with his affective, intellectual life". Minkowski [50] summarized this lack of coherence in schizophrenia in the following statement:

Expressions like "discordance" (Chaslin), "intrapsychic ataxia" (Stransky), "intrapsychic disharmony" (Urstein), "loss of inner unity" (Kraepelin), "schizophrenia" (Bleuler) point to the idea that it is not *this* or *that* function that is disturbed, but much more their *cohesion*, their harmonious interplay, in their globality. To make use of an image, the essential disorder does not alter one or many faculties, whatever their order in the hierarchy of functions, but rather resides *between* them, in the "interstitial space" [italics added].

A few years later, Hoch and Polatin [42] described the "pseudoneurotic forms of schizophrenia" (which other psychiatrists called "borderline cases"). They emphasized their similarity to psychopathological pictures observed in recovered schizophrenics and in biological relatives of schizophrenics. In these forms of illness, "the basic mechanisms of schizophrenia" were present, differing "qualitatively and quantitatively from mechanisms seen in the true psychoneuroses". They emphasized that no single symptom was diagnostic of schizophrenia and its pseudoneurotic forms; rather the diagnosis rests on a "constellative evaluation", taking into account quantitative aspects and the simultaneous occurrence of several symptoms. They emphasized the autistic orientation of these patients (yet admitting that "there is no objective way to demonstrate it clinically"), a diffuse and widespread ambivalence, inappropriate emotional connections ("many of these patients show the cold, controlled, and at the same time, hypersensitive reactions to emotional situations"), pan-anxiety, frequent depressions, and anhedonic states, and the presence of subtle formal thought disorder. Hoch and Polatin also noted a chaotic organization of their patients' sexuality with "polymorphous perverse manifestations". Pseudo-neurotic patients may suffer from micro-psychotic episodes characterized by hypochondriac ideas, ideas of reference, and depersonalization.

A "pseudo-psychopathic" variant of these disorders [56], typically encountered in forensic psychiatric contexts, was later described. It applied to seemingly antisocial offenders, who, on a closer evaluation, appeared to harbor autistic features, that also transpired through the nature of their offence, which was typically senseless, illogical or bizarre, and without (even a short-term) personal gain, normally characteristic of criminal conduct.

The US-DK Adoption Studies of Schizophrenia, conducted by Seymour Kety and his collaborators [46], played a decisive role in the formation of

TABLE 1.2. Kety *et al.*'s clinical criteria for borderline or latent schizophrenia

---

Thinking: strange or atypical mentation; the ignoring of reality, logic or experience; fuzzy, murky, vague speech

Experience: brief episodes of cognitive distortion (e.g. transient delusional ideas), feelings of depersonalization, strangeness or unfamiliarity with or towards the familiar; micropsychosis

Affectivity: anhedonia (i.e. never experiences extreme pleasure, never happy); no deep involvement with anyone

Interpersonal: may appear poised, but lacking in depth ("as if" personality); sexual maladjustment (i.e. chaotic fluctuation, mixture of hetero- and homosexuality)

Psychopathology: multiple neurotic manifestations, which shift frequently (obsessive concerns, phobias, conversion, psychosomatic symptoms, etc.); severe widespread anxiety

---

the DSM-III criteria for SPD [30]. Kety introduced the concept of a "spectrum" of pathological conditions aetiologically (genetically) related to schizophrenia:

> We had recognized certain qualitative similarities in the features that characterized the diagnoses of schizophrenia, uncertain schizophrenia, and inadequate personality, which suggested that these syndromes formed a continuum: this we called the schizophrenia spectrum of disorders [46].

Kety's criteria used in the Danish Adoption Study for "borderline schizophrenia" were strongly influenced by Hoch and Polatin's "pseudo-neurotic schizophrenia" [30,46] and are presented in detail in Table 1.2.

The Search for Psychological Organization

Minkowski and the Notion of "Generative Disorder"

Eugène Minkowski was a French psychiatrist influenced by Bleuler (at whose clinic he trained) and by the philosopher Henri Bergson, who, together with William James, provided the first modern (proto-phenomenological) accounts of the structure of consciousness. Minkowski's psychopathological efforts aimed at "bringing back all the richness of symptoms and clinical pictures contained within dementia præcox to a fundamental disorder, and specifying its nature" [50]. This was a task that many, including Bleuler, had already attempted without great success, perhaps because of inadequate conceptual resources. It was a search for something unifying and specific to the schizophrenic disorders. Most psychiatrists agreed on the existence of this something that conferred a conceptual-clinical validity on these disorders in the first place, even though they all had difficulty specifying it in non-trivial propositional terms.

Minkowski rightly realized that such an organizing principle could not be found on the level of symptoms or even symptom complexes. In order to serve as a symptom unifier, it had to be searched for on a deeper level, in the basic infrastructures of the life of consciousness. Minkowski claimed that a mental state was never an isolated free-floating fragment, because it is always a part expressing the whole from which it originates. This whole is the overall structure of subjectivity (life of consciousness). Each anomalous mental state is a condensed presentation of the more basic experiential and existential alterations, comprising, for example, changes in the organization of lived subjective space, in temporalization, or in the elementary relatedness between the subject and his/her world. Each major psychiatric syndrome, says Minkowski, such as schizophrenia or a mood disorder, is characterized by a specific pattern of such basic changes that constitutes its generative disorder ("trouble générateur"). The generative disorder is a subtle phenomenal core transpiring through the individual symptoms, shaping them, keeping them meaningfully interconnected, and constraining their long-term evolution. Minkowski considered autism to be the "trouble générateur" of schizophrenia. But autism was not considered to be a withdrawal to splendid solitude (it cuts across the categories of extra- and introversion), but as a deficit in the basic, non-reflective attunement between the person and his/her world, i.e. a lack of "vital contact with reality". Minkowski defined the vital contact as the ability to "resonate with the world", to empathize with others, the ability to become affected and to act suitably, as a fluid pre-reflective immersion in the intersubjective world: "Without being ever able to formulate it, we know what we have to do; and it is that that makes our activity infinitely malleable and human" [57]. Manifestations of autism involve a peculiar distortion of the relationship of the person to him/herself, and of the person to the world and to other people. There is a decline in the dynamic, flexible, and malleable aspects of these relations, and a corresponding or supervening domination of the fixed, static, rational, and objectified or spatialised elements. Autism is not limited to peculiar expressivity (e.g. lack of emotional rapport or inadequate affective modulation), but transpires as well through the patient's acting and attitudes, reflecting a profoundly changed existential pattern. "Autistic activity" shows itself not so much through its content or purpose as such, but more through an inappropriate manner by which such content or purpose is enacted, a certain friction or inappropriateness with the situational context. The pure form of autism ("autisme pauvre"—poor or empty autism) manifests itself as sterility, lack of attunement to the world, and emptiness, sometimes accompanied by a supervening "morbid rationalism" (abnormal, inflexible or rigid hyper-rational attitude; tendency to hyper-reflectivity, and incapacity for intuitive grasp of the world), whereas autism, as defined by Bleuler ("autisme riche"), is a secondary form, associated with compensatory fantasizing mental activity [58,59]. Minkowski, anticipating the diathesis-stress model, considered schizoidia to be a "constitutionally determined" core phenotype; a transition into overt schizophrenia could be induced by noxious and non-specific environmental hazards.

The Schizotypal Organization by Rado and Meehl

In the midst of massive psychoanalytic domination, Sandor Rado [43] and Paul Meehl [15] pointed to certain limits of the psychodynamic understanding of schizophrenia and its attenuated conditions: both drew attention to the phenotypic manifestations that were so basic that they resisted any further psychological reduction or explanation. Rado coined the term "schizotype" as an abbreviation of "schizophrenic phenotype". Neither Rado nor Meehl viewed schizotypy as inherited, as such. It is therefore a mistake to ascribe to Rado (as is too often the case, e.g. numerous websites, and [30,60]) the coining of the term as an abbreviation of schizophrenic genotype. Within a proposal for a new general conceptual framework for classifying mental disorders, which he called "adaptational psychodynamics", Rado [43] suggested that:

> When we subject (the) gross manifestations of the open (schizophrenic) psychosis to minute psychodynamic analysis, we discover an underlying ensemble of psychodynamic traits that (...) is demonstrable in the patient during his whole life. This finding will define him as a schizotype from birth to death, and will allow us to view his life history as a sequence of schizotypal changes. The ensemble of psychodynamic traits peculiar to the schizotypes may be called *schizotypal organization*.

Two basic inherited deficiencies were underlying schizotypy: an "integrative pleasure deficiency" and a "proprioceptive diathesis". "The first defect manifests itself in a weakness of the motivating power of pleasure; the second, in a propensity to a distorted awareness of bodily self". These defects are viewed "not merely as symptoms, but as the *two central axes of an organization sui generis*". Rado ascribes a central role to the "action-self", "the highest integrative system of the organism, and the very basis of its self-awareness" [44]. Integrative pleasure deficiency reduces the coherence of the action-self, further damaged by the proprioceptive diathesis. Depending on the severity of these innate deficits, on the one hand, and on the extent of the individual adaptive resources over changing life circumstances, on the other hand, schizotypal disorders can manifest various developmental stages of schizotypal organization: (1) compensated schizo-adaptation, similar to schizoidia; (2) de-compensated schizo-adaptation, with the clinical picture of "pseudoneurotic schizophrenia"; (3) schizotypal disintegration, i.e. a schizophrenic psychosis; (4) schizotypal deterioration, i.e. "cessation of certain functions indicative of a progressive withdrawal from any adaptive concern" [44]. At the first manifestations of decompensation, "the organism (...) ceases to have a definite selfhood; (...) the psychodynamic life is now the interaction of a *fragmented* organism with a *fragmented* environment" [43].

Meehl [15] listed four core traits and symptoms as indicators of schizophrenia: formal thought disorder ("cognitive slippage"), interpersonal aversiveness, anhedonia, and ambivalence (all traits being diluted Bleulerian fundamental symptoms). Meehl suggested [15] that an "integrative neural defect" or "schizotaxia" was "the only direct phenotypic consequence produced by the genic mutation" (Meehl maintained a preference for a monogenic theory of schizophrenia). This defect was viewed [13] as "a (ubiquitous) slight quantitative aberration in the synaptic control over the spiking of a neuron".

> I hypothesize that the statistical relation between schizotaxia, schizotypy, and schizophrenia is a class inclusion: all schizotaxics become, *on all actually existing social learning regimes*, schizotypic in personality organization; but most of them remain compensated. (...) What makes schizotaxia etiologically specific is its role as a *necessary* condition. I postulate that a non-schizotaxic individual, whatever his other genetic makeup and whatever his learning history, would at most develop a character disorder or a psychoneurosis; but he would not become a schizotype and therefore could never manifest its decompensated form, schizophrenia [15].

Exploring the First Person Perspective

Although all of the authors mentioned so far certainly paid attention to their patients' spontaneous complaints, only a few specifically embarked on more systematic projects of exploring and describing the patients' typical ways of self-experience and of experiencing the world. Paul Meehl, in one of his last publications [61], drew attention to an "unmistakable phenomenon showing up in a sizable minority of pseudoneurotic patients and in the majority of disintegrated schizotypes":

> I have treated bright, introspective, and psychologically sophisticated individuals with Hoch-Polatin syndrome who complained of an acutely unpleasant mental state but steadfastly refused to accept my proffered labels (e.g. "anxiety", "shame", "guilt", "grief" [object loss], "depression"). I am persuaded that this is not a semantic or defensive matter; rather it reveals the existence of a special kind of negative mental state that I (...) cannot empathize with because I have never experienced anything close to it in a phenomenal space. (...) Here are some [examples] that I can recall: "My whole mind just hurts" (this from a woman—a psychology student—in whom I first noted the symptom some 45 years ago); "It's a bad pressure in the head" (query: a headache?), "No, in my mind, a stress". (...) I conjecture the phenomenon to be *pathognomonic of schizophrenia*, deserving to be listed along with such signs as Bleuler's associative loosening, schizophasia, thought deprivation, bizarre somatic delusions, and extreme perceptual aberrations as nearly sure indicators of the disease [italics added].

Numerous authors considered various phenomena of "depersonalization" to be potential manifestations of schizoidia or "degraded schizophrenia". These phenomena were, and are, typically seen as mere contingent "symptoms". It is only in the writings of those authors who try to comprehend mental disorders from a more overarching framework (e.g. informed by philosophy of mind or phenomenology) that anomalous subjective experiences and distortions of self-awareness are both described in phenomenological detail and related to a more comprehensive approach to pathological alterations in the structure of consciousness. What seemed to Meehl as a novelty, in fact, has been thoroughly described both in early French [62,63] and German literature on schizophrenia and its subclinical variants. The Viennese psychiatrist Josef Berze published a monograph, in 1914 [64], with rich clinical material (vignettes and quotations) to support his claim that the basic disorder of the schizophrenic conditions was to be found in a diminished sense of self-awareness, usually also associated with a panoply of subjective cognitive and perceptual aberrations ("hypophrenia"). Similar ideas were proposed by a Swedish psychiatrist, Gadelius [38], who provided the following quote, illustrative of the disorder of the self:

> "My head is quite choked, when I look down at the paper, it is not as it used to be, it is as if I had to push through my whole head to get down to the paper. All the back of my head received all impressions and

movements instead of being insensible as it ought to be. (...) When it is morning it ought to be felt, but I never have the real feeling of morning. Formerly when I woke up I had the feeling of a new day. I have no ordinary perception. I have only the *thinking process* left."

Gadelius commented:

In the most unmistakable manner she gives expression to her incapability of living fully. "She is only half". She envies other people who can move freely without having to think of their movements, who can walk and stand, dress and have intercourse with their neighbours naturally and freely without giving constant heed to themselves. (...) She is worried by continual uncertainty and embarrassment and feels that she cannot do the simplest thing or make the simplest movement spontaneously and naturally. Everything she does, she has to follow with her thoughts, and accordingly feels uncomfortable and stiff.

Berze and Gruhle, in a remarkable monograph on the "Psychology of schizophrenia" from 1929 [65], considered diminished sense of automatic self-awareness (immediate first person perspective) as the very core feature of the schizophrenia spectrum disorders, ascribing to it the status of the "schizophrenic basic mood" ("schizophrene Grundstimmung"). We describe these phenomena in more detail in the section on the clinical manifestations of SPD.

An important contribution in this particular domain is the work of Wolfgang Blankenburg [66]. His concern, as it was for Minkowski, is to capture the essential features of the transformed experience in schizophrenia. One can characterize Blankenburg's project as an attempt to describe autism from the first person perspective, from the patient's own view and subjective experience. Blankenburg's work integrates contributions of many of his predecessors, especially Bleuler, Minkowski, Berze, and Gruhle.

Blankenburg [66,67] conceives the essence of schizophrenia and its spectrum as a "crisis of common sense" or a "loss of natural self-evidence". He considers common sense or natural self-evidence to be a non-conceptual and non-reflective "indwelling" in the intersubjective world, an automatic pre-understanding of the context and the background, which is a necessary condition for a fluid grasp of the significance of objects, situations, events, and other people. Common sense and basic sense of selfhood are complementary aspects of the subject-world relatedness, and both aspects are typically affected in the schizophrenia spectrum disorders. When natural self-evidence is absent or when the basic sense of selfhood no longer tacitly permeates all experiencing, the world ceases to function as a stable background; the patient lives unnaturally, in a constant interrogative and insecure attitude, and becomes intersubjectively displaced.

Gerd Huber, Joachim Klosterkötter, and their colleagues in Germany have continued systematically this subjectivity-oriented line of research (but with a nomothetic orientation) for the last decades. In a series of long-term studies, they identified not-yet-psychotic, qualitative experiential anomalies in the domain of emotion, cognition, perception, and bodily experience, which they designated as the "basic symptoms". These symptoms were considered "basic" because they precede the psychosis temporally and were believed to be more proximate to the biological substrate than the psychotic symptoms [68–71]. In English-speaking psychiatry, McGhie and Chapman [72] described non-psychotic experi-ential anomalies in young patients with beginning schizophrenia (dividing them into categories nearly isomorphic with the classes of basic symptoms). This work attracted widespread attention and incited an explosive interest in perceptual–attentional disorders in schizophrenia, stimulating efforts to develop psychometric scales for measuring anhedonia and perceptual aberrations.

What was common to the views of Minkowski, Rado and Blankenburg was to link the conceptual validity of the schizophrenia spectrum disorders to the trait-like alterations of closely interdependent infrastructures of consciousness: (a) self-awareness, (b) relatedness to the other, and (c) relatedness to the world (in phenomenological terms: self-awareness, intersubjectivity and intentionality [73]). Although they differed in terminology and in the accent that they assigned to each of these three basic aspects, they all agreed that the conceptual validity of schizophrenia could not be based alone on single clinical symptoms, signs, nor their combinations.

DSM-III: Transforming Prototypes into Categories

In the creation of the DSM-III [74], the psychopathologic content of the classic notion of schizoidia was channelled into the following categories of disorders of personality: schizotypal (peculiar-odd), schizoid ("hypo-esthetic" introvert), avoidant ("hyper-esthetic").

Figure 1.1 schematizes the sources of DSM-III-R "Cluster A" person-ality disorders. DSM-III created three distinct diagnoses to catch the sub-psychotic part of what Kety et al. [46] called the schizophrenia spectrum of disorders; the elimination, during the mid-1970s, of one small word ("of") shifted the view of the relatedness of these disorders, from a prototypical, dimensional conception to that of discrete, categorical entities [75].

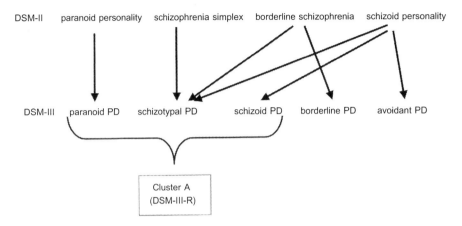

Figure 1.1   Sources of the DSM-III-R Cluster A personality disorders (PD)

Paranoid personality was a well-established concept in classic psychiatry, overlapping schizoidia in some respects, but also very different (e.g. exhibiting a confrontational-combative attitude, keeping the patient attached to the shared world), and it was retained in the DSM-III. Kendler [30], noting that PPD is more common in biological relatives of schizophrenics than in controls (see Table 1.3), wondered whether the features of PPD should be incorporated in the concept of SPD, so that "the latter diagnosis (would) cover all the deviant relatives of schizophrenic patients".

The creation of the SPD criteria by Spitzer *et al.* [76] was based on the clinical descriptions of "borderline schizophrenia" in the US-DK adoption studies [46] (see Table 1.3 for the latest of these studies). From detailed reviews of 36 cases diagnosed as borderline schizophrenia, via a consensus of the principal researchers, research assistants extracted 17 diagnostic items that occurred frequently across the vignettes. These items were then reapplied to these 36 vignettes. Using the eight most frequent items, a cut-off of at least 3 items correctly identified 30 of the 36 patients, but only picked up 2 out of 43 cases unanimously considered by Kety *et al.* to be outside the schizophrenia spectrum (sensitivity, 86%; specificity, 95%). In the first revision of the DSM-III, a ninth item was added to the list of SPD criteria [77].

Kendler [30] pointed out two major "traditions" that have influenced the conceptualization of SPD in DSM-III: a familial approach, emphasizing the traits found in the non-psychotic relatives of schizophrenics, and a clinical approach, focusing on patients demonstrating attenuated phenotypic resemblance to schizophrenia. He argued that the SPD criteria "represent a hybrid including symptoms from both the clinical and familial traditions", mainly because "these criteria were created in an attempt to operationalize the judgments used by Kety and coworkers in diagnosing borderline schizophrenia and not primarily to identify biological relatives of schizophrenic adoptees". However, the distinction between a clinical tradition and a familial tradition does not reflect a historically precise division of scientific labor. In the first half of the 20th century, research and clinical work were very intimately interwoven, and nearly all of the presented authors seem to have based their observations both on the patient studies and the interviews (or conversations) with the relatives. Nevertheless, Kendler's framework raises related important issues, such as trait vs. state and personality vs. syndrome, which are briefly addressed in the concluding section of this review.

GENETIC-EPIDEMIOLOGICAL FINDINGS AND THE DIATHESIS-STRESS MODEL

In a certain sense, a genetic relationship between schizophrenia and the disorders considered to represent its attenuated forms was built into the concept of the "schizophrenic spectrum", because, as noted already, the very concept of spectrum emerged from descriptions of relatives of schizophrenic patients. As early as the first systematic family studies by Rüdin and Kallmann in Germany, it was observed that substantial proportions of biological relatives of patients with schizophrenia exhibited a range of other psychiatric abnormalities in addition to schizophrenia itself.

Table 1.3 summarizes the results from representative twin, adoption, family and high-risk studies with reasonable sample sizes. It also includes two older studies antedating the creation of the DSM-III, but deserving special interest. Thus, in the very first adoption study, Heston [88] observed a familial aggregation not only of schizophrenia but of "schizoid sociopaths" as well. In the famous Maudsley twin study, meticulously analysed and reported by Gottesman and Shields [78], the assessments performed by Essen-Möller (a Swedish psychiatrist invited to join the study because of his widely acknowledged expertise in the domain of "schizoidia") showed nearly complete concordance rates in monozygotic twins, if the schizophrenia spectrum concept was widened to include the deviations considered by Essen-Möller to bear an intrinsic relationship to schizophrenia (deviations which Essen-Möller was unable to operationalize).

Nearly all other studies show a significant relationship between schizophrenia and SPD. There are, however, findings that deviate from the main line of evidence: Coryell and Zimmerman [80] failed to detect familial aggregation of schizophrenia and SPD altogether, whereas two other studies showed similar risks for SPD in the relatives of schizophrenic and affective probands [10,87,91]. However, in the sample B of the New York High-Risk Project, the SPD aggregated selectively in the relatives of schizophrenia (morbid risk: subjects at high risk for schizophrenia = 14.1% [5 out of 35]; subjects at high risk for affective disorders = 3.1% [1 out of 32]; controls = 3.3% [2 out of 61]) [92]. Apart from the above discrepant findings—most likely methodologically determined (the most important factor probably being the degree of sensitivity of psychiatric assessment: e.g. in the Coryell and Zimmerman study, 70% of the subjects were assessed through telephone questioning; see also Kendler's review [93])—the majority of studies point to a clear and specific familial relationship between SPD and schizophrenia. In general, the studies seem to indicate that SPD is more frequent than schizophrenia itself. PPD and, especially, SdPD appear to be so infrequent in the relatives of index probands and control populations that they often elude the possibility of statistical comparisons. Some of the studies in Table 1.3 show, however, a statistically significant familial link between schizophrenia and PPD. In addition, one study showed a significant familial link between PPD and SPD [94], whereas a reanalysis of the earlier data from the Copenhagen part of the US-DK adoption studies, using DSM-III diagnoses, revealed a significant familial connection between chronic schizophrenia and PPD [95].

One important issue to consider when evaluating the recent studies applying the DSM criteria is whether they conform to or waive the distress-dysfunction criterion, which is the first requirement for any personality disorder diagnosis (the DSM is primarily a clinical tool). The studies in question typically do not address this issue, but it is most likely that they have incorporated this entry criterion. This has probably attenuated the rates, because well-functioning subjects with full symptomatic schizotypal picture would not be included as informative cases.

A strong confirmation of the purported genetic relationship between schizophrenia and SPD stems from two studies that show an elevated frequency of schizophrenia in the relatives of SPD probands [81] and two other studies that show increased risk of schizophrenia in the siblings of schizophrenia index probands, if the parental diagnosis is SPD [9,84,96]; a similar finding was reported in the Copenhagen High-Risk Study [97], which demonstrated increased risk for the schizophrenia spectrum disorders in the offspring as a function of parental assortative mating.

Finally, findings from the emerging molecular genetic studies that show positive linkage results when using SPD as an informative phenotype, in addition to schizophrenia itself, add to the validity of a schizophrenia-SPD genetic connection [98,99].

A recent, thorough, and the most extensive of the family studies (the Roscommon Family Study), carefully conducted in Ireland by Kenneth

Kendler and his Irish and US collaborators [100], provides perhaps the most solid and detailed information on the issue of the composition and the nature of the schizophrenia spectrum disorders (see Table 1.3). We will therefore present some of the conclusions from this study in detail, as being, in a provisional sense, the most informative on the issues concerning the genetics of the schizophrenia spectrum of disorders:

(1) The Roscommon Study does not support the idea that affective illness and schizophrenia are on a single aetiologic continuum [101].
(2) SPD belongs to a spectrum of disorders related to schizophrenia, with a strong familial transmission [8].
(3) The liability to schizophrenia spectrum disorders in probands and their first-degree relatives is 0.36, a correlation that (assuming the genetic factors to be mainly responsible for familial aggregation) is approximately half of the heritability of the disorder (typically estimated to be around 0.70). This liability correlation was found to converge with independently obtained results in four family studies [102,103].
(4) The model of transmission that best fits the Roscommon data is a multifactorial threshold model of the same underlying vulnerability. The threshold for manifesting SPD is lower than the threshold for typical schizophrenia, but is not clearly distinguishable from the thresholds for other, non-affective psychoses and the schizo-affective disorder. The conclusions on the mode of inheritance are concordant with the predominant views on the mechanisms of genetic transmission that are derived from the joint evidence stemming from family, twin and adoption studies [104].

Alternative, monogenic or mixed transmission models have surfaced regularly in the literature. Heston [105] spoke of a dominantly transmitted "schizoid disease". More recently, the so-called "latent trait model" (LTM) has been proposed by Holzman and his colleagues to account for the distribution of schizophrenia and eye movement disorders in a Norwegian twin sample (more specifically, to account for the fact that eye tracking disorder and schizophrenia segregate in partial independence [106]). According to the LTM, the transmission mode is autosomal dominant with low penetrance and results in a "latent trait", a hypothetical underlying neural deficit that is inherited, but which may remain phenotypically mute or manifest itself pleiotropically as partially independent phenotypes, such as eye movement dysfunction, schizophrenia, or schizotypy.

One framework for aetiological consideration, compatible with several genetic models, is based on Meehl's paradigmatic triad: schizotaxia (inherited)—SPD (core phenotype)—schizophrenia (de-compensated schizotypy). In this paradigm, SPD is considered to be the core clinical phenotype that all schizotaxic individuals acquire regardless of rearing regimes. Schizophrenia, on the other hand, is considered a condition caused by additional polygenetic influences and environmental stress factors, in brief (and for pragmatic purposes), as largely an environmentally decompensated schizotypy. This model was successfully applied to the data analyses in the Copenhagen HR study: in schizophrenia-SPD comparisons, the SPD cases had fewer obstetric complications, had less exposure to institutional rearing in childhood, had no cerebral ventricular enlargement, but equalled schizophrenia in cortical abnormalities [107–111]. Moreover, the study suggested a second-order interaction between the level of genetic risk for schizophrenia and the effect of obstetric complications on the origins of adult ventricular enlargement [112]. Cannon *et al.* [113] replicated the high-risk morphological findings in a Finnish family study (schizophrenia exhibited cortical deficits and ventricular enlargements, whereas non-schizophrenic relatives were spared from ventriculomegaly, but displayed cortical anomalies similar to those found in schizophrenics). In the Finnish adoption study [114], the risk of adult schizophrenia spectrum disorder in the adoptee was a function of an interaction between genetic vulnerability and dysfunctional rearing environment.

An important question confronted by this paradigm is the extent to which a patient with schizophrenia is premorbidly deviant, in the sense of resembling an SPD patient (which was one of the main assumptions behind the original concept of schizoidia). Data analyses from the Copenhagen High-Risk Study support such temporal evolution: disorders of affect and emotional rapport, isolation, and subtle formal thought disorder distinguished adolescent high-risk offspring who later developed schizophrenia spectrum disorders from those who did not [107,115,116]. Pre-schizotypal subjects were especially characterized by passivity, disengagement, and hypersensitivity [117]. In the New York High-Risk Project, premorbidly measured attentional deficits were found to predict later anhedonia, which in turn antedated schizotypal features [118]. Moreover, elevated levels of formal thought disorder and negative features predicted schizophrenia-related adult psychoses [119]. In an Israeli draft study [120], an SPD diagnosis at the time of draft assessment (a very rare occurrence) predicted later schizophrenia, and in Klosterkötter *et al.*'s [71] prospective study of non-psychotic patients, an SPD diagnosis (also an infrequent event) was likewise predictive of subsequent schizophrenia. Retrospective studies of schizophrenic patients [121] show that the vast majority of patients with schizophrenia exhibit personality deviations with avoidant, paranoid, schizoid, and schizotypal traits. There is also evidence that specific premorbid dimensions may selectively associate with dimensions of adult psychopathology, e.g. schizoid or schizotypal traits with negative

TABLE 1.3 Summary of selected genetic-epidemiologic findings

Study	Sample characteristics	Diagnosis	Main results
Gottesman and Shields [78]	24 MZ and 33 DZ twin pairs (114 individuals)	Blind diagnoses of case summaries by Essen-Möller, using his own continental concept of schizophrenia spectrum	For typical schizophrenia and schizophrenia-like psychosis, MZ pair-wise concordance 67%, DZ pair-wise concordance 11%. All unaffected co-twins of MZ index twins with typical schizophrenia exhibited "schizoid character traits" without inflating DZ concordance.
Torgersen [79]	44 SPD, 15 mixed SPD-BPD, and 10 BPD twin probands and 69 control twins	DSM-III criteria. Interviews performed by the author and consisting of the PSE and a personality questionnaire	Concordance for SPD was 33% in MZ co-twins of SPD index twins and 4% in DZ co-twins of SPD index twins. No co-twin of SPD index twin had BPD.
Frangos et al. [7]	572 FDR of schizophrenia probands and 694 FDR of controls	DSM-III criteria. Unstructured clinical interviews performed by psychiatrists	MR among FDR of probands: schizophrenia = 3.97%, cluster A = 5.23% compared respectively to controls: 0.58% ($p = 0.005$) and 1.68% ($p = 0.005$)
Baron et al. [9]	376 FDR of schizophrenia and 374 FDR of controls	RDC and DSM-III criteria. Interviews by "mental health professionals" with the SADS-L	MR for schizophrenia 5.8–7.4%. MR for definite SPD (values for control relatives in brackets): 14.6% (2.1), probable SPD: 12.2% (6.5), SdPD: 1.6% (0), PPD: 7.3% (2.7). Probable, definite SPD and PPD aggregate significantly among relatives of patients with schizophrenia.
Baron et al. [9]	Proband-sample identified through a screening of college students. 576 FDR of SPD probands, mixed SPD-BPD, pure BPD and controls	RDC and DSM-III criteria. SADS and Schedule for Interviewing Borderlines, performed by "mental health professionals". Unavailable subjects assessed by Family History Method.	SPD and BPD breed true (MR 12% and 11.7% respectively). No schizophrenia among 56 relatives of pure SPD probands

Study	Sample	Methods	Results
Coryell and Zimmerman [80]	Group 1: 120 FDR of psychotically depressed; Group 2: 188 FDR of depressed schizoaffectives; Group 3: 80 FDR of schizophrenics; Group 4: 185 FDR of control subjects free of any mental illness	DSM-III criteria. DIS and SIDP Lay interviewers, interviews mainly by telephone (70%)	MR for Cluster A (SPD in brackets) in groups 1 = 1.9 (1.9); 2 = 7.6 (5.3); 3 = 5.6 (2.8); 4 = 2.5 (2.5). Differences are non-significant. Lack of significant familial aggregation of schizophrenia (MR = 1.4%)
Battaglia et al. [81]	93 FDR of 21 SPD clinical probands, 111 FDR relatives of 21 non-SPD clinical probands and 201 FDR of 42 medical controls. SPD and non-SPD probands were matched for Axis I disorder	DSM-III criteria. SADS-L and SIDP interviews performed by psychiatrists and residents	MR for schizophrenia was 4.64% in relatives of SPD probands; 1.06% in relatives of non-SPD probands and 0.6% among control relatives. Among 21 SPD clinical probands, 5 (23.8%) were co-morbid for PPD; 2 (9.5%) non-SPD clinical probands had PPD diagnosis
Onstad et al. [82]	215 FDR (parents and siblings) of 88 index twins (59 with schizophrenia, 20 with mood disorder and 9 with non-affective psychosis)	DSM-III-R criteria. SCID-I and II interviews by trained non-clinicians (?) taped for assessment of reliability	MR in relatives of schizophrenics: schizophrenia = 7.4% ($p<0.001$ vs. relatives of mood disordered twins), SdPD = 1%, PPD = 5%, SPD = 7% ($p<0.05$ vs. relatives of mood disordered twins)
Torgersen et al. [83]	176 non-schizophrenic co-twins and other FDR of schizophrenic probands were compared with 101 co-twins and other FDR of probands with major depression	DSM-III-R criteria. SCID-I and II. No information on the raters' training	MR (MR for relatives of depressed in brackets) for cluster A: PPD = 6.8% (4%), SdPD = 2.3% (2%), SPD = 9.7 (1%, $p = 0.01$)
Maier et al. [10]	Probands in-patients ($n = 330$) with schizophrenia, schizophreniform disorder, schizoaffective disorder and unipolar depression, 109 control families. A total of 1257 FDR face-to-face examination	DSM-III-R criteria. SADS-L and SCID-II, administered by trained lay persons	MR for schizophrenia = 5.2% in FDR of schizophrenic probands (RDC diagnosis). MR for relatives of schizophrenic probands (values for control relatives in brackets): PPD: 1.7% (0.9), SdPD: 0.7% (0.5), SPD: 2.1% (0.3) $p<0.05$. No difference in MR for SPD between FDR of schizophrenic and depressed patients

(continued)

TABLE 1.3 *(continued)*

Study	Sample characteristics	Diagnosis	Main results
Kendler *et al.* [84]	534 probands (415 face-to-face interview) and 2043 living FDR (1753 face-to-face interview) and a random sample of 150 unscreened control families (580 subjects face-to-face interview)	DSM-III-R criteria. SCID and SIS. Probands assessed by psychiatrists. Relatives assessed by trained non-clinicians	MR for schizophrenia is 6.5% in relatives of schizophrenic probands and 6.9% in relatives of SPD probands. In relatives of schizophrenic probands MR for SPD = 6.9%, for PPD = 1.4 (in comparisons with controls p values are <0.001 and 0.05). The risk for schizophrenia and SPD in the siblings of probands with a spectrum disorder increased if a parental diagnosis was SPD
Asarnow *et al.* [85]	148 FDR of probands with childhood onset schizophrenia (COS), 369 FDR of ADHD patients and 206 community controls	DSM-III-R criteria. DIS and SADS mainly performed by clinicians	MR for schizophrenia and SPD among parents of COS 4.95% and 4.21% respectively, compared to MR among parents of ADHD 0.45% ($p = 0.02$) and 0.9% ($p = 0.05$) respectively, and to no schizophrenia or SPD in community controls ($p = 0.01$; $p = 0.02$). No differences for PPD
Parnas *et al.* [86]	207 offspring of severely schizophrenic mothers (HR) and 104 control children (LR) matched on age, sex, paternal socioeconomic status and amount of time spent in institutional rearing	DSM-III-R criteria. Samples systematically examined at 15, 20, 25, 33 years of age (only a HR subsample) and 40 years. Senior clinicians with the PSE, SADS-L and PDE performed the three most recent follow-ups. Follow-ups were nearly complete with respect to attrition.	Life-time hierarchical diagnoses: HR: schizophrenia = 16.2%, total Cluster A = 21.9%. LR: schizophrenia = 1.9% ($p = 0.0001$), total Cluster A = 2.9% ($p = 0.0001$). Non-hierarchical Cluster A disorders among HR and LR groups: SPD = 20.8% vs. 5%, $p = 0.0001$; SdPD = 10.9% vs. 0%, $p = 0.01$; PPD = 4.2% vs. 0%, $p = 0.05$. In hierarchical diagnosis 20 out of 21 SdPD and 1 out of 2 PPD were absorbed by the SPD category. Paternal spectrum diagnosis increased the likelihood of spectrum disorders in the offspring

Study			
Erlenmeyer-Kimling et al. [87]	63 offspring of at least one schizophrenic parent and 43 offspring of affective (unipolar and bipolar) parent, and 100 controls geographically matched. Families had to be intact at inclusion	DSM-III-R criteria. Six examinations, the latest at the age of 31; the three most recent follow-ups with SADS-L and the latest with PDE as well. Lay interviewers	HR for schizophrenia: schizophrenia = 11.1%; affective disorders = 3.7%; SPD = 4.5%, PPD = 6.8%, SdPD = 6.8%. HR for affective disorders: schizophrenia = 0%; affective disorders = 4.9%; SPD = 2.8%, PPD = 8.3%, SdPD = 0%. Controls: schizophrenia = 1.1%; SPD = 0%, PPD = 1.1%, SdPD = 0%
Heston [88]	47 adopted away offspring of chronic schizophrenia mothers (separated within 3 days after birth) and 50 adopted away offspring (matched to index adoptees on sex, type of placement, and amount of institutional rearing) of mothers with no psychiatric history	Clinical follow-up until the age of 36 by the author ("pre-operational" clinical diagnoses)	Offspring of schizophrenics: schizophrenia = 5 (10.6%), "schizoid sociopath" = 8 (15%), "sociopathic personality" = 1 (2%), neurotic personality = 13 (27%). Offspring of controls: schizophrenia = 0, "schizoid sociopath" = 0, "sociopathic personality" = 2 (4%), neurotic personality = 7 (14%)
Kety et al. [89]	279 biological and 111 adoptive relatives of 47 adoptees with chronic schizophrenia, 237 biological and 117 control adoptees	Interviews performed by senior clinicians using SADS-L as well as additional checklists. Final diagnoses (Bleulerian criteria) assigned at a consensus discussion between interviewers and principal investigators	MR among relatives of chronic schizophrenics (values for the adoptive relatives of chronic schizophrenia appear in brackets): chronic schizophrenia = 5% (0), latent schizophrenia = 10.8% (1.8), SdPD (not equivalent to DSM-III concept) = 5.7% (0.9), PPD = 1.4% (0)
Tienari et al. [90]	186 adopted away offspring of schizophrenic/paranoid mothers (76% fulfilling DSM-III-R criteria for schizophrenia) and 203 adopted away offspring of 201 unscreened mothers (3.5% had a spectrum diagnosis)	DSM-III-R criteria. Adoptees examined twice, latest at median age of 36 years, by face-to-face interviews performed by psychiatrists using the PSE, SCID-II and SIS	MR for offspring of schizophrenics (corresponding values for control offspring in brackets): schizophrenia = 6.7% (2%; $p = 0.027$), schizoaffective disorder = 0.6% (0), schizophreniform disorder = 0.6% (0), SPD = 2.4% (0). Subtotal narrow spectrum 10.4% vs. 2%, $p < 0.001$. SdPD = 2.4% (1%), PPD = 0.6% (0.5%)

ADHD, attention-deficit/hyperactivity disorder; BPD, borderline personality disorder; DIS, Diagnostic Interview Schedule; DZ, dizygotic; FDR, first-degree relatives; HR, high risk; LR, low risk; MR, morbid risk; MZ, monozygotic; PDE, Personality Disorders Examination; PPD, paranoid personality disorder; PSE, Present State Examination; RDC, Research Diagnostic Criteria; SADS-L, Schedule for Affective Disorders and Schizophrenia, Lifetime; SCID-I, Structured Clinical Interview for DSM-IV Axis I Disorders; SCID-II, Structured Clinical Interview for DSM-IV Axis II Personality Disorders; SdPD, schizoid personality disorder; SIDP, Semistructured Interview for DSM-III Personality Disorders; SIS, Structured Interview for Schizotypy; SPD, schizotypal personality disorder symptoms; antisocial traits with disorganization [122–124]. Some clinical studies point to a symptomatic overlap between pre-schizotypal states in childhood and the Asperger's syndrome [125,126].

Unfortunately, the studies in this group are not directly comparable. Yet, a conclusion can be drawn nevertheless: a substantial proportion of patients with schizophrenia premorbidly displays (a) some of the SPD features in different degrees and combinations, or (b) the features of the neighbouring personality disorders (SdPD, PPD, and avoidant personality disorder).

DIMENSIONS OF PSYCHOPATHOLOGY

Table 1.4 presents in detail selected factor or cluster analytic studies of the dimensionality of schizotypy. This approach was first applied to psychiatric data (a correlational matrix) in 1930. In 1948 it was proposed [146] that schizophrenic symptomatology could be accounted for by 3 factors: (1) "schizoid withdrawal", (2) "paranoid projection" and (3) "heboid regression". These correspond to the contemporary designations of negative, positive, and disorganized symptoms. It needs to be noted that mathematically derived dimensions of psychopathology are often less a discovery than a confirmation of the clinically motivated reiterations of essential or major psychopathological facets, considered in the first place by clinicians to reflect or define the nature of the disorder in question (unless the analysed item pool also contains non-clinical data).

Most of the recent studies agree about the presence of three or four factors. Researchers largely agree on the presence of a positive dimension, characterized by unusual perceptual experiences and magical ideation, as well as a negative dimension, with varying composition and characterized mainly by anhedonia (social and/or physical). The content of the third and fourth factors is more disputed (with some agreement that disorganization and suspiciousness are the third and fourth dimensions, respectively). There is thus a parallelism between the dimensional models of schizotypy and those of schizophrenia. However, the designating labels of a given dimension may be misleading. For example, the so-called "negative dimension" of schizotypy is frequently tapped by Chapman *et al.*'s scales of anhedonia (Physical Anhedonia Scale and Revised Social Anhedonia Scale), whereas the negative symptomatology of schizophrenia comprises many more features. Moreover, anhedonia is not actually part of the diagnostic criteria of schizotypy (for a discussion, see [143]). Variability of findings is largely related to the use of different instruments (Tables 1.5 and 1.6), and to the composition of the investigated samples (ranging from normal students to severely ill psychiatric patients). One recent study of relatives of schizophrenic probands ([137]; see Table 1.4) included neurocognitive measures in the factor analysis. They detected a disorganization dimension composed of odd or eccentric behaviour and deficits in attention and perception.

Many studies on the dimensions of schizotypal symptomatology emphasize the heritability of the so-called "negative" schizotypy (pioneered by Gunderson et al. [168]), rather than its "positive", subpsychotic or cognitive-perceptual features (however, Vollema et al. [169] suggest that positive dimensions of Schizotypal Personality Questionnaire reflect the genetic vulnerability to schizophrenia). Results from such studies should be viewed with caution: the pattern of results that emerges will always depend on the size of the studied samples and on the phenomenological detail and scope of the investigated phenomena.

Also in this research domain, the Roscommon study presents detailed information [170]. In a multivariate analysis of six (factor analytically derived) dimensions of SPD, four dimensions remained significant when tested together: "negative" (poor rapport, aloofness-coldness, guardedness, odd behaviour), social dysfunction (lack of motivation, occupational status below expected), social isolation (isolation, social anxiety, and hypersensitivity), and formal thought disorder (odd speech, cognitive slippage). These four dimensions accurately characterized relatives of schizophrenic probands compared with the relatives of matched controls. Of the 12 items composing these dimensions, nine were signs and three were (self-reported) symptoms. Kendler et al. concluded that signs observed by trained interviewers were more powerful at detecting personality traits related to schizophrenia than were self-report measures. In a separate analysis, Fanous et al. [171], using the Roscommon data, concluded that positive and negative symptoms in schizophrenic probands respectively correspond to positive and negative schizotypal features in their relatives, suggesting perhaps that these factors are aetiologically distinct from each other. Moreover, negative symptoms in probands predicted more schizotypal features in their relatives, which is coherent with the generally accepted notion that negative symptoms have a stronger familial basis than positive symptoms.

Torgersen et al. [172] compared 14 subjects with SPD who were monozygotic co-twins or first-degree relatives of schizophrenic patients with 29 subjects with SPD who were not related to schizophrenics. All schizotypal features were found in both schizotypal groups. However, negative, eccentric schizotypy was more frequent in the familial group and positive schizotypy in the second group. Additional observations on schizotypal features were made on monozytic and dizygotic twins, and other first-degree relatives of schizophrenics ($n = 195$), schizotypes who were not relatives of schizophrenics ($n = 70$), and patients with other psychiatric disorders ($n = 349$). In these comparisons, inadequate rapport,

TABLE 1.4 Main factor or cluster analytic studies of schizotypy

Study	Measure(s)	Sample	Factors type
Battaglia et al. [11]	SIDP-R	538 outpatients 225 controls	1. cognitive/perceptual; 2. interpersonal; 3. oddness
Bentall et al. [127]	(a) CSTQ (b) CSTQ+DSSI	180 subjects from general population	(a) 1. positive psychotic symptomatology; 2. negative psychotic symptomatology; 3. cognitive disorganization/social anxiety (b) idem + 4. disinhibited or asocial schizotypy
Bergman et al. [128]	SIDP	213 patients	1. cognitive perceptual; 2. interpersonal; 3. paranoid
Claridge et al. [129]	CSTQ (420 items)	1095 subjects from general population	1. aberrant perceptions and beliefs; 2. cognitive disorganization; 3. introvertive anhedonia; 4. asocial behaviour
Fossati et al. [23]	SCID-II	564 patients	(latent class analysis of criteria for SPD) 1. no close friends or confidants, odd thinking, suspiciousness, inappropriate affect; 2. ideas of reference, magical thinking, unusual perceptual experiences, suspiciousness; 3. suspiciousness, ideas of reference, no close friends
Gruzelier et al. [130]	SPQ	122 medical students	1. no close friends, social anxiety, blunted affect, suspiciousness; 2. unusual perceptual experience, odd beliefs, ideas of reference, suspiciousness; 3. eccentric behaviour, odd speech
Gruzelier [131]	(a) SPQ, (b) SPQ+EPQ+PhA	(a) 151 medical students (b) idem+sample of Gruzelier et al. [144]	(a) 1. no close friends, social anxiety, constricted affect, suspiciousness; 2. unusual perceptual experience, odd beliefs, ideas of reference, suspiciousness; 3. eccentricity, odd speech. (b) Idem + 4. neuroticism, social anxiety, suspiciousness
Handest and Parnas [132]	Semi-structured interview with various scales	100 non psychotic patients, among them 50 with ICD-10 schizotypal disorders	(ICD-10 criteria) 1. interpersonal/negative; 2. disorganized; 3. perceptual/positive; 4. paranoid
Kendler et al. [133]	SIS + SRQ	29 twin pairs from general population	SIS: 1. positive symptom schizotypy; 2. negative symptom schizotypy. SRQ 1. positive trait schizotypy; 2. trait anhedonia. Correlations between SIS 1 and SRQ 1, as well as between SIS 2 and SRQ 2
Kendler and Hewitt [134]	SRQ	400 twins from general population	1. positive trait schizotypy; 2. nonconformity; 3. social schizotypy

Study	Instrument	Sample	Factor solution
Livesley and Schroeder [135]	Own scales	274 subjects from general population, 133 outpatients with PD	1. social avoidance; 2. perceptual-cognitive distortion
Mason [136]	CSTQ	1095 subjects from general population	1. unusual experiences; 2. cognitive disorganization; 3. impulsive nonconformity; 4. introversive anhedonia
Nuechterlein et al. [137]	SCID-II and neurocognitive assessment	313 relatives of schizophrenic probands	7 factor solution: 1. borderline, 2. schizoid, 3. avoidant, 4. negative schizotypy, 5. paranoid symptoms, 6. positive schizotypy, 7. cognitive disorganization (containing odd speech and bad performance on Trail B speed and span 10-letter target detection and odd, eccentric behaviour)
Raine et al. [138]	SPQ	822 undergraduates 102 subjects from general population	1. cognitive perceptual; 2. interpersonal; 3. disorganization
Reynolds et al. [139]	SPQ	1201 subjects from general population	1. cognitive perceptual; 2. interpersonal; 3. disorganized
Rossi and Daneluzzo [140]	SPQ	175 psychiatric patients (among them 93 schizophrenics)+172 controls	1. cognitive perceptual; 2. interpersonal; 3. disorganized
Suhr and Spitznagel [141]	SPQ, PAS, MIS	(a) 1366 undergraduates (b) 348 of those in the top 10th percentile	(a) 1. positive symptoms; 2. negative symptoms; 3. disorganized (b) 1. positive; 2. negative; 3. disorganized; 4. paranoid thinking
Venables and Bailes [142]	SAE	437 adults and 333 adolescents from general population	1. unusual perceptual experience, paranoid and magical ideation; 2. social anxiety, disorganization; 3. physical anhedonia; 4. social anhedonia
Venables and Rector [143]	SAE improved	330 college students	1. positive schizotypy; 2. negative schizotypy; 3. social impairment
Vollema and Hoijtink [144]	SPQ	418 "mild" psychiatric patients	1. positive schizotypy; 2. negative schizotypy; 3. disorganization
Wolfradt and Straube [145]	STA	1362 adolescents	1. magical ideation and unusual experiences; 2. ideas of reference and social anxiety; 3. suspiciousness

CSTQ, Combined Schizotypal Traits Questionnaire; DSSI, Delusions Symptoms States Inventory; EPQ, Eysenck Personality Questionnaire; MIS, Magical Ideation Scale; PAS, Perceptual Aberration Scale; PhA, Physical Anhedonia Scale; SAE, Survey of Attitudes and Experiences; SCID-II, Structured Clinical Interview for DSM-IV Axis II Personality Disorders; SIDP, Semistructured Interview for DSM-III Personality Disorders; SIDP-R, Semistructured Interview for DSM-III-R Personality Disorders; SIS, Structured Interview for Schizotypy; SPQ, Schizotypal Personality Questionnaire; SRQ, Self-Report Questionnaire for Schizotypy; STA, Schizotypal Personality Scale.

TABLE 1.5 Main instruments to measure or assess schizotypy and/or psychosis-proneness: self-report scales

Name	Reference
Impulsive Nonconformity Scale (IN)	Chapman *et al.* [147]
Magical Ideation Scale (MIS)	Eckblad and Chapman [148]
Perceptual Aberration Scale (PAS)	Chapman *et al.* [149]
Peters *et al.* Delusions Inventory (PDI)	Peters *et al.* [150]
Physical Anhedonia Scale (PhA)	Chapman *et al.* [151]
Psychoticism Subscale (P)	Eysenck and Eysenck [152]; Eysenck *et al.* [153]
Revised Social Anhedonia Scale (SA-R)	Eckblad *et al.* [154]
Rust Inventory of Schizoid Cognitions (RISC)	Rust [155]
Schizoidia Scale (GM)	Golden and Meehl [156]
Schizophrenism and Anhedonia Scale (SAE)	Venables *et al.* [157]
Schizophrenism (NP)	Nielsen and Petersen [158]
Schizotypal Personality Questionnaire (SPQ)	Raine [159]
Schizotypal Personality Scale (STA)	Claridge and Broks [160]
Schizotypy Scale (SS)	Venables *et al.* [157]

TABLE 1.6 Main instruments to measure or assess schizotypy and/or psychosis-proneness: (semi)structured interviews

Name	Reference
Personality Disorders Examination (PDE)	Loranger *et al.* [161]
Schedule for Schizotypal Personalities (SSP)	Baron *et al.* [162]
Semistructured Interview for DSM-III Personality Disorders (SIDP)	Pfohl *et al.* [163]
Semistructured Interview for DSM-III-R Personality Disorders (SIDP-R)	Pfohl *et al.* [164]
Structured Clinical Interview for DSM-IV Axis II Personality Disorders (SCID-II)	First *et al.* [165]
Structured Interview for Schizotypy (SIS)	Kendler *et al.* [166]
Structured Interview for Schizotypy-Revised (SIS-R)	Vollema and Ormel [167]

odd communication, social isolation and delusions and hallucinations appear to represent the genetic core of schizophrenia-related schizotypy. Interestingly, "identity disturbance" distinguished familial and non-familial SPD from other psychiatric disorders and normal controls. Although familial SPD scored numerically lower than non-familial SPD, the difference was not statistically significant.

A specific effort has been devoted to studying familial aggregation of formal thought disorder (corresponding to "odd speech"), considered as a dimension, yet with qualitative aspects as well—usually measured by the

Rorschach-derived Thought Disorder Index (TDI) [173]. A handful of studies using the TDI have shown quantitative and qualitative differences in the thinking of biological relatives of schizophrenic patients compared to relevant control groups [174,175]. Shenton *et al.* [176] reported differences in the qualitative categories seen in families, suggesting that specific consistent qualitative patterns of thought disorder run in families.

Although the majority of authors working with samples of the normal population advocate a dimensional model of schizotypy, there are still discussions concerning whether this model is "fully" or "quasi" dimensional [60]; moreover, some researchers suggest, in line with ideas of Meehl [15], that schizotypy is taxonic [116,177]. This debate is reminiscent of the controversies raised by Kretschmer and Bleuler in the first half of 20th century on the continuity or discontinuity in the transitions from normality to a full-blown schizophrenia [178].

BIOLOGICAL AND NEUROPSYCHOLOGICAL CORRELATES

There are three basic approaches to the study of the neuropsychological and biological aspects of SPD (and the other Cluster A disorders to a lesser extent). The first approach uses the pool of individuals with the diagnosis of SPD with the objective to understand the underlying mechanisms of schizophrenia and associated psychotic disorders. The majority of the published research following this approach states, for example, that "cognitive deficits have been identified as one of the central abnormalities found in schizophrenic patients". The logic then proceeds that it is hard to control for the "well-known third-variable confounds" [179]—deterioration, medication, institutionalization, long-term hospitalization, poor motivation, psychotic states, etc.—thus using individuals with SPD is the best way to control for these otherwise uncontrollable confounding effects. The assumption is that if the same type of deficits shows up in subjects with SPD, this confirms the deficits found in the schizophrenia patients, and also confirms their assumed underlying common pathology. As Roitman *et al.* [180] have suggested, people with SPD are the ideal population for studying "the cognitive impairments thought to characterize the schizophrenia spectrum".

The second approach addresses issues more directly associated with the construct of a schizophrenia spectrum of disorders. The assumption is that people with SPD (and to a lesser degree PPD and SdPD) are members of a spectrum of disorders, which is often characterized as a continuum, with schizophrenia at the severe end and SPD at the milder end ("There is a gradient of disorders related to schizophrenia [e.g. schizotypal personality disorder, quasi-psychotic conditions]; each of these related disorders may, in part, have its origins in errors of fetal development" [181]). The main goal of this approach is to find markers for the spectrum, that is, behavioural deficits or biological indices that people with SPD have in common with the other spectrum members. Thus, reliable findings from research with schizophrenia samples are used as a jumping off point to develop research models predicting that people with SPD will have similar deficits or biological markers. Moreover, those deficits or biological markers that are exhibited by people with schizophrenia but not by people with SPD are presumed to be associated with whatever it is that causes the psychosis that distinguishes schizophrenia from SPD, a paradigm alluded to by Meehl's diathesis-stress model. Likewise, deficits or strengths that people with SPD exhibit compared to normal control samples, but which are different from the schizophrenic participants, are often considered to be protective factors (i.e. protective from psychosis). Other similar approaches assume that the schizophrenia spectrum is aetiological in nature, and that "the features of schizotypal personality disorder parallel the prodromal signs of schizophrenia and have been shown to occur in preadolescents and adolescents. It is assumed that a subgroup of persons with schizotypal personality disorder will progress to schizophrenia" [182].

The third approach to the study of SPD can more correctly be described as a body of research that uses samples of individuals who are psychometrically defined as high schizotypy (e.g. high scores on scales measuring magical ideation, psychosis proneness) and high-risk individuals (e.g. relatives [with and without schizophrenia spectrum disorders] of schizophrenic probands). Thus, research is conducted to explore the above-mentioned behavioural deficits and biological markers, because these types of samples are presumed to include members of the schizophrenia spectrum and they are predicted to be at greater risk for schizophrenia than is the general population. There is general agreement that the psychometrically-defined schizophrenia spectrum members greatly increase the heterogeneity of the schizophrenia spectrum. Further, as suggested by Lencz and Raine [183], because college samples are preselected on the basis of sound intellectual functioning, it is more difficult to uncover cognitive impairments.

Somewhat surprisingly, there appears to be relatively little interest in studying SPD from a basic research perspective, i.e. to understand the disorder in and of itself. There is even less interest in SdPD and PPD.

Due to the space limitations, the following review of the research literature will be restricted for the most part to studies that include samples of clinically diagnosed individuals with SPD (a search of the Medline database using the keywords schizotypal or schizotypy resulted in references to 1359 articles). Further, the review is limited, primarily, to research published since 1998 (for further reviews, see [184,185]).

Structural Brain Differences

One of the most consistent findings in schizophrenia research is that the brains of schizophrenic patients are structurally different from those of non-schizophrenic patients (as compared to normal individuals and individuals with other psychiatric disorders) (Table 1.7). Findings from structural neuroimaging indicate that the most consistent neuroanatomical changes found in schizophrenia (e.g. cortical sulcal, lateral, and third ventricular enlargement) appear to be associated with genetic liability to schizophrenia, but that environmental insult (e.g. perinatal complications) also influence ventricular size [228]. The hope is that evaluation of the brain structure of people with SPD will offer insight into the endophenotypes common to SPD and schizophrenia. Differences that are found between SPD and schizophrenia might suggest the brain changes in schizophrenia that are contributing to the development of psychoses.

The relatively consistent findings in the structural imaging of the brains of schizophrenic individuals have led researchers to consider the implications regarding the brains of individuals within the schizophrenia spectrum, and in particular people with SPD. The hypotheses in general are that: (a) the brain structure of people with SPD will be different from normal comparison groups and people with other personality disorders, (b) that these changes will generally be grossly similar to those of schizophrenic individuals.

Dickey et al. [189] recently reviewed 17 structural imaging studies of SPD and reported that individuals with SPD had been shown to have abnormalities that were similar in nature (although generally of lesser magnitude) to those found in people with schizophrenia, including reduction of gray matter in the superior temporal gyrus, asymmetry of the parahippocampal gyrus, larger left anterior and temporal horn, and the splenium region of corpus callosum, thalamus, and the total cerebrospinal fluid volume intermediate to schizophrenia and normal subjects. Buchsbaum et al. [199] suggest that findings regarding the brains of people with SPD indicate that there is "less severe anatomical alteration in SPD patients than in schizophrenia. Findings appear to be somewhat more consistent for temporal than frontal regions".

However, reported results from the majority of these studies of structural abnormalities in SPD should be interpreted cautiously, due to problems with small sample sizes, samples that are predominantly male, multiple comparisons with inadequate control for familywise error, and vague or absent hypotheses. Further, because the studies are correlational in nature, the direction of the cause is always in question.

Functional Brain Differences

Even fewer studies have been done examining the functional differences of the brains of individuals with SPD (Table 1.7). The majority of studies that examined differences between SPD and normal controls reported some differences. For example, Siever *et al.* [229], in a review of studies from their group (e.g. [192, 196, 198]), suggested that there was evidence that "cognitive impairment in schizophrenia and schizotypal personality disorder may be associated in part with anomalous prefrontal cortical activity, activity which is diminished overall in schizophrenia but may reflect islands of preserved or compensatory function in schizotypal personality disorder." They further suggested that there is evidence for "reduced subcortical dopaminergic activity in schizotypal personality disorder compared to schizophrenic patients during cognitive task performance." These conclusions were supported by their findings from studies on regional neurotransmitter activity.

However, as with the research on the structure of the brain, due to small sample sizes, the predominant use of male participants, and vague or lacking hypotheses, conclusions should be drawn with caution.

Minor Physical Abnormalities

The search for a link between minor physical abnormalities and SPD has primarily been motivated by findings that individuals with schizophrenia are more likely to have minor physical abnormalities than control groups (see Table 1.7). Thus, the assumption is that people with Cluster A disorders and/or family members of schizophrenic patients should also have minor physical abnormalities. The hypothesis is that they share an underlying (perhaps neurological) vulnerability that may be evident in these shared physical anomalies. Several researchers have attempted to find links between minor deviations in external physical characteristics and the Cluster A disorders. For example, Weinstein *et al.* [182] reported that adolescents with SPD had increased minor physical anomalies and fluctuating dermatoglyphic asymmetries compared to normal control adolescents.

Because of the paucity of research in this area, drawing conclusions is not recommended. Nevertheless, Kelly [230] provides a reasonable synthesis of the research literature, suggesting that "minor physical anomalies in people with schizophrenia (1) are more numerous than those of comparison subjects, (2) are more numerous than, and are different from, those in unaffected people with high-risk genetic inheritance (e.g. offspring, siblings), and (3) are different from those in people with certain quasi-psychotic phenomena." He also suggests that "while a variety of psychotic and quasi-psychotic conditions may indeed belong on a clinical schizo-phrenia spectrum, they may well have arrived there by significantly different routes."

Motor Function

Motor dysfunction, or "neurological soft signs" as termed by Meehl [13], in schizophrenia has been the subject of considerable study, thus researchers have also examined the same in Cluster A personality disorders (see Table 1.7). For example, Walker *et al.* [208] reported that adolescents with SPD had more involuntary movements of arms, hands, head, etc. than did normal adolescents. However, overall conclusions are hard to make because of the scarcity of replication.

Attention, Perception and Information Processing

Information-processing deficits have been suggested as viable markers of vulnerability to schizophrenia and/or membership in the schizophrenia spectrum. The types of markers proposed have included measures of, for example, smooth pursuit eye movement, sustained attention, span of apprehension, selective attention, and various indices of distractibility. Since attentional dysfunctions have been consistently reported in schizo-phrenia patients, to control for third-variable confounds, many researchers have attempted to replicate these findings using samples of schizotypal individuals and normal control groups (see Table 1.7).

In one study, SPD-diagnosed first admitted patients, tentatively considered to be in the prodromal pre-schizophrenic stages [231], performed *better* than both chronic schizophrenic patients and normal controls on the Müller-Lyer's illusion task (less sensitive to illusion) and on a figure detection task; they were better at detecting a figure popping out from the randomly distributed line segments of the background; this particular test was originally proposed as paradigmatic for the intra-modal perceptual binding [232]. These results (apart from the possibility of type I error) were interpreted as pointing to a less context-bound perceptual performance in SPD.

Event-Related Activity in Brain

In this research, attention and information processing are assessed by testing the event-related potentials (ERPs) (e.g. P50 suppression in response to auditory clicks, prepulse inhibition, startle response). The overall hypothesis is that presumed inhibitory functioning deficits make it more difficult for individuals within the schizophrenia spectrum to filter out trivial internal and external stimuli. As can be seen in Table 1.7, this is a comparatively well-studied area using SPD individuals as research subjects. The general finding is that there are attenuated differences between SPD and normal controls (attenuated compared to findings with schizophrenia subjects), and that the measured indices of SPD subjects are generally intermediate between schizophrenia and normal control groups. For example, Niznikiewicz *et al.* [221] found that the N400 amplitude was reduced for related words with shorter stimulus-onset asynchrony in females with SPD compared to a normal control group of females, but only in the left frontal area. The authors suggested that their findings supported the general theory that there is an overactivation of semantic networks in SPD.

Perceptual-Motor Speed

Research on visual search and motor speed has been conducted in individuals with SPD. These tests of selective attention are often administered in the context of a battery of tests, and include, for example, digit symbol (Wechsler scale), cancellation tests, Stroop Color-Word Test, Trail Making Test (A and B). Findings regarding perceptual speed have been consistent with hypotheses: SPD individuals have deficits inter-mediate between normal controls and individuals with schizophrenia. Cadenhead *et al.* [210], for example, found that SPD subjects had an intermediate performance (although not necessarily with statistically signifi-cant differences) between normal controls and schizophrenia subjects on the Stroop task.

Verbal Learning and Memory

Dysfunctions in short-term verbal and visual memory are evident in schizophrenia. The problems are generally greater for recall than for recognition, which has been suggested to indicate that the problem is in the encoding process (e.g. slowed processing, mnemonic organization).

According to Roitman *et al.* [180], "impaired working memory is hypothesized to be a central component of several of these more complex cognitive deficits" (e.g. "ability to identify and maintain a shifting cognitive set in response to verbal feedback", Verbal Fluency Test, Stroop Color Word Test).

Although there is substantial evidence of deficits in learning and memory in schizophrenia patients, there has been relatively little published work on verbal learning and memory functioning in SPD.

Overall, the findings from recent studies (see Table 1.7) suggest that individuals with SPD, although exhibiting some deficits in cognitive functioning, do not have the same generalized intellectual impairment as often found in individuals with schizophrenia.

Executive Functioning

Findings regarding measures of executive functioning (e.g. abstraction, concept formation, executive control) are fairly consistent in schizophrenia samples; individuals with schizophrenia perform worse on tasks of executive functioning (e.g. Wisconsin Card Sorting Test (WCST)) than do normal control subjects. This poor performance is theorized to be associated with frontal cortical dysfunction. Nevertheless, the findings regarding SPD and executive functioning are much less consistent (see Table 1.7) [233]. Individuals with SPD have been found to have poorer performance on measures of executive function than normal controls in some studies, but in other studies their performance is comparable to normal control samples.

Battaglia *et al.* [199] have suggested that perhaps the inconsistent findings regarding WCST performance, in particular, are due to two issues: (a) poor performance is more a function of the disease process of schizophrenia than it is a trait marker of the liability to schizophrenia; (b) different types of samples are being studied, i.e. SPD versus high schizotypy.

COURSE

There are five basic time-frame variables that appear to form the basis of the concept of course of illness: age of onset, mode of onset, duration or chronicity, episodicity, and progression [234]. The DSM definition of personality disorders indicates that

> ... a personality disorder is an *enduring* pattern of inner experience and behaviour that deviates markedly from the expectations of the individual's culture, is pervasive and inflexible, has an *onset in adolescence* or *early adulthood*, is *stable over time*, and leads to distress or impairment [1] [italics added].

TABLE 1.7   Recent neurobiological and neuropsychological findings in schizotypal personality disorder (SPD)

Study	Sample	Differences between SPD and normal subjects
Structural Differences in the Brain		
Byne et al. [186]	SZ, SPD, norm	Pulvinar reduced in SPD
Cannon et al. [113]	Cluster A, no-Cluster A	Differences in cortical gray matter and cerebrospinal fluid volume
Dickey et al. [187]	SPD, norm	In SPD, reduced gray matter of left superior temporal gyrus. No differences in medial temporal lobe
Dickey et al. [188]	SPD, norm	Cerebrospinal fluid volume greater in SPD. No difference in overall intracranial contents or white matter
Dickey et al. [189]	SPD, norm	Gray matter volume in left Heschl's gyrus smaller in SPD. Planum temporale not different
Downhill et al. [190]	SZ, SPD, norm	Splenium bigger in SPD. Genu area larger in SPD. No differences in total callosal area
Downhill et al. [191]	SZ, SPD, norm	In SPD, smaller gray matter volume in temporal lobe, reduced volume of whole temporal lobe
Hazlett et al. [192]	SZ/SZA, SPD, norm	In SPD, fewer pixels in right mediodorsal nucleus. No differences in thalamus volume
Kurokawa et al. [193]	SZ spectrum, OCD, norm	In SZ spectrum (SZ and SPD), enlarged ventricular system
Kwon et al. [194]	SZ, affective, SPD, norm	No differences regarding cavum septi pellucidi
Levitt et al. [195]	SPD, norm	Left and right caudate nucleus relative volumes smaller in SPD
Shihabuddin et al. [196]	SZ, SPD, norm	In SPD, smallest putamen volume. No differences in caudate nucleus
Takahashi et al. [197]	SZ, SPD (ICD), norm	No differences on volume of gray and white matter of anterior cingulate gyrus
Functional/Metabolic Differences in Brain		
Buchsbaum et al. [198]	SPD, norm	In SPD, more activation in middle frontal gyrus. In normals, more activation in precentral gyrus
Buchsbaum et al. [199]	SZ, SPD, norm	In SPD, higher cortical metabolic rates in medial frontal and temporal, Broadmann area 10
Fukusako et al. [200]	SPD, norm	Decreased phosphomonoesters in left temporal lobe of SPD
Hazlett et al. [192]	SZ/SZA, SPD, norm	No differences on thalamic glucose metabolic rate
Kirrane et al. [201]	SSPD, OPD	In SPD, improvement on visuospatial working memory under amphetamine administration
Kirrane et al. [202]	SPD	After infusion of physostigmine, weak trend toward improving visuospatial working memory.

Shihabuddin et al. [196]	SZ, SPD, norm	In SPD, higher glucose metabolic rate in ventral putamen
Siegal et al. [203]	SPD	Under amphetamine challenge, improvement in WCST task performance
Minor Physical Abnormalities		
Grove et al. [204]	SZ, SPD*, not SPD	No relationship between small/dysmorphic head size and SPD*
Schiffman et al. [205]	SZ spectrum, OMI, NMI	Greater number of physical anomalies (11–13 yrs) differentiated SZ spectrum diagnosis from NMI (at 31–33 yrs)
Weinstein et al. [182]	Adolescents: SPD, OPD, norm	In SPD, more minor physical anomalies and dermatoglyphic asymmetries
Motor Function		
Neumann and Walker [206]	SPD, OPD, No PD	SPD more excessive in motor force. Motor overflow and negative symptoms linked to higher salivary cortisol levels
Thaker et al. [207]	Relatives: SPD*, non-SPD*; Community: SPD*, non-SPD*	In SPD* relatives, more errors than community SPD* on antisaccade task. SPD* relatives same as normals on error rates
Walker et al. [208]	Adolescents: SPD, OPD, norm	In SPD, more involuntary movements of head, trunk. Salivary cortisol levels associated with involuntary movements
Attention and Information Processing		
Brenner et al. [209]	SZ, SPD, norm	SPD more similar to normals than to SZ on antisaccade and ocular motor delayed response.
Cadenhead et al. [210]	SZ, SPD, norm	SPD intermediate (effect size only) between normal and SZ on measures of attention, cognitive inhibition
Cadenhead et al. [211]	SPD, norm	No difference in amplitude or latency of P50 wave, but SPD had impaired suppression
Cadenhead et al. [212]	SZ, SPD, relatives of SZ, norm	SPD had deficit in right-side prepulse inhibition. No differences in startle reactivity, latency, habituation rate
Cadenhead et al. [213]	SPD	P50 and antisaccade task deficits moderately linked
Granholm et al. [214]	SPD, norm	SPD had abnormal global processing advantage, SPD faster at global relative to local targets
Harvey et al. [215]	SPD, OPD, norm	SPD impairment in ability to discriminate target and non-target information (degraded CPT)
Laurent et al. [216]	SZ, SSPD, non-SSPD, norm	Performance of SSPD relatives and non-SSPD relatives did not differ on any measures
Moran et al [217]	SSPD, norm	In SSPD, longer reaction time to right visual field invalid targets. No difference in left visual field target performance

(continued)

TABLE 1.7 *(continued)*

Study	Sample	Differences between SPD and normal subjects
Moriarty et al. [218]	SPD, OPD, norm	In SPD, more errors of omission on CPT tasks in the dual-task conditions due to resource limitations
Niznikiewicz et al. [219]	SPD, norm	More negative N400 amplitude in SPD in congruent condition (visual and auditory). Longer N400 latency in visual modality for SPD
Niznikiewicz et al. [220]	SPD, norm	P3 amplitude smaller in SPD at midline electrodes. At lateral electrodes small reduction of P3 amplitude in SPD on left side compared to right side
Niznikiewicz et al. [221]	SPD, norm	In SPD, less negative N400 amplitude (left frontal area) for related words with short stimulus-onset asynchrony
Raine et al. [222]	SPD, norm	In SPD, more abnormal orienting with amplitude increasing across trials of skin conductance response habituation
Salisbury et al. [223]	SPD, norm	In SPD, asymmetrical P3, with smaller amplitudes over left posterior temporal lobe
Voglmaier et al. [224]	SPD, norm	In SPD, deficit in verbal attention and memory processing with more difficult tasks and/or interference
Verbal Learning and Memory		
Bergman et al. [225]	SPD, OPD	SPD learned fewer total numbers of words and at a slower rate. Retention not different
Cadenhead et al. [210]	SZ, SPD, norm	SPD intermediate (trends) to normal and SZ on verbal working memory, general intelligence
Farmer et al. [226]	SPD, norm	SPD performed more poorly on recognition memory tests. No difference on contrast sensitivity or discrimination
Roitman et al. [180]	SPD, OPD, norm	SPD had greater working memory deficit that was not attributable to differences in immediate recall condition
Voglmaier et al. [224]	SPD, norm	In SPD mild general cognitive deficit, deficit on verbal fluency, short-term verbal retention
Executive Functioning/Abstract Reasoning		
Cadenhead et al. [210]	SZ, SPD, norm	No significant differences on abstract reasoning (WCST)
Diforio et al. [227]	SPD, OPD, norm	SPD performed worse on modified WCST

CPT, Continuous Performance Task; NMI, no mental illness; OCD, obsessive-compulsive disorder; OMI, other mental illness; OPD, other personality disorder; PD, personality disorders; SPD*, SPD based on Schedule for Schizotypal Personalities; SSPD, schizophrenia spectrum personality disorder; SZ, schizophrenia; SZA, schizoaffective disorder; WCST, Wisconsin Card Sorting Test.

And in reference specifically to the Cluster A personality disorders, the DSM observes that

Particularly in response to stress, individuals with this disorder may experience very brief psychotic episodes (lasting minutes to hours) [1].

Further, of the three Cluster A disorders in the DSM, only SPD warrants a subsection called "Course", although this is only one sentence long:

Schizotypal Personality Disorder has a relatively stable course, with only a small proportion of individuals going on to develop Schizophrenia or another psychotic disorder [1].

Thus, according to the DSM definition of Cluster A personality disorders, the course of the illness entails information about the age of onset (adolescence, early adulthood), mode of onset (implies that it is insidious), duration (from adolescence to time of diagnosis), episodicity (implies continuous, with possible brief psychotic episodes), and progression (stable).

However, there is little empirical evidence to support (or refute) the DSM course description of the Cluster A personality disorders. For example, in a systematic review of the literature spanning the years from 1970 to 1989 (including the period in which the DSM definition of SPD was being formulated), Mezzich and Jorge [234] found 75 papers that specifically referred to the course of psychiatric disorders. Of these, they cited only one study that included a focus on the course of personality disorders (age range of the sample was 49–93 years old). Maier *et al.* [184], in their more recent review of the literature (up to 1998), reported that empirical evidence regarding the long-term course of the Cluster A personality disorders [235,236] was scarce, and that there were no systematic follow-up studies in non-clinical, naturalistic samples. Further, they reported that the examination of the stability of Cluster A disorders was also a rarity, and that there were no prospective studies examining the purported transitional relationship between Cluster A disorders and schizophrenia.

A more recent search of the literature (from 1998 to 2003) in the current review indicates that there is still relatively little empirical work focusing on the course of the Cluster A personality disorders. Although some researchers have examined test-retest reliability of assessment measures, this obviously does not adequately examine the issue of course/stability. However, there are a handful of studies that have been/are being conducted to explore the stability of personality disorders in general (i.e. not necessarily focusing on the Cluster A disorders alone).

For example, Lenzenweger [237] followed 250 college students for four years in a prospective longitudinal study examining the stability of personality disorder characteristics and reported that personality disorder "features display relatively high levels of individual difference stability and appreciable mean level stability, with some change occurring over time." However, "categorical diagnoses could not be reliably evaluated for stability owing to a low prevalence…" Lenzenweger concludes that "the overall theoretical implication of these mean level data suggests *continuity* consistent with the DSM definition of personality disorder".

According to findings from the Children in the Community Study, a community-based longitudinal study, the prevalence of personality disorder traits tended to decline during adolescence and early adulthood [18]. There were significant declines (55%) in the Cluster A traits from the youngest test age (age 9 to 12 years) to the oldest (age 25 to 28 years). Nevertheless, adolescents diagnosed with SPD and PPD had elevated personality disorder traits (of the same kind) as young adults.

One of the main purposes of the Collaborative Longitudinal Personality Disorders Study [238] is to examine the purported stability (short- and long-term) of four of the DSM-IV Axis II disorders (schizotypal, borderline, avoidant, and obsessive–compulsive personality disorders) with a multisite, prospective naturalistic approach. The authors reported on the short-term stability of these four DSM disorders using data from the first year of prospective follow-up. In comparison to participants with major depressive disorder, a larger proportion of the personality disorder subjects (4% versus 44%, respectively) remained at or above diagnostic thresholds for the 12-month period. However, the authors note that "whether personality disorders appear stable depends upon how stability is defined". As such, they concluded that, although the personality disorder subjects were more diagnostically stable than people with major depressive disorder, the majority of the personality disorder subjects did not retain DSM-IV criteria thresholds (i.e. 56% fell below threshold) and that there was a significant decrease in the average number of criteria for each of the four personality disorder groups. They concluded that "while individuals are very consistent in terms of their rank order of personality disorder features, they may fluctuate in the severity or amount of personality disorder features present at any given point".

TREATMENT

Although it is virtually impossible to substantiate, one of the often-repeated statements regarding treatment of the Cluster A personality disorders is that individuals with these diagnoses do not seek psychiatric treatment for the traits and characteristics that define the disorders. If the epidemiological estimates of prevalence are accurate, up to 5% of the population might be suffering from the untreated symptoms, which by definition are causing distress or impairment, associated with a Cluster A personality disorder. This notwithstanding, it is often suggested that they seek treatment for associated symptoms (e.g. depression, anxiety, substance-related disorders). Thus, the study of the treatment of Cluster A personality disorders is difficult because it is problematic to disentangle the effects of treatment approaches and their targets (i.e. the associated symptom versus the characteristics of the disorder itself). The absence of people with Cluster A personality disorders seeking treatment and the associated difficulties with confounding symptoms are perhaps some of the reasons that contribute to the paucity of empirical work studying treatment effects. There is virtually no empirical work examining the impact of drug therapies or psychotherapies on PPD and SdPD specifically. In their review of the literature prior to 1998, Maier *et al.* [184] could find no investigations of drug therapy or psychotherapeutic interventions for SdPD. Although they reported that case studies have been published regarding treatments of PPD, there were no well-controlled studies on either pharmacotherapy or psychotherapy.

In one comprehensive review [239], the goal was to determine whether personality disorders are changeable, and whether this changeability can be influenced by treatment. As a general conclusion, the authors reported, "there is evidence that effective treatments exist to alleviate symptoms and reduce symptomatic behaviours that accompany personality disorders". However, they only found two longitudinal or naturalistic studies that included samples of individuals with SPD, and one that examined Cluster A diagnoses. Not surprisingly, of the 28 outcome studies of psychopharmacological treatment, a relatively high proportion (8/28) included samples of patients with SPD (but 5 of these 8 studies included patients co-morbid with BPD). The primary target of these studies was the reduction of low-level psychotic symptoms (e.g. odd thinking, ideas of reference). The authors reported that the use of antipsychotics "...demonstrated a moderate degree of efficacy that was primarily limited to the symptom realm". On the other hand, "tricyclic antidepressants (...) do not appear warranted". Finally, none of the studies of psychosocial treatment targeted Cluster A disorders.

Similarly, Maier *et al.* [184] reported no controlled studies examining the effect of psychotherapy in SPD. However, there were a handful of controlled studies that examined the use of pharmacotherapy (i.e. antipsychotics, anxiolytics) with SPD patients. Placebo-controlled studies found a range of therapeutic effects from moderate to significant improvement concerning thiothixene, haloperidol, clozapine, etc. However, few studies had carefully examined the use of anxiolytics or tricyclic agents, monoamine oxidase inhibitors, lithium, etc. Maier *et al.* [184] concluded "there is preliminary evidence that low doses of antipsychotic medication (1–2 mg per day of haloperidol equivalent) are effective in, at least temporarily, reducing or relieving the psychotic-like symptoms of schizotypal PD. In psychotherapy there is only clinical experience available...".

Our more recent review of the literature (from 1999 to 2003) indicated that there is still a paucity of empirical work examining the treatment of Cluster A personality disorders. There were apparently no new studies examining the treatment of SdPD and PPD. Nevertheless, one of the only additions to the literature was a placebo-controlled, double-blind study by Koenigsberg *et al.* [240], which examined the use of risperidone in treating patients with SPD. The results indicated that low doses of risperidone can reduce symptom severity (negative, positive, and general symptoms) in patients with SPD.

THE CLINICAL PHENOMENOLOGY OF SCHIZOPHRENIA SPECTRUM DISORDERS

Here we address the psychopathological issues that have direct relevance for the clinical application of the SPD diagnosis, including diagnostic ambiguities and differential diagnostic considerations. Table 1.8 lists the DSM-IV diagnostic criteria: any combination of a total of 5 criteria is necessary and sufficient for making the SPD diagnosis.

The Single Diagnostic SPD Criteria in a Clinical-Phenomenological Perspective

The SPD diagnostic criteria are only laconically presented in the DSM-IV (and ICD-10 alike). The following elaboration is anchored in the classic and

TABLE 1.8 DSM-IV criteria for schizotypal personality disorder

---

1. Ideas of reference (excluding delusions of reference)
2. Odd beliefs or magical thinking that influences behaviour and is inconsistent with subcultural norms
3. Unusual perceptual experiences, including bodily illusions
4. Odd thinking and speech
5. Suspiciousness or paranoid ideation
6. Inappropriate or constricted affect
7. Behaviour or appearance that is odd, eccentric, or peculiar
8. Lack of close friends or confidants other than first-degree relatives
9. Excessive social anxiety that does not diminish with familiarity and tends to be associated with paranoid fears rather than negative judgments about self

---

recent phenomenological-empirical accounts of the schizophrenia spectrum conditions, as well as in our own clinical and research experience. There are several issues to emphasize regarding such clinical elaboration. First, all of the SPD symptoms and signs can also be present in individuals with schizophrenia—as indicated already, the concepts of SPD and schizophrenia are reciprocally connected. It is also necessary to note that some SPD criteria represent trait features, reflecting a person's style of being (e.g. eccentricity or constricted or manneristic expressivity), whereas other criteria appear more clearly as state features (e.g. paranoid ideation) that may intra-individually wax and wane. Certain criteria contain *both* trait and state components (e.g. odd speech), which perhaps accounts for a portion of the variability of results in the psychometric studies of SPD dimensions (Table 1.4). Finally, although there have been many attempts to organize the features of SPD into a coherent whole, none has been extremely successful. In the following description, we have tried to organize the symptoms using a clinical-phenomenological rationale and approach. In the contemporary operational paradigm it is sometimes forgotten that psychopathological features (symptoms or signs) are only rarely well demarcated and well-defined, thing-like entities. Typically, when explored in the individual patient, psychopathological features are phenomenologically interrelated and therefore partly overlapping. These interdependencies are not of a causal-mechanical nature. Rather they form a network of meaning, originating in intentional intertwining, motivation and mutual implication, that subtends and contributes to a certain sense of coherence (unity) of normal and abnormal consciousness [241].

Fundamental Expressive Features

Criteria 4, 6, 7, and 8 of the DSM system (see Table 1.8) represent attenuated fundamental (mainly "autistic") expressive features of schizophrenia, described by Bleuler [40] and numerous other authors. These criteria are reflective of a fundamental intersubjective disturbance that was central to the conceptual validity of schizophrenia and its spectrum disorders. It should also be noted that these features are all traditionally depicted as "third-person" phenomena or observable "signs".

Odd thinking and speech. This criterion refers to varieties of subtle formal thought disorder (or "cognitive slippage" using Meehl's terminology). Formal thought disorder in this context is considered to be a trait phenomenon, although it can have the potential for being both a trait and a state feature, because it becomes accentuated during symptomatic exacerbations. Moreover, the degree of manifestation of the disorder by a given patient is not independent of the technique of psychiatric interviewing (see below). The formal thought disorder in the definition of SPD is delineated at a level of severity that is much more discreet than the equivalent criterion for schizophrenia (for which features such as incoherence, neologisms, and gross interpolations of thought are included).

In the case of the schizophrenia spectrum, there are at least three major aspects of formal thought disorder: disorganization/looseness, semantic disturbances, and logical slippage. The disorganized characteristic refers to fluidity of conceptual boundaries with a tendency to combine distant elements that have little in common. Instead of simply being a failure to stay focused on a particular topic, theme, or object of awareness (as in mania), it refers to a more fundamental failure to stay anchored within a single frame of reference, perspective or orientation [242–244]. Normally, a train of thoughts or a discourse is always in a reciprocal relation to its dispositional framework: e.g. when chatting about the price of tomatoes, we are typically in a mundane rather than in an abstract-philosophical frame of mind. In the schizophrenia spectrum, a lack of perspectival stability leads to shifts or jumps across conceptual levels, including hyper-abstract as well as hyper-concrete (or hyper-literal) perspectives. Thus, whereas the formal thought disorder in manic or hypo-manic patients is "extravagantly combinatory, usually with humour, flippancy, and playfulness", pointing to an acceleration and dis-inhibition of thought processes, the schizophrenia spectrum formal thought disorder appears "disorganized and ideationally fluid", with "interpenetrations of one idea by another [and by] unstable verbal referents" that "convey an impression of bewilderment, and may cause confusion in the listener as well" [243,245].

The unstable semantics (disorder of meaning/reference) is manifested in a private, idiosyncratic use of existing words or terms (metonymy), use of metaphor in an excessively concrete or abstract manner, and excessive use of symbols, all of which typically happens in an involuntary manner and is unnoticed by the patient him/herself—in contradistinction to creative or poetic violations of language rules. Entire sentences or phrases may seem vague, hyper-abstract, or hyper-concrete (in contrast, organic circumstantial thinking is stably concrete, without perspectival shifts or semantic peculiarities). The transitions between thought sequences may be oblique and slightly beside the point (i.e. tangential). The overall impression of the patient's thinking and speech is that of vagueness: despite a normal conversational engagement ("speech production"), the patient may convey very little concrete or well-structured information (it may be impossible afterwards to summarize in writing the content of such an interview). Finally, the person's thinking may exhibit subtle flaws of logic, partly related to the disorganization described above (such as combining two distant, barely related themes on the basis of a single, inessential element).

The disturbances of language (regarding purely linguistic aspects) characteristic of the schizophrenia spectrum disorders are distinct from the aphasias, because they particularly affect what is called the pragmatic dimension of speech [244,246]. There is a subtle and shifting relationship between what can be asserted and what would normally be presupposed—that is, between what emerges as the shared focus at a given moment of a conversation and what normally serves as the taken-for-granted background. Moreover, the patient may tend to ignore deictic coordinates of speech, as if taking for granted that all background information is somehow available to the listener ("deixis" is a Greek word meaning "pointing to"). Typical deictic coordinates are spatial, temporal and personal. An example of a total lack of deixis would be a sentence written on a piece of paper found in a bottle floating in the ocean: "Meet me here tomorrow" [247]. These types of language disorder appear to be reflective of a pervasive disorder of intersubjective attunement. Finally, some patients manifest speech-mannerisms, for example, talking in an affected, professorial or drawn style (the term mannerism referring to a goal-directed action performed with inappropriately exaggerated expressivity). The manneristic expressive style in a schizophrenia spectrum patient strikes the psychiatrist as a kind of affliction, i.e. more as something that happens to the patient, in contrast to a histrionic theatricality, which typically conveys an aura of something willfully intended, purposeful or subtly manipulative [248].

In general, the formal thought disorder becomes clearly manifest or conspicuous only during unstructured conversation, where the patient has both possibility and time to elaborate his thoughts and ideas in a spontaneous manner. Moreover, the level of formal thought disorder may flare up if the conversation's theme is emotionally dramatic or taxing or if it touches the patient's deepest personal convictions of political, metaphysical, religious, or spiritual nature. Andreasen [249] published a scale targeting clinically descriptive aspects of the formal thought disorder. Johnston and Holzman [135] have developed, so far, the most sophisticated, quantitative and qualitative Rorschach-based system for the assessment of formal thought disorder [250].

Inappropriate or constricted affect. As noted earlier, this criterion belongs to the group of intersubjective disturbances. The patient's expressivity is monotonous and rarely changes throughout a conversation (constricted affect), or he/she has a constant smile or other expression that is unrelated to the changing emotional and cognitive content of his/her communication (inappropriate modulation). Affective expression may also appear inadequate because it is disorganized (paramimia)—with different emotional tags in different parts of the face (typically with a tendency to immobility of expressive muscles of the upper part of the face and a more lively expressivity in the lower part, with a consequent discordant expressivity of the two parts). There may be a very subtle tendency to grimacing (parakinetic movements, i.e. non-goal directed, involuntary, irregular, tick-like movements), such as, repeatedly closing or squinting the eyes; momentarily opening the eyes very wide with a retraction of the upper eyelid revealing the normally invisible part of the sclera above the iris (Meehl called this "scleral flash"); stereotyped and peculiar lip or oral movements. Eye contact may be diminished in frequency or duration; in other patients the gaze may be penetrating, watchfully observing or glancing suspiciously; there may be fixed staring and the ocular axes may exhibit excessive rigid parallelism; or gaze may be wandering or unanchored in the interlocutor, conferring on the latter a sentiment of redundancy, of not being truly present for the patient. Disordered expressivity may also manifest itself in posture, gait and other movements (e.g. relative immobility of the head, extremely straight or stiff posture of the spinal column, often with a curious bend of the upper part of the spine and bent arms [251]; diminished gestures; stereotyped movements i.e. repetitive, non-goal directed, regular/monotonous movements that may be voluntarily suppressed, such as a repeated scratching of a part of the body, strange circular hand movements, etc.).

Emotional contact or rapport, that is, a sense of reciprocal empathy and joint emotional modulation felt in the encounter with the patient, is typically diminished (disturbances of affective expression contribute to, but do not exhaust, the origins of this feeling). The patient may appear inaccessible, indifferent, or somehow disinterested, as if disengaged or not fully present.

Behaviour or appearance that is odd, eccentric, or peculiar. Eccentricity is a diagnostic feature that is impossible to spell out in objective terms because it is a normative, highly contextual notion, reflecting the psychiatrist's own subjective experience. The sentiment of eccentricity refers to a global and pre-reflective (direct/un-mediated) experience of a strange disharmony or disproportion in the perceived Gestalt of a fellow human: the patient appears as peculiar and strange, as if somehow slightly displaced from the shared (intersubjective) space (etymologically, eccentricity literally means being "out, or away from the centre or the axis"). All of the expressive abnormalities (but especially disorganization) described so far may induce such sentiment. What the patient says, how he says it, how he behaves, how he dresses, etc. may in different ways constitute this disharmonious Gestalt. The psychiatrist, in explicit reflection, may be able to reduce this global sentiment into its more concrete constituent components (e.g. specific distortions of expressivity or behaviour). Sometimes, however, this sentiment defies reflective scrutiny and one remains with a global, subjective impression that is atmospheric and nearly ineffable, a sense of strangeness (Bleuler) or "anthropological disproportion" emphasized in the phenomenological literature as being one of the important diagnostic indicators of the schizophrenia spectrum conditions [252] (for a clinical description of the notion of "anthropological disproportion", see [58]).

Lack of close friends or confidants other than first-degree relatives. Although this criterion is mainly defined in the DSM in the third person perspective as a sign (apart from a casual remark on a diminished desire for interpersonal contact), it usually involves or stems from specific subjective experiences, such as extreme sensitivity or a paranoid, suspicious attitude, leading to excessive social anxiety (criterion 9) and avoidant behaviour. Interpersonal anxiety may also be founded on a more fundamental insecurity, where it is one's own self and existence that are felt to be at stake ("ontological anxiety", see below). Quite often, social isolation is a consequence of a pervasive deficit in the normally automatic, un-reflected (un-mediated) understanding of the significance of the world, other people, social rules, and situations ("lack of natural evidence" [58,66,73]). The patient is bewildered by the world and other people and tends to reflect on matters normally unnoticed, taken for granted, or presupposed by other people: e.g. why are there three colours in traffic lights or why is the grass green, etc. This condition of low-grade perplexity [66,253] and hyper-reflexivity isolates the patient because interpersonal interactions (e.g. unstructured "small talk" situations) feel arduous and unbearably taxing. Some patients consider other people as spiritually or intellectually inferior, thus exhibiting a kind of grandiose attitude (see below) that may detach them from the social world.

Subtle Psychotic-like Phenomena

Criteria 1, 2, and 5 (see Table 1.8) reflect subtle psychotic-like phenomena, which to a certain extent have a clear state or occurrent character (e.g. paranoid ideation) and sometimes intensify into very brief psychotic episodes (described in the ICD-10 as micropsychoses). However, other features, such as magical thinking, may be of a more habitual or dispositional character. The DSM definitions of the individual criteria in this group are far from satisfactory. Thus, paranoid ideation is defined as "ideation of less than delusional proportions", whereas an overvalued idea is defined as an "unreasonable belief maintained with less than delusional intensity". Both definitions are vague and have very limited pragmatic value (e.g. in the assessment of a dissimulating, suspicious patient). It seems that most of these criteria point to very transient psychotic episodes. As an example, a woman looking around in a shoe shop hears a telephone start to ring. She gets a sudden thought that it is the police calling, to check upon her whereabouts. A few minutes later she is already able to distance herself from this idea that she now considers to be complete nonsense. Magical thinking (defined as thinking violating the normative understanding of causality), if only assessed on the basis of its content, is quite non-specific and prevalent in the society. Yet, magical beliefs that are linked to or derived from altered structure of subjective experiencing (see below) possess more important diagnostic significance, because under these circumstances they are more like a dispositional feature. Something similar applies to ideas of reference: these may be based on suspiciousness or variable paranoid mental contents. However, certain patients experience a sort of primary (i.e. psychologically not reducible) sentiment of being at the center of attention. Others may fleetingly experience an even more articulated feeling of centrality and direct connectedness to the surrounding world. In these cases, the self-reference derives from an altered structure of conscious experience manifest through a semi-constant sentiment of living in an immediate resonance with the surrounding world (which, in the schizophrenic psychosis, may become associated with the experiences of possessing omnipotent influence or of being influenced, or both simultaneously).

First Person Perspective

Unusual perceptual experiences (criterion 3) is the only criterion that reflects the patient's subjective (first person) perspective. However, also here we are confronted with a mixture of state features and features that may be more stable, habitual, or dispositional. In general, this domain is ignored and typically unknown in English-speaking psychiatry (but see [72] and the Chapmans' work on anhedonia and perceptual disorders).

Schizotypal patients, no matter if diagnosed by the DSM-III-R [254] or the ICD-10 [132], experience a whole panoply of non-psychotic (without delusional elaboration) subjective experiential anomalies in the domains of affectivity, perception, cognition, and movement and body experience (Table 1.9). These "basic symptoms" [69] are thoroughly described in an interview schedule [255], which is translated into several languages, including a shortened English-language version, available upon request from the authors [71].

One important aspect of distorted subjectivity in the schizophrenia spectrum conditions, linked to the basic symptoms, comprises a pervasive sense of self-distance [256–258]. The core phenomenon here is a diminished sense of the very basic, pre-reflective selfhood ("ipseity", from Latin ipse = self, itself). In normal experience, no matter in which modality (e.g. seeing a

TABLE 1.9 Selected basic symptoms

Affect-emotion	Anhedonia, diminished vitality, apathy = feeling of a lack of feelings, ambivalence, loss of naturalness of the world
Perceptual	Qualitative and quantitative changes of vision (e.g. micro-macropsia, seeing faces changed) and audition, heightened perception
Cognitive	Thought-block, thought pressure, thought interference, audible thoughts restricted to inner space, perplexity, unclear differentiation of modalities of experience (e.g. perception vs. fantasy or remembrance and fantasy), hyper-reflectivity, pseudo-obsessive ruminations
Motor and bodily	Sudden sense of motor paralysis, loss of automaticy of movement, strange sensations from the inside of the body (pulling, shrinking) or from the body surface (e.g. "electrical" or "migrating" sensations)

house, thinking about vacation, or being in love or tired, etc.), the experience always happens in a first person perspective, as *my* experience, with me as a tacitly self-coinciding perspective on the world. Experience and self-awareness are not separate entities; rather, ipseity is the mode in which experience articulates itself. In the schizophrenia spectrum disorders, this basic sense of self, or sense of being a subject, becomes diminished or distorted and there is an increasing gap between the sense of self and the experiencing. A patient so afflicted said: "I have a slightly strange experience of a lacking relation between myself and what I am thinking". Another complained that "It is as if I am not a part of this world; I have a strange ghostly feeling as if I were from another planet. I am almost non-existent". Yet another patient told us that he always tried hard to "gain his human dignity" by setting for himself difficult attainable tasks in life. He further explained that the expression of "lacking human dignity" referred to a peculiar feeling that he lived his existence "as if" he were a dispensable physical object, just a thing, e.g. a refrigerator, and not really as a living or spiritual subject. This lack of self-presence is typically accompanied by a sense of inner void or a lacking "inner nucleus" (i.e. very elementary forms of identity disturbance), hyper-reflectivity, perplexity, occasional feelings of disturbed transparency of consciousness (feeling "half-awake" or "being 70% conscious"), and diminished immersion or presence in the world. The patient often lives in a reality that is grasped in purely cognitive or intellectual terms ("Realität") rather than in a reality that is felt and lived naturally (["Wirklichkeit"]; see also the vignette by Gadelius in the section on Conceptual evolution). In many patients, the self disorders have a continuous, persisting, trait-like status and they appear to underlie other complaints (such as ambi- or poly-valence, anhedonia or a pervasive, all embracing existential or "ontological" anxiety [259]; see [257] for detailed clinical exposition of the self disorders).

In some patients, the entire existential orientation may be altered into a quasi-solipsistic position: the world appears less real and objective, and it may be fleetingly experienced as somehow relying on one's own consciousness. Such a solipsistic dispositional orientation is often at the bottom of schizotypal grandiosity and may generate occurrent beliefs that we, as psychiatrists, classify on the basis of their content as odd or magical.

Symptoms Omitted from the DSM Diagnostic Criteria

Naturally, in the process of reducing Kety *et al.*'s clinical data into operational format, many features, widely considered to be characteristic of sub-schizophrenic conditions, disappeared and are being increasingly forgotten by clinicians and researchers as well. This progressively spreading amnesia functions as a driving force behind many of the so-called co-morbidity studies, rediscovering sometimes the links already described in the prototypical approach to diagnosis (for a recent theoretical contribution on the issue of comorbidity, see [260]). One such important domain is the "pseudo-neurotic" aspect: at the first medical contact, many patients present symptoms that were once considered as "neurotic", e.g. anxiety and phobias, hypochondria, histrionic conversions, psychosomatic syndromes, eating disorders and obsessive–compulsive symptoms. Unusual combinations of these symptoms, their temporal transformations from one type to another, or their failure to prevent the upsurge of pre-psychotic disintegrative panic or of primitively aggressive and sexual impulses and mental contents, were considered as being potentially indicative of an underlying sub-schizophrenic psychological organization. The same applies to chaotic sexuality, potentially signaling underlying disorganization. The ICD-10 contains one of the "pseudo-neurotic" features in its list of schizotypal criteria: pseudo-obsessive ruminations, often with dysmorphophobic concerns. Obsessions in schizotypy lose their immediate ego-dystonic quality: although recurring, painful and unwelcome, they cease to be strongly and automatically resisted, and convert into a more habitual type of ideation or intense pictorial fantasizing in which the patient may become absorbed, sometimes with a participating or curious attitude. The affective symptoms such as anxiety and depression are not mentioned in the operational context of schizotypy, although these features are quite prevalent in the clinical, treated samples because they constitute some of the reasons for treatment seeking [261]. Anhedonia and ambivalence are mentioned neither in the DSM nor in the ICD—but, as already indicated, both are crucial features of the schizophrenia spectrum disorders, linked, in our view, to the more fundamental anomalies of self-awareness. As already noted, abuse is a common co-morbidity, due to multiple causal pathways [262].

Another important issue is the differential diagnosis between schizotypy and affective illness, although formally speaking it is less a problem for the DSM (where schizotypy is an Axis II disorder) than it is for the ICD (where it is a syndrome, listed just after schizophrenia). This problem is partly related to the phenomenological vacuity and non-specificity of the defining criteria of major depression and partly related to the fact that many schizotypal (and pre-schizophrenic) states are marked by chronic and pervasive anhedonia, lack of existential meaning, and diminished self-presence, that may be mistaken for genuine, primary depressive complaints [146].

It seems to us that the difference between the prototypical and the operational approach to diagnosis [263] accounts for at least some of the problems encountered in contemporary diagnosing, including the issues of co-morbidity. In the prototypical approach, the entire diagnostic process relies on the dialectic between pattern recognition and specific and focused explorations of psychopathology. Schizophrenia spectrum diagnosis is very much dependent on the presence of autistic Gestalt, further investigated by assessment of thought structure, emotional rapport, interpersonal relatedness and the structure of subjective experience. Typically, a single presenting complaint needs an in-depth exploration because it has a widely polysemic meaning. For example, when the patient complains of "being tired and depressed", these terms may signify a whole panoply of subjectively very different mental and bodily states. Unfortunately, such psychopathologic considerations have largely vanished from contemporary psychiatry. Moreover, they are difficult to reconcile with structured interviewing, typically performed by non-clinicians.

THE PARANOID AND SCHIZOID PERSONALITY DISORDERS

The introduction of SPD into DSM-III drained the interest of clinicians and researchers from PPD and SdPD towards SPD, and the former are now "dying" or "dead" entities [264]. This lack of controversy, however, is not indicative of a large consensus within the scientific community. Rather, PPD and SdPD are simply understudied [265].

PPD is defined solely by distrust and suspiciousness, and the DSM-IV criterion A simply lists some of the ways suspiciousness may be enacted; one may wonder why such paraphrasing is limited to seven items rather than, for example, two or twenty. This criterion is also included in the SPD diagnosis, which limits the PPD to more or less purely suspiciousness driven conditions. SdPD is defined by two traits: detachment from social relationships and

TABLE 1.10 DSM-IV Criterion A for paranoid personality disorder (PPD) and schizoid personality disorder (SdPD)

PPD	SdPD
Suspects, without sufficient basis, that others are exploiting, harming, or deceiving him or her	Neither desires nor enjoys close relationships, including being part of a family
Is preoccupied with unjustified doubts about the loyalty or trustworthiness of friends or associates	Almost always chooses solitary activities
Is reluctant to confide in others because of unwarranted fear that the information will be used maliciously against him or her	Has little, if any, interest in having sexual experiences with another person
Reads hidden demeaning or threatening meanings into benign remarks or events	Takes pleasure in few, if any, activities
Persistently bears grudges, i.e. is unforgiving of insults, injuries, or slights	Lacks close friends or confidants other than first-degree relatives
Perceives attacks on his or her character or reputation that are not apparent to others and is quick to react angrily or to counterattack	Appears indifferent to the praise or criticism of others
Has recurrent suspicions, without justification, regarding fidelity of spouse or sexual partner	Shows emotional coldness, detachment, or flattened affectivity

restricted emotional expressivity; criterion A is also limited to a paraphrasing of such traits. In fact, the evacuation of all ego-dystonic features from the SdPD makes it questionable that it is a personality disorder at all. These two SdPD diagnostic features taken at their face value induce an overlap with the SPD criteria (constricted affect and social isolation).

SUMMARY

This review emphasizes SPD as the main area of scientific interest within the recent years, with SdPD and PPD being only occasionally investigated. It appears that SdPD has lost its affinity to schizophrenia after having been converted into an ego-syntonic introversion. PPD is now homogeneously defined by suspiciousness and its behavioural enactments. Epidemiological data from non-genetic studies show a wide prevalence range of these disorders, perhaps suggestive of methodological differences despite the use of operational criteria and structured interviews.

The search for the boundaries of diagnostic entities, such as the schizophrenia spectrum of disorders, does not happen out of the blue or in a theoretical void (no matter how much that is desired), but always starts somewhere. This primary and basic component of validity is its "non-empirical" [32] or conceptual aspect [73]: it refers to what the diagnostic category is supposed to reflect in the very first place, its distinctive original clinical "raison d'être", a precursor of construct validity. In philosophical terms [266], it does not refer to "symptoms" (which may be, but need not be present), but to "criteria", i.e. more basic phenomenal structures defining the nature of a given disorder (e.g. the concepts of autism, generative disorder, or structures of consciousness). This validity aspect of the schizophrenia spectrum disorders is seriously neglected and nearly absent from contemporary discussions. Examples of this absence of considerations on the conceptual validity are the eternal debate on the diagnostic status of K. Schneider's first rank symptoms, and the debate over the diagnosis (affective illness vs schizophrenia) of President Schreber [267–270]. Yet the frequency of the schizophrenia diagnosis varies by a factor of three when the same patients are diagnosed with different, equally reasonable, diagnostic criteria [31]. By extension, similar problems apply to the domain of spectrum disorders, and it seems unlikely that adding or removing one or another symptom in a diagnostic list can resolve this issue. The SPD construct does not have clear and consistent empirical contours (partly because of different ways of recruiting the study subjects). In fact, when preparing this report, we were struck by the disproportion between the massive quantity of empirical effort invested in this domain and the quite provisional validity of the eight original DSM-III SPD criteria that nonetheless have rigidly structured all these empirical efforts. It seems that the operational criteria became reified to the point of a nearly complete and premature extinction of exploratory phenomenological studies, especially concerning subjective experience, psychological structures and, *a fortiori*, the conceptual validity of the schizophrenia spectrum of disorders [241]. Instead, a lot of work has been devoted to creating psychometric scales and interview schedules, typically solely compatible to the existing criteria, and then used in a self-enclosed and self-perpetuating research paradigm (with the work of the Chapmans being one of the notable exceptions). We are like Plato's cavemen who only see shadows and take them to be forms.

In current research, an assumption is implicitly made that neurocognitive dysfunctions may causally underlie or be closely associated with the origins of the clinical symptoms. Tsuang *et al.* [271] suggested recently to expand the schizophrenia spectrum with "schizotaxia" (in the sense of Meehl); an entity marked by subtle cognitive deficits and mild non-specific psychiatric symptoms, on the assumption that such cases may have a potential to progress towards more symptomatic conditions and may be responsive to low-dose antipsychotic treatment. It seems to us, however, that a study of links between neurocognitive profiles and clinical features demands more sophisticated psychopathological descriptions than the current notions of negative, positive, and disorganized symptoms are able to offer, and that the patient's subjectivity and first person perspective need to regain their scientific significance (with the methodological implications that follow from studying the first person perspective [241]). A similar argument applies for the studies of brain-structure/function-clinical symptoms relation.

The classic debate on the continuities and discontinuities in the transitions from normality to full-blown schizophrenia (Bleuler, Kretschmer) repeats itself occasionally in the current literature. There is no decisive information on this issue, and, more precisely, on which transitions, i.e. normality > schizotypy or schizotypy > schizophrenia, are of kind or of degree. During the heydays of operationalism, it was believed that the diagnosis should ultimately reflect distinct, objective and natural illness categories, "carving the nature at its joints" [272]. This so-called "essentialist" view of mental disorders, defined by fixed and intrinsic biological properties, is less vocal today [273]. The more realistic multifactorial threshold models undermine the very notion of natural kind as a well-demarcated ontological entity. Discrete categories may emerge due to nonlinear interactions among multiple causal influence or threshold phenomena. "Discontinuity is often less a joint than it is a bend or graded inflection" [273]. Continuous dimensional phenotypic transitions between entities do not preclude underlying taxonic discontinuity; yet the notion of a taxon should not be confused with the notion of natural kind.

Not unexpectedly, when subjected to mathematical analyses, the SPD construct reveals a variable number of dimensions, usually dependent on the composition of the initial item pool. We have noted Kendler's [30] distinction between the familial and clinical origins of the schizotypy concept: "although the syndromes described by these two traditions share certain important symptoms, they are *not* fundamentally the same". It is often argued that the familial criteria, best reflected in the variously defined "negative" dimension of schizotypy, should have more specific diagnostic importance than the more contingent, clinically derived features.

However, it seems to us that a trait-state distinction is perhaps a better framework to address these issues. Typically, trait dimensions are more likely to display familial aggregation, but state dimensions are a natural component of the clinical picture, and in a certain sense are heritable as well. Viewed in this perspective, the current SPD construct is a mixture of trait and state features; to complicate the matter even more, this mixture is also detectable within the single criteria. As such, the SPD appears less as a personality disorder and more as a syndrome, as it is considered in the ICD-10.

Consistent Evidence

SdPD is rare in clinical settings and does not appear to bear a genetic relation to schizophrenia. SPD is clearly related to schizophrenia on the shared dimension of underlying genetic vulnerability.

Incomplete Evidence

SPD is not a homogenous phenotypic entity. PPD, although rather infrequent in genetic samples, appears to form a part of the schizophrenia spectrum of disorders.

Areas Still Open to Research

There is an urgent need to explore the phenomenology of SPD-related conditions, especially in the domain of subjective experience, relation between experience and expression, and potential shifts of anomalies of subjective experience into psychotic symptoms.

Research is needed on the long-term evolutions of Cluster A conditions and their treatment. There is a need for neurobiological and neuropsychological SPD research, including studies of associations between clinical phenotypes, neurocognitive profiles, brain structure, and function.

Molecular genetic studies may contribute to our understanding of the composition of the so-called schizophrenia spectrum disorders.

REFERENCES

1. American Psychiatric Association (1994) *Diagnostic and Statistical Manual of Mental Disorders*, 4th edn. American Psychiatric Association, Washington.
2. Siever L., Bernstein D.P., Silverman J.M. (1996) Schizotypal personality disorder. In *DSM-IV Sourcebook*, Vol. 4 (Eds T.A. Widiger, A.J. Frances, H.A. Pincus, R. Ross, M.B. First, W. Davis, M. Kline), pp. 682–702. American Psychiatric Association, Washington.
3. Bernstein D.P., Useda D., Siever L.J. (1996) Paranoid personality disorder. In *DSM-IV Sourcebook*, Vol. 4 (Eds T.A. Widiger, A.J. Frances, H.A. Pincus, R. Ross, M.B. First, W. Davis, M. Kline), pp. 665–674. American Psychiatric Association, Washington.
4. World Health Organization (1992) *The ICD-10: International Statistical Classification of Diseases and Related Health Problems* (10th edn.). World Health Organization, Geneva.

5. Ottosson H., Ekselius L., Grann M., Kullgren G. (2002) Cross-system concordance of personality disorder diagnoses of DSM-IV and diagnostic criteria for research of ICD-10. *J. Personal. Disord.*, **16**: 283–292.
6. Torgersen S., Kringlen E., Cramer V. (2001) The prevalence of personality disorders in a community sample. *Arch. Gen. Psychiatry*, **58**: 590–596.
7. Frangos E., Athanassenas G., Tsitourides S., Katsanou N., Alexandrakou P. (1985) Prevalence of DSM-III schizophrenia among the first-degree relatives of schizophrenic probands. *Acta Psychiatr. Scand.*, **72**: 382–386.
8. Kendler K.S., McGuire M., Gruenberg A.M., O'Hare A., Spellman M., Walsh D. (1993) The Roscommon Family Study. III. Schizophrenia-related personality disorders in relatives. *Arch. Gen. Psychiatry*, **50**: 781–788.
9. Baron M., Gruen R., Rainer J.D., Kane J., Asnis L., Lord S. (1985) A family study of schizophrenic and normal control probands: implications for the spectrum concept of schizophrenia. *Am. J. Psychiatry*, **142**: 447–455.
10. Maier W., Lichtermann D., Minges J., Heun R. (1994) Personality disorders among the relatives of schizophrenia patients. *Schizophr. Bull.*, **20**: 481–493.
11. Battaglia M., Cavallini M.C., Macciardi F., Bellodi L. (1997) The structure of DSM-III-R schizotypal personality disorder diagnosed by direct interviews. *Schizophr. Bull.*, **23**: 83–92.
12. Koenigsberg H.W., Kaplan R.D., Gilmore M.M., Cooper A.M. (1985) The relationship between syndrome and personality disorder in DSM-III: experience with 2,462 patients. *Am. J. Psychiatry*, **142**: 207–212.
13. Meehl P.E. (1989) Schizotaxia revisited. *Arch. Gen. Psychiatry*, **46**: 935–944.
14. Bleuler M. (1978) *The Schizophrenic Disorders. Long-term Patient and Family Studies.* Yale University Press, New Haven.
15. Meehl P.E. (1962) Schizotaxia, schizotypy, schizophrenia. *Am. Psychol.*, **17**: 827–838.
16. Torgersen S., Alnæs R. (1992) Differential perception of parental bonding in schizotypal and borderline personality disorder patients. *Compr. Psychiatry*, **33**: 34–38.
17. Johnson J.G., Cohen P., Smailes E.M., Skodol A.E., Brown J., Oldham J.M. (2001) Childhood verbal abuse and risk for personality disorders during adolescence and early adulthood. *Compr. Psychiatry*, **42**: 16–23.
18. Johnson J.G., Cohen P., Kasen S., Skodol A.E., Hamagami F., Brook J.S. (2000) Age-related change in personality disorder trait levels between early adolescence and adulthood: a community-based longitudinal investigation. *Acta Psychiatr. Scand.*, **102**: 265–275.
19. Hoek H.W., Susser E., Buck K.A., Lumey L.H., Lin S.P., Gorman J.M. (1996) Schizoid personality disorder after prenatal exposure to famine. *Am. J. Psychiatry*, **153**: 1637–1639.
20. Venables P.H. (1996) Schizotypy and maternal exposure to influenza and to cold temperature: the Mauritius Study. *J. Abnorm. Psychol.*, **105**: 53–60.
21. Parnas J., Cannon T., Schulsinger F., Mednick S.A. (1995) Early predictors of onset and course of schizophrenia: results from the Copenhagen High-Risk Study. In *Search for the Causes of Schizophrenia*, Vol. 3 (Eds H. Häfner, W.F. Gattaz), pp. 67–86. Springer, Berlin.
22. Stuart S., Pfohl B., Battaglia M., Bellodi L., Grove W., Cadoret R. (1998) The cooccurences of DSM-III-R personality disorders. *J. Person. Disord.*, **12**: 302–315.
23. Fossati A., Maffei C., Battaglia M., Bagnato M., Donati D., Donini M., Fiorilli M., Novella L. (2001) Latent class analysis of DSM-IV schizotypal personality disorder criteria in psychiatric patients. *Schizophr. Bull.*, **27**: 59–71.

24. Nestadt G., Romanoski A.J., Samuels J.F., Folstein M.F., McHugh P.R. (1992) The relationship between personality and DSM-III Axis I disorder in the population: results from an epidemiological survey. *Am. J. Psychiatry*, **149**: 1228–1233.
25. Alnaes R., Torgersen S. (1998) DSM-III symptom disorders (Axis I) and personality disorders (Axis II) in an outpatient population. *Acta Psychiatr. Scand.*, **78**: 348–355.
26. Sobin C., Blundell M.L., Weiller F., Gavigan C., Haiman C., Karayiorgou M. (2000) Evidence of a schizotypy subtype in OCD. *J. Psychiatr. Res.*, **34**: 15–24.
27. Jansson L., Parnas J. (2000) Schizophrenia spectrum diagnoses in 100 consecutive first admissions to a psychiatric department: problems of sampling. Presented at the 2nd International Conference on Early Psychosis, New York.
28. Kalus O., Bernstein D.P., Siever L.J. (1996) Schizoid personality disorder. In *DSM-IV Sourcebook*, Vol. 4 (Eds T.A. Widiger, A.J. Frances, H.A. Pincus, R. Ross, M.B. First, W. Davis, M. Kline), pp. 675–684. American Psychiatric Association, Washington.
29. Millon T. (1981) *Disorders of Personality. DSM-III: Axis II.* Wiley, New York.
30. Kendler K.S. (1985) Diagnostic approaches to schizotypal personality disorder: a historical perspective. *Schizophr. Bull.*, **11**: 538–553.
31. Jansson L., Handest P., Nielsen J., Saebye D., Parnas J. (2002) Exploring boundaries of schizophrenia: a comparison of ICD-10 with other diagnostic systems in first-admitted patients. *World Psychiatry*, **1**: 109–114.
32. Kendler K.S. (1990) Towards a scientific psychiatric nosology. *Arch. Gen. Psychiatry*, **47**: 969–973.
33. Morel B.A. (1860) *Traité des maladies mentales.* Masson, Paris.
34. Kraepelin E. (1909–1915) *Psychiatrie*, 8. Auflage. Barth, Leipzig.
35. Berze J. (1910) *Die hereditären Beziehungen der Dementia præcox: Beitrag zur Hereditätslehre.* Deuticke, Leipzig.
36. Hoch A. (1910) Constitutional factors in the Dementia præcox group. *Rev. Neurol. Psychiatry*, **8**: 463–474.
37. Kahlbaum K. (1890) Über Heboidophrenie. *Allg. Z. Psychiatrie*, **46**: 461–474.
38. Gadelius B. (1933) *Human Mentality in the Light of Psychiatric Experience.* Levin and Munksgaard, Copenhagen.
39. Diem O. (1903) Die einfach demente Form der Dementia praecox (Dementia simplex). Ein klinischer Beitrag zur Kenntniss der Verblödungspsychosen. *Arch. Psychiat. Nervenkrt.*, **37**: 111–187.
40. Bleuler E. (1911) Dementia præcox oder Gruppe der Schizophrenien. In *Handbuch der Psychiatrie* (Ed G. Aschaffenburg). Deuticke, Leipzig.
41. Zilboorg G. (1941) Ambulatory schizophrenias. *Psychiatry*, **4**: 149–155.
42. Hoch P.H., Polatin P. (1949) Pseudoneurotic forms of schizophrenia. *Psychiatr. Q.*, **23**: 248–276.
43. Rado S. (1953) Dynamics and classification of disordered behavior. *Am. J. Psychiatry*, **110**: 406–416.
44. Rado S., Buchenholz B., Dunton H., Karlen S.H., Senescu R. (1956) Schizotypal organization. Preliminary report on a clinical study of schizophrenia. In *Changing Concepts of Psychoanalytic Medicine* (Eds S. Rado, G.E. Daniels), pp. 225–241. Grune and Stratton, New York.
45. Frosch J. (1964) The psychotic character. Clinical psychiatric consideration. *Psychiatr. Q.*, **38**: 1–16.

46. Kety S.S., Rosenthal D., Wender P.H., Schulsinger F. (1968) The types and prevalence of mental illness in the biological and adoptive families of adopted schizophrenics. In *The Transmission of Schizophrenia* (Eds D. Rosenthal, S.S. Kety), pp. 345–362. Pergamon Press, Oxford.

47. Binswanger K. (1920) Über schizoide Alkoholiker. *Z. ges. Neurol. Psychiat.*, **60**: 127–159.

48. Kretschmer E. (1921) *Körperbau und Charakter: Untersuchungen zum Konstitutionsproblem und zur Lehre von den Temperamenten*. Springer, Berlin.

49. Bleuler E. (1922) Die Probleme der Schizoidie und der Syntonie. *Z. ges. Neurol. Psychiat.*, **78**: 373–399.

50. Minkowski E. (1927) *La schizophrénie. Psychopathologie des schizoïdes et des schizophrènes*. Payot, Paris.

51. Kasanin J., Rosen Z.A. (1933) Clinical variables in schizoid personalities. *Arch. Neurol. Psychiatry*, **30**: 538–566.

52. Kallman F.J. (1938) *The Genetics of Schizophrenia*. Augustin, New York.

53. Nannarello J.J. (1953) Schizoid. *J. Nerv. Ment. Dis.*, **118**: 237–249.

54. Deutsch H. (1942) Some forms of emotional disturbance and their relationship to schizophrenia. *Psychoanal. Q.*, **11**: 301–321.

55. Fairbairn W.R.D. (1952) *An Object Relations Theory of Personality*. Basic Books, New York.

56. Dunaif S.L., Hoch P.H. (1955) Pseudopsychopathic schizophrenia. In *Psychiatry and the Law* (Eds P.H. Hoch, J. Zubin), pp. 169–195. Grune and Stratton, New York.

57. Minkowski E. (1933) *Le Temps vécu. Etudes phénoménologiques et psychopathologiques*. Coll. de l'Evolution psychiatrique, Paris.

58. Parnas J., Bovet P. (1991) Autism in schizophrenia revisited. *Compr. Psychiatry*, **32**: 1–15.

59. Urfer A. (2001) Phenomenology and psychopathology of schizophrenia: the views of Eugène Minkowski. *Philos. Psychiatry Psychol.*, **8**: 279–289.

60. Claridge G. (1997) Theoretical background and issues. In *Schizotypy. Implications for Illness and Health* (Ed. G. Claridge), pp. 3–18. Oxford University Press, Oxford.

61. Meehl P.E. (2001) Primary and secondary hypohedonia. *J. Abnorm. Psychol.*, **110**: 188–193.

62. Janet P. (1903) *Les obsessions et la psychasthénie*. Alcan, Paris.

63. Hesnard A.L.M. (1909) *Les troubles de la personalité dans les états d'asthénie psychique. Étude de psychologie clinique*. Thèse de médecine. Université de Bordeaux, Bordeaux.

64. Berze J. (1914) *Über die primäre Insuffizienz der psychischen Aktivität*. Deuticke, Leipzig.

65. Berze J., Gruhle H.W. (1929) *Psychologie der Schizophrenie*. Springer, Berlin.

66. Blankenburg W. (1971) *Der Verlust der natürlichen Selbstverständlichkeit: Ein Beitrag zur Psychopathologie symptomarmer Schizophrenien*. Enke, Stuttgart.

67. Blankenburg W. (1969) Ansätze zu einer Psychopathologie des "common sense" *Confin. Psychiatr.*, **12**: 144–163.

68. Huber G., Gross G., Schuettler R. (1979) *Schizophrenie. Eine Verlaufs- und sozialpsychiatrische Langzeitstudie*. Springer, Berlin.

69. Huber G. (1983) Das Konzept substratnaher Basissymptome und seine Bedeutung für Theorie und Therapie schizophrener Erkrankungen. *Nervenarzt*, **54**: 23–32.

70. Klosterkötter J. (1988) *Basissymptome und Endphänomene der Schizophrenie. Eine empirische Untersuchung der psychopathologischen Übergangsreihen zwischen defizitären und produktiven Schizophreniesymptomen.* Springer, Berlin.
71. Klosterkötter J., Hellmich M., Steinmeyer E.M., Schultze-Lutter F. (2001) Diagnosing schizophrenia in the initial prodromal phase. *Arch. Gen. Psychiatry,* 58: 158–164.
72. McGhie A., Chapman J. (1961) Disorders of attention and perception in early schizophrenia. *Br. J. Med. Psychol.,* 34: 103–116.
73. Parnas J., Bovet P., Zahavi D. (2002) Schizophrenic autism: clinical phenomenology and pathogenetic implications. *World Psychiatry,* 1: 131–136.
74. American Psychiatric Association (1980) *Diagnostic and Statistical Manual of Mental Disorders,* 3rd edn. American Psychiatric Association, Washington.
75. Bovet P., Gamma F. (2002) Vulnerability to schizophrenia: relevance of patients' subjective experience for empirical and clinical work. *Am. J. Med. Gen. (Neuropsychiatr. Gen.),* 114: 923–926.
76. Spitzer R.L., Endicott J., Gibbon M. (1979) Crossing the border into borderline personality and borderline schizophrenia: the development of criteria. *Arch. Gen. Psychiatry,* 36: 17–24.
77. American Psychiatric Association (1987) *Diagnostic and Statistical Manual of Mental Disorders,* 3rd edn, revised. American Psychiatric Association, Washington.
78. Gottesman I.I., Shields J. (1972) *Schizophrenia and Genetics: A Twin Study Vantage Point.* Academic Press, New York.
79. Torgersen S. (1984) Genetic and nosological aspects of schizotypal and borderline personality disorders. *Arch. Gen. Psychiatry,* 41: 546–554.
80. Coryell W., Zimmerman M. (1988) The heritability of schizophrenia and schizoaffective disorder. A family study. *Arch. Gen. Psychiatry,* 45: 323–327.
81. Battaglia M., Gasperini M., Sciuto G., Scherillo P., Diaferia G., Bellodi L. (1991) Psychiatric disorders in the families of schizotypal subjects. *Schizophr. Bull.,* 17: 659–668.
82. Onstad S., Skre I., Edvardsen J., Torgersen S., Kringlen E. (1991) Mental disorders in first-degree relatives of schizophrenics. *Acta. Psychiatr. Scand.,* 83: 463–467.
83. Torgersen S., Onstad S., Skre I., Edvardsen J., Kringlen E. (1993) "True" schizotypal personality disorder: a study of co-twins and relatives of schizophrenic probands. *Am. J. Psychiatry,* 150: 1661–1667.
84. Kendler K.S., McGuire M., Gruenberg A.M., O'Hare A., Spellman M., Walsh D. (1993) The Roscommon Family Study. III. Schizophrenia-related personality disorders in relatives. *Arch. Gen. Psychiatry,* 50: 781–788.
85. Asarnow R.F., Nuechterlein K.H., Fogelson D., Subotnik K.L., Payne D.A., Russell A.T., Asamen J., Kuppinger H., Kendler K.S. (2001) Schizophrenia and schizophrenia-spectrum personality disorders in the first-degree relatives of children with schizophrenia: the UCLA family study. *Arch. Gen. Psychiatry,* 58: 581–588.
86. Parnas J., Cannon T., Jacobsen B., Schulsinger H., Schulsinger F., Mednick S.A. (1993) Life-time DSM-III-R diagnostic outcomes in offspring of schizophrenic mothers: the results from the Copenhagen High Risk Study. *Arch. Gen. Psychiatry,* 50: 707–714.
87. Erlenmeyer-Kimling L., Squires-Wheeler E., Adamo U.H., Bassett A.S., Cornblatt B.A., Kestenbaum C.J., Rock D., Roberts S.A., Gottesman I.I. (1995) The New York High-Risk Project: psychoses and cluster A personality

disorders in offspring of schizophrenic patients at 23 years of follow-up. *Arch. Gen. Psychiatry*, **52**: 857–865.

88. Heston L.L. (1966) Psychiatric disorders in foster home reared children of schizophrenic mothers. *Br. J. Psychiatry*, **112**: 819–825.

89. Kety S.S., Wender P.H., Jacobsen B., Ingraham L.J., Jansson L., Faber B., Kinney D.K. (1994) Mental illness in the biological and adoptive relatives of schizophrenic adoptees. Replication of the Copenhagen Study in the rest of Denmark. *Arch. Gen. Psychiatry*, **51**: 442–455.

90. Tienari P., Wynne L.C., Moring J., Läksy K., Nieminen P., Sorri A., Lahti I., Wahlberg K.E., Naarala M., Kurki-Suonio K. *et al.* (2000) Finnish adoptive family study: sample selection and adoptee DSM-III-R diagnoses. *Acta Psychiatr. Scand.*, **101**: 433–443.

91. Squires-Wheeler E., Skodol A.E., Friedman D., Erlenmeyer-Kimling L. (1988) The specificity of DSM-III schizotypal personality traits. *Psychol. Med.*, **18**: 757–765.

92. Erlenmeyer-Kimling L. (2003) Personal communication.

93. Kendler K.S. (1988) Familial aggregation of schizophrenia and schizophrenia spectrum disorders. Evaluation of conflicting results. *Arch. Gen. Psychiatry*, **45**: 377–383.

94. Siever L.J., Silverman J.M., Horvath T.B., Klar H.M., Coccaro E., Keefe R.S., Pinkham L., Rinaldi P., Mohs R.C., Davis K.L. (1990) Increased morbid risk for schizophrenia-related disorders in relatives of schizotypal personality disordered patients. *Arch. Gen. Psychiatry*, **47**: 634–640.

95. Kendler K.S., Gruenberg A.M. (1982) Genetic relationship between paranoid personality disorder and the "schizophrenic spectrum" disorders. *Am. J. Psychiatry*, **139**: 1185–1186.

96. Kendler K.S., Walsh D. (1995) Schizotypal personality disorder in parents and the risk for schizophrenia in siblings. *Schizophr. Bull.*, **21**: 47–52.

97. Parnas J. (1985) Mates of schizophrenic mothers: a study of assortative mating from the American-Danish high risk study. *Br. J. Psychiatry*, **146**: 490–497.

98. Straub R.E., MacLean C.J., Ma Y., Webb B.T., Myakishev M.V., Harris-Kerr C., Wormley B., Sadek H., Kadambi B., O'Neill F.A. *et al.* (2002) Genome-wide scans of three independent sets of 90 Irish multiplex schizophrenia families and follow-up of selected regions in all families provides evidence for multiple susceptibility genes. *Mol. Psychiatry*, **7**: 542–559.

99. Lewis C.M., Levinson D.F., Wise L.H., DeLisi L.E., Straub R.E., Hovatta I., Williams N.M., Schwab S.G., Pulver A.E., Faraone S.V. *et al.* (2003) Genome scan meta-analysis of schizophrenia and bipolar disorder, part II: Schizophrenia. *Am. J. Hum. Genet.*, **73**: 34–48.

100. Kendler K.S., McGuire M., Gruenberg A.M., O'Hare A., Spellman M., Walsh D. (1993) The Roscommon Family Study. I. Methods, diagnosis of probands, and risk of schizophrenia in relatives. *Arch. Gen. Psychiatry*, **50**: 527–540.

101. Kendler K.S., McGuire M., Gruenberg A.M., O'Hare A., Spellman M., Walsh D. (1993) The Roscomon Family Study. IV. Affective illness, anxiety disorders, and alcoholism in relatives. *Arch. Gen. Psychiatry*, **50**: 952–960.

102. Kendler K.S., Neale M.C., Walsh D. (1995) Evaluating the spectrum concept of schizophrenia in the Roscommon Family Study. *Am. J. Psychiatry*, **152**: 749–754.

103. Kendler K.S., Gardner C.O. (1997) The risk for psychiatric disorders in relatives of schizophrenic and control probands: a comparison of three independent studies. *Psychol. Medicine*, **27**: 411–419.

104. Gottesman I.I. (1994) Schizophrenia epigenesis: past, present, and future. *Acta Psychiatr. Scand.*, **90**: 26–33.
105. Heston L.L. (1970) The genetics of schizophrenic and schizoid disease. *Science*, **167**: 249–256.
106. Holzman P.S., Kringlen E., Matthysse S., Flanagan S.D., Lipton R.B., Cramer G., Levin S., Lange K., Levy D.L. (1988) A single dominant gene can account for eye tracking dysfunctions and schizophrenia in offspring of discordant twins. *Arch. Gen. Psychiatry*, **45**: 641–647.
107. Parnas J., Schulsinger F., Schulsinger H., Mednick S.A., Teasdale T.W. (1982) Behavioral precursors of schizophrenia spectrum: a prospective study. *Arch. Gen. Psychiatry*, **39**: 658–664.
108. Parnas J., Teasdale T.W., Schulsinger H. (1985) Institutional rearing and diagnostic outcome in children of schizophrenic mothers: a prospective high risk study. *Arch. Gen. Psychiatry*, **42**: 762–769.
109. Carter J.W., Schulsinger F., Parnas J., Cannon T., Mednick S.A. (2003) A multivariate prediction model of schizophrenia. *Schizophr. Bull.*, **28**: 649–682.
110. Schulsinger F., Parnas J., Petersen T.E., Schulsinger H., Teasdale T.W., Mednick S.A., Møller L. (1984) Cerebral ventricular size in offspring of schizophrenic mothers: a preliminary study. *Arch. Gen. Psychiatry*, **41**: 602–606.
111. Cannon T.D., Mednick S.A., Parnas J., Schulsinger F., Præstholm J., Vestergaard Å. (1993) Developmental brain abnormalities in the offspring of schizophrenic mothers: I. Contributions of genetic and perinatal factors. *Arch. Gen. Psychiatry*, **50**: 551–564.
112. Cannon T.D., Mednick S.A., Parnas J., Schulsinger F., Praestholm J., Vestergaard Å. (1994) Developmental brain abnormalities in the offspring of schizophrenic mothers. II. Structural brain characteristics of schizophrenia and schizotypal personality disorder. *Arch. Gen. Psychiatry*, **51**: 955–962.
113. Cannon T.D., van Erp T.G., Huttunen M., Lonnqvist J., Salonen O., Valanne L., Poutanen V.P., Standertskjold-Nordenstam C.G., Gur R.E., Yan M. (1998) Regional gray matter, white matter, and cerebrospinal fluid distributions in schizophrenic patients, their siblings, and controls. *Arch. Gen. Psychiatry*, **55**: 1084–1091.
114. Tienari P., Wynne L.C., Sorri A., Lahti I., Läksy K., Moring J., Naarala M., Nieminen P., Wahlberg K.E., Miettunen J. (2002) Genotype-environment interaction in the Finnish adoptive family study. Interplay between genes and environment? In *Risk and Protective Factors in Schizophrenia. Towards a Conceptual Model of the Disease Process* (Ed. H. Häfner), pp. 29–38. Steinkopff, Darmstadt.
115. Parnas J., Jørgensen Å. (1989) Premorbid psychopathology in schizophrenia spectrum. *Br. J. Psychiatry*, **155**: 623–627.
116. Tyrka A.R., Cannon T.D., Haslam N., Mednick S.A., Schulsinger F., Schulsinger H., Parnas J. (1995) The latent structure of schizotypy. I. Premorbid indicators of a taxon of individuals at risk for schizophrenia spectrum disorders. *J. Abnorm. Psychol.*, **104**: 173–183.
117. Olin S.S., Raine A., Cannon T.D., Parnas J., Schulsinger F., Mednick S.A. (1997) Childhood behavior precursors of schizotypal personality disorder. *Schizophr. Bull.*, **23**: 93–103.
118. Freedman L.R., Rock D., Roberts S.A., Cornblatt B.A., Erlenmeyer-Kimling L. (1998) The New York High-Risk Project: attention, anhedonia and social outcome. *Schizophr. Res.*, **30**: 1–9.

119. Ott S.L., Allen J., Erlenmeyer-Kimling L. (2001) The New York High-Risk Project: observations on the rating of early manifestations of schizophrenia. *Am. J. Med. Genet.*, **105**: 25–27.
120. Weiser M., Reichenberg A., Rabinowitz J., Kaplan Z., Mark M., Bodner E., Nahon D., Davidson M. (2001) Association between nonpsychotic psychiatric diagnoses in adolescent males and subsequent onset of schizophrenia. *Arch. Gen. Psychiatry*, **58**: 959–964.
121. Rodriguez Solano J.J., Gonzalez De Chavez M. (2000) Premorbid personality disorders in schizophrenia. *Schizophr. Res.*, **44**: 137–144.
122. Jørgensen Å., Parnas J. (1990) The Copenhagen High-Risk Study: premorbid and clinical dimensions of maternal schizophrenia. *J. Nerv. Ment. Dis.*, **178**: 370–376.
123. Cannon T.D., Mednick S.A., Parnas J. (1990) Antecedents of predominantly negative- and predominantly positive-symptom schizophrenia in a high-risk population. *Arch. Gen. Psychiatry*, **47**: 622–632.
124. Cuesta M.J., Peralta V., Caro F. (1999) Premorbid personality in psychoses. *Schizophr. Bull.*, **25**: 801–811.
125. Wolff S. (1991). 'Schizoid' personality in childhood and adult life. I: The vagaries of diagnostic labelling. *Br. J. Psychiatry*, **159**: 615–620.
126. Wolff S., Townshend R., McGuire R.J., Weeks D.J. (1991). 'Schizoid' personality in childhood and adult life. II: Adult adjustment and the continuity with schizotypal personality disorder. *Br. J. Psychiatry*, **159**: 620–629.
127. Bentall R.P., Claridge G.S., Slade P.D. (1989) The multidimensional nature of schizotypal traits: a factor analytic study with normal subjects. *Br. J. Clin. Psychol.*, **28**: 363–375.
128. Bergman A.J., Harvey P.D., Mitropoulou V., Aronson A., Marder D., Silverman J., Trestman R., Siever L.J. (1996) The factor structure of schizotypal symptoms in a clinical population. *Schizophr. Bull.*, **22**: 501–509.
129. Claridge G., McCreery C., Mason O., Bentall R., Boyle G., Slade P., Popplewell D. (1996) The factor structure of schizotypal traits: a large replication study. *Br. J. Clin. Psychol.*, **35**: 103–115.
130. Gruzelier J., Burgess A., Stygall J., Irving G., Raine A. (1995) Patterns of cognitive asymmetry and syndromes of schizotypal personality. *Psychiatry Res.*, **56**: 71–79.
131. Gruzelier J.H. (1996) The factorial structure of schizotypy: Part I. Affinities with syndromes of schizophrenia. *Schizophr. Bull.*, **22**: 611–620.
132. Handest P., Parnas J. (in press) Clinical characteristics of 50 first admitted ICD-10 schizotypal patients. *Br. J. Psychiatry*.
133. Kendler K.S., Ochs A.L., Gorman A.M., Hewitt J.K., Ross D.E., Mirsky A.F. (1991) The structure of schizotypy: a pilot multitrait twin study. *Psychiatry Res.*, **36**: 19–36.
134. Kendler K.S., Hewitt J. (1992) The structure of self-report schizotypy in twins. *J. Personal. Disord.*, **6**: 1–17.
135. Livesley W.J., Schroeder M.L. (1990) Dimensions of personality disorder. The DSM-III-R cluster A diagnoses. *J. Nerv. Ment. Dis.*, **178**: 627–635.
136. Mason O. (1995) A confirmatory factor analysis of the structure of schizotypy. *Eur. J. Personal.*, **9**: 271–281.
137. Nuechterlein K.H., Asarnow R.F., Subotnik K.L., Fogelson D.L., Payne D.L., Kendler K.S., Neale M.C., Jacobson K.C., Mintz J. (2002) The structure of schizotypy: relationships between neurocognitive and personality disorder

features in relatives of schizophrenic patients in the UCLA family study. *Schizophr. Res.*, **54**: 121–130.

138. Raine A., Reynolds C., Lencz T., Scerbo A., Triphon N., Kim D. (1994) Cognitive-perceptual, interpersonal, and disorganized features of schizotypal personality. *Schizophr. Bull.*, **20**: 191–201.

139. Reynolds C.A., Raine A., Mellingen K., Venables P.H., Mednick S.A. (2000) Three-factor model of schizotypal personality: invariance across culture, gender, religious affiliation, family adversity, and psychopathology. *Schizophr. Bull.*, **26**: 603–618.

140. Rossi A., Daneluzzo E. (2002) Schizotypal dimensions in normals and schizophrenic patients: a comparison with other clinical samples. *Schizophr. Res.*, **54**: 67–75.

141. Suhr J.A., Spitznagel M.B. (2001) Factor versus cluster models of schizotypal traits. I: Comparison of unselected and highly schizotypal samples. *Schizophr. Res.*, **52**: 231–239.

142. Venables P.H., Bailes K. (1994) The structure of schizotypy, its relation to subdiagnoses of schizophrenia and to sex and age. *Br. J. Clin. Psychol.*, **33**: 277–294.

143. Venables P.H., Rector N.A. (2000) The content and structure of schizotypy: a study using confirmatory factor analysis. *Schizophr. Bull.*, **26**: 587–602.

144. Vollema M.G., Hoijtink H. (2000) The multidimensionality of self-report schizotypy in a psychiatric population: an analysis using multidimensional Rasch models. *Schizophr. Bull.*, **26**: 565–575.

145. Wolfradt U., Straube E.R. (1998) Factor structure of schizotypal traits among adolescents. *Person. Individ. Diff.*, **24**: 201–206.

146. Wittman P., Sheldon W. (1948) A proposed classification of psychotic behavior reactions. *Am. J. Psychiatry*, **105**: 124–128.

147. Chapman L.J., Chapman J.P., Numbers J.S., Edell W.S., Carpenter B.N., Beckfield D. (1984) Impulsive nonconformity as a trait contributing to the prediction of psychotic-like and schizotypal symptoms. *J. Nerv. Ment. Dis.*, **172**: 681–691.

148. Eckblad M., Chapman L.J. (1983) Magical ideation as an indicator of schizotypy. *J. Consult. Clin. Psychol.*, **51**: 215–225.

149. Chapman L.J., Chapman J.P., Raulin M.L. (1978) Body-image aberration in schizophrenia. *J. Abnorm. Psychol.*, **87**: 399–407.

150. Peters E.R., Joseph S.A., Garety P.A. (1999) Measurement of delusional ideation in the normal population: introducing the PDI (Peters *et al.* Delusions Inventory). *Schizophr. Bull.*, **25**: 553–576.

151. Chapman L.J., Chapman J.P., Raulin M.L. (1976) Scales for physical and social anhedonia. *J. Abnorm. Psychol.*, **85**: 374–382.

152. Eysenck H.J., Eysenck S.B.G. (1975) *Manual of the Eysenck Personality Questionnaire*. Hodder and Stoughton, London.

153. Eysenck S.B.G., Eysenck H.J., Barrett P. (1985) A revised version of the psychoticism scale. *Person. Indiv. Diff.*, **6**: 21–29.

154. Eckblad M.L., Chapman L.J., Chapman J.P., Mishlove M. (1982) *The Revised Social Anhedonia Scale*. Unpublished test. University of Wisconsin, Madison.

155. Rust J. (1988) The Rust Inventory of Schizotypal Cognition (RISC). *Schizophr. Bull.*, **14**: 317–322.

156. Golden R.R., Meehl P.E. (1979) Detection of the schizoid taxon with MMPI indicators. *J. Abnorm. Psychol.*, **88**: 217–233.

157. Venables P.H., Wilkins S., Mitchell D.A., Raine A., Bailes K. (1990) A scale for the measurement of schizotypy. *Person. Indiv. Diff.*, **11**: 481–495.
158. Nielsen T.C., Petersen N.E. (1976) Electrodermal correlates of extraversion, trait anxiety, and schizophrenism. *Scand. J. Psychol.*, **17**: 73–80.
159. Raine A. (1991) The SPQ: A scale for the assessment of schizotypal personality based on DSM-III-R criteria. *Schizophr. Bull.*, **17**: 555–564.
160. Claridge G.S., Broks P. (1984) Schizotypy and hemisphere function: I. Theoretical considerations and the measurement of schizotypy. *Person. Indiv. Diff.*, **5**: 633–648.
161. Loranger A.W., Sussman V.L., Oldham J.M., Russakoff L.M. (1985) *Personality Disorder Examination: A Structured Interview for Making Diagnosis of DSM-III-R Personality Disorders.* Cornell Medical College, White Plains.
162. Baron M., Asnis L., Gruen R. (1981) The Schedule for Schizotypal Personalities (SSP): a diagnostic interview for schizotypal features. *Psychiatry Res.*, **4**: 213–228.
163. Stangl D., Pfohl B., Zimmerman M., Bowers W., Corenthal C. (1985) A structured interview for the DSM-III personality disorders. A preliminary report. *Arch. Gen. Psychiatry*, **42**: 591–596.
164. Pfohl B., Blum N., Zimmerman M., Stangl D. (1989) *Structured Interview for DSM-III-R Personality Disorders—Revised (SIDP-R).* University of Iowa, Iowa City.
165. First M.B., Spitzer R.L., Gibbon M., Williams J.B.W., Benjamin L. (1994) *Structured Clinical Interview for DSM-IV Axis II Personality Disorders (SCID-II).* New York State Psychiatric Hospital, New York.
166. Kendler K.S., Lieberman J.A., Walsh D. (1989) The Structured Interview for Schizotypy (SIS): a preliminary report. *Schizophr. Bull.*, **15**: 559–571.
167. Vollema M.G., Ormel J. (2000) The reliability of the Structured Interview for Schizotypy—Revised. *Schizophr. Bull.*, **26**: 619–629.
168. Gunderson J.G., Siever L.J., Spaulding E. (1983) The search for a schizotype. Crossing the border again. *Arch. Gen. Psychiatry*, **40**: 15–22.
169. Vollema M.G., Sitskoorn M.M., Appels M.C.M., Kahn R.S. (2002) Does the Schizotypal Personality Questionnaire reflect the biological-genetic vulnerability to schizophrenia? *Schizophr. Res.*, **54**: 39–45.
170. Kendler K.S., McGuire M., Gruenberg A.M., Walsh D. (1995) Schizotypal symptoms and signs in the Roscommon family study. Their factor structure and familial relationship with psychotic and affective disorders. *Arch. Gen. Psychiatry*, **52**: 296–303.
171. Fanous A., Gardner C., Walsh D., Kendler K.S. (2001) Relationship between positive and negative symptoms of schizophrenia and schizotypal symptoms in nonpsychotic relatives. *Arch. Gen. Psychiatry*, **58**: 669–673.
172. Torgersen S., Edvardsen J., Øien P.A., Onstad S., Skre I., Lygren S., Kringlen E. (2002) Schizotypal personality disorder inside and outside the schizophrenic spectrum. *Schizophr. Res.*, **54**: 33–38.
173. Johnston M.H., Holzman P.S. (1979) *Assessing Schizophrenic Thinking. A Clinical and Research Instrument for Measuring Thought Disorder.* Jossey-Bass, San Francisco.
174. Arboleda C., Holzman P.S. (1985) Thought disorder in children at risk for psychosis. *Arch. Gen. Psychiatry*, **42**: 1004–1013.
175. Kinney D.K., Holzman P.S., Jacobsen B., Jansson L., Faber B., Hildebrand W., Kasell E., Zimbalist M.E. (1997) Thought disorder in schizophrenic and control adoptees and their relatives. *Arch. Gen. Psychiatry*, **54**: 475–479.

176. Shenton M.E., Solovay M.R., Holzman P.S., Coleman M., Gale H.J. (1989) Thought disorder in the relatives of psychotic patients. *Arch. Gen. Psychiatry*, **46**: 897–901.

177. Korfine L., Lenzenweger M.F. (1995) The taxonicity of schizotypy: a replication. *J. Abnorm. Psychol.*, **104**: 26–31.

178. Essen-Möller E. (1946) The concept of schizoidia. *Mtschrft. Psychiatr. Neurol.*, **112**: 258–271.

179. Lenzenweger M.F. (2000) Two-point discrimination thresholds and schizotypy: illuminating a somatosensory dysfunction. *Schizophr. Res.*, **42**: 111–124.

180. Roitman S.E., Mitropoulou V., Keefe R.S., Silverman J.M., Serby M., Harvey P.D., Reynolds D.A., Mohs R.C., Siever L.J. (2000) Visuospatial working memory in schizotypal personality disorder patients. *Schizophr. Res.*, **41**: 447–455.

181. Schiffman J., Ekstrom M., LaBrie J., Schulsinger F., Sorensen H., Mednick S. (2003) Dr. Schiffman and colleagues reply. *Am. J. Psychiatry*, **160**: 394.

182. Weinstein D.D., Diforio D., Schiffman J., Walker E., Bonsall R. (1999) Minor physical anomalies, dermatoglyphic asymmetries, and cortisol levels in adolescents with schizotypal personality disorder. *Am. J. Psychiatry*, **156**: 617–623.

183. Lencz T., Raine A. (1995) Schizotypal personality: synthesis and future directions. In *Schizotypal Personality* (Eds A. Raine, T. Lencz, S.A. Mednick), pp. 429–459. Cambridge University Press, New York.

184. Maier W., Falkai P., Wagner M. (1999) Schizophrenia spectrum disorders: a review. In *Schizophrenia* (Eds M. Maj, N. Sartorius), pp. 311–371. Wiley, Chichester.

185. O'Flynn K.O., Gruzelier J., Bergman A., Siever L.J. (2003) The schizophrenia spectrum personality disorders. In *Schizophrenia. Part One. Descriptive Aspects* (Eds S.R. Hirsch, D. Weinberger), pp. 80–100. Blackwell, Oxford.

186. Byne W., Buchsbaum M.S., Kemether E., Hazlett E.A., Shinwari A., Mitropoulou V., Siever L.J. (2001) Magnetic resonance imaging of the thalamic mediodorsal nucleus and pulvinar in schizophrenia and schizotypal personality disorder. *Arch. Gen. Psychiatry*, **58**: 133–140.

187. Dickey C.C., McCarley R.W., Voglmaier M.M., Niznikiewicz M.A., Seidman L.J., Hirayasu Y., Fischer I., Teh E.K., Van Rhoads R., Jakab M. *et al.* (1999) Schizotypal personality disorder and MRI abnormalities of temporal lobe gray matter. *Biol. Psychiatry*, **45**: 1393–1402.

188. Dickey C.C., Shenton M.E., Hirayasu Y., Fischer I., Voglmaier M.M., Niznikiewicz M.A., Seidman L.J., Fraone S., McCarley R.W. (2000) Large CSF volume not attributable to ventricular volume in schizotypal personality disorder. *Am. J. Psychiatry*, **157**: 48–54.

189. Dickey C.C., McCarley R.W., Voglmaier M.M., Frumin M., Niznikiewicz M.A., Hirayasu Y., Fraone S., Seidman L.J., Shenton M.E. (2002) Smaller left Heschl's gyrus volume in patients with schizotypal personality disorder. *Am. J. Psychiatry*, **159**: 1521–1527.

190. Downhill J.E. Jr., Buchsbaum M.S., Wei T., Spiegel-Cohen J., Hazlett E.A., Haznedar M.M., Silverman J., Siever L.J. (2000) Shape and size of the corpus callosum in schizophrenia and schizotypal personality disorder. *Schizophr. Res.*, **42**: 193–208.

191. Downhill J.E. Jr., Buchsbaum M.S., Hazlett E.A., Barth S., Lees-Roitman S., Nunn M., Lekarev O., Wei T., Shihabuddin L., Mitropoulou V. *et al.* (2001) Temporal lobe volume determined by magnetic resonance imaging in

schizotypal personality disorder and schizophrenia. *Schizophr. Res.*, **48**: 187–199.

192. Hazlett E.A., Buchsbaum M.S., Byne W., Wei T.C., Spiegel-Cohen J., Geneve C., Kinderlehrer R., Haznedar M.M., Shihabuddin L., Siever L. J. (1999) Three-dimensional analysis with MRI and PET of the size, shape, and function of the thalamus in the schizophrenia spectrum. *Am. J. Psychiatry*, **156**: 1190–1199.

193. Kurokawa K., Nakamura K., Sumiyoshi T., Hagino H., Yotsutsuji T., Yamashita I., Suzuki M., Matsui M., Kurachi M. (2000) Ventricular enlargement in schizophrenia spectrum patients with prodromal symptoms of obsessive-compulsive disorder. *Psychiatry Res.*, **99**: 83–91.

194. Kwon J.S., Shenton M.E., Hirayasu Y., Salisbury D.F., Fischer I.A., Dickey C.C., Yurgelun-Todd D., Tohen M., Kikinis R., Jolesz F.A. *et al.* (1998) MRI study of cavum septi pellucidi in schizophrenia, affective disorder, and schizotypal personality disorder. *Am. J. Psychiatry*, **155**: 509–515.

195. Levitt J.J., McCarley R.W., Dickey C.C., Voglmaier M.M., Niznikiewicz M.A., Seidman L.J., Hirayasu Y., Ciszewski A.A., Kikinis R., Jolesz F.A. *et al.* (2002) MRI study of caudate nucleus volume and its cognitive correlates in neuroleptic-naive patients with schizotypal personality disorder. *Am. J. Psychiatry*, **159**: 1190–1197.

196. Shihabuddin L., Buchsbaum M.S., Hazlett E.A., Silverman J., New A., Brickman A.M., Mitropoulou V., Nunn M., Fleischman M.B., Tang C. *et al.* (2001) Striatal size and relative glucose metabolic rate in schizotypal personality disorder and schizophrenia. *Arch. Gen. Psychiatry*, **58**: 877–884.

197. Takahashi T., Suzuki M., Kawasaki Y., Kurokawa K., Hagino H., Yamashita I., Zhou S.Y., Nohara S., Nakamura K., Seto H. *et al.* (2002) Volumetric magnetic resonance imaging study of the anterior cingulate gyrus in schizotypal disorder. *Eur. Arch. Psychiatry Clin. Neurosci.*, **252**: 268–277.

198. Buchsbaum M.S., Trestman R.L., Hazlett E., Siegel B.V. Jr., Schaefer C.H., Luu-Hsia C., Tang C., Herrera S., Solimando A.C., Losonczy M. *et al.* (1997) Regional cerebral blood flow during the Wisconsin Card Sort Test in schizotypal personality disorder. *Schizophr. Res.*, **27**: 21–28.

199. Buchsbaum M.S., Nenadic I., Hazlett E.A., Spiegel-Cohen J., Fleischman M.B., Akhavan A., Silverman J.M., Siever L.J. (2002) Differential metabolic rates in prefrontal and temporal Brodmann areas in schizophrenia and schizotypal personality disorder. *Schizophr. Res.*, **54**: 141–150.

200. Fukuzako H., Kodama S., Fukuzako T. (2002) Phosphorus metabolite changes in temporal lobes of subjects with schizotypal personality disorder. *Schizophr. Res.*, **58**: 201–203.

201. Kirrane R.M., Mitropoulou V., Nunn M., New A.S., Harvey P.D., Schopick F., Silverman J., Siever L.J. (2000) Effects of amphetamine on visuospatial working memory performance in schizophrenia spectrum personality disorder. *Neuropsychopharmacology*, **22**: 14–18.

202. Kirrane R.M., Mitropoulou V., Nunn M., Silverman J., Siever L.J. (2001) Physostigmine and cognition in schizotypal personality disorder. *Schizophr. Res.*, **48**: 1–5.

203. Siegel B.V. Jr., Trestman R.L., O'Flaithbheartaigh S., Mitropoulou V., Amin F., Kirrane R., Silverman J., Schmeidler J., Keefe R.S., Siever L.J. (1996) D-amphetamine challenge effects on Wisconsin Card Sort Test. Performance in schizotypal personality disorder. *Schizophr. Res.*, **20**: 29–32.

204. Grove W.M., Lebow B.S., Medus C. (1991) Head size in relation to schizophrenia and schizotypy. *Schizophr. Bull.*, **17**: 157–161.

205. Schiffman J., Ekstrom M., LaBrie J., Schulsinger F., Sorensen H., Mednick S. (2002) Minor physical anomalies and schizophrenia spectrum disorders: a prospective investigation. *Am. J. Psychiatry*, **159**: 238–243.

206. Neumann C.S., Walker E.F. (1999) Motor dysfunction in schizotypal personality disorder. *Schizophr. Res.*, **38**: 159–168.

207. Thaker G.K., Ross D.E., Cassady S.L., Adami H.M., Medoff D.R., Sherr J. (2000) Saccadic eye movement abnormalities in relatives of patients with schizophrenia. *Schizophr. Res.*, **45**: 235–244.

208. Walker E., Lewis N., Loewy R., Palyo S. (1999) Motor dysfunction and risk for schizophrenia. *Dev. Psychopathol.*, **11**: 509–523.

209. Brenner C.A., McDowell J.E., Cadenhead K.S., Clementz B.A. (2001) Saccadic inhibition among schizotypal personality disorder subjects. *Psychophysiology*, **38**: 399–403.

210. Cadenhead K.S., Perry W., Shafer K., Braff D.L. (1999) Cognitive functions in schizotypal personality disorder. *Schizophr. Res.*, **37**: 123–132.

211. Cadenhead K.S., Light G.A., Geyer M.A., Braff D.L. (2000) Sensory gating deficits assessed by the P50 event-related potential in subjects with schizotypal personality disorder. *Am. J. Psychiatry*, **157**: 55–59.

212. Cadenhead K.S., Swerdlow N.R., Shafer K.M., Diaz M., Braff D.L. (2000) Modulation of the startle response and startle laterality in relatives of schizophrenic patients and in subjects with schizotypal personality disorder: evidence of inhibitory deficits. *Am. J. Psychiatry*, **157**: 1660–1668.

213. Cadenhead K.S., Light G.A., Geyer M.A., McDowell J.E., Braff D.L. (2002) Neurobiological measures of schizotypal personality disorder: defining an inhibitory endophenotype? *Am. J. Psychiatry*, **159**: 869–871.

214. Granholm E., Cadenhead K., Shafer K.M., Filoteo J.V. (2002) Lateralized perceptual organization deficits on the global-local task in schizotypal personality disorder. *J. Abnorm. Psychol.*, **111**: 42–52.

215. Harvey P.D., Keefe R.S.E., Mitropoulou V., DuPre R., Lees Roitman S., Mohs R.C., Siever L.J. (1996) Information-processing markers of vulnerability to schizophrenia: performance of patients with schizotypal and nonschizotypal personality disorders. *Psychiatry Res.*, **60**: 49–56.

216. Laurent A., Biloa-Tang M., Bougerol T., Duly D., Anchisi A.M., Bosson J.L., Pellat J., d'Amato T., Dalery J. (2000) Executive/attentional performance and measures of schizotypy in patients with schizophrenia and in their nonpsychotic first-degree relatives. *Schizophr. Res.*, **46**: 269–283.

217. Moran M.J., Thaker G.K., Laporte D.J., Cassady S.L., Ross D.E. (1996) Covert visual attention in schizophrenia spectrum personality disordered subjects: visuospatial cuing and alerting effects. *J. Psychiatr. Res.*, **30**: 261–275.

218. Moriarty P.J., Harvey P.D., Mitropoulou V., Granholm E., Silverman J.M., Siever L.J. (2003) Reduced processing resource availability in schizotypal personality disorder: evidence from a dual-task CPT study. *J. Clin. Exp. Neuropsychol.*, **25**: 335–347.

219. Niznikiewicz M.A., Voglmaier M., Shenton M.E., Seidman L.J., Dickey C.C., Rhoads R., Teh E., McCarley R.W. (1999) Electrophysiological correlates of language processing in schizotypal personality disorder. *Am. J. Psychiatry*, **156**: 1052–1058.

220. Niznikiewicz M.A., Voglmaier M.M., Shenton M.E., Dickey C.C., Seidman L.J., Teh E., Van Rhoads R., McCarley R.W. (2000) Lateralized P3 deficit in schizotypal personality disorder. *Biol. Psychiatry*, **48**: 702–705.

221. Niznikiewicz M.A., Shenton M.E., Voglmaier M., Nestor P.G., Dickey C.C., Frumin M., Seidman L.J., Allen C.G., McCarley R.W. (2002) Semantic dysfunction in women with schizotypal personality disorder. *Am. J. Psychiatry*, **159**: 1767–1774.

222. Raine A., Benishay D., Lencz T., Scarpa A. (1997) Abnormal orienting in schizotypal personality disorder. *Schizophr. Bull.*, **23**: 75–82.

223. Salisbury D.F., Voglmaier M.M., Seidman L.J., McCarley R.W. (1996) Topographic abnormalities of P3 in schizotypal personality disorder. *Biol. Psychiatry*, **40**: 165–172.

224. Voglmaier M.M., Seidman L.J., Niznikiewicz M.A., Dickey C.C., Shenton M.E., McCarley R.W. (2000) Verbal and nonverbal neuropsychological test performance in subjects with schizotypal personality disorder. *Am. J. Psychiatry*, **157**: 787–793.

225. Bergman A.J., Harvey P.D., Roitman S.L., Mohs R.C., Marder D., Silverman J.M., Siever L.J. (1998) Verbal learning and memory in schizotypal personality disorder. *Schizophr. Bull.*, **24**: 635–641.

226. Farmer C.M., O'Donnell B.F., Niznikiewicz M.A., Voglmaier M.M., McCarley R.W., Shenton M.E. (2000) Visual perception and working memory in schizotypal personality disorder. *Am. J. Psychiatry*, **157**: 781–788.

227. Diforio D., Walker E.F., Kestler L.P. (2000) Executive functions in adolescents with schizotypal personality disorder. *Schizophr. Res.*, **42**: 125–134.

228. Wickham H., Murray R.M. (1997) Can biological markers identify endophenotypes predisposing to schizophrenia? *Int. Rev. Psychiatry*, **9**: 355–364.

229. Siever L.J., Koenigsberg H.W., Harvey P., Mitropoulou V., Laruelle M., Abi-Dargham A., Goodman M., Buchsbaum M. (2002) Cognitive and brain function in schizotypal personality disorder. *Schizophr. Res.*, **54**: 157–167.

230. Kelly B.D. (2003) Physical anomalies and schizophrenia spectrum disorders. *Am. J. Psychiatry*, **160**: 393.

231. Parnas J., Vianin P., Sæbye D., Jansson L., Larsen A.V., Bovet P. (2001) Visual binding abilities in the initial and advanced stages of schizophrenia. *Acta Psychiatr. Scand.*, **103**: 171–180.

232. Singer W. (1995) Development and plasticity of cortical processing architectures. *Science*, **270**: 758–764.

233. Battaglia M., Abbruzzese M., Ferri S., Scarone S., Bellodi L., Smeraldi E. (1994) An assessment of the Wisconsin Card Sorting Test as an indicator of liability to schizophrenia. *Schizophr. Res.*, **14**: 39–45.

234. Mezzich J.E., Jorge M.R. (1997) Patterns of course of illness. In *DSM-IV Sourcebook* (Vol. 3) (Eds T.A. Widiger, A.J. Frances, H.A. Pincus, R. Ross, M.B. First, W. Davis), pp. 459–486. American Psychiatric Association, Washington.

235. Fulton M., Winokur G. (1993) A comparative study of paranoid and schizoid personality disorders. *Am. J. Psychiatry*, **150**: 1363–1367.

236. McGlashan T.H. (1986) Schizotypal personality disorder. Chestnut Lodge follow-up study: VI. Long-term follow-up perspectives. *Arch. Gen. Psychiatry*, **43**: 329–334.

237. Lenzenweger M.F. (1999) Stability and change in personality disorder features: the longitudinal study of personality disorders. *Arch. Gen. Psychiatry*, **56**: 1009–1015.

238. Shea M.T., Stout R., Gunderson J., Morey L.C., Grilo C.M., McGlashan T., Skodol A.E., Dolan-Sewell R., Dyck I., Zanarini M.C. *et al.* (2002) Short-term diagnostic stability of schizotypal, borderline, avoidant, and obsessive-compulsive personality disorders. *Am. J. Psychiatry*, **159**: 2036–2041.

239. Sanislow C.A., McGlashan T.H. (1998) Treatment outcome of personality disorders. *Can. J. Psychiatry*, **43**: 237–250.
240. Koenigsberg H.W., Reynolds D., Goodman M., New A.S., Mitropoulou V., Trestman R.L., Silverman J., Siever L.J. (2003) Risperidone in the treatment of schizotypal personality disorder. *J. Clin. Psychiatry*, **64**: 628–634.
241. Parnas J., Zahavi D. (2002) The role of phenomenology in psychiatric classification and diagnosis. In *Psychiatric Diagnosis and Classification* (Eds M. Maj, W. Gaebel, J.J. Lopez-Ibor, N. Sartorius), pp. 137–162. Wiley, Chichester.
242. Angyal A. (1964) Disturbances of thinking in schizophrenia. In *Language and Thought in Schizophrenia* (Ed. J.S. Kasanin), pp. 115–123. Norton, New York.
243. Holzman P.S., Shenton M.E., Solovay M.R. (1986). Quality of thought disorder in differential diagnosis. *Schizophr. Bull.*, **12**: 360–372.
244. Sass L. (1992) *Madness and Modernism: Insanity in the Light of Modern Art, Literature, and Thought*. Basic Books, New York.
245. Solovay M.R., Shenton M.E., Holzman P.S. (1987) Comparative studies of thought disorder: mania and schizophrenia. *Arch. Gen. Psychiatry*, **44**: 13–20.
246. Schwartz S. (1982) Is there a schizophrenic language? *Behav. Brain Sci.*, **5**: 579–588.
247. Rosenbaum B., Sonne H. (1987) *The Language of Psychosis*. NY University Press, New York.
248. Tatossian A. (1999) Le problème du diagnostic dans la clinique psychiatrique. In *L'Approche Clinique en Psychiatrie* (Eds P. Pichot, W. Rein), pp. 171–188. Institut Synthélebo, Le Plessis-Robinson.
249. Andreasen N.C. (1986) Scale for the Assessment of Thought, Language, and Communication (TLC). *Schizophr. Bull.*, 12: 473–482.
250. Kleiger J.H. (1999) *Disordered Thinking and the Rorschach*. Analytic Press, London.
251. Sigmund D., Mundt C. (1999) The cycloid type and its differentiation from core schizophrenia: a phenomenological approach. *Compr. Psychiatry*, **40**: 4–18.
252. Kraus A. (1999) The significance of intuition for the diagnosis of schizophrenia. In *Schizophrenia* (Eds M. Maj, N. Sartorius), pp. 47–49. Wiley, Chichester.
253. Störring G. (1939/1987) Perplexity. In *The Clinical Roots of the Schizophrenia Concept* (Eds J. Cutting, M. Shepherd), pp. 79–82. Cambridge University Press, Cambridge.
254. Parnas J. (1994) Basic disorder concept from the viewpoint of family studies in schizophrenia. In *Perspektiven psychiatrischer Forschung und Praxis* (Ed. G. Gross), pp. 65–68. Schattauer, Stuttgart.
255. Gross G., Huber G., Klosterkotter J., Linz M. (1987) *BSABS, Bonner Skala für die Beurteilung von Basissymptome*. Springer, Berlin.
256. Møller P., Husby R. (2000) The initial prodrome in schizophrenia: searching for naturalistic core dimensions of experience and behavior. *Schizophr. Bull.*, 26: 217–232.
257. Parnas J., Handest P. (2003) Phenomenology of anomalous self-experience in early schizophrenia. *Compr. Psychiatry*, **44**: 121–134.
258. Sass L.A., Parnas J. (2004) Schizophrenia, consciousness and the self. *Schizophr. Bull.* 29: 427–444.
259. Laing R.D. (1959) *The Divided Self*. Tavistock, London.
260. Cloninger R.C. (2002) Implications of comorbidity for the classification of mental disorders: the need for a psychobiology of coherence. In *Psychiatric*

Diagnosis and Classification (Eds M. Maj, W. Gaebel, J.J. Lopez-Ibor, N. Sartorius), pp. 79–106. Wiley, Chichester.
261. Parnas J., Teasdale T.W. (1987) Treated versus untreated schizophrenia spectrum cases: a matched paired high risk population study. *Acta Psychiatr. Scand.*, **75**: 44–50.
262. Mass R., Bardong C., Kindl K., Dahme B. (2001) Relationship between cannabis use, schizotypal traits, and cognitive function in healthy subjects. *Psychopathology*, **34**: 209–214.
263. Schwarz M.A., Wiggins O.P. (1987) Diagnosis and ideal types: a contribution to psychiatric classification. *Compr. Psychiatry*, **28**: 277–291.
264. Blashfield R.K., Intoccia V. (2000) Growth of the literature on the topic of personality disorders. *Am. J. Psychiatry*, **157**: 472–473.
265. Akhtar S. (1990) Paranoid personality disorder: a synthesis of developmental, dynamic, and descriptive features. *Am. J. Psychother.*, **44**: 5–25.
266. Wittgenstein L. (1958) *The Blue and the Brown Books*. Basil Blackwell, Oxford.
267. Kendler K.S., Spitzer R.L. (1985) A reevaluation of Schreber's case. *Am. J. Psychiatry*, **142**: 1121–1123.
268. Lipton A.A. (1984) Was the "nervous illness" of Schreber a case of affective disorder? *Am. J. Psychiatry*, **141**: 1236–1239.
269. Sass L.A. (1994) *The Paradoxes of Delusion: Wittgenstein, Schreber, and the Schizophrenic Mind*. Cornell University Press, Ithaca.
270. Schreber D.P. (1903) *Denkwürdigkeiten eines Nervenkranken*. Oswald Mutze, Leipzig.
271. Tsuang M.T., Stone W.S., Faraone S.V. (2000) Towards reformulating the diagnosis of schizophrenia. *Am. J. Psychiatry*, **157**: 1041–1050.
272. Robins L., Barrett J. (1989) Preface. In *The Validity of Psychiatric Diagnosis* (Eds L. Robins, J. Barrett). Raven Press, New York.
273. Haslam N. (2002) Kinds of kinds: a conceptual taxonomy of psychiatric categories. *Philos. Psychiatry Psychol.*, **9**: 203–217.

Commentaries

1.1
Paul E. Meehl's Model of Schizotypy and Schizophrenia
Mark F. Lenzenweger[1]*

With Paul E. Meehl's passing in 2003, the world of clinical psychology and psychiatry lost perhaps its most luminous star and the firmament has dimmed unmistakably. As many of us prepared our pieces for this impressive WPA volume, discussion via the internet led many of us to express the sentiment that this volume should be dedicated in Paul's honour. In that spirit, Professor Mario Maj has graciously allowed me to focus my piece on Meehl's model of schizotypy. Paul was both a colleague and friend with whom I enjoyed many intellectually stimulating exchanges over the years, many of which focused on schizotypy, taxometrics, and the genetics of schizophrenia.

Meehl's model of schizotaxia, schizotypy, and schizophrenia has been the guiding beacon for research in this area for over 40 years and his primary position papers on this model have been cited over 1000 times. Although well-known, Meehl's model is not always well understood—a view Meehl himself expressed to me and others (see [1])—and, therefore, this context represents a useful one in which to review his model as well as common misunderstandings of the model.

Both Kraepelin and Bleuler noted the existence of schizophrenia-like, but non-psychotic, phenomenology in relatives of schizophrenia patients and, later, many clinicians in office practice described patients who seemed to have subtle thought disorder and interpersonal oddities that suggested a relation to schizophrenia. However, many of the early depictions of schizotypic pathology were merely descriptive in nature. While the peculiarities of the relatives of schizophrenics or the symptoms of schizophrenic-like outpatients were noted and thought to be related to schizophrenia in some manner, none of the early workers advanced a model that unambiguously posited a genetic diathesis for schizophrenia

[1] Department of Psychology, State University of New York at Binghamton, Science IV, Binghamton, NY 13902-6000, USA

* Portions of this commentary are abridged and adapted with permission from Lenzenweger M.F. (2002) *Paul E. Meehl's Model of Schizotypy.*

and traced its influence through neurodevelopmental and behavioural paths to a variety of clinical (and non-clinical) outcomes. Unlike his predecessors, Meehl [2] proposed a model which was (and is) clearly neurodevelopmental in nature and came to have a profound impact on the manner in which informed psychologists and psychiatrists would think about schizophrenia, being reflected in nearly all contemporary models of the disorder (e.g. "dysmentia", "developmentally reduced synaptic connectivity", "neurodevelopmental disease process").

Meehl's model of schizotypy was first articulated in the classic [2] position paper titled "Schizotaxia, schizotypy, schizophrenia". Elaboration on and refinement of the original [2] theory can be found in later papers (e.g. [3,4]). The theory was updated and described fully in a subsequent extended position paper, which appeared in the *Journal of Personality Disorders* [5] and the origins of some of his more speculative assertions are discussed elsewhere ([6]; see also [7]).

In brief, Meehl's [2,5–7] model of schizotypy holds that a single major gene (what he termed the "schizogene") exerts its influence during brain development by coding for a specific "functional parametric aberration of the synaptic control system" in the central nervous system (CNS) [5]. The aberration, present at the neuronal level, is termed "hypokrisia" and suggests a neural integrative defect characterized by an "insufficiency of separation, differentiation, or discrimination" in neural transmission. Meehl argued that his conceptualization of schizotaxia should not be taken to represent a simple defect in basic sensory or information retrieval capacities, nor a CNS inhibitory function deficit [5]. The defect in neural transmission amounts to the presence of "slippage" at the CNS synapse and such slippage at the synapse has its behavioural counterparts (at the molar level) in the glaring clinical symptomatology of actual schizophrenia. Hypokrisia was hypothesized to characterize the neuronal functioning throughout the brain of the affected individual, thus producing what amounts to a rather ubiquitous CNS anomaly [5] termed "schizotaxia".

Thus, according to the model, schizotaxia is the "genetically determined integrative defect, predisposing to schizophrenia and a sine qua non for that disorder" and is conjectured to have a general population base rate of 10% (see [5] for derivation of the base rate estimate; see also [8] for consistent support). It is essential to note that schizotaxia essentially describes an aberration in brain functioning characterized by pervasive neuronal slippage in the CNS—it is not a behaviour or observable personality pattern. The schizotaxic brain, however, becomes the foundation which other factors will build upon and interact aversively with to possibly produce clinically diagnosable schizophrenia. The other factors which interact with the schizotaxic brain, so to speak, and influence individual development (as well as clinical status) are the social learning history of an individual as well as other genetic factors termed "polygenic potentiators".

Meehl [2,5,7] generally held that all (or nearly all) schizotaxic individuals develop "schizotypy" (i.e. a schizotypal personality organization) on existing social reinforcement schedules. Schizotypy, therefore, refers to the psychological and personality organization resulting from the schizotaxic individual interacting with and developing within the world of social learning influences. An individual who displays schizotypy is considered a "schizotype". In this context it is essential to note that Meehl's "schizotypal personality organization" is not the same as the DSM-IV Axis II disorder schizotypal personality disorder (a point that is frequently misunderstood). He [5] considered the possibility that a schizotaxic individual might not develop schizotypy if reared in a sufficiently healthful environment, but such an outcome was not viewed as very probable.

The second major set of factors influencing the development of clinical schizophrenia in the schizotypic individual is a class of genetically determined factors (or dimensions) termed polygenic potentiators. According to Meehl [5], "a potentiator is any genetic factor which, given the presence of the schizogene and therefore of the schizotypal personality organization, raises the probability of clinical decompensation". Potentiators include personality dimensions (independent of schizotaxia), such as social introversion, anxiety proneness, aggressivity, hypohedonia, and others. Such potentiators do not modify (in the technical genetic sense of the term) the expression of the putative schizogene, but rather interact with the established schizotypic personality organization and the social environment to facilitate (or, in some cases, "depotentiate") the development of decompensated schizotypy, namely schizophrenia. Meehl [5] stresses: "It's not as if the polygenes for introversion somehow 'get into the causal chain' between the schizogene in DNA and the parameters of social reinforcement". Rather the potentiators push the schizotype toward psychosis. In this context it is interesting to note that Meehl's model encompassed the idea of a "mixed" model of genetic influence, namely a single major gene (i.e. an autosomal diallelic locus) operating against a background due to an additive polygenic (or cultural) component. Meehl maintained his view of a major locus playing a key role in the aetiology of schizophrenia throughout his career, although the full model is best viewed as a "mixed model". Thus, reviewing briefly, according to Meehl [2,5], the development of clinically diagnosable schizophrenia is the result of a complex interaction among several crucial factors: (a) a schizotaxic brain characterized by genetically determined hypokrisia at the synapse; (b) environmentally mediated social learning experiences (that bring about a schizotypal personality organization); and (c) the polygenic potentiators.

The modal schizotype does not decompensate into diagnosable schizo-phrenia. However, Meehl suggested that all schizotypes reveal the influence of their latent diathesis through aberrant psychological and social functioning. This simple yet core assumption, that of a latent liability that necessarily manifested itself subtly in neurocognitive processes, would direct years of research on laboratory risk markers of and endophenotypes [9] for schizophrenia liability. Meehl [2] described what he believed were the four fundamental clinical signs and symptoms of schizotypy: cognitive slippage (or mild associative loosening), interpersonal aversiveness (social fear), anhedonia (pleasure capacity deficit), and ambivalence. Later, in 1964 [10], he developed a clinical checklist for schizotypic signs, which included rich clinical descriptions of not only these four signs/symptoms, but also several others which he suggested were valid schizotypy indicators (the manual remains a treasure trove of clinical observation to this day). Basically, all aspects of the core clinical phenomenology and psychological functioning seen in the schizotype were hypothesized to derive fundamen-tally from the aberrant CNS functioning (i.e. hypokrisia) as determined by the schizogene. For example, primary cognitive slippage gives rise to observable secondary cognitive slippage in thought, speech, affective integration, and behaviour, while primary aversive drift (i.e. the steady developmental progression toward negative affective tone in personality functioning across the lifespan) gives rise to social fear, ambivalence, and anhedonia.

It is important to indicate that the role anhedonia has played in Meehl's model has changed over the years. In the 1962 [2] model, anhedonia was hypothesized to represent a fundamental and aetiologically important factor in the development of schizotypy, actually falling somewhat "between" the genetic defect hypokrisia and the other schizotypic sign/symptoms interpersonal aversiveness, cognitive slippage, and ambivalence. As of 1990, Meehl de-emphasized anhedonia (termed hypohedonia; but see also [10]) as a fundamental aetiologic factor in the development of schizotypy and schizophrenia. Hypohedonia was now viewed as playing an aetiologic role in the development of schizotypy by functioning as a nontaxonic (i.e. dimensional) polygenic potentiator (i.e. not deriving from the core genetically determined schizophrenia diathesis). The reconfigura-tion of hypohedonia's role in the 1990 [5] model was rather major and was discussed further elsewhere [6,11]. Meehl [5] noted that many schizotypes indeed display what he termed "secondary" hypohedonia, namely clinically observable symptoms of a low hedonic capacity that derive from either a primary hedonic deficit or aversive drift. He noted [11] that the schizotypy taxon (i.e. core, true schizotypy) "will generate hypohedonic taxonicity in the adult population". Furthermore, in the 1990 [5] revision, Meehl strongly suggested associative loosening and aversive drift are those psychological processes (deriving from hypokrisia) that genuinely determine the behavioural and psychological characteristics of the schizotype. What does the schizotype look like? The answer to this question is "it depends on the level of compensation that characterizes the individual". A most important assumption in Meehl's model is that schizotypy, as a personality organization reflective of a latent liability (i.e. not directly observable) for schizophrenia, can manifest itself phenotypically (i.e. behaviourally and psychologically) in various degrees of clinical compensation. This personality organization gives rise to schizotypic psychological and behavioural manifestations [2,5,10], such as subtle thought disorder (cognitive slippage) or excessive interpersonal fear, yet it may be manifested relatively "quietly", so to speak, through deviance detectable only on laboratory measures as endophenotypes (e.g. eye tracking dysfunction, sustained attention deficits, psychomotor impairment, somatosensory dysfunction). In short, the schizotype may be highly compensated (showing minimal signs and symptoms of schizotypic functioning), or may reveal transient failures in compensation, or may be diagnosably schizophrenic. A crucial implication of this assumption is that not all schizotypes develop diagnosable schizophrenia (i.e. one could genuinely be at risk yet never develop a psychotic illness), however all schizotypes will display some evidence of their underlying liability in the form of aberrant psychobiologic and/or psychological functioning. This particular implication of the model has guided nearly 40 years of research directed at developing methods for the valid and efficient detection of schizotypy endophenotypes (through clinical, psychometric, or other means) and it articulated the heart of the "diathesis-stressor" model/approach for psychopathology.

In discussing Meehl's model of schizotypy, it is important to point out several misconceptions of the model and the resultant fallacies which often underlie the misunderstandings:

Fallacy #1: Schizotypy is the same as DSM-IV schizotypal personality disorder. Meehl was quite clear that his conceptualization of schizotypy was not synonymous with the DSM-IV diagnosis of schizotypal personality disorder (see [5]). Although there is some degree of phenomenologic similarity between schizotypic symptoms and signs and the diagnostic criteria for DSM-IV schizotypal personality disorder, important differences exist between the two concepts. Schizotypy refers to a latent personality organization and is essentially a broader construct linked to a developmental theory. DSM-IV schizotypal personality disorder is a cluster of observable signs and symptoms which tend to aggregate, and the disorder is described in an atheoretical manner. It is quite conceivable that Meehl's schizotypy construct may underlie or encompass several of the personality disorder diagnoses on Axis II. For example, the schizotype may display not only some schizotypal symptoms, but also may reveal paranoid, compulsive, avoidant, and/or schizoid phenomenology. The term schizotypy should never be taken to imply solely phenotypic manifestations of schizotypal personality pathology. In this context, it should be noted that the European (ICD-10) concept of "schizoid personality disorder" is also not isomorphic with either Meehl's schizotypy or DSM-IV schizotypal personality disorder.

Fallacy #2: All aspects of schizotypy are heritable. Meehl has been quite clear on this point. Schizotypy *per se* (i.e. a personality organization) is not inherited, all that can be spoken of as heritable is the defect of hypokrisia and, by definition, the "schizotaxic brain" [5]. Although most schizotaxics develop schizotypy on existing social learning regimes, there is the theoretical possibility that a schizotaxic will not become schizotypic (although the prevalence of such cases is probably rather small). Schizotaxia is genetically determined and is therefore heritable, whereas schizotypy develops in interaction with (non-heritable) environmental influences and, therefore, cannot be spoken of as heritable.

Fallacy #3: Meehl's schizotaxia, schizotypy, schizophrenia model is entirely genetic. Such a misconception could not be farther from the truth. Meehl's model is one in which the role of environmental influences in the development of schizotypy and schizophrenia is unequivocal (see [5]). Just as he speculated on the nature of the CNS pathology in schizotaxia, so Meehl speculated on the role of environment in the development of *both* schizotypy and schizophrenia. Meehl [5] unambiguously reveals his support for environmental influences in statements such as "environmental factors *must* be potent determiners of which schizotypes decompensate". The reader is encouraged to consult Meehl's position statements on the schizotypy model [2,5] as well as his classic "High School Yearbooks" paper [12] for elegant descriptions of plausible causal chains in the development of schizophrenia that incorporate environmental influences.

Fallacy #4: The term schizotype can only be used for those cases identified by observable schizotypal feature. This fallacy is a relatively common misunderstanding of the term schizotype. Meehl's model holds that schizotypy can manifest itself in different manners, ranging from full-blown schizophrenia to schizotypic psychopathology (e.g. DSM-IV schizotypal or paranoid personality disorder) to deviance on valid laboratory measures of schizotypy (endophenotypes). Thus, the schizotype, *per se*, can be identified on the basis of deviance on laboratory measures (e.g. psychometric or neurocognitive measures) or on the basis of observable signs and symptoms. It is also defensible, on the basis of theory and genetic expectancies, to term the first-degree biological relative of a validly diagnosed schizophrenia case as a schizotype (the likelihood of being a liability carrier in this population is enhanced on average irrespective of one's preferred model of transmission). Thus, anyone who restricts the term schizotype to only those cases showing schizotypal features is making a conceptual mistake and the same is true for those who fail to appreciate that the biological relative of a schizophrenia case is a valid schizotype.

Fallacy #5: All (or nearly all) schizotypes should develop schizophrenia. This assumption is simply incorrect. Meehl's model makes it abundantly clear that not all schizotypes will develop clinical schizophrenia during the life-course. What proportion of schizotypes develops clinical schizophrenia across the life-span? This remains an open question with very little empirical data available that speak to it.

REFERENCES

1. Lenzenweger M.F. (2003) On thinking clearly about taxometrics, schizotypy, and genetic influences: Correction to Widiger (2001). *Clin. Psychol. Science & Practice*, **10**: 367–369.
2. Meehl P.E. (1962) Schizotaxia, schizotypy, schizophrenia. *Am. Psychol.*, **17**: 827–838.
3. Meehl P.E. (1972) Specific genetic etiology, psychodynamics and therapeutic nihilism. *Int. J. Ment. Health*, **1**: 10–27.
4. Meehl P.E. (1975) Hedonic capacity: some conjectures. *Bull. Menninger Clin.*, **39**: 295–307.
5. Meehl P.E. (1990) Toward an integrated theory of schizotaxia, schizotypy, and schizophrenia. *J. Person. Dis.*, **4**: 1–99.
6. Meehl P.E. (1993) The origins of some of my conjectures concerning schizophrenia. In *Progress in Experimental Personality and Psychopathology Research* (Eds L.J. Chapman, J.P. Chapman, D.C. Fowles), pp. 1–10. Springer, New York.
7. Meehl P.E. (1989) Schizotaxia revisited. *Arch. Gen. Psychiatry*, **46**: 935–944.
8. Lenzenweger M.F., Korfine L. (1992) Confirming the latent structure and base rate of schizotypy: a taxometric analysis. *J. Abnorm. Psychol.*, **101**: 567–571.
9. Gottesman I.I., Gould T.D. (2003) The endophenotype concept in psychiatry: etymology and strategic intentions. *Am. J. Psychiatry*, **160**: 636–645.
10. Meehl P.E. (1964) *Manual for use with Checklist of Schizotypic Signs*. University of Minnesota, Minneapolis.
11. Meehl P.E. (2001) Primary and secondary hypohedonia. *J. Abnorm. Psychol.*, **110**: 188–193
12. Meehl P.E. (1971) High school yearbooks: a reply to Schwarz. *J. Abnorm. Psychol.*, **77**: 143–148.

1.2
Whatever Happened to Healthy Schizotypy?
Gordon Claridge[1]

In a robust review Parnas *et al.* give a critical clinicians' account of the historical origins, evolution, and diagnostic status of (mostly) schizotypal personality disorder (SPD) as part of the Cluster A personality disorders, together with an opinion on schizotypy as a theoretical construct for explaining the schizophrenia spectrum disorders, and a selective survey of the empirical literature on the topic. My comments are confined to a single theme. This is one that Parnas *et al.* scarcely touch upon but is worth airing, to supplement their otherwise comprehensive account.

I refer to the two different ways of construing the dimensionality which (most agree) connects, along the schizophrenia spectrum, schizotypy in non-clinically diagnosed individuals, SPD, and schizophrenia [1]. One, the "quasi-dimensional" (Meehl) view, which Parnas *et al.* favour, states that schizotypy is inherently a "defect state" that accounts for the variation in severity of illness along the schizophrenia spectrum, but has no true reference in healthy personality; if it appears to have such a connection this is because of compensation for the defect, or mimicking of the phenotypic features. The other, "fully dimensional", view, proposes that—like, say, trait anxiety in relation to anxiety disorders—schizotypy is a substantially biologically based personality dimension which, though predisposing to SPD and schizophrenia, is actually neutral with respect to outcome: the consequence of high schizotypy is either healthy (creative, adaptive) or pathological, according to circumstances.

Parnas *et al.* discuss this distinction briefly and dismiss its relevance on two grounds: (a) it is merely a re-run of an earlier debate that goes back to Bleuler and Kretschmer (hardly a valid reason. Does God exist?!); (b) the issue is out of time because (insofar I understand what they are writing) they claim that appreciation of the relationship between continuity and discontinuity has now become more sophisticated, rendering the distinction unnecessary. I suspect that they are being deliberately artless here. Their comment that "Continuous dimensional phenotypic transitions between entities do not preclude underlying taxonic discontinuity..." could equally well be replaced by: "Taxonic discontinuities do not preclude continuous underlying dimensional phenotypes". The point is that the debate is still very much alive: the proposition that illness entities can be held responsible for a *major part* of the observed variation in healthy personality is no more,

---

[1] Department of Experimental Psychology, University of Oxford, UK

and I would suggest less, plausible than the notion that healthy personalities might occasionally disintegrate into illness.

Reluctance to recognise the above distinction has some impact on the slant of the Parnas et al. paper. For example, in their Table 5, they fail to include the O-LIFE, the four-scale "schizotypy" questionnaire that Mason developed from what is still the largest factor analysis of data in this area, in terms of items and sample size [2]. The footnote to Table 5 suggests that the authors have confused O-LIFE with CSTQ, which was merely the data base from which the former was constructed, in order to produce a more personality, and less symptom, based set of scales for measuring the various aspects of schizotypy [3].

A more significant omission is the failure to include any reference to experimental investigations of psychometrically defined schizotypy; instead they confine their review to studies of diagnosed SPD patients. Yet some of the most cogent findings have come from work using the former strategy [4]. If, as Parnas et al. state, one reason for studying a condition further down the spectrum than full-blown schizophrenia is to avoid the confounding influence of severe illness and medication, then surely psychometrically defined schizotypes would be the optimal subjects to choose, rather than SPD patients. To suggest, as the authors do, that using such individuals (who because of sampling are sometimes of high intelligence) decreases the likelihood of finding cognitive impairments prematurely forecloses the debate on the normal biological variation/deficit issue. Signs of schizotypy do not have to be deficits. There are a number of examples where differences found in schizophrenia and SPD have been extrapolated to healthy, high functioning schizotypes, where it would be unconvincing to construe these as the result of impairment. Reduced brain asymmetry (e.g. mixed handedness) is a case in point [5].

Another consequence of ignoring the healthy end of the schizophrenia spectrum is that it makes it easier for Parnas and his co-authors to conclude that SPD is not a personality disorder at all, but a psychiatric syndrome. This would be a foreign idea to those of us who see disorders of the personality as precisely that: extreme aberrations of otherwise normal individual variations, though certainly with discontinuities of function that result, as Parnas et al. rightly point out, from an interaction of trait and state, as well as other causes. In that regard, there seems no reason to make an exception of SPD, while of course recognising the latter's multi-faceted nature.

Finally, an irony of this critique is that in their final remarks Parnas et al. call for more attention to be paid to the subjective experience of SPD and related conditions. It is an opinion that would be fully endorsed by those who take a "fully" dimensional view of the schizophrenia spectrum, as a counterweight to the overmedicalisation of the personality disorders.

REFERENCES

1. Claridge G., Davis C. (2003) *Personality and Psychological Disorders*. Arnold, London.
2. Mason O., Claridge G., Jackson M. (1995) New scales for the assessment of schizotypy. *Personal. Indiv. Diff.*, **18**: 7–13.
3. Claridge G., McCreery C., Mason O., Bentall R., Boyle G., Slade P., Popplewell D. (1996). *Br. J. Clin. Psychol.*, **35**: 103–115.
4. Claridge G. (Ed.) (1997) *Schizotypy: Implications for Illness and Health*. Oxford University Press, Oxford.
5. Shaw J., Claridge G., Clark K. (2001) Schizotypy and shift from dextrality: a study of handedness in a large non-clinical sample. *Schizophr. Res.*, **50**: 181–189.

1.3
Genetic Enhancements to Schizotypy Theorizing

Irving I. Gottesman[1] and L. Erlenmeyer-Kimling[2]

Parnas *et al.* provide a rock-solid foundation for launching further inquiries into the comprehensive understanding of the so-called Cluster A personality disorders, set in their historic context and following the strategies of the time-honored Handbuch, by digesting no fewer than 274 references (in multiple languages) on the field's behalf. Their breadth and depth of scholarship, plus their challenges to received wisdom, help to highlight the tasks for the current and next generations of psychopathologists with various values and allegiances. Our own preferences, non-exclusively, are for a broad complex adaptive systems context for examining the roles of genetic, experiential, neurobehavioural, and epigenetic factors, as well as their interactions, in studying schizotypy and schizophrenia [1–4]. Varieties of family (prospective high-risk studies on offspring of schizophrenic parents) and twin strategies (reared-together, concordant or not, and their offspring)—approaches most likely to cast light on components of the aetiologies of schizophrenia—have focused our energies since our youthful mentoring by P.E. Meehl, F.J. Kallmann and E.T. Slater, some 4 decades ago.

Research into Cluster A personality disorders on Axis II of the DSM requires a certain abeyance of scientific standards for such research to move forward, warts and all. The canons of construct validity [5] would require

[1] *Department of Psychiatry, University of Minnesota School of Medicine, Minneapolis, USA*
[2] *Department of Medical Genetics, New York State Psychiatric Institute, and Departments of Psychiatry and of Genetics and Development, College of Physicians and Surgeons, Columbia University, New York, USA*

much more evidence than currently exists for the first two axes to be separated so neatly. A similar stricture would apply to delineating the three personality disorder clusters in the absence of formal searches for clusters. Criteria for membership within and between clusters are a cause for concern [6], absent a hierarchical, empirically-based stipulation. Some family and adoption studies of schizophrenia count avoidant personalities as hits for a schizophrenia spectrum with impunity (e.g. [7]), and who can say whether that is alright at this stage of our understanding? Others are concerned as to the arbitrariness of the DSM in demanding, without a body of research, that a person meet 5/9 criteria before obtaining a diagnosis of schizotypal personality, while 4/7 will suffice for a diagnosis of paranoid personality. And, what is the likelihood that all criteria deserve equal weighting?

Parnas *et al.* are inclined to omit schizoid and paranoid personalities from the schizophrenia spectrum and point to the research findings as support. However, sufficient positive findings exist from relatives of schizophrenics, whether reared with them or not, to suggest that the jury is still out [8]. False negatives reduce the power of gene-finding efforts, as do false positives. Morey ([9], cf. [10]) provided co-occurrence rates for patients meeting DSM-III-R criteria for personality disorders without imposing any hierarchy rules. Among the disquieting findings were the following: of 64 criterion paranoid patients, 23% and 25% also met criteria for schizoid personality disorder (SdPD) and schizotypal personality disorder (SPD) respectively, and 48% for avoidant personality disorder. Of 32 SdPD patients, 47% were diagnosed paranoid personality disorder (PPD) and 53% avoidant personality disorder. Of 26 SPD, 44% had SdPD and 59% PPD. In the New York High Risk Project (NYHRP), the addition of avoidant personality disorder would not have added any cases to the offspring at high risk for schizophrenia, but a few to the offspring at high risk for affective disorders. Clearly, rules of the DSM and ICD diagnostic game are conventions agreed to by a majority of committee members, for the time being, while awaiting better signs and symptoms [11].

Given the rapid developments in the neurosciences generally and in molecular genetics in particular as they relate to psychopathology, frustrations over the lack of success in identifying causal gene variants have also developed. It is impossible to avoid the observation that intervening variables mediating between the implicated genes themselves and the phenotypes of interest—termed "endophenotypes"—have attracted attention recently in schizophrenia research programs [1,12] to complement strategies for the "endgame". Such variables would include the pattern of neurocognitive tests separating the offspring who developed schizophrenia-related psychoses from their two control groups [13] in the

NYHRP, glial cell abnormalities [14], and psychological test indicators of schizotypy [15], among many others.

Every time a new gene or gene region is implicated by linkage or association strategies in schizophrenia [16], the door is opened to examining schizophrenia-spectrum relatives or members of the general population for polymorphisms in those genes. Painting with a very broad brush, and taking advantage of the advanced state of bioinformatics and proteonomics, the Chinese National Human Genome Center [17] in Beijing has compiled an online-accessible database dedicated to the observed variation in schizophrenia "candidate genes" derived from their search of genetic databases around the world. So far, they have identified 23 648 variations, most of them single nucleotide polymorphisms (SNPs), assigned to a total of 186 genes. For anyone interested in working from the bottom up in the complex pathways between genomes and phenotypes, with schizophrenia-associated endophenotypes including schizotypy indicators in the middle, this represents nirvana. Let the thinking and the race begin.

REFERENCES

1. Gottesman I.I., Gould T.D. (2003) The endophenotype concept in psychiatry: etymology and strategic intentions. *Am. J. Psychiatry*, **160**: 636–645.
2. Erlenmeyer-Kimling L. (2000) Neurobehavioral deficits in offspring of schizophrenic parents: liability indicators and predictors of illness. *Am. J. Med. Genet. (Semin. Med. Genet.)*, **97**: 65–71.
3. Gottesman I.I. (2001) Psychopathology through a life span-genetic prism. *Am. Psychol.*, **56**: 867–878.
4. Erlenmeyer-Kimling L., Roberts S.A., Rock D. (in press) Longitudinal prediction of schizophrenia in a prospective high-risk study. In *Behavior Genetics Principles: Perspectives in Development, Personality, and Psychopathology* (Ed. L.F. DiLalla). American Psychological Association, Washington.
5. Cronbach L., Meehl P.E. (1955) Construct validity in psychological tests. *Psychol. Bull.*, **52**: 281–302.
6. Widiger T.A. (1993) Issues in the validation of the personality disorders. *Progr. Exper. Personal. Psychopathol. Res.*, **16**: 117–136.
7. Tienari P., Wynne L.C., Läksy K., Moring J., Nieminen P., Sorri A., Lahti I., Wahlberg K.E. (2003) Genetic boundaries of the schizophrenia spectrum: evidence from the Finnish adoptive family study of schizophrenia. *Am. J. Psychiatry*, **160**: 1587–1594.
8. Kendler K.S. (2003) The genetics of schizophrenia: chromosomal deletions, attentional disturbances, and spectrum boundaries. *Am. J. Psychiatry*, **160**: 1549–1553.
9. Morey L.C. (1988) Personality disorders in DSM-III and DSM-III-R: convergence, coverage, and internal consistency. *Am. J. Psychiatry*, **145**: 573–577.
10. Widiger T.A., Frances A., Warner L., Bluhm C. (1986) Diagnostic criteria for the borderline and schizotypal personality disorders. *J. Abnorm. Psychol.*, **95**: 43–51.

11. Cloninger C.R. (2004) *The Science of Well-Being: Biopsychosocial Foundations.* Oxford University Press, New York.
12. Manji HK, Gottesman I.I., Gould T.D. (2003) Signal transduction and genes-to-behaviors pathways in psychiatric diseases. *Sci. STKE*, **49**: 1–7.
13. Erlenmeyer-Kimling L., Rock D., Roberts S.A., Janal M., Kestenbaum C., Cornblatt B., Adamo U.H., Gottesman, I.I. (2000) Attention, memory, and motor skills as childhood predictors of schizophrenia-related psychoses: the New York high-risk project. *Am. J. Psychiatry*, **157**: 1416–1422.
14. Moises H.W., Zoega T., Gottesman I.I. (2002) The glial growth factors deficiency and synaptic destabilization hypothesis of schizophrenia. *BMC Psychiatry*, **2**: 8.
15. Bolinskey P.K., Gottesman I.I., Nichols D.S. (2003) The schizophrenia proneness (*SzP*) scale: an MMPI-2 measure of schizophrenia liability. *J. Clin. Psychol.*, **59**: 1031–1044.
16. Owen M.J., Williams N.M., O'Donovan C.C. (2004) The molecular genetics of schizophrenia: new findings promise new insights. *Mol. Psychiatry*, **9**: 14–27.
17. Zhou M., Zhuang Y.-L., Xu Q., Li Y.-D., Shen Y. (2004) VSD: a database for schizophrenia candidate genes focusing on variations. *Hum. Mutation*, **23**: 1–7.

1.4
Cluster A Personality Disorders: Unanswered Questions about Epidemiological, Evolutionary and Genetic Aspects

Matti Isohanni and Pekka Tienari[1]

The basic epidemiology of Cluster A personality disorders is relatively unknown. Cases are rarely detected and entered into clinical, register or population based databanks—after the 31-year follow-up of 11 017 persons in the register-based Northern Finland 1966 Birth Cohort we have only four hospital-treated cases! Study samples are usually biased in many respects, not representative and non-epidemiological and consequently the results of different studies show considerable variation.

Cluster A disorders are usually harmful and partly hereditary. So why do these "odd" diseases not disappear through natural selection? Do they have some advantage and some carriers act as "reformers of the world, philosophers, writers, and artists" as Bleuler expressed? The hypotheses and minimal data suggesting a role of schizoid and schizotypal conditions in some creative individuals are succinctly reviewed by Lauronen *et al.* [1]. The social advantage hypothesis argues that even extremely deviant behaviour may have led to high social achievements. A talented person who shows divergent thinking, or vulnerability for psychosis, can succeed as a mystic, shaman, saint, prophet or leader.

[1] *Department of Psychiatry, University of Oulu, P.O. Box 5000, 90014 Oulu, Finland*

Diagnostic boundaries in relation to genetically related disorders represent an unresolved problem. The Finnish Adoptive Family Study of Schizophrenia [2], designed to disentangle genetic and environmental factors of schizophrenia, lends some support to the hypothesis of a broad schizophrenia spectrum. In adopted-away offspring of mothers with schizophrenia spectrum disorders, the genetic liability for schizophrenia-related disorders is broadly dispersed not only for narrowly defined, typical schizophrenia but also for schizotypal and schizoid personality disorders (perhaps including avoidant personality disorder) and nonschizophrenic nonaffective psychoses. In an earlier adoptees' study [3] Lowing *et al.* reanalysed Danish adoptees and found an increase of DSM-III schizotypal personality disorder (6/39 vs. 3/39) and schizoid personality disorder (4/39 vs. 1/39) in the offspring of schizophrenic mothers. In the Roscommon Family study [4], schizotypal personality disorder had a significant familial relationship with schizophrenia, as did paranoid, schizoid and avoidant personality disorders. Also in the UCLA Family Study [5], in addition to schizotypal personality disorder, risk for avoidant personality disorder was increased in parents of childhood-onset schizophrenic probands. Paranoid personality disorder and delusional disorder may share the same liability and overlap with schizophrenia-related disorders. Similarities between schizoid personality disorder and the prodromal and residual phases of schizophrenia raise questions. Also the evidence supporting genetic transmission of negative rather than positive symptoms and the prominence of negative symptoms in schizoid personality disorder suggests a possible link between schizophrenia and schizoid personality disorder [6].

Using the Thought Disorder Index (TDI) and Communication Deviance (CD) scored from individual Rorschach test protocols, Wahlberg *et al.* [7] showed that fluid thinking and idiosyncratic verbalization were more frequent in high risk adoptees as compared with adoptees without genetic risk. When Rorschach CD of adoptive parents was introduced as a continuous predictor variable, the odds ratio for the idiosyncratic verbalization component of the TDI of the high-risk adoptees was higher than for the control adoptees. In another study, conducted in a sample of Finnish twins, schizotypy symptoms were associated with increased risk for cognitive deficits only in those with genetic risk for schizophrenia [8].

In the Finnish Adoptive Family Study, for adoptees at high but not low genetic risk, adoptive family ratings were significantly predictive of schizophrenia spectrum diagnoses at long-term follow-up [9]. This indicates that adoptees at high genetic risk are more sensitive to adverse (or protective) environmental effects in an adoptive rearing than are adoptees at low genetic risk.

REFERENCES

1. Lauronen E., Veijola J., Isohanni I., Jones P.B., Nieminen P., Isohanni M. (in press) Links between creativity and mental disorders. *Psychiatry*.
2. Tienari P., Wynne L.C., Läksy K., Moring J., Nieminen P., Sorri A., Lahti I., Wahlberg K.-E. (2003) Genetic boundaries of the schizophrenia spectrum: evidence from the Finnish adoptive family study. *Am. J. Psychiatry*, 160: 1587–1594.
3. Lowing P.A., Mirsky A.F., Pereira R. (1983) The inheritance of schizophrenia spectrum disorders: a reanalysis of the Danish adoptee study data. *Am. J. Psychiatry*, 140: 1167–1171.
4. Kendler K.S., McGuire M., Gruenberg A.M., O'Hare A., Spellman M., Walsh D. (1993) The Roscommon Family Study. III. Schizophrenia-related personality disorders in relatives. *Arch. Gen. Psychiatry*, 50: 781–788.
5. Asarnow R.F., Nuechterlein K.H., Fogelson D., Subotnik K.L., Payne D.A., Russel A.T., Asamen J., Kuppinger H., Kendler K.S. (2001) Schizophrenia and schizophrenia-spectrum personality disorders in the first-degree relatives of children with schizophrenia. *Arch. Gen. Psychiatry*, 58: 581–588.
6. Gunderson J.G., Siever L.J., Spaulding E. (1983) The search for a schizotype: crossing the border again. *Arch. Gen. Psychiatry*, 40: 15–22.
7. Wahlberg K.-E., Wynne L.C., Oja H., Keskitalo P., Anias-Tanner H., Koistinen P., Tarvainen T., Hakko H., Lahti I., Moring J. *et al.* (2000) Thought Disorder Index of Finnish adoptees and communication deviance of their adoptive parents. *Psychol. Med.*, 30: 127–136.
8. Johnson J.K, Tuulio-Henriksson A., Pirkola T., Huttunen M.O., Lönnqvist J., Kaprio J., Cannon T. (2003) Do schizotypal symptoms mediate the relationship between genetic risk for schizophrenia and impaired neuropsychological performance in co-twins of schizophrenic patients? *Biol. Psychiatry*, 54: 1200–1204.
9. Tienari P., Wynne L., Sorri A., Lahti I., Läksy K., Moring J., Nieminen P., Wahlberg K.-E. (in press) Genotype-environment interaction in schizophrenia spectrum disorder: long-term follow-up study of Finnish adoptees. *Br. J. Psychiatry*.

1.5
Schizotypy and Schizophrenia

Joachim Klosterkötter[1]

Parnas *et al.*'s review on Cluster A personality disorders highlights that, of the three included subtypes, schizotypal personality disorder (SPD) is of outstanding interest in research. The reasons for this interest and the development of the schizophrenia spectrum and schizotypy concepts are retraced in extenso by the authors. This allows an understanding of the historical development of the discrepancies between the ICD-10 syndrome

[1] *Department of Psychiatry and Psychotherapy, University of Cologne, Germany*

diagnosis "schizotypal disorder" and the DSM-IV Axis II diagnosis "SPD", which poses difficulties for current research.

When Emil Kraepelin first integrated the independent syndromes "dementia paranoides", "hebephrenia" and "catatonia" into "dementia praecox", he mentioned a common durable core syndrome that, besides paranoid-hallucinatory, hebephrenic or catatonic episodes, seemed to exist by itself and was termed "dementia simplex" by Diem. Eugen Bleuler defined the durable core features of this syndrome as fundamental symptoms and emphasised one, the "breaking of associative threads", as the primary origin of the disorder accounting for the majority of other symptoms. He introduced the term "latent schizophrenia" for mild forms of fundamental symptoms below the threshold of "schizophrenia simplex" and postulated that these various and scarcely describable expressions were far more common than the overt forms and especially frequent in affected families and in the pre-psychotic stages of the manifest disorder.

In line with Bleuler's original schizophrenia concept, the ICD-10 category of schizotypal disorder—although defined in accordance to the DSM—is traditionally regarded as a syndrome within the schizophrenia spectrum rather than a personality disorder. Already the pioneers in this field described peculiarities in the personality of biological relatives of schizo-phrenia patients, yet these were regarded as an expression of "latent schizophrenia" and not as a personality disorder in terms of a mid-position between normal personality and mental illness on Kretschmer's later postulated dimensional continuum. On the other hand, the DSM-III definition of SPD was influenced by the psychoanalytical tradition in American psychiatry and the conceptualization of a psychodynamic organization of the schizotypal personality structure in terms of an adaptation to the congenital integrative neuronal deficit of "schizotaxia". In consequence, schizoid personality disorder, borderline schizophrenia and "schizophrenia simplex" were pooled, and SPD allocated to Axis II. Hence, the current DSM definition of SPD was developed in close association to genetic high-risk research on rather stable vulnerability factors and trait markers in schizophrenia, whereas a more clinical approach to chronic, yet quantitatively fluctuating aberrations and symptoms in family members of schizophrenics was taken in ICD-10. An interesting intermediate position between ICD-10 and DSM-IV is taken by the schizotypy concept of the Chapman group and the psychometric high risk paradigm drawn upon this, because they are conceptualized in a psychopathologically broader and more detailed way than DSM SPD and, as such, are closer to the ICD-10 concept.

All known genetic, neurobiological and psychometric risk factors defining the so-called schizotropic vulnerability also occur in persons who never develop schizophrenia. Thus, the predictive value of vulnerability markers for psychoses still is too small to base a selective prevention upon them, and the central questions of how the frank disorder develops from a given vulnerability and what biological and psychosocial factors mediate the progression to schizophrenia remain [1].

To investigate these factors thoroughly, samples in different stages of the early, pre-psychotic course are needed. The conclusions of Parnas et al.'s review offer starting points for this aim. The authors suggest a revision of the schizotypy concept returning to its primarily non-empirical validity and incorporating more subtle psychopathologic analyses, also of anomalies of subjective experiences and their potential shifts into psychotic symptoms. Thereby, a disintegration of the unfortunate mixture of trait and state features in current SPD concept and more clarity as regards its classification as personality disorder or syndrome might be reached. Interestingly, besides transient psychotic symptoms and the combination of risk factor plus recent functional deterioration, certain SPD criteria, i.e. attenuated psychotic symptoms, are utilized in current early detection and intervention research as definition criteria of high risk mental states [2]. Currently available prospective data of such defined at-risk persons show an average transition rate to a first psychotic episode of about 37% during 12 months [3]. In addition, in the Cologne Early Recognition study, basic symptoms showed a transition rate of more than 70% in 3 years, which suggests that they can be used to define an early prodromal state, whereas attenuated psychotic symptoms can be used to define a late prodromal state [4].

As first-episode schizophrenia generally seems to develop in defined sequences of risk states, research on Cluster A personality disorders and on prodromes should become more linked to be able to dissolve the trait-state mixture of SPD and to develop valid criteria of each state. Only then, more distinct samples could be investigated for the factors determining the transition from predisposition to frank psychosis.

REFERENCES

1. Parnas J. (1999) From predisposition to psychosis: progression of symptoms in schizophrenia. Acta Psychiatr. Scand., 99 (Suppl. 395): 20–29.
2. Yung A.R., McGorry P.D., McFarlane C.A., Jackson H.J., Patton G.C., Rakkar A. (1996) Monitoring and care of young people at incipient risk of psychosis. Schizophr. Bull., 22: 283–303.
3. Schultze-Lutter F. (in press) Prediction of psychosis is necessary and possible. In Schizophrenia: Challenging the Orthodox (Eds C. McDonald, K. Schulze, R. Murray, P. Wright). Taylor and Francis, London.
4. Klosterkötter J., Hellmich M., Steinmeyer E.M., Schultze-Lutter F. (2001) Diagnosing schizophrenia in the initial prodromal phase. Arch. Gen. Psychiatry, 58: 158–164.

1.6
Parsing the Schizophrenia Spectrum
Loring J. Ingraham[1]

The seeds for the present discussion of the nature of syndromes related to schizophrenia were sown by Eugen Bleuler in his 1911 monograph "Dementia Praecox, or the Group of Schizophrenias" [1]. After describing schizophrenia-like syndromes observed among the relatives of patients with schizophrenia, Bleuler noted: "There is also a latent schizophrenia, and I am convinced that this is the most frequent form, although admittedly these people hardly ever come for treatment. It is not necessary to give a detailed description of the various manifestations of latent schizophrenia. In this form, we can see *in nuce* all the symptoms and all the combinations of symptoms which are present in the manifest types of the disease".

Nearly one hundred years later, we are working to provide valid, empirically based detailed descriptions of the various manifestations of non-psychotic syndromes associated with schizophrenia initially sketched by Bleuler. Despite considerable efforts directed toward investigating the components of these syndromes, we are as yet unable to specify the necessary and sufficient signs or symptoms for a syndrome to be unequivocally part of the schizophrenia spectrum. Likewise, despite reports of gene-environment interactions in the risk for psychopathology (e.g. [2,3]), the interplay between genes and the environments they influence and are influenced by is as yet insufficiently characterized for the schizophrenia spectrum.

As Parnas *et al.* note, the strongest empirical support for a schizophrenia spectrum of disorders is the clear and specific familial relationship between schizophrenia and schizotypal personality disorder (SPD). Converging data from several research groups support this observation, and provide initial evidence for the validity of the diagnosis of SPD [4–6]. While large-scale studies of schizophrenia revealed an empirical association between schizophrenia and the less severe SPD, parallel large-scale studies of SPD have not been conducted. Characterization of the relationship between SPD and less severe schizoid personality disorder (and non-pathological dimensions of personality) remains uncertain. In particular, the lack of evidence linking schizoid personality disorder to schizophrenia may reflect limitations in the definition (and clinical vs. non-clinical status) of schizoid personality disorder rather than setting a firm limit on the range of personality characteristics associated with schizophrenia [7]. In this

[1] *Center for Professional Psychology, George Washington University, 2300 M Street NW, Washington, DC 20037, USA*

conjunction, it is worth noting that Meehl [8] viewed introversion as a potential polygenic potentiator of schizophrenia.

Parnas and his colleagues [9,10] have asked the field to continue to focus attention on alterations in self-experience in schizophrenia; broadening that effort to include SPD and other potentially schizophrenia-related disorders is apposite. Renewed attention to self-experience will build on the relatively underused earlier work of the International Pilot Study of Schizophrenia [11] that identified lack of insight as the most frequently observed symptom of schizophrenia in a trans-national series of samples.

In brief, I concur with Parnas *et al.* that there is clear and consistent evidence for a genetically mediated link between schizophrenia and SPD, but that additional attention must be paid to the phenomenology (particularly course) and validity of the Cluster A personality disorders. While schizoid personality disorder has not been shown to have a clear genetic relationship to schizophrenia, the specific nature of the genetic mechanism remains unknown, and there is insufficient evidence that SPD and paranoid personality disorder are the sole characteristic changes in personality influenced by the heritable genetic risk associated to schizophrenia. Continued phenomenological (including self-experiential) investigation in combination with neurobiological, neuropsychological, and molecular genetic studies is necessary. With persistence and good fortune, perhaps by the 100th anniversary of Bleuler's Dementia Praecox [1], we will successfully complete a detailed description of the schizophrenia spectrum of disorders.

REFERENCES

1. Bleuler E. (1911) Dementia praecox oder Gruppe der Schizophrenien. In *Handbuch der Psychiatrie*, Part 4 (Ed. G. Aschaffenburg). Deuticke, Leipzig.
2. Mirsky A.F., Ingraham L.J., Lowing P.L. (1992) Childhood stressors, parental expectation, and the development of schizophrenia. *Progr. Exper. Person. Psychopathol. Res.*, **15**: 110–130.
3. Caspi A., Sugden K., Moffitt T.E., Taylor A., Craig I.W., Harrington H., McClay J., Mill J., Martin J., Braithwaite A. *et al.* (2003) Influence of life stress on depression: moderation by a polymorphism in the 5-HTT gene. *Science*, **301**: 386–389.
4. Kety S.S. (1985) Schizotypal personality disorder: an operational definition of Bleuler's latent schizophrenia? *Schizophr. Bull.*, **11**: 590–594.
5. Ingraham L.J., Kety S.S. (1988) Schizophrenia spectrum disorders. In *Nosology, Epidemiology and Genetics of Schizophrenia* (Eds M.T. Tsuang, J.C. Simpson), pp. 117–139. Elsevier, Amsterdam.
6. Kety S.S., Wender P.H., Jacobsen B., Ingraham L.J., Jansson L., Faber B., Kinney D.K. (1994) Mental illness in the biological and adoptive relatives of schizophrenic adoptees: replication of the Copenhagen study in the rest of Denmark. *Arch. Gen. Psychiatry*, **51**: 442–455.

7. Ingraham L.J. (1999) Genetic influences on personality characteristics of schizophrenia patients' relatives. *Schizophr. Res.*, **36**: 21.
8. Meehl P.E. (1989) Schizotaxia revisited. *Arch. Gen. Psychiatry*, **46**: 935–944.
9. Parnas J., Bovet P., Zahavi D. (2002) Schizophrenic autism: clinical phenomenology and pathogenetic implications. *World Psychiatry*, **1**: 131–136.
10. Parnas J., Handest P. (2003) Phenomenology of anomalous self-experience in early schizophrenia. *Compr. Psychiatry*, **44**: 121–134.
11. World Health Organization (1973) *The International Pilot Study of Schizophrenia*. World Health Organization, Geneva.

1.7
The Future of Cluster A Personality Disorders

Ming T. Tsuang[1,2,3,4] and William S. Stone[1,2]

Parnas *et al.*'s review of Cluster A personality disorders underscores the point that their phenomenology is considerably broader than the clinical criteria used to define them (e.g. DSM-IV). An important implication of this view is that conceptualizations of individual disorders in the cluster will be constricted artificially, which then leads to distorted conceptions about the schizophrenia spectrum to which these disorders may belong (especially schizotypal personality disorder). This is an issue that has influenced genetic research on the schizophrenia spectrum, for at least two related reasons. First, if clinical diagnostic criteria provide unnecessarily limited or otherwise inadequate reflections of their underlying aetiologies, then the genetic (and other biological) bases of the disorders will be more difficult to identify. Second, decisions about which disorders or syndromes belong in the schizophrenia spectrum will also be harder to make accurately. Both of these points are particularly relevant to attempts to identify the nature of the liability to schizophrenia in order to facilitate strategies for therapeutic intervention.

It should be emphasized that the use of clinical symptoms in the DSM and ICD classification systems remains quite useful, and has allowed the field to develop to this point [1]. The question now is, where do we go from here? Parnas *et al.* emphasize the importance of subjective experience, such as the "basic symptoms" [2], in providing sophisticated and nuanced descriptions of psychopathology. On the other hand, they describe recent

[1] *Harvard Medical School Department of Psychiatry at Massachusetts Mental Health Center, Boston, MA, USA*
[2] *Harvard Institute of Psychiatric Epidemiology and Genetics, Boston, MA, USA*
[3] *Institute of Behavioral Genomics, Department of Psychiatry, University of California at San Diego, La Jolla, CA, USA*
[4] *Psychiatry Service, Massachusetts General Hospital, Boston, MA, USA*

attempts to reformulate Paul Meehl's notion of "schizotaxia" [3,4], using negative symptoms and specific neuropsychological deficits [5,6], into a proposed syndrome of liability to schizophrenia, as not sophisticated enough to capture the relevant psychopathology ("...a study of links between neurocognitive profiles and clinical features demands more sophisticated psychopathological descriptions than the current notions of negative, positive and disorganized symptoms are able to offer..."). Setting issues of sophistication aside, the approaches are not necessarily exclusive of each other, and have a number of common goals. Among the most important of these is to find reliable and valid ways of identifying membership in schizophrenia spectrum disorders, using that information to form relatively homogenous groups for additional study, and developing effective strategies for therapeutic intervention. Moreover, both approaches rest on the assumption that clinical diagnostic symptoms in DSM and ICD do not capture the essence of Cluster A personality disorders, or of schizophrenia itself.

Regardless of the approach that is used, there is a need to identify syndromes that denote membership in the schizophrenia spectrum, and delineate the liability to develop schizophrenia. While schizotaxia is not the only available conceptualization of the nature of membership in the schizophrenia spectrum, the approach it embodies is a promising one, for several reasons. First, the proposed syndrome is defined empirically on the basis of research diagnostic criteria, which makes it amenable to experimental confirmation or disconfirmation. Second, its amenability to treatment with low doses of antipsychotic medication [7] and its relationships to independent measures of social and clinical function [8], provide initial evidence for concurrent validation of the syndrome. Third, schizotaxia fills a need by providing an initial working model of a syndrome that has a biological relationship to schizophrenia, and that addresses the relationship of that syndrome to the development of psychosis.

If the proposed syndrome is validated, the concept will likely evolve in a number of ways, and come to include additional features associated with schizophrenia and with Cluster A personality disorders. Recently, for example, we proposed conceptual similarities between schizotaxia and the notion of "negative schizotypy" [9,10]. Quite possibly, relationships between schizotaxia and basic symptoms will be identified, as well. From a genetic perspective, the current formulation of schizotaxia is consistent with a multifactorial polygenetic model of schizophrenia [11], in which multiple genes contribute to the liability for the disorder. Although the latent trait model proposed by Holzman and colleagues emphasizes an autosomal dominant mode of transmission [12], the notion that genes that confer susceptibility to schizophrenia might have pleiotropic actions that express themselves as interrelated phenotypes (e.g. eye tracking dysfunction) is also consistent with the current formulation of schizotaxia. An important implication of this point is that conceptualizations of schizophrenia, schizophrenia-related cluster A personality disorders, and schizotaxia will likely evolve to include behaviours, measures of clinical, social and neuropsychological function, and measures of biology that are not predictable based solely on observable or self-reported aspects of psychopathology.

In regard to the latter point, for example, we demonstrated recently that at least three genes that control glycolysis showed significant evidence of genetic linkage to schizophrenia in a Caucasian-American sample obtained through the National Institute of Mental Health (NIMH) Genetics Initiative for Schizophrenia [13]. One of those genes showed significant evidence of linkage in a combined European- and African-American sample. Weissman *et al.* demonstrated evidence for a syndrome based on a genetic linkage study of panic disorder, which involved bladder problems (urinary interstitial cystitis), migraine headaches, thyroid problems and/or mitral valve prolapse in addition to the symptoms of panic [14]. These findings underscore the view that the symptoms used to diagnose mental disorders may represent significantly constricted representations of broader underlying syndromes.

The target paper by Parnas *et al.* makes clear that there is still a considerable theoretical distance to traverse before the boundaries of psychiatric disorders, including those in the schizophrenia spectrum, will be established with confidence. It is clear, however, that the development and utilization of reliable, valid alternative phenotypes to diagnostic clinical symptoms (including clinical, neuropsychological, phenomenological, social and biological levels of function) will advance us towards that goal.

ACKNOWLEDGMENT

The preparation of this commentary was supported in part by the National Institute of Mental Health grants 1 R01MH4187901, 5 UO1 MH4631802, 1R37MH4351801 and R25 MH 60485 to Ming T. Tsuang.

REFERENCES

1. Tsuang M.T., Stone W.S., Faraone S.V. (2000) Towards reformulating the diagnosis of schizophrenia. *Am. J. Psychiatry*, **147**: 1041–1050.
2. Klosterkotter J., Ebel H., Schultze-Lutter F., Steinmeyer E.M. (1996) Diagnostic validity of basic symptoms. *Eur. Arch. Psychiatry Clin. Neurosci.*, **246**: 147–154.

3. Meehl P.E. (1962) Schizotaxia, schizotypy, schizophrenia. *Am. Psychol.*, **17**: 827–838.
4. Meehl P.E. (1989) Schizotaxia revisited. *Arch. Gen. Psychiatry*, **46**: 935–944.
5. Faraone S.V., Green A.I., Seidman L.J., Tsuang M.T. (2001) "Schizotaxia": clinical implications and new directions for research. *Schizophr. Bull.*, **27**: 1–18.
6. Tsuang M.T., Stone W.S., Faraone S.V. (2002) Understanding predisposition to schizophrenia: toward intervention and prevention. *Can. J. Psychiatry*, **47**: 518–526.
7. Tsuang M.T., Stone W.S., Tarbox S.I., Faraone S.V. (2002) Treatment of nonpsychotic relatives of patients with schizophrenia: six cases studies. *Am. J. Med. Genet.*, **114**: 943–948.
8. Stone W.S., Faraone S.V., Seidman L.J., Green A.I., Wojcik J.D., Tsuang M.T. (2001) Concurrent validation of schizotaxia: a pilot study. *Biol. Psychiatry*, **50**: 434–440.
9. Gunderson J.G., Siever L.J., Spaulding E. (1983) The search for a schizotype: crossing the border again. *Arch. Gen. Psychiatry*, **40**: 15–22.
10. Tsuang M.T., Stone W.S., Tarbox S.I., Faraone S.V. (2002) An integration of schizophrenia with schizotypy: identification of schizotaxia and implications for research on treatment and prevention. *Schizophr. Res.*, **54**: 169–175.
11. Gottesman I.I. (2001) Psychopathology through a life-span genetic prism. *Am. Psychol.*, **56**: 864–878.
12. Holzman P.S. (2000) Eye movements and the search for the essence of schizophrenia. *Brain Res. Rev.*, **31**: 350–356.
13. Stone W.S., Faraone S.W., Su J., Tarbox S.I., Van Eerdewegh P., Tsuang M.T. (2004) Evidence for linkage between regulatory enzymes in glycolysis and schizophrenia in a multiplex sample. *Am. J. Med. Genet.*, **127**: 5–10.
14. Weissman M.M., Gross R., Fyer A., Heiman G.A., Gameroff M.J., Hodge S.E., Kaufman D., Kaplan S.A., Wickramaratne P.J. (2004) Interstitial cystitis and panic disorder. *Arch. Gen. Psychiatry*, **61**: 273–279.

1.8
Schizotypal Personality Disorder and Phenotype Specification for Genetic Studies of Schizophrenia

Jeremy M. Silverman[1]

As Parnas *et al.* note, surprisingly little research effort has focused on studying schizotypal personality disorder (SPD) for itself. Instead, research has been primarily motivated by several other inter-related but conceptually distinct aims: (a) understanding the "underlying mechanisms of schizophrenia and associated psychotic disorders"; (b) delineating the genetic boundaries of the "construct of the schizophrenia spectrum of disorders"; (c) focusing on specific schizotypal dimensions or traits

[1] *Department of Psychiatry, Mount Sinai School of Medicine, One Gustave L. Levy Place, New York, NY 11201, USA*

and using individuals who are "psychometrically defined as high schizotypy....'' All of these aims are connected to schizophrenia (albeit the third much less directly so than the first two). The characteristics or associated features of SPD that are key, however, will vary depending on which of these aims is driving the research.

In the first of these, what matters most about SPD is its phenomenological similarity to schizophrenia. The individual symptoms in SPD are categorically related to those in schizophrenia but fall at the milder, more attenuated end of the severity continuum. As Parnas *et al.* note, investigators taking this approach emphasize this strong phenomenological relationship and capitalize on the overall absence in SPD of a large variety of common confounding variables present in schizophrenia (e.g. the effects of medication, hospitalization, and psychosis itself). From this perspective, a focus on SPD phenomenology potentially provides the opportunity to identify original biological mechanisms associated with unconfounded clinical traits closely approximating the more frequently contaminated traits found in schizophrenia.

Interestingly, some of the same impetus that leads schizophrenia investigators to SPD can also lead them to the opposite end of the severity continuum, i.e. the most severe chronic forms of schizophrenia—e.g. Kraepelinian schizophrenia [1]. While such cases are typically riddled with all the confounding variables that are absent in SPD, a focus on the most chronic cases may also reveal something essential about schizophrenia. Studying both ends of this continuum and finding commonalities that are distinct from non-schizophrenia related populations may be an especially telling strategy for revealing the biological mechanisms associated with schizophrenia.

A focus on delineating schizophrenia phenotypes (item (b) above) is also an aim that is directly tied to schizophrenia but in a different way than the first. Here, the central concern is not the similar clinical phenomenology but the presumed shared underlying heritability between schizophrenia and SPD. SPD, from this perspective, would be no less interesting if, however unlikely, its features were phenomenologically orthogonal to schizophrenia. The task would still be to best characterize these features in an effort to identify the shared underlying genetic traits.

Both of these different approaches, essentially the "familial" versus "clinical traditions" described by Kendler in 1985 [2], were used to conceptualize and define SPD. However, more rapid progress toward achieving either aim would arguably follow from releasing them from their *a priori* ties to one another via the single SPD category. For example, uncoupling models of affectedness from DSM categories, without abandoning the reproducibility that DSM-III and its successors provided, toward more precise schizophrenia related phenotypes, would strengthen the individual genetic studies of schizophrenia that used them. For over twenty years, using a variety of genetic epidemiological strategies, improved specification of SPD features with a familial/genetic relationship to schizophrenia has been pursued. With respect to molecular genetic studies of schizophrenia, relatively few have used even DSM defined SPD in their affectedness classifications—with, however, some notable successes [3,4]. Even fewer are the genetic studies that have attempted to use a refined SPD-associated entity based on genetic epidemiological evidence [5]. This is likely in part due to the substantial added effort involved in assessment of SPD-related personality traits and the increased diagnostic rigor required to make these diagnostic distinctions.

Another legitimate concern is that heterogeneity, already a major problem in schizophrenia alone, may be increased by including as affected those with milder schizophrenia related personality traits. Yet schizophrenia is a genetically complex disorder, and those with the illness probably carry multiple genetic liability factors. Each of these factors may result in specific protein changes leading by themselves to relatively subtle traits and ones that are more discrete than schizophrenia and/or SPD. Honing in on the specific, reliably measurable SPD personality traits with strong familial associations to schizophrenia (and well characterized neurobiological endophenotypes) may help lead to discovery of the underlying genes in schizophrenia.

REFERENCES

1. Keefe R.S.E., Mohs R.C., Losonczy M.F., Davidson M., Silverman J.M., Kendler K.S., Horvath T.B., Nora R., Davis K.L. (1987) Characteristics of very poor outcome schizophrenia. *Am. J. Psychiatry*, **144**: 889–895.
3. Kendler K.S. (1985) Diagnostic approaches to schizotypal personality disorder: a historical perspective. *Schizophr. Bull.*, **11**: 538–553.
4. Straub R.E., MacLean C.J., O'Neall F.A., Burke J., Murphy B., Duke F., Shinkwin R., Webb B.T., Zhang J., Walsh D. *et al.* (1995) A potential vulnerability locus for schizophrenia on chromosome 6p24-22: evidence for genetic heterogeneity. *Nature Gene*, **11**: 287–292.
5. Brzustowicz L.M., Honer W.G., Chow E.W., Little D., Hogan J., Hodgkinson K., Bassett A.S. (1999) Linkage of familial schizophrenia to chromosome 13q32. *Am. J. Hum. Genet.*, **65**: 1096–1103.
6. Silverman J.M., Greenberg D.A., Altstiel L.D., Siever L.J., Mohs R.C., Smith C.J., Zhou G., Hollander T., Yang X.-P., Kedache M. *et al.* (1996) Evidence of a locus for schizophrenia and related disorders on the short arm of chromosome 5 in a large pedigree. *Am. J. Med. Genet. (Neuropsychiatr. Genet.)*, **67**: 162–171.

1.9
A Developmental, Behavioural Genetic Look at Schizotypal Disorder

Marco Battaglia[1]

The advent of operational criteria to diagnose mental disorders, including the personality disorders (PDs), has remarkably boosted research, but has unavoidably generated some problematic issues. Parnas *et al.* provide a comprehensive and crispy review of how the Cluster A PDs can be conceptualized today and what are the controversial issues that remain open to discussion, and hint that subjective experiences may constitute a domain warranting further research. Schizotypal PD (SPD) is the most extensively investigated Cluster A PD: the effort has proven worthwhile, since this category has shown value in expanding our comprehension of the schizophrenia spectrum [1–4]. As schizophrenia is more and more conceptualized as a neurodevelopmental disorder, whose determinants are partially genetic and partially environmental, a developmental view of SPD becomes desirable [5].

From this vantage point, several questions are at issue. Is there clinical/descriptive evidence that SPD begins early in life? Which among the different traits of SPD appear first and why? What are the similarities and differences from the already-existing categories of developmental psychopathology, such as the Asperger syndrome?

In asking these questions we cannot ignore two important methodological issues. First, SPD is not a unitary construct. At the psychometric, genetic, neurofunctional levels, SPD is multidimensional, and there are many different combinations of traits by which a subject can meet a DSM-IV SPD diagnosis. Therefore, there are likely to be several alternative developmental pathways by which SPD may manifest itself in life, or remain unexpressed even in presence of higher-than-average liability. Second, phenomenological continuity/discontinuity must be addressed separately from causative continuity/discontinuity [6]. Some SPD traits are likely to show phenomenological continuity in life (i.e. they may well manifest early in childhood and remain substantially stable), while other traits may not appear before adolescence–early adulthood, or are perhaps more likely to show heterotypic continuity, which is a relative change of surface behavioral manifestations in front of unaltered sources of liability. For instance, a subject as a child may well appear introverted and clumsy, but manifest no overt aloofness or oddness before adolescence/early adulthood. On the other hand, while SPD as a category runs in families [7], some dimensions of SPD are more heritable (i.e. more strongly influenced by

[1] *Department of Psychology, San Raffaele Vita-Salute University, Milan, Italy*

genetic determinants) than others [8,9]. It should be remembered that "heritable" and "manifesting early in life" should not necessarily be equated, since the relative contribution of genetic and non-genetic determinants upon the same trait can vary widely across two time-point observations [10].

In addressing the question of early descriptors of SPD, it should be noted that there are few studies on the precursors of SPD, mostly based on high risk samples, and very rare prospective studies [11] that address the question of what can be the risk/protective factors for developing SPD in community subjects. The Olin *et al.* study [12] analysed teachers' reports of children from the Copenhagen high-risk sample who later received a diagnosis of schizophrenia, SPD, or no diagnosis, and who were born to well mothers or mothers with schizophrenia. Factor analysis showed four factors, that the authors named: passive-unengaged, hypersensitive to criticism, socially anxious, disruptive. Children who later developed SPD were found to be more passive and unengaged and more interpersonally sensitive than the non-schizophrenic group, while future SPD children were less disruptive than the future schizophrenic children, with 74% ability to predict adults SPD diagnosis. While these data are precious and quite impressive, one may wonder whether community—instead of high-risk— studies would yield similar results, at least at the psychometric level. Unfortunately, there are no questionnaires/interviews to assess possible SPD traits in childhood/adolescence, even though the DSM-IV provides a tentative list of childhood equivalents of adults SPD traits. It could be argued that most such traits are in fact tapped relatively well in already-existing popular childhood psychometric questionnaires like the Child Behavior Checklists (CBCL) [13], even though they are scattered across several dimensions of the current CBCL narrow band scales. In an exploratory study of 648 community children, we found that a group between 14 and 20 CBCL items—several of which belonging to the Withdrawn scale—could fit reasonably well the DSM-IV childhood equivalent of SPD traits. A factor analysis explaining 45% of variance revealed three independent factors closely resembling three factors of SPD commonly extracted from adult samples.

Beyond early identification of SPD traits, it would be important to understand how and why some SPD traits appear first, and some others are to follow later in time. For instance, Torgersen *et al.* [9] suggested that a young subject who is primarily aloof and isolated is likely to develop beliefs and intuitions that—as a consequence of isolation—are more likely to be idiosyncratic compared to his/her cultural milieu, and which in turn form the basis for later magical thinking. While this hypothesis is very plausible, we lack longitudinal studies to show how such phenomena take place.

Finally, to address the issue of possible coincidence of early manifestations of SPD with other constructs, such as the Asperger syndrome, much
more writing would be needed than a short paragraph like this. The paucity
of empirical literature and systematic research on the possible relationships
between SPD and Asperger syndrome calls for a much closer contact and
collaboration between adult and childhood psychopathologists. Many traits
are likely to coincide between SPD and Asperger syndrome, and even more
likely in a longitudinal perspective. On the other hand, no data available
show that there is a clear familial-genetic relationship between SPD and the
autism spectrum, and vice versa.

REFERENCES

1. Freedman R., Adler L.E., Olincy A., Waldo M.C., Ross R.G., Stevens K.E.,
   Leonard S. (2002) Input dysfunction, schizotypy, and genetic models of
   schizophrenia. *Schizophr. Res.*, **54**: 25–32.
2. Nuechterlein K.H., Asarnow R.F., Subotnik K.L., Fogelson D.L., Payne D.L.,
   Kendler K.S., Neale M.C., Jacobson K.C., Mintz J. (2002) The structure of
   schizotypy: relationships between neurocognitive and personality disorder
   features in relatives of schizophrenic patients in the UCLA Family Study.
   Schizophr. Res., **54**: 121–130.
3. Parnas J. (2000) Genetics and psychopathology of spectrum phenotypes. *Acta
   Psychiatr. Scand.*, **101**: 413–415.
4. Battaglia M., Torgersen S. (1996) Schizotypal disorder: at the crossroads of
   genetics and nosology. *Acta Psychiatr. Scand.*, **94**: 303–310.
5. Raine A., Venables P.H., Mednick S., Mellingen K. (2002) Increased psychophysiological arousal and orienting at ages 3 and 11 years in persistently
   schizotypal adults. *Schizophr. Res.*, **54**: 77–85.
6. Hewitt J.K., Eaves L.J., Neale M.C., Meyer J.M. (1988) Resolving the causes of
   developmental continuity or 'tracking': longitudinal twin studies during
   growth. *Behav. Genet.*, **18**: 133–151.
7. Battaglia M., Bernardeschi L., Franchini L., Bellodi L., Smeraldi E. (1995) A
   family study of schizotypal disorder. *Schizophr. Bull.*, **21**: 33–45.
8. Battaglia M., Fossati A., Torgersen S., Bertella S., Bajo S., Maffei C., Bellodi L.,
   Smeraldi E. (1999) A psychometric-genetic study of schizotypal disorder.
   Schizophr. Res., **37**: 53–64.
9. Torgersen S., Edvardsen P., Øien P.A., Onstad S., Skre I., Lygren S., Kringlen E.
   (2002) Schizotypal personality disorder inside and outside the schizophrenic
   spectrum. *Schizophr. Res.*, **54**: 33–38.
10. Goldsmith H.H., Gottesman I.I. (1996) Heritable variability and variable
    heritability in developmental psychopathology. In *Frontiers of Developmental
    Psychopathology* (Eds M. Lenzenweger, J. Haugaard), pp. 5–43. Oxford
    University Press, New York.
11. Raine A., Mellingen K., Liu J., Venables P., Mednick S.A. (2003) Effects of
    environmental enrichment at ages 3–5 years on schizotypal personality and
    antisocial behavior at ages 17 and 23 years. *Am. J. Psychiatry*, **160**: 1627–1635.

12. Olins S.S., Raine A., Cannon T.D., Parnas J., Schulsinger F., Mednick S.A. (1997) Childhood behavior precursors of schizotypal personality disorder. *Schizophr. Bull.*, **23**: 93–103.
13. Achenbach T.M. (1991) *Manual for the CBCL4-18 and 1991 profile.* Department of Psychiatry, University of Vermont, Burlington.

1.10
The Premorbid Personality Background of Psychotic Disorders
Victor Peralta and Manuel J. Cuesta[1]

In their very detailed review of Cluster A personality disorders (PDs), Parnas *et al.* provide not only a comprehensive summary of the literature, but also a heuristic conceptual framework for describing and investigating these disorders. They mainly focus on schizotypal personality disorder and on its relationship to schizophrenia, given that, as they correctly state, paranoid and schizoid personality disorders remain largely understudied. In this commentary we wish to discuss the relationship between premorbid PDs and the whole spectrum of psychotic disorders.

Over the last century, authors have debated on whether there is a continuity or discontinuity between premorbid personality and psychosis, with some authors (i.e. Bleuler and Kretchmer) supporting the continuity hypothesis, and others (i.e. Jaspers and Schneider) supporting the discontinuity hypothesis. We report here on data from a large clinical study on psychotic disorders, in which premorbid personality was diagnosed using DSM-III-R criteria, and Axis I disorders were defined according to a polydiagnostic approach including, among others, DSM-III-R criteria.

The study sample comprised 660 consecutively admitted psychotic inpatients (see [1] for details). The DSM-III-R Axis I diagnostic breakdown was: schizophrenia ($n = 352$), schizophreniform disorder ($n = 88$), schizoaffective disorder ($n = 37$), bipolar disorder ($n = 62$), major depression ($n = 21$), delusional disorder ($n = 25$), brief reactive psychosis ($n = 25$), and atypical psychotic disorder ($n = 50$). The DSM-III-R Axis II diagnostic breakdown was: no PD ($n = 335$), paranoid PD ($n = 31$), schizoid PD ($n = 147$), schizotypal PD ($n = 18$), antisocial PD ($n = 22$), borderline PD ($n = 2$), histrionic PD ($n = 9$), narcissistic PD ($n = 0$), avoidant PD ($n = 6$), dependent PD ($n = 4$), obsessive–compulsive PD ($n = 10$), passive–aggressive PD ($n = 0$), and mixed/unspecified PD ($n = 76$). To examine the association between premorbid PD and specific diagnoses of psychotic disorders, we conducted a series of logistic regression analyses in which the

[1] *Psychiatric Unit, Virgen del Camino Hospital, Irunlarrea 4, 31008 Pamplona, Spain*

dependent variable was the presence or absence of a specific psychotic disorder and the independent variables all the personality disorders.

Table 1.10.1 shows that a relatively specific pattern of associations exists between Axis I and Axis II disorders: schizotypal, schizoid and antisocial PD were related to schizophrenia, avoidant PD was related to schizophreniform disorder, obsessive-compulsive PD was related to major depression, paranoid PD was related to delusional disorder, hystrionic PD was related to brief reactive psychosis, and dependent PD was related to atypical psychosis. The presence of a premorbid schizoid PD decreased the probability of a diagnosis of schizoaffective and bipolar disorders. These data suggest that the relationship between personality and psychotic disorders is disorder-specific, in that type of premorbid personality may predispose in a relatively specific way to type of psychotic disorder.

Regarding the association between PDs and schizophrenia, it is interesting to note that a similar pattern of associations was found by our group using a dimensional assessment of personality in an independent sample of psychotic disorders [2]. Furthermore, in this study, it was shown that schizoid, schizotypal and antisocial premorbid traits were differentially related to the schizophrenic positive, negative and disorganization dimensions of psychopathology.

The nature of the association between premorbid PD and psychosis remains an obscure question and the involved mechanisms appear to be heterogeneous. A number of hypotheses have been proposed to explain the ways in which Axis I and Axis II disorders may interact [3,4], and here we will mention those hypotheses that are potentially relevant to explain the observed associations between premorbid PD and psychosis. These are: (A) premorbid personality may constitute a predisposing (i.e. risk) factor for the psychoses; (B) premorbid personality and psychosis can represent overlapping manifestations of one underlying disorder; (C) premorbid personality can have pathoplastic effects on the clinical manifestations and course of the psychotic disorder.

Hypothesis A seems to be the most parsimonious explanation of the observed associations, and it is compatible with previous reports indicating relatively consistent associations of premorbid PDs with different types of psychoses [4].

Compatible with hypothesis B is the existing phenomenological continuity between some PDs and some psychotic disorders. The association of schizoid and schizotypal PD with the deficit syndrome suggest a phenomenological continuity between these PDs and the negative symptomatology of schizophrenia [5]. Such a phenomenological relatedness seems also to underlie the observed association between paranoid PD and delusional disorder. In these cases premorbid personality may be viewed as an integral part of the psychotic disorder, in which abnormal personality traits represent an

TABLE 1.10.1   Association between diagnoses of psychotic disorder and premorbid personality

	Premorbid personality	OR (95% CI)	p
DSM-III-R Axis I diagnosis			
Schizophrenia	Schizotypal	5.03 (1.43–17.69)	0.000
	Schizoid	2.28 (1.51–3.43)	0.012
	Antisocial	2.68 (1.02–7.02)	0.044
Schizophreniform disorder	Avoidant	6.28 (1.23–32.07)	0.027
Schizoaffective disorder	Schizoid	0.31 (0.11–0.92)	0.036
Bipolar disorder	Schizoid	0.30 (0.14–0.63)	0.001
Major depression	Obsessive–compulsive	10.50 (2.74–40.23)	0.001
Delusional disorder	Paranoid	19.46 (6.95–54.47)	0.000
Brief reactive psychosis	Histrionic	12.38 (2.78–55.10)	0.001
Atypical psychosis	Dependent	14.22 (1.91–105.8)	0.010
Other diagnoses			
Cycloid psychosis	Histrionic	10.71 (2.74–41.77)	0.001
	Schizoid	0.42 (0.18–0.98)	0.047
Deficit state	Schizoid	3.02 (1.84–4.95)	0.000
	Schizotypal	3.00 (1.01–8.89)	0.047

attenuated manifestation of the psychotic illness. Hypothesis B would also explain the well-established common genetic liability for both schizotypal PD and schizophrenia. However, a common genetic liability has not been demonstrated for other psychotic and personality disorders.

Compatible with hypothesis C is the finding of a relationship between some PDs and the chronicity of psychotic disorders. Those disorders in which a phenomenological continuity with premorbid personality was evident (i.e. schizophrenia and delusional disorder) do have a mainly chronic nature. This contrasts with the other psychotic disorders, which are characterized by essentially a phasic or non-chronic character. We can, therefore, speculate that PDs, in addition to (or instead of) being a predisposing factor for the development of psychosis, may also have a pathoplastic effect influencing the clinical manifestations and course of the psychosis. In that way schizotypal, schizoid, antisocial and paranoid PDs are linked to chronic forms of the psychotic illness, whereas all other PDs are linked to remitting psychotic disorders.

The three hypotheses mentioned here are not incompatible among themselves, and they may interact to influence the complex phenomenological manifestations of the psychotic illness. Furthermore, predisposing, patho-plastic, and overlapping manifestations may converge in a given patient or disorder, as would be the case for the PDs associated with schizophrenia and delusional disorder. It may be, therefore, that the continuity vs. discontinuity debate between premorbid personality and psychosis is ill-founded, since the association between Axis I and Axis II may be mediated by factors other than the phenomenological relatedness or continuity.

REFERENCES

1. Peralta V., Cuesta M.J. (1999) Dimensional structure of psychotic symptoms: an item-level analysis of SAPS and SANS symptoms in psychotic disorders. *Schizophr. Res.*, **38**: 13–26.
2. Cuesta M.J., Peralta V., Caro F. (1999) Premorbid personality in psychoses. *Schizophr. Bull.*, **25**: 801–811.
3. Akiskal H.S., Hirschfield R.M.A., Yerevanian B.I. (1983) The relationship of personality to affective disorders. *Arch. Gen. Psychiatry*, **40**: 801–810.
4. Hulbert C.A., Jackson H.J., McGorry P.D. (1996) Relationship between personality and course and outcome in early psychosis: a review of the literature. *Clin. Psychol. Rev.*, **16**: 707–727.
5. Peralta V., Cuesta M.J., de Leon J. (1991) Premorbid personality and positive and negative symptoms in schizophrenia. *Acta Psychiatr. Scand.*, **84**: 336–339.

1.11
Changing Boundaries at Different Levels of Validity

Erik Simonsen[1]

The Cluster A personality disorders (often referred to as the "odd cluster") have attracted much less attention among clinicians than the "dramatic" and "anxious" clusters. This may be attributed to the lower level of subjective distress reported by patients from within this cluster; they therefore tend not to seek treatment [1]. Within Cluster A, the terms schizoid and paranoid personalities have the longest history. Through the last century, they were among the most-used and well-accepted personality terms in clinical psychiatry. They both have clear clinical characteristics and face validity, well represented in the descriptive psychiatry and psychoanalytic literature. They have continued to be used in clinical practice in spite of their quite limited external (criterion-based) validity [2]. On the contrary, it is schizotypy (belonging to the schizophrenia group in ICD-10) that is now the best investigated in research.

[1] *Institute of Personality Theory and Psychopathology, Smedegade 10-16, DK-4000 Roskilde, Denmark*

Boundaries with normality and cultural factors. The epidemiological data concerning Cluster A personality disorders, as described by Parnas *et al.*, vary greatly from study to study. It is also hard to get a reliable measure, as the criteria set has changed in recent years (most notably for the schizoid), but even more so due to the role played by cultural factors in defining and assessing cut-off levels for abnormal behaviour. Reliability in using semi-structured instruments is monitored within the local research group, but each group is biased by its own norms. The boundaries of normality are not clear across cultures; rather, they differ over time and context. Factors such as moral beliefs, religion, age, ethnicity, and gender will influence the epidemiological data and lead to labeling and stereotypes of personalities in the society. The construction of self-concept will, for example, differ in each part of the world, as will the balance between accepted egocentric versus sociocentric behaviour. This self-other dimension is an important factor in defining the threshold of abnormal behaviour. Each particular culture obviously facilitates particular personality types and pathology. For instance, a grandiose, detached, solitary asceticism highly valued in the Orient may be regarded as schizoid personality in the West. Even subcultures differ within a society, each having their own norms. In Denmark the most prevalent personality categories for inpatients are the schizotypal, emotionally unstable (impulsive and borderline) and "the rest" (as mixture of other personality disorders), with each of these accounting for approximately one third of the diagnoses. Cultural factors among professionals also play an important role. Earlier studies have shown that the prevalence of personality diagnoses is very dependent on conceptual fashions and school orientations [3].

Changing diagnostic approach, changing demands on validity. The current debate on personality disorders questions the validity and clinical utility of the ICD-10 and DSM-IV categories. Clinicians rarely assign a personality disorder diagnosis to any psychiatric patient and, if they do, they will most frequently diagnose only one personality disorder. This occurs in spite of the fact that the research data shows that most personality-disordered patients have two or more personality disorders, a finding consistent with the polythetic approach.

The DSM-III prompted use of the polythetic approach to the study of diagnostic categories in psychiatry; this method outdated the idiographic. Reliability in research became a more important issue than clinical utility of well-established terms, and this allowed for a new category to be developed. The Danish–American high-risk study coined the term schizotypal person-ality disorder, the only personality disorder to have been derived from empirical studies rather than from clinical consensus. However, it remains somewhat odd that diagnostic criteria are coined on the basis of a genetic relatedness to schizophrenia. This is not very useful information for clinicians, where a diagnosis rather should incorporate a much broader context, including data on aetiology, assessment and delineation from other diagnoses, prognosis and course, treatment, and outcome.

It is not surprising, then, that the Cluster A personality disorders have very little validity in this regard. Parnas *et al.*'s excellent review highlights this important problem. Simply put, beyond schizotypy, very little has been investigated. It is relatively easy to get comparable samples and reliable research data for schizotypy across sites, while schizoid and paranoid personality disorders have failed to show any important empirical data that might warrant their status as a clinical diagnosis. Very little information is given about these terms besides what we know from thoughtful portrayals of these personalities from early theorists. Furthermore, given the empirical data, one might argue that schizotypal personality disorder is better characterized as a syndrome within the schizophrenia group (as it is in ICD-10), even if it has still only little data qualifying it as a valid diagnosis. These patients feel ill, their state is ego-dystonic, biology plays an important role in aetiology, they more easily accept a traditional doctor–patient relationship and therapeutic alliance, and there is less question of the demarcation of normality versus abnormality. It is the condition itself, rather than related complications, that leads these patients to treatment. This description seems closer to an Axis I syndrome.

Changing criteria set, changing validity. Schizoid personality disorder is a threatened category, and has lost its earlier status, its applicability, and its significance since it was divided into schizotypal, schizoid and avoidant personality disorders. Social isolation and emotional distance (lack of tender feelings) is, to a large extent, more a defence towards involvement or a consequence of other factors (such as a symptom of another illness) than a discrete personality disorder. The original concept of schizoid personality in childhood has shown its validity as a predictor of later disorders, in particular schizoid personality disorder and schizophrenia [4]. Owing to the current more narrow definition, an important part of the original concept has been placed in the avoidant and schizotypal personality disorders, and less has been incorporated into the paranoid personality disorder. As pointed out by Parnas *et al.*, the consequences of introducing the schizotypal and avoidant personality disorders in the DSM-III in 1980 were never considered. It seems that we have lost subtypes and variants of the original schizoid (also described by Manfred Bleuler in his investigation of the premorbid personalities in schizophrenia [5]), and there is currently a confusion on what is left. Interestingly enough, Peter Tyrer's studies on a dimensional approach to personality description shows that the schizoid personality scores high on aloofness, introspection, eccentricity, and suspiciousness (i.e. a mixture of schizoid and schizotypal features) [5].

Categories vs. dimensions. One of the main problems in the current diagnostic system is the redundancy of the criteria that undoubtedly influences diagnostic validity. The more criteria, the more risk of overlapping definitions. A dimensional approach might solve this problem and ease the discussion of boundaries towards normality. To achieve a better acceptance of personality ratings from clinicians, one might supplement the categorically-based classification system by one derived from empirically-based dimensions. The most well studied dimensional systems containing terms related to DSM and ICD personality disorder categories are the ones by Tyrer, Clark and Livesley [6,7]. In relation to the Cluster A categories, the following dimensions might be highlighted as belonging to the schizophrenia personality disorder spectrum: Tyrer's aloofness, suspiciousness, eccentricity, vulnerability, anxiousness, sensitivity, introspection; Clark's detachment, negative temperament, mistrust, eccentric perceptions; Livesley's suspiciousness, perceptual cognitively distortion, restricted expression, intimacy avoidance.

Conclusion. Schizotypal personality disorder belongs to schizophrenia disorders and shares much of its validity with the same kind of empirical data. Its delineation from other disorders and other kinds of validation stems mainly from genetics, family studies, biological and neuropsychological data. The "leftover" criteria for the schizoid and paranoid personality disorders seem unlikely to be clinically useful, while these disorders may still be accepted as traditional "face valid" categories. From a clinician's viewpoint, one may be better off by having an additional dimensional approach, which contains the same basic Cluster A features as those included in the DSM/ICD diagnostic criteria set, like aloofness/detached/restricted expression/intimacy avoidance and mistrust/suspiciousness/sensitivity. Such an approach would be more fruitful for clinical practice purposes, but would open up for other kinds of problems like how to define dimensions. Which dimensions to choose would depend on further comparative studies. At the same time, to have the dimensions, categories and subtypes rooted in biology and test their clinical validity (like prediction of treatment response, course, outcome validation) is a major challenge for the future.

REFERENCES

1. Tyrer P., Mitchard S., Methuen C., Ranger M. (2003) Treatment rejecting and treatment seeking personality disorders: type R and type S. *J. Person. Disord.*, **17**: 263–268.
2. Kendell R.E. (1989) Clinical validity. *Psychol. Med.*, **19**: 45–55.
3. Simonsen E., Mellergaard M. (1988) Trends in the use of the borderline diagnosis in Denmark from 1975 to 1985. *J. Person. Disord.*, **2**: 102–108.
4. Wolff S., Chick J. (1991) Schizoid personality in child and adult life. *Br. J. Psychiatry*, **159**: 615–635.

5. Bleuler M. (1941) *Course of Illness, Personality and Family History in Schizophrenics*. Thieme, Leipzig.
6. Tyrer P. (2000) *Personality Disorders—Diagnosis, Management and Course*, 2nd edn. Butterworth-Heinemann, Oxford.
7. Clark L.A., Livesley W.J., Morey L. (1997) Personality disorder assessment: the challenge of construct validity. *J. Person. Disord.*, **11**: 205–231.

1.12
Finding The Right Level of Analysis
Richard P. Bentall[1]

Since the mid 19th century, English-speaking psychopathologists have sought to differentiate personality disorders from mental illnesses on the grounds that, in the former, the mental state of the patient remains normal whereas, in the latter, it is abnormal; the personality disordered patient has therefore been regarded as retaining personal responsibility for his or her actions [1]. Many attempts to define the personality disorders also suggest that they are enduring or trait-like, whereas the mental illnesses are presumed to be more episodic. For example, in the DSM-IV, the definition of personality disorder makes reference to "an enduring pattern of inner experience and behaviour" that "is pervasive and inflexible" and "stable over time".

Consistent with these assumptions, the DSM-IV places personality disorders on a separate axis to the psychiatric disorders. However, this approach is far from satisfactory, and fudges the question of whether they are attenuated forms of mental illness, extreme variants of normal personality, both or neither. As the DSM-IV acknowledges, patients diagnosed with some personality disorders may experience brief psychotic episodes, so it is by no means clear that the mental state of such patients should always be regarded as normal. Although very little evidence is available about the long-term stability of personality disorder characteristics, there is some evidence that Cluster A traits decline with age, as Josef Parnas notes. However, schizotypal personality characteristics have been successfully combined with other criteria to predict onset of psychosis over the short term [2], spawning a number of attempts to prevent severe mental illness by offering treatment to individuals in the high-risk category [3–5]. At the same time, epidemiological studies suggest that the psychotic disorders are best described by dimensional models that place them at the extreme end of normal functioning, rather than as discrete illnesses [6]. Taken together,

[1] *Department of Psychology, University of Manchester, UK*

these observations suggest that it should be possible to accommodate psychiatric disorders, personality disorders and normal personality within a single explanatory framework.

One way of attempting this would be to map the psychiatric conditions onto a taxonomy of normal personality characteristics. Recent personality research has converged on the "big five" dimensions of extraversion (talkative, sociable vs. quiet, passive), agreeableness (good natured, trusting vs. irritable, ruthless), neuroticism (worrying, anxious vs. calm, self-controlled), openness (creative, imaginative vs. uncreative, preferring routine), and conscientiousness (conscientious, hardworking vs. negligent, aimless) and a number of self-report measures are available to locate individuals on them (most famously, Costa and McCrae's NEO inventories [7]). Not surprisingly, a number of researchers have selected individuals meeting the criteria for various DSM personality disorders and have then attempted to identify a big five profile corresponding with each diagnosis [8].

Saulsman and Page [9] have recently reported a meta-analysis of studies of this kind. Data were available from 12 studies yielding 15 independent samples, including personality disorder patients, substance abusers, sex offenders, relatives of psychotic patients, war veterans, students and adults living in the community. The most important finding was that the personality disorders as a whole were associated with high levels of neuroticism and low levels of agreeableness. Less importantly, perhaps, some of the other personality dimensions help to discriminate between the different categories (for example, paranoid personality is associated with introversion whereas the schizoid and schizotypal personality disorders are moderately associated with extraversion). As Saulsman and Page [10] note in a commentary on their own work, most researchers addressing the "big five" profile of the different personality disorder categories have hoped to find ways of improving diagnosis and more accurately assigning patients to categories. However, given the well known comorbidity between the different categories, discussed in Parnas' review, and the relative failure of the "big five" to discriminate between them (despite discriminating between personality disordered patients in general and other people), it makes more sense to think in terms of a dimensional model that could ultimately replace the categorical system. On this way of thinking, future research should be directed towards understanding why some people manifest the high-neuroticism, low-agreeableness personality profile.

There are several problems that are likely to face this kind of approach. First, as critics of the "big five" model have pointed out [11], the "big five" dimensions have been derived empirically, mostly from factor analytic studies, and are not anchored to a theoretical understanding of underlying psychological or biological processes. It is accepted that the traits comprising the five main dimensions may be under partial genetic control [12], but it seems likely that experience plays some role in shaping these traits in the developing child. Kagan's [13] research on fearful infants has shown that early experience affects the likelihood that vulnerable children will develop neurotic traits during the course of development. However, almost nothing is known about the origins of agreeableness.

A second problem with this approach is that it has little to say about the actual behaviour and experiences of patients. For example, the fact that some people are abnormally suspicious (thereby attracting a diagnosis of paranoid personality disorder) whereas others are more inclined to magical thinking (thereby being more likely to attract the diagnosis of schizotypal personality disorder) raises questions about the psychological mechanisms underlying these two characteristics. Research studying the psychological mechanisms underlying specific psychotic symptoms may be relevant here. For example, hallucinatory experiences have been attributed to source monitoring deficits (deficits in the ability to discriminate between self-generated experiences and perceptions) and meta-cognitive biases (catastrophic beliefs about one's own mental processes, leading to dysfunctional strategies for controlling them) [14]. Paranoid thinking, on the other hand, has been associated with attachment difficulties and an abnormal style of reasoning about the causes of events [15]. Importantly, a common strategy employed by researchers investigating these processes is to study individuals selected by means of various schizotypal trait measures. In the case of hallucinatory experiences, the results obtained have usually paralleled those obtained from psychotic patients [16,17], but it is so far unclear whether the same will be true for paranoid traits [18].

In summary, it seems that a full understanding of the personality disorders will require progress at several levels. Research on broad ranging personality dimensions will be required to identify processes conferring liability to a wide range of abnormal behaviours and experiences. Research on those specific behaviours and experiences will be required to identify specific, underlying psychological processes. Research on personality disorder categories such as those in the DSM-IV is unlikely to achieve either of these ends.

REFERENCES

1. Tyrer P. (1993) Personality disorder in perspective. In *Personality Disorder Reviewed* (Eds P. Tyrer, G. Stein), pp. 1–16. Gaskell, London.
2. Yung A.R., Phillips L.J., McGorry P.D., McFarlane C.A., Francey S., Harrigan S., Patton G.C., Jackson H.J. (1998) Prediction of psychosis: a step towards indicated prevention of psychosis. *Br. J. Psychiatry*, **172** (Suppl. 33): 14–20.

3. Morrison A.P., Bentall R.P., French P., Walford L., Kilcommons A., Knight A., Kreutz M., Lewis S.W. (2002) A randomised controlled trial of early detection and cognitive therapy for preventing transition to psychosis in high risk individuals: study design and interim analysis of transition rate and psychological risk factors. *Br. J. Psychiatry*, **181** (Suppl. 43): s78–s84.
4. McGorry P.D.. Yung A.R., Phillips L.J., Yuen H.P., Francey S., Cosgrave E.M., Germano D., Bravin J., McDonald T., Blair A. *et al.* (2002) Randomized controlled trial of interventions designed to reduce the risk of progression to first-episode psychosis in a clinical sample with subthreshold symptoms. *Arch. Gen. Psychiatry*, **59**: 921–928.
5. Rosen J.L., Woods S.W., Miller-Tandy J., McGlashan T.H. (2002) Prospective observations of emerging psychosis. *J. Nerv. Ment. Dis.*, **190**: 133–141.
6. Morrison A.P., French P., Walford L., Lewis S.W., Kilcommons A., Green J., Lomax S., Bentall R.P. (in press) A randomised controlled trial of cognitive therapy for the prevention of psychosis in people at ultra-high risk. *Br. J. Psychiatry*.
7. Costa P.T., McCrae R.R. (1992) *Revised NEO Personality Inventory (NEO-PI-R) and NEO Five-Factor Inventory (NEO-FFI) Professional Manual.* Psychological Assessment Resources, Odessa.
8. Costa P.T., Widiger T.A. (Eds) (2002) *Personality Disorders and the Five-Factor Model of Personality.* American Psychological Association, Washington.
9. Saulsman L.M., Page A.C. (2004) The five-factor model and personality disorder empirical literature: a meta-analytic review. *Clin. Psychol. Rev.*, **23**: 1055–1085.
10. Saulsman L.M., Page A.C. (2003) Can trait measures diagnose personality disorders? *Curr. Opin. Psychiatry*, **16**: 83–88.
11. Block J. (1995) A contrarian view of the five-factor approach to personality description. *Psychol. Bull.*, **117**: 187–215.
12. Loehlin J.C., McCrae R.R., Costa P.T. (1998) Heritabilities of common and measure-specific components of the big five personality factors. *J. Res. Personal.*, **32**: 431–453.
13. Kagan J. (1994) *Galen's Prophecy: Temperament in Human Nature.* Westview Press, New York.
14. Bentall R.P. (2000) Hallucinatory experiences. In *Varieties of Anomalous Experience: Examining the Scientific Evidence* (Eds E. Cardena, S.J. Lynn, S. Krippner), pp. 85–120. American Psychological Association, Washington.
15. Bentall R.P., Corcoran R., Howard R., Blackwood N., Kinderman P. (2001) Persecutory delusions: a review and theoretical integration. *Clin. Psychol. Rev.*, **21**: 1143–1192.
16. Bentall R.P., Slade P.D. (1985) Reality testing and auditory hallucinations: a signal-detection analysis. *Br. J. Clin. Psychol.*, **24**: 159–169.
17. Morrison A.P., Wells A., Nothard S. (2000) Cognitive factors in predisposition to auditory and visual hallucinations. *Br. J. Clin. Psychol.*, **39**: 67–78.
18. Martin J.A., Penn D.L. (2001) Social cognition and subclinical paranoid ideation. *Br. J. Clin. Psychol.*, **40**: 261–265.

1.13
Search for a Systematic Approach to the Diagnosis of Personality Disorders
Jan Libiger[1]

Psychiatric diagnoses are moving targets. The same words mean different concepts over time. The same words denote entities that were defined by different methods in different populations. Psychiatric diagnostic concepts survive under cultural selective pressures and their meaning reflects the complex history of psychiatry in a society. There is a considerable blurring of concept boundaries and the impact of a diagnosis varies in different settings: research, clinical or administrative.

Recently, we observed a widening gap between the surviving prototypical approach and the operational approach to diagnosis in psychiatry. This is also reflected in heuristic and rational approaches to treatment. Whereas pharmacoepidemiological findings detect an increasing trend to polypharmacy [1], the regulatory authorities and professional organizations offer algorithms, standards and guidelines that usually recommend combinations of psychoactive agents only under specified circumstances [2]. How can we explain this difference between theory and practice?

Monotherapy is based on the traditional assumption of the usefulness of a specific treatment for a well defined categorical psychiatric disease. This approach works in most usual situations and fails in non-typical cases. Operational criteria were meant to improve the exactness of diagnostic process and reveal the structure of psychiatric taxonomy by the use of universal criteria and rules. They were intended to improve communication among clinicians and remove the burden of vague and historical meanings that most psychiatric concepts are associated with. Their success was partial and there was a price to pay. The increased reliability of an operational diagnosis worked nicely for bureaucratic purposes (insurance, organization, planning). However, operational criteria shattered the validity of some diagnostic concepts. This may have been one of the reasons for an increase in using multiple diagnoses, which provides a rational justification for polypharmacy.

Schizotypal disorder became a new taxonomic entity in the group of schizophrenias, describing patients who do not develop a florid schizophrenia, but share the same genetic liability of patients with schizophrenia. It may be considered as a premorbid phase, before the psychopathological adaptations to basic subjective experiences of schizophrenia develop. It may also be considered as a low activity schizophrenia with changes in cognitive

[1] *Department of Psychiatry, Charles University Medical School, Hradec Králové, Czech Republic*

abilities which are intermediate between adaptive mental health and psychosis. The clinician has difficulties to consider schizotypal personality disorder as equal to the other two Cluster A diagnoses. These are stable, with little relationship to an active psychopathological process. They are present in persons who hardly ever look for psychiatric care. This may be the reason for the lack of research interest in these diagnostic concepts and their "retreat from glory".

There is an alternative to prototypical and operational approaches to diagnoses, that seems to fit personality disorders better than other groups of psychiatric diagnoses. Diagnoses of personality disorders can be thought of as extreme positions in a systematic dimensional personality description [3]. In the attempt to relate diagnoses of personality disorders to a systematic psychometric description of personality, Svrakic et al. [4] found characteristic profiles of correlations between schizoid and schizotypal personality disorders and scores on Cloninger's Temperament and Character Inventory (TCI) Questionnaire.

The dimensions can be derived from psychometric instruments, but they may also have a purely clinical origin. In addition to empirical clinical clusters, they may include, for instance, the rate of progression or fluctuation of a disorder or the stability of psychopathology. These dimensions may represent evolutionary adaptive responses to stressful conditions. The individual profile of these adaptive processes, together with the profile of protective (genetic, environmental tolerance) or facilitating factors (developmental insult, trauma, psychosocial adversity) can be potentially clustered in a system of diagnostic concepts that would go beyond description and provide a theoretical framework for hypotheses to be falsified and to advance the knowledge.

REFERENCES

1. Tempier R.P., Pawliuk N.H. (2003) Conventional, atypical and combination antipsychotic prescriptions: a 2-year comparison. *J. Clin. Psychiatry*, **64**: 673–679.
2. Kane J.M., Leucht S., Carpenter D., Docherty J.P. (2003) Optimizing pharmacologic treatment of psychotic disorders. Expert consensus guideline series. *J. Clin. Psychiatry*, **64**: Suppl. 12.
3. Blashfield R.K. (1984) *The Classification of Psychopathology*. Plenum Press, New York.
4. Svrakic D.M., Whitehead C., Przybeck T.R., Cloninger R.C. (1993) Differential diagnosis of personality disorders by the seven-factor model of temperament and character. *Arch. Gen. Psychiatry*, **50**: 991–999.

1.14
Schizotypal Personality Disorder—
a Minor Variant of Schizophrenia?
Ana Cristina Chaves[1]

After reading the impressive review by Parnas *et al.*, I agree with the authors that there seems to be little interest in studying schizotypal personality disorder (SPD) from a basic research perspective, i.e. in understanding the disorder in itself. The investigators in this area seem to be more interested in finding clues to identify underlying mechanisms of schizophrenia than in the personality disorder itself. There are few community studies about SPD and most of the SPD samples come from clinical settings, relatives of schizophrenic patients and college students.

Based on their clinical and research experience, Parnas *et al.* elaborated criteria for SPD from a clinical-phenomenological perspective. For them, all of the SPD symptoms and signs can also be present in individuals with schizophrenia, and the concepts of SPD and schizophrenia are reciprocally connected, but the study of links between neurocognitive profiles and clinical features demands more sophisticated psychopathological descriptions than the current notions of negative, positive and disorganized symptoms are able to offer.

This issue could be illustrated by a study conducted by Corin and Lauzon [1] in Montreal, Canada. Using a model based on anthropology and European phenomenology, they explored the coping strategies developed by schizophrenic patients in order to remain in community. The aim of the study was to describe the mode of being-in-the-world that the patients had developed and experienced. Forty-five schizophrenic patients were randomly selected and divided in two groups according to their history of hospitalization in the last 4 years. An open interview was used to collect the data and qualitative and quantitative analyses were carried on. Unexpectedly, the authors discovered that features indicating a position "outside" of the social world significantly characterized the group of non-rehospitalized patients. For them, this seems to correspond to an attitude of "detachment", rather than a perceived dynamics of exclusion as in the group of frequently rehospitalized patients. The frequently rehospitalized patients perceived themselves as excluded from the family and social relationships. This was felt as negative and was followed by an expectation of having more social contacts. The other group had few social contacts, but they did not want to have more. Thus, the position of these patients towards

[1] *Schizophrenia Program, Federal University of São Paulo, Rua Botucatu 740, CEP 04023-900, São Paulo, Brazil*

the "world" seems be characterized by a general tendency to "disinvest" the interpersonal and the social fields, and a tendency to stay at a distance from the environment. Both groups feel as if they are out of the social world, but only the rehospitalized patients have a feeling of exclusion. In the other group the more appropriate term is "detachment".

Could the same model be applied for a person with SPD? The SPD negative dimension resembles the schizophrenia negative syndrome. One of the few community studies about Cluster A [2] showed that the prevalence is higher in men over 50 years and living alone in the centre of the cities. Maybe the above-mentioned model is relevant to these men.

One of the theories about SPD is that it is a first step in the development of schizophrenia. The reverse is not mentioned: may some remitted schizophrenia patients suffer from a minor variant of schizophrenia resembling SPD?

REFERENCES

1. Corin E., Lauzon G. (1990) Positive withdrawal and the quest for meaning: the reconstructions of experience among schizophrenics. *Psychiatry*, **55**: 266–278.
2. Torgensen S., Kringlen E., Cramer V. (2001) The prevalence of personality disorders in a community sample. *Arch. Gen. Psychiatry*, **58**: 590–596.

1.15
Diagnosis Versus Classification in Psychiatry

Robert Cancro[1]

Parnas *et al.* have written an excellent review on the cluster A personality disorders. The product is Herculean. Perhaps another Greek reference might be more accurate by describing the project as Sisyphean. This comment is not meant sardonically but rather to recognize simultaneously the importance of utilizing phenomenologic approaches for the present, while also recognizing that the future of psychiatric diagnosis lies in the establishment of an aetiopathogenic classification of illness. The issues evoked in this commentary are directed to personality disorders, but are generalizable to the whole range of psychiatric disorders.

In practice, to a great extent, the psychiatrist has two sources of information. The first is observation, which is usually referred to as the

[1] *Department of Psychiatry, New York University School of Medicine, 550 First Avenue, New York, NY 10016-6481, USA*

recognition of signs. The second, the complaints of the patient, which are labelled the symptoms. These data may be conceptualized in various ways as dimensions or categories, but in fact, patients are grouped according to their signs and symptoms. With the exception of certain dementing disorders, pathophysiology does not enter into the labelling process. The groupings of patients that have been created by this methodology can then be studied in various ways. One can do imaging studies and find, for example, that certain structural changes are statistically more common in one category than in another. This is not equivalent to a pathognomonic finding that creates a pathophysiologic grouping. Similarly, one can look at the frequency of similar clinical pictures in first- and second-degree relatives. An obvious limitation of this methodology is that the family member must in fact show some symptomatology in order to be included. If that symptomatology is latent, that individual does not get included. It would be similar to looking for a diabetic propensity in individuals who have not shown clinical signs of diabetes. If we are utilizing markedly elevated blood sugars as the admission criterion to the group called diabetes, then having the predisposition, in the absence of the manifestation, prevents the individual from being counted, although the genetic predisposition is still there.

The problem of using linguistic distinction in an effort to find differences has been long recognized and has been described by artists as well as scientists. Herman Melville [1], shortly before his death, wrote the following quote: "Who in the rainbow can draw the line where the violet tint ends and the orange tint begins? Distinctly we see the difference of the color, but where exactly does the first one visibly enter into the other? So with sanity and insanity. In pronounced cases there is no question about them. But in some cases, in various degrees supposedly less pronounced, to draw the line of demarcation few will undertake, though for a fee some professional experts will. There is nothing namable but that some men will undertake to do for pay. In other words, there are instances where it is next to impossible to determine whether a man is sane or beginning to be otherwise". The answer to Melville's conundrum would be basing the colour distinction on the frequency of the light, rather than the eye of the observer. In this fashion one moves from subjectivity to objectivity.

There is a fundamental difference between diagnosis and classification. The word diagnosis means a thorough understanding and it is a statement of what is troubling an individual at a given time, in a given context, in a particular manner. It is an attempt to unite general knowledge concerning illness with particular knowledge concerning an individual. The purpose is to help that individual. The use of a particular diagnostic schema may or may not deepen our understanding of the basis of the disorder that is being described. It may simply be useful to the individual being treated.

Classification, on the other hand, is an essential method of science. It intends to bring order out of disorder by arranging the data in a logical fashion. It is meant to help our conceptualization and allow a more profound understanding of the nature of that which is being studied [2]. The classification of disease on the basis of aetiopathogenesis is the goal of all of medicine, but has not yet been achieved in psychiatry.

Parnas *et al.* should be congratulated for continuing to struggle with the methods that are available to us at this time. It would be foolish to merely shrug our shoulders and say let us wait until someone understands the pathophysiology better, then we can do the job properly. Later efforts are always based on what came before. The struggle to improve what we are able to do with observation and self-report is to be praised and not dammed. Nevertheless, it should not be seen as the goal, but rather as a transient way-station until we achieve medical classification based on aetiology and pathology.

The imaging techniques offer considerable hope that the day is not too far in the future when our ability to identify functional abnormalities will have improved sufficiently so that we can group people on the basis of the malfunction rather than on the presenting symptoms. The case of thalamocortical dysrhythmia is an excellent example of just this process [3,4]. Abnormal theta wave activity in the thalamus can be associated with a range of symptoms that can be described as neurologic, pain, or psychiatric. Yet all of these patients suffer from the same pathophysiology, although the manifestations of the pathophysiology differ depending on the cortical distribution of the thalamic disorder. This is a model of how one can identify functional abnormalities, localize them in the brain, study their distribution, and classify patients accordingly. Until this goal is achieved more broadly, it is essential that we continue to labour in the field of phenomenology, with all of the frustration that is inherent in that effort. Those who do this good work should be praised. Hopefully, at some point that work will no longer be necessary.

REFERENCES

1. Melville H. (1962) *Billy Budd, Sailor* (1891). University of Chicago, Chicago.
2. Cancro R., Pruyser P.W. (1970) A historical review of the development of the concept of schizophrenia. In *The Schizophrenic Reactions* (Ed. R. Cancro), pp. 3–12. Brunner/Mazel, New York.
3. Llinas R., Ribary U., Jeanmonod D., Cancro R., Kronberg E., Schulman J.J., Zonenshayn M., Magnin M., Morel A., Siegemund M. (2001) Thalamocortical dysrhythmia I: Functional and imaging aspects. *Thalamus and Related Systems*, 1: 237–244.

4. Jeanmonod D., Magnin M., Morel A., Siegemund M., Cancro R., Lanz M., Llinas R., Ribary U., Kronberg E., Schulman J.J. et al. (2001) Thalamocortical dysrhythmia II: Clinical and surgical aspects. *Thalamus and Related Systems*, 1: 245–254.

1.16
Cluster A Personality Disorders:
Conundrums and New Directions

David L. Braff[1]

Parnas et al.'s paper is an extensive review of schizoid, paranoid and schizotypal personality disorders, which together form the Cluster A personality disorders. The authors have decided to concentrate on the literature on schizotypal personality disorder (SPD), and parse SPD subjects into three groups: (a) patients identified in clinical settings, (b) persons diagnosed in genetic family studies, and (c) "psychometric" samples who are usually college students or people recruited via advertisements. The latter group of individuals are quite different from patients, because they are recruited on the basis of "volunteering" for research and then scoring high on self report questionnaires targeting "presumed schizotypal dimensions".

The epidemiology of these disorders represents a very complicated area, and the recent figure of 4.1% for all Cluster A personality disorders seems like a reasonable but general estimate. Still, as Torgersen et al. [1] note, there is tremendous variation between reported incidences of Cluster A personality disorders, partly because of the ambiguous criteria used to define them and the fact that there may be three different "subgroups", even of a disorder that appears as "unitary" as SPD.

When one adds to this the fact that Cluster A personality disorders are less clearly defined and have more "fuzzy" boundaries than schizophrenia itself, there is a profound problem in trying to define the limitations of the diagnosis. Minkowski [2] went far beyond what modern psychiatrist do with DSM-IV, or what even Bleuler [3] did in terms of descriptive psychiatry, and searched for the "deeper level" which would act as a symptom unifier for the structure of subjectivity and the life consciousness. From an intellectual perspective this work is extremely interesting. From an epidemiological perspective, it raises profound problems in trying to create reliable and stable criteria.

[1] *Department of Psychiatry, University of California, San Diego, 9500 Gilman Drive, La Jolla, CA 92093-0804, USA*

Parnas *et al.* segue way into Meehl's seminal work on the four core traits and symptoms of schizophrenia [4]. Minkowski, Rado, Blankenburg, Meehl and others have created very complex schemata for defining Cluster A personality disorders. Although the authors concentrate on SPD, it remains unclear that these Cluster A personality spectrum disorders have shared underlying neurocognitive, attentional, and even perhaps genetic substrates. These findings are bundled together in a diathesis stress model, which is usually applied to schizophrenia *per se* but can be (tentatively) applied to the Cluster A disorders. Here we run into a major conceptual problem which the authors wrestle with: should one derive the Cluster A personality disorders from high risk studies, family studies, or schizotypal personality questionnaires? More data are needed on this challenging conundrum.

Treatment is also a very difficult issue, since people with Cluster A personality disorders (as with many other personality disorders) often do not seek treatment, and treatment frequently fails. It is thus virtually impossible at this time to substantiate whether or not treatments of various kinds are very effective across the entire spectrum of SPD individuals, a point of great import.

I agree with the authors that "we are like Plato's cavemen who only see shadows and take them to be forms", when we are trying to understand and define schizotypy and SPD. Therefore, there is a real need to look at SPD-related conditions in a scientifically robust manner. Perhaps the best way to start in this complex and difficult area is to select SPD patients who are genetically related to schizophrenia patients. Thus, by taking the "purest" and most easily defined form of the disorder (SPD patients), one could characterize these individuals genetically, cognitively, neurobiologically, and via functional brain imaging. This is very akin to what scientists did with the family of hyperlipidaemias, which is to concentrate on the most clear and severe forms of a particular disorder and then "reason backwards" into the lesser and more ambiguous forms, such as sub-syndromal or marginal hyperlipidaemia. Since SPD itself is so difficult to study, by selecting the most genetically and clinically "loaded" and pure cases, we probably have the best chance of resolving many dilemmas that are posed by SPD as well as the other cluster A personality disorders.

REFERENCES

1. Torgersen S., Kringlen F., Cramer V. (2001) The prevalence of personality disorders in a community sample. *Arch. Gen. Psychiatry*, **58**: 590–596.
2. Minkowski E. (1933) *Le Temps Vecu. Etudes Phenomenologiques et Psychopathologiques*. Coll. de l'Evolution Psychiatrique, Paris.
3. Bleuler E. (1911) Dementia praecox oder Gruppe der Schizophrenien. In: *Handbuch der Psychiatrie* (Ed. G. Aschaffenburg). Deuticke, Leipzig.

4. Meehl P.E. (1962) Schizotaxia, schizotypy, schizophrenia. *Am. Psychol.*, **17**: 827–838.

1.17
Have Paranoid and Schizoid Personality Disorders Become Dispensable Diagnoses?

David P. Bernstein[1]

Parnas *et al.* have written a rich and informative review of the literature on schizotypal personality disorder (SPD). However, the other two Cluster A personality disorders, paranoid (PPD) and schizoid (SdPD) personality disorders, which have been largely neglected in empirical studies, receive scant attention in the review. Parnas *et al.* raise the question of whether PPD and SdPD are moribund, having been rendered superfluous by the diagnostic restructuring that occurred in the DSM-III. In this commentary, I will attempt to address this question.

The DSM-III diagnostic criteria for the odd cluster disorders were based on classic descriptions of psychiatric patients and other individuals (e.g. relatives of schizophrenic patients) who were thought to bear a phenomenological resemblance to schizophrenics, but without the presence of overt psychotic symptoms. Subsequent research has largely supported the idea of a genetic link between SPD and schizophrenia. On the other hand, there is much less evidence that PPD, as it is currently defined, is a schizophrenia-spectrum disorder, and little or no evidence that SdPD is related to schizophrenia [1,2]. Moreover, the high degree of comorbidity among these disorders has led some authors to conclude that PPD and SdPD are redundant with SPD [3]. These findings raise the question of whether PPD and SdPD deserve to be retained in the diagnostic nomenclature.

There are several reasons to question the reputed demise of PPD and SdPD. First, PPD and SdPD are diagnosed as frequently or more frequently than SPD in studies using DSM-III or later diagnostic criteria [1,2]. Second, a substantial proportion of individuals with PPD or SdPD do not meet diagnostic criteria for SPD [1,2]. Finally, although PPD and SdPD bear some phenomenological resemblance to SPD, the aetiologies of these disorders may be partially or completely distinct from that of SPD or schizophrenia [4].

Psychoanalytic object relations theorists have viewed severe personality disorders, including PPD and SdPD, in terms of pervasive ego deficits, impaired object relations, and primitive defence mechanisms, stemming

[1] Department of Psychology, Fordham University, Dealy Hall, Bronx, NY 10458, USA

from noxious childhood experiences [5]. For example, when early caregivers are abusive, shaming, or depriving, the result can be "splitting"—an inability to integrate the positive and negative attributes of other people, resulting in the tendency to view others as either "all good" or as persecutory "bad objects" [5].

More recent cognitive and evolutionary theories suggest that severe personality disorders result from an interaction of a child's innate temperament and the toxic and frustrating or facilitating aspects of his caregiving environment. For example, Jeffrey Young's integrative cognitive model [6] conceives of personality disorders in terms of early maladaptive schemas—enduring themes or patterns that originate in the interplay between noxious childhood experiences and childhood temperament. For example, in Young's model [6], early maladaptive schemas, such as defectiveness/shame and abuse/mistrust, can arise when caregivers are habitually shaming and abusive. Such schemas, and maladaptive coping mechanisms, such as counter-attacking, are responsible for the paranoid patient's habitual belief that others are out to humiliate and abuse him, his over-sensitivity to slights and perceived insults, and his guarded and antagonistic stance towards others.

In Theodore Millon's biopsychosocial model [4], personality disorders can result from a poor fit between a child's innate temperament and his caregiving environment. For example, a child who inherits a passive temperament may require a greater than average degree of sensitivity from caregivers. Because the child's lack of responsiveness is experienced as unrewarding, the parent frequently withdraws attention; the child becomes more passive and withdrawn, provoking further parental disengagement. This vicious cycle reinforces the child's innate passivity, eventually producing the emotional and interpersonal detachment that is the hallmark of SdPD.

Aaron Beck's cognitive-evolutionary model [7] emphasizes the adaptive aspect of personality disorders. Beck speculates that in mankind's evolutionary past, personality traits like suspiciousness conferred an adaptive advantage—suspicious individuals were better equipped to anticipate and protect themselves against threats from others, increasing their inclusive fitness (i.e. the likelihood of transmitting their genes to subsequent generations). Thus, suspiciousness and other seemingly maladaptive personality traits conferred an adaptive advantage on our evolutionary ancestors.

Although these theoretical models of PPD and SdPD hold considerable promise, empirical research to test them has been sorely lacking. Phenomenological, laboratory, longitudinal, and treatment studies are needed to test the various aetiological hypotheses about PPD and SdPD, and to develop more effective means of treating them. Useda [8] has recently developed a modified criteria set and diagnostic instrument for PPD that has good preliminary reliability and validity, and may represent an improvement over the PPD criteria in the DSM-IV. Studies are also needed to investigate whether PPD and SdPD represent true diagnostic categories, or whether they are better conceptualized as dimensions such as "suspiciousness" and "detachment", that may explain some of the comorbidity between the odd cluster diagnoses.

As Parnas *et al.* suggest, PPD and SdPD need not be seen as moribund. These disorders are merely understudied. PPD and SdPD cause considerable impairment in interpersonal functioning. PPD also exacts a substantial societal cost in terms of violence; such individuals are overrepresented among perpetrators of spousal abuse and other forms of violence [9]. The future of research on PPD and SdPD will depend on the efforts of investigators who seize the opportunity represented by these understudied, but important, diagnostic entities.

REFERENCES

1. Bernstein D.P., Useda D., Siever L.J. (1996) Paranoid personality disorder. In *DSM-IV Sourcebook* (Eds T.A. Widiger, A.J. Frances, H.A. Pincus, R. Ross, M.B. First, W. Davis, M. Kline), pp. 665–674. American Psychiatric Association, Washington.
2. Kalus O., Bernstein D.P., Siever L.J. (1996) Schizoid personality disorder. In *DSM-IV Sourcebook*, Vol. 4 (Eds T.A. Widiger, A.J. Frances, H.A. Pincus, R. Ross, M.B. First, W. Davis, M. Kline), pp. 675–684. American Psychiatric Association, Washington.
3. Blashfield R.K., Intoccia V. (2000) Growth of the literature on the topic of personality disorders. *Am. J. Psychiatry*, 157: 472–473.
4. Millon T., Davis R.O. (1996) *Disorders of Personality: DSM-IV and Beyond*, 2nd edn. Wiley, Chichester.
5. Kernberg O. (1984) *Severe Personality Disorders*. Yale University Press, New Haven.
6. Young J.E., Klosko J.S., Weishaar M.E. (2003) *Schema Therapy: A Practitioner's Guide*. Guilford, New York.
7. Pretzer J.L., Beck A.T. (1996) A cognitive theory of personality disorders. In *Major Theories of Personality Disorder* (Eds J.F. Clarkin, M.F. Lenzenweger), pp. 36–105. Guilford Press, New York.
8. Useda J.D. (2002) The construct validation of the Paranoid Personality Disorder Features Questionnaire (PPDFQ): a dimensional assessment of paranoid personality disorder. Dissertation Abstracts International, Section B: The Sciences & Engineering. Vol. 62(9-B), p. 4240.
9. Dutton D.G. (1998) *The Abusive Personality: Violence and Control in Intimate Relationships*. New York: Guilford.

2

Antisocial Personality Disorder: A Review

C. Robert Cloninger

Washington University School of Medicine,
Department of Psychiatry and Sansone
Center for Well-Being, Campus Box 8134, 660 S. Euclid,
St. Louis, MO 63110, USA

INTRODUCTION

The essential feature of antisocial personality disorder (ASPD) is a pattern of recurrent antisocial, delinquent, and criminal behaviour that begins in childhood or early adolescence and pervades every aspect of a person's life, including school, work, and social relationships. ASPD is the best validated and most extensively studied disorder of personality, because criminality has always been a common and serious problem for all human communities [1–3]. Large-scale and controlled trials of many psychosocial and neurobiological treatments of criminals with ASPD have clearly demonstrated the rarity of complete spontaneous remission of ASPD without treatment, as well as the weak and incomplete effectiveness of most conventional approaches to treatment [4–9]. Fortunately, these studies also help to identify the particular biopsychosocial conditions needed for a radical transformation of a person with ASPD to healthy well-being, thereby serving as a model for the assessment and treatment of disorders of personality in general [10].

Before the 18th century, criminals were considered sinners and were treated by harsh punishment, execution, or banishment. James Pritchard's description of "moral insanity" in 1835 may be the first description of what is now called ASPD [11]. He described moral insanity in this way: "The intellectual faculties appear to have sustained little or no injury, while the disorder is manifested principally or alone in the state of the feelings, temper, or habits. In cases of this description the moral and active principles of the mind are strongly perverted and depraved, the power of self

Personality Disorders. Edited by Mario Maj, Hagop S. Akiskal, Juan E. Mezzich and Ahmed Okasha.
©2005 John Wiley & Sons Ltd: ISBN 0-470-09036-7

government is lost or impaired and the individual is found to be incapable...of conducting himself with decency and propriety..." Similarly, in 1812 Benjamin Rush described individuals with good intellect and a lifelong history of irresponsibility without capacity for guilt or empathy for the suffering of others as having "derangement of the moral faculties" [12].

As late as the end of the 19th century, the adjective "psychopathic" meant "psychopathological" and referred to any form of mental disorder. Koch introduced the term "psychopathic inferiority" to refer to deviations of personality [13]. Kraepelin, Kahn and Schneider proposed alternative classifications of personality disorders [14–16]. Kurt Schneider's definition of personality disorder included "all those abnormal personalities who suffer from their abnormalities or cause society to suffer". Subsequently, the term "psychopathy" was used inconsistently to refer to all personality disorders or to a subgroup of antisocial or aggressive personalities. To avoid confusion, in 1952 the American Psychiatric Association (APA) adopted the term "sociopathic personality disturbance" in DSM-I to refer to ASPD. Nevertheless, some people continued to use the terms "sociopathy" and "psychopathy" interchangeably, whereas others used "sociopathy" as the antisocial type of psychopathy. Consequently, the term "antisocial personality" was introduced in later editions of the APA's DSM. The term "dissocial personality disorder" was adopted in ICD-10 to include "amoral, antisocial, asocial, psychopathic, and sociopathic personality disorders".

Studies of criminal psychopaths during the 20th century distinguished "primary psychopaths", who were callous, calm, cold-blooded, and remorseless, from "secondary psychopaths", who were anxious and emotionally unstable [17]. Both groups were impulsive and antisocial, but the secondary or neurotic psychopaths were also affectively labile. Neurotic psychopaths correspond to patients who are today usually classified as borderline personality disorder (BPD) in DSM-IV and as emotionally unstable personality disorder in ICD-10. ICD-10 further subdivides the emotionally unstable personality disorder into an impulsive type, including explosive and aggressive personality disorders, and the borderline type, who also experience chronic feelings of emptiness, intense and unstable relationships with alternating idealization and devaluation, and recurrent acts of self-mutilation. In 1941 Hervey Cleckley described psychopathy as "the mask of sanity" in ways reminiscent of Pritchard's ideas of moral insanity with defective mental self-government [18]. Robert Hare closely followed Cleckley's description of psychopathy in the development of his Psychopathy Checklist (PCL) [19].

Factor analyses of PCL scores in groups of criminals confirm the presence of two factors [20]. The first factor includes items characteristic of primary psychopathy, including glibness or superficial charm, grandiose sense of self-worth, pathological lying, conning or manipulation, lack of remorse or guilt, shallow affect, callousness or lack of empathy, and failure to accept responsibility for own actions. The content of the first PCL factor is identical with the features of primary narcissism, as has been well described in ego and self psychology [21]. Empirically, the first PCL factor correlates positively with narcissistic and histrionic personality disorder and negatively with avoidant and dependent personality disorder according to DSM criteria [22]. The first factor also correlates moderately with the adventurous or antisocial triad of high Temperament and Character Inventory (TCI) novelty seeking, *low* TCI harm avoidance, and low TCI reward dependence in criminals [23].

The second PCL factor includes items characteristic of secondary psychopathy (i.e. borderline, emotionally unstable personality), including need for stimulation or proneness to boredom, parasitic lifestyle, poor behavioural control, early behavioural problems, lack of realistic long-term goals, impulsivity, and irresponsibility. It correlates with borderline and antisocial personality disorder as defined in DSM [22]. The second factor correlates moderately with the explosive or borderline triad of high TCI novelty seeking, *high* TCI harm avoidance, and low TCI reward dependence in criminals [23]. The second PCL factor also correlates positively with sensation seeking and impulsivity and negatively with nurturance [20], as expected from the overlap between the TCI and these scales [24].

Likewise, family and adoption studies of individuals with ASPD demonstrate an excess of ASPD, somatization disorder, and substance dependence in relatives. ASPD is more prevalent in the male relatives and somatization disorder is more prevalent in the female relatives in the same families, and there is an excess of both disorders in probands (i.e. comorbidity) and in their relatives (i.e. familial aggregation) [25–27]. ASPD, somatization disorder, and type 2 alcoholism and substance dependence share common personality factors observed in cluster B personality disorders (i.e. high novelty seeking, low self-directedness, and low cooperativeness as measured by the TCI). In addition, individuals with BPD and somatization disorder are high in harm avoidance (i.e. anxiety-prone, fearful, worried, and shy), whereas primary psychopathy and ASPD are low in harm avoidance (i.e, risk-taking, over-confident, denying real problems, and narcissistic or grandiose). The distinctions among putative subgroups of personality disorder were originally based largely on behavioural or psychodynamic descriptions, but studies of the genetic epidemiology and psychobiology of such patients are now providing a strong foundation for a scientific understanding of personality, its disorders, and ways of developing well-being [10].

GENETIC EPIDEMIOLOGY

The lifetime prevalence of ASPD in samples of the general population based on interviews by psychiatrists is 3.3% in men and 0.9% in women [25]. The prevalence in the Epidemiologic Catchment Area (ECA) study using the Diagnostic Interview Schedule (DIS) administered by non-psychiatrists was 4.5% in men and 0.8% in women, with little difference according to race (2.6% whites, 2.3% blacks) but a decreasing gradient with increasing age [28], presumably due to excess early mortality from accidents, violence, and cardiovascular disease in ASPD [5,29]. The National Comorbidity Survey estimated that 5.8% of men and 1.2% of women reported features diagnostic of ASPD, with approximately half reporting ongoing antisocial behaviour in the year prior to interview [30]. According to behavioural criteria of DSM for ASPD, most convicted felons and forensic cases have ASPD, with the prevalence varying from about 50% to 80% depending on the setting [1]. In contrast, only about 15% to 30% of the same individuals meet the criteria for psychopathy as defined by Hare, but nearly 90% of psychopaths satisfy behavioural criteria for ASPD [20]. Thus ASPD can be roughly subdivided into primary psychopaths with prominent narcissistic traits and secondary psychopaths with prominent borderline traits.

Demographic studies using crime statistics or broad diagnoses of ASPD (i.e. combining ASPD and BPD) indicate that ASPD is associated with low educational achievement, occupational instability, marital instability, and little or no religious affiliation [2,3,23]. However, these associations are confounded by diagnostic criteria that include school, work, and marital problems as the basis for diagnosis. When personality dimensions were measured directly using the TCI in the St. Louis Health Survey (SLHS), borderline personality was associated with failure to graduate from high school (30% in BPD versus 12% in others), but ASPD was not (8%). Likewise, underemployment (i.e. part-time or no job) was associated with borderline and other impulsive personality disorders in the SLHS but not antisocial personality. Those with ASPD were usually employed full time, although not continuously at the same job. In the SLHS, ASPD was most strongly associated with having never been married (46% versus 18%), particularly before age 30 years. The SLHS excluded prisoners and institutionalized subjects, so it may underestimate the association of ASPD with extreme social deviance in some people. It can be concluded, nevertheless, that much of the association of broad behaviourally-defined ASPD with social deviance may actually be characteristic of secondary psychopaths, who have BPD and not primary psychopathy or narrowly-defined ASPD based on multidimensional personality profiles. Social deviance, as defined by the second factor of Hare's PCL, and by measures of social dysfunction in school, work, and marriage, is associated with the combination of predispositions to basic negative emotions of anxiety (i.e. high harm avoidance), anger (i.e. high novelty seeking), disgust and aloofness (i.e. low reward dependence), and laziness (i.e. low persistence), which is the temperament profile leading to the emotional instability of BPD or secondary psychopathy when combined with immature character development [31,32].

Family studies of ASPD reveal strong aggregation in the same families of ASPD, somatization disorder, and substance dependence, including alcohol and a variety of drugs. Relevant family data for ASPD and somatization are summarized in Table 2.1 [25,27]. The substance dependence in these families is primarily early in onset (i.e. before 25 years and usually in adolescence) and associated with high novelty seeking; in other words, it is type-2 substance dependence or polysubstance abuse [33,34]. Hence, common vulnerability to each of these disorders is explained primarily by the heritable personality traits of high novelty seeking and low self-directedness [33–37]. The risk of illness in relatives varies inversely with the prevalence of the disorder in the general population: that is, antisocial women have the lowest population prevalence and highest familial loading, somatizing women have the highest population prevalence and lowest family loading, and antisocial men are intermediate in prevalence and family loading, as shown in Table 2.1. This pattern is typical of complex multifactorial inheritance in which there is non-linear interaction of multiple genetic and environmental variables [10,25].

Subsequent work to understand the structure of personality disorder revealed that low levels of character development (particularly low TCI self-directedness and low TCI cooperativeness) distinguished individuals

TABLE 2.1   Familial aggregation of antisocial personality and somatization disorder

| Diagnosis and sex of probands | Observed prevalence in general population | | Observed prevalence of illness in first-degree relatives | | | | | |
| | | | Antisocial men | | Antisocial women | | Somatizer women | |
	n	%	n	%	n	%	n	%
Antisocial men	329	3.3	54	25.9	79	6.3	79	9.9
Antisocial women	318	0.9	5	40.0	13	15.4	13	24.0
Somatizer women	153	2.4	20	15.0	56	0	56	25.8

Note: Prevalence of somatization disorder and antisocial personality are age-corrected.
Source: Cloninger et al. [25] (1975). The multifactorial model of disease transmission: II Sex differences in the familial transmission of sociopathy (Antisocial Personality). Br. J. Psychiatry, 127, 11–22. [27] The multifactorial model of disease transmission: III Familial relationship between sociopathy and hysteria (Briquet's syndrome). Br. J. Psychiatry, 127: 23–32, data obtained from interviews with subjects; all subjects were white.

TABLE 2.2   Descriptors of individuals who score high and low on the three character dimensions of the Temperament and Character Inventory (Source: Cloninger (2004) Feeling Good: The Sciences of Well-being, Oxford University Press, New York [10])

	Descriptors of extreme variants	
Character dimension	High	Low
Self-directedness	responsible purposeful resourceful self-accepting hopeful	blaming aimless inept vain deliberating
Cooperative	reasonable empathic helpful compassionate principled	prejudiced insensitive hostile revengeful opportunistic
Self-transcendent	judicious idealistic transpersonal faithful spiritual	repressive practical dualistic sceptical materialistic

who had a personality disorder from those who did not, regardless of subtype of personality disorder [31,38]. The temperament profile distinguished subtypes, such as ASPD and BPD, but all personality disorders are characterized by their lack of self-awareness. Lack of self-awareness is another way of describing deficient mental self-government, much as originally described by Pritchard in 1835. The TCI provides reliable quantitative measures of the three branches of mental self-government: executive functions are measured by self-directedness, legislative functions by cooperativeness, and judicial functions by self-transcendence. Descriptors of the three character dimensions corresponding to each of five subscales of each aspect of mental self-government are summarized in Table 2.2. One subscale of each TCI character dimension is designed as the mental reflection of the modulation of a particular step in thought [10]. Each of the four temperament dimensions and the three character dimensions of the TCI are moderately heritable (broad heritabilities are each about 50%), each has unique genetic variability, are modulated by different brain networks, and carry out distinct psychological functions [10].

Each dimension of human personality is about equally influenced by genetic variability and by variability unique to each individual [39]. Each dimension appears to be a complex adaptive system maintained by stabilizing selection, so that intermediate values are most common for each dimension and either extreme (high or low) increases susceptibility to mental disorder, as expected for complex or quantitative traits [10]. Personality disorder and related psychopathology is expected to be the result of non-linear interactions among multiple personality dimensions, which produce the complex patterns of multifactorial inheritance and comorbidity observed in the families of individuals with ASPD and other complex mental disorders [40].

These expectations have been confirmed by replicated observations in family, twin, and adoption studies of ASPD and criminality, which have been thoroughly reviewed elsewhere [26]. For example, in the most complete population-based study, Christiansen's twins born on the Danish Islands (1881–1910), the correlation in liability to criminality was 0.74 (± 0.07) in 712 pairs of monozygotic (MZ) twins, 0.46 (± 0.06) in 1390 same-sex dizygotic (DZ) twins, and 0.23 (± 0.10) in 2073 opposite-sex twins [26]. Criminality was defined as the illegal acts sanctioned by loss of liberty after the age of 15 years, which was the legal age of responsibility in Denmark at the time. The lifetime prevalence of criminality was 9.9% in male twins and 1.5% in female twins in this population. These results indicated a substantial heritability for adult criminality, estimated as about 56% from twice the difference between the MZ and DZ correlations. The lower concordance between opposite sex pairs suggested that sex-specific determinants of adult criminality were important. Furthermore, both crimes against property and crimes against person were heritable, but the predisposition to crimes of violence was largely independent of that to crimes against property [26]. Subsequently, it was shown that hostile aggression, as seen in suspicious and paranoid loners, is more strongly correlated with low TCI cooperativeness than with scores on other temperament or character traits, including high novelty seeking and low self-directedness [24]. TCI cooperativeness has substantial genetic determinants that are not shared with other traits [39], thereby helping to explain the different genetic causes of crimes against property and against persons.

In contrast, there is little or no evidence of heritability of juvenile delinquency, as shown by the absence of differences in concordance between MZ and DZ twins [26]. Juvenile delinquency appears to be largely determined by powerful situational influences, such as role models and neighbourhoods that encourage delinquency or discourage responsibility and hope. More generally, the continuation of recurrent criminal behaviour from adolescence into adulthood is unusual in the absence of personality disorder, substance dependence, and powerful situational influences, such as loyalty and identification with other criminals in a gang, neighbourhood, or prison [9,35,41]. A criminal career, like pathological gambling, is an occupational role, mask, or façade that disguises the underlying lack of self-directedness and impulse control of individuals with impulsive personality disorders, including some, but not all individuals, with narcissistic, histrionic, antisocial, and borderline personality configurations [42]. The incoherent wish for short-term gratification leads to chronic self-defeating behaviour.

Adoption studies of ASPD and criminality in the USA [43–45], psychopathy in Denmark [46], and criminality in Sweden [35] and Denmark [47] confirmed the importance of biological parents, adoptive parents, and rearing environment in the development of adult antisocial behaviour. Genetic influences were moderate as measured by the characteristics of the biological parents, which is consistent with the moderate heritability of quantitative personality traits in twin and adoption studies. Unstable environments in the first year of life, low socioeconomic status of the rearing home, and criminal behaviour or substance abuse by adoptive parents increased the later risk of adult antisocial behaviour in adopted children weakly, creating powerful situations and models that individuals with impulsive personality disorders are poorly prepared to resist [41].

Molecular genetic studies on novelty seeking have confirmed the expected importance of nonlinear gene–gene and gene–environment interactions in novelty seeking. A polymorphism of the dopamine transporter is associated with individual differences in initiating and continuing to smoke cigarettes, an effect which is mediated by the joint association of cigarette smoking and the dopamine transporter with novelty seeking [48]. In addition, the dopamine receptor DRD4 exon 3 seven-repeat allele has been associated with high novelty seeking and increased risk of opiate dependence [49]. Other work has shown that novelty seeking is associated with the ten-repeat allele of the dopamine transporter DAT1 when the DRD4 seven-repeat allele is absent [50].

Novelty seeking also depends on the three-way interaction of DRD4 with cathecol-O-methyl-transferase (COMT) and the serotonin transporter locus promoter's regulatory region (5-HTTLPR). In the absence of the short 5-HTTLPR allele (5HTTLPR L/L genotype) and in the presence of the high activity COMT Val/Val genotype, novelty seeking scores are higher in the presence of the DRD4 seven-repeat allele than in its absence [51]. Furthermore, within families, siblings who shared identical genotype groups for all three polymorphisms (COMT, DRD4, and 5-HTTLPR) had significantly correlated novelty seeking scores (intraclass correlation $= 0.39$ in 49 subjects, $p < 0.008$). In contrast, sibs with dissimilar genotypes in at least one polymorphism showed no significant correlation for novelty seeking (intraclass coefficient $= 0.18$ in 110 subjects, $p = 0.09$). Similar interactions were also observed between these three polymorphisms and novelty seeking in an independent sample of unrelated subjects [51] and have been replicated by independent investigators [52].

Gene–environment interaction has also been demonstrated for TCI novelty seeking in prospective population-based studies [53–55]. The TCI was administered to two large birth cohorts of Finnish men and women, and the individuals who scored in the top 10% and bottom 10% of TCI novelty seeking were genotyped for the exon 3 repeat polymorphism of DRD4. The four-repeat and seven-repeat alleles were most common in the Finnish sample [53,54], as is usual throughout the world [56]. The two-repeat and five-repeat alleles, which are rare in the Americas and Africa, were more than three times as frequent (16% versus 5%) in Finns who were very high in novelty seeking than in those who were very low in novelty seeking [53,54], and this difference was replicated in an independent sample [54]. The association with the two-repeat and five-repeat alleles was strongest for the two most adaptive aspects of novelty seeking, exploratory excitability and impulsive decision making [54]. Finnish men and women with the two-repeat and five-repeat alleles were higher in novelty seeking as adults if they had experienced a hostile childhood environment, as measured by maternal reports of emotional distance and a strict authoritarian disciplinary style with physical punishment [55]. The effect of a hostile childhood environment on novelty seeking was significant for the total novelty seeking score and for the spiritual aspect of novelty seeking (exploratory excitability) but not for the intellectual aspect of novelty seeking (impulsive decision making). The mothers' reports of childhood environment were obtained when the children were aged 18 to 21 years, and genotyping and personality assessment of novelty seeking was done independently 15 years later. If children had the two-repeat or five-repeat alleles of the DRD4 polymorphism, their TCI novelty seeking scores were high if they were reared in a hostile childhood environment and their novelty seeking scores were low if they were reared in a kind and cooperative environment. Children with certain genotypes are likely to evoke a characteristic pattern of responses from their parents and others, and to select for themselves certain aspects from the available environments [57]. However, therapeutic environments, such as kind and cooperative parenting or psychotherapy, can evoke positive adaptation by modifying gene expression, which depends on the orchestrated interaction of many genes and environmental influences [55].

CLINICAL PICTURE AND COMPLICATIONS

No natural boundaries have been identified that distinguish subtypes of personality disorder by descriptive, biological, or genetic procedures [40,58,59]. There are no points of rarity in admixture analysis, for example, that separate patients into discrete taxons or disease entities. Consequently, in the absence of a definitive procedure or test, the clinical picture of ASPD depends on the procedure used to make the diagnosis. For example, DSM-IV emphasizes behavioural criteria that have been well-validated by the work of Lee Robins and others in St. Louis, including Sam Guze and myself [1]. When the diagnosis is based on a history of recurrent antisocial behaviour beginning by 15 years of age, it necessarily follows that the patients show recurrent antisocial behaviour, such as running away from home, fighting, and getting into trouble at school (truancy, suspension, expulsion) during adolescence and then frequent criminality, poor job performance, and marital instability during adulthood [1]. However, when the diagnosis is based on their multidimensional personality profile, the associations with social deviance remain but are much weaker, as described in the prior section. Such artifacts of diagnostic procedures do not mean that all features of patient subgroups are artifactual, but only that natural boundaries between subtypes are lacking, so that differentiation is never sharp and is influenced substantially by ascertainment and assessment procedures. Nevertheless, the validity of the clinical associations of ASPD with male gender and with somatization disorder and substance abuse can be supported by quantitative genetic analyses of family, twin, and adoption data. These show that these features are not only correlated within individuals (which could be artifacts of diagnostic procedures) but are also correlated between individuals within the same family (which cannot be artifactual when there is population-based ascertainment of all families containing a proband).

Some aspects of the clinical picture are robust regardless of procedural variables and are confirmed by family studies. Personality traits diagnostic of ASPD are measurable in childhood and moderately stable throughout life in most individuals [33,60]. Such childhood onset is an intrinsic feature of personality development, not an artifact of diagnostic criteria for ASPD.

The number and severity of childhood antisocial behaviours, such as runaway, fighting, and school problems, is a robust predictor of the risk of adult antisocial behaviour [2,3], so this is a natural feature of personality development and the power of adolescent socialization, not an artifact of diagnostic criteria. Most people with recurrent antisocial behaviour as a child or adolescent do *not* persist in antisocial behaviour as adults. The variables that are predictive of chronic delinquency and adult criminality are the frequency of antisocial behaviour, its variety, its early age of onset, and its occurrence in more than one setting [61]. These factors predispose to adult ASPD, substance abuse, and a higher rate of violent death [3,5]. Perhaps it is most accurate to regard the stability of severe antisocial behaviour, when it does occur, as an indicator of the power of dissocial experiences on adolescents, as suggested by ICD-10 adopting the name "dissocial personality", not antisocial personality. In population-based samples, most individuals with uncomplicated ASPD commit a small number of petty property offences during early childhood and adolescence and show little overt criminal behaviour after middle age [35]. Those who commit repeated or violent crimes often have alcohol or drug abuse as a complication of the personality disorder.

Longitudinal studies also show that substantial numbers of individuals with ASPD do "mature" in character, "burn out" or stop their criminal behaviour by middle age, mostly between the ages of 30 and 40 years [2,5,62]. Robins found that in 82 individuals with ASPD followed from childhood into adulthood (mostly in their mid-40s), 12% were completely in remission, 27% had "burned out" with greatly reduced range and severity of antisocial behaviour, and 61% showed little improvement. Improvement occurred in each decade when it occurred at all, but most often between the ages of 30 and 40. It is important to distinguish between "maturity" and "burn out" [63]. Some individuals actually do mature in the sense that they experience a radical transformation of their thinking, goals, and values. Matured individuals may develop satisfying social relationships, recognize criminal activity as foolish and self-defeating, redirect their goals and values to legitimate work, and become less self-centred, rebellious, and hedonistic. In contrast, others may be tired of criminal activity but remain irresponsible and lacking in impulse control and self-awareness. The burn-out of overt criminal behaviour does not usually permit the individual with ASPD to make up for their earlier socioeconomic problems ("the lost years"), and they may continue to have impulsive–aggressive temperamental traits even if they mature in character [2]. Furthermore, individuals who are intelligent and socially successful may still have ASPD, as vividly described by Cleckley [18] and population-based epidemiological studies [23].

When individuals are diagnosed as having ASPD based on behavioural criteria, they nevertheless are observed to have particular personality traits that can be quantified in terms of temperament and character development. For example, primary psychopathy or ASPD has been consistently associated with impulsivity (as in high novelty seeking), risk-taking and autonomic underarousal (as in low harm avoidance), aloofness and social detachment (as in low reward dependence) [31,64]. In addition, individuals with ASPD are immature in character, with low scores on TCI self-directedness and cooperativeness. Lying, conning, and other features of primary narcissism (i.e. grandiosity without self-awareness) are characteristic of ASPD, primary psychopathy, and other personality disorders with a similar severity of character deficit [1,21] or level of thought [10].

Recent work has suggested a natural boundary between the presence or absence of self-aware consciousness that can be precisely and reliably quantified in psychological and biological terms [10]. Human beings are uniquely capable of self-aware recollection and this ability matures with the development of a capacity for self-efficacy in the terms of social psychology, initiative in the terms of Erikson's ego psychology, or the phallic phase in Freud's psychosexual theory [10]. Consequently, a personality disorder can be defined as a description of someone whose thoughts and human relationships are usually lacking in self-awareness (which is defined specifically as awareness of one's own initiative and self-efficacy). In addition, the person with the antisocial subtype of personality disorder is someone who also has an adventurous temperament, which is character-ized by high novelty seeking, low harm avoidance, and low reward dependence. Such a multidimensional definition allows everyone to be assigned to mutually exclusive groups by explicit quantitative rules, as has been described in detail elsewhere [65,66]. When this procedure is followed, precise statements can be made about the clinical picture of ASPD and its complications and neighbouring conditions. There is no need to assume that ASPD is a discrete disease entity in order for the diagnosis of the syndrome to be useful as a dimensional configuration that is quasi-stable during development [67].

DIFFERENTIAL DIAGNOSIS AND MOTIVATION FOR TREATMENT

The possible configurations of the three temperament dimensions of harm avoidance, novelty seeking, and reward dependence can be visualized as a cube, as shown in Figure 2.1. The corners of the cube correspond to extreme combinations of the temperament dimensions, with ASPD characterized by the adventurous temperament with high novelty seeking, low harm avoidance, and low reward dependence. The three neighbouring tempera-ment subtypes each differ from the adventurous subtype in terms of one dimension, sharing the features of the other two temperament dimensions. The adventurous (antisocial) temperament configuration is low in harm avoidance, low in reward dependence, and high in novelty seeking. The neighbours of the adventurous (antisocial) subtype are the explosive (borderline) subtype that is high in harm avoidance, the passionate (histrionic) subtype that is high in reward dependence, and the indepen-dent (schizoid) subtype that is low in novelty seeking. The temperament subtypes are labelled according to what most strongly motivates their behaviour, which is crucial to recognize in order to motivate therapy: adventure and curiosity (the ''adventurous''), attention and approval (the ''passionate''), appeasement and nurturance (the ''explosive''), and compe-tition (the ''independent''). When these motives are not integrated with

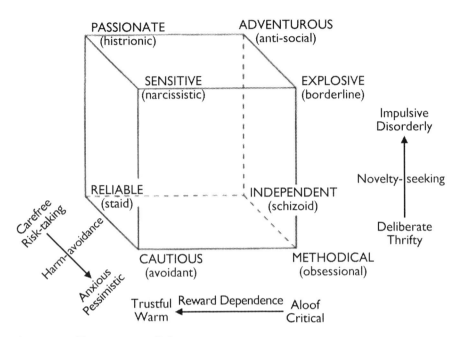

Figure 2.1   Temperament Cube

coherent goals and values in a mature character, they become maladaptive and are described as antisocial, histrionic, borderline, and schizoid traits, respectively. Motivating patients with ASPD usually requires that they view the context of their situation as an adventure in which they are trusted and respected as free agents. Of course, a prison or jail is a powerful situation that is the antithesis of what is needed to motivate the development of responsibility and self-efficacy in a person with an adventurous temperament, as is discussed later [41,68].

Any of these temperament configurations can occur in people with either mature or immature characters. Consequently, the clinical presentation of these neighbouring temperament configurations depends on the level of character development, which is measured by the three TCI dimensions of self-directedness, cooperativeness, and self-transcendence. For example, low scores on TCI self-directedness and cooperativeness indicate the presence of a personality disorder [31]. Nevertheless, immature character development is associated with poor modulation of attention, affect, and behaviour, so impulsive personality disorders can be easily confused with bipolar disorder based on cross-sectional behaviour, particularly when the bipolar disorder presents with chronic irritability, distractibility, and grandiosity. The longitudinal history of recurrent antisocial behaviour without periods of remission usually indicates a personality disorder.

Family history and mental status features, such as flight of ideas and ego inflation in mania, usually allow a definite diagnosis. Clinicians may erroneously create a long miscellaneous list of psychiatric diagnoses for a patient with ASPD or BPD by careless differential diagnosis or by the "good intention" of suggesting a diagnosis they believe to be more treatable than ASPD. A long list of diagnoses including ASPD, substance dependence, psychoses and mood disorders suggests the need for careful differential diagnosis and review of records to determine what was documented on mental status examination and by objective information in the past. Clinicians must remember that people with personality disorders may have other mental disorders, and vice versa. However, long lists of different diagnoses are usually the result of the non-specificity of behavioural criteria and lack of knowledge and skill in the assessment of the structure of thought, the facilitation of healthy development of psychological maturity, or both.

Detailed assessment of the structure of a person's thought and the level of his or her psychological maturity is a more definitive basis for differential diagnosis than behavioural or psychological checklist criteria. The level of psychological maturity can be measured quantitatively in terms of the degree of coherence of character functions. Learning ability in human beings has evolved in seven major steps that can be described as (1) instinct, (2) habit, (3) ritual, (4) emotion, (5) intellect, (6) culture, and (7) intuition or self-aware consciousness. There are individual differences in human thought processes for five of these steps, excluding instinct and culture, which do not involve distinct processes of self-aware consciousness. Consequently, there are five steps in human (i.e. self-aware) thought processes, which are modulated by subscales of the TCI character dimensions, as shown in Table 2.3. For example, the first step in thought is intuitive recognition, which is modulated by TCI character subscales measuring degree of responsibility versus feeling controlled and victimized (SD1), tolerance versus prejudice and hatred (CO1), and sensibility versus hysterical repression (ST1). The initial intuition (i.e. cognitive schema) may be mature and coherent when these modulatory processes are mature (i.e. responsible, tolerant, and sensible), or it may be maladaptive when the processes are immature (i.e. victimized, prejudiced, and repressive).

The result of all these processes leads to variability in the level of coherence of thought that can be precisely quantified and reliably measured [10]. Furthermore, the same method of measurement can be used to quantify maturation over years as well as variability in the coherence of thought from moment to moment in the same individual. The five major steps in the evolution of thought give rise to variation in five planes of thought involving sexuality, materiality, emotion, intellect, and spirituality. Each plane is partially reflected in the others in self-aware consciousness, so

TABLE 2.3   Five steps in thought and their modulation by processes measured by the subscales of TCI character dimensions of Self-directedness (SD), Cooperativeness (CO), and Self-Transcendence (ST) (adapted from Cloninger [10])

Step in Self-aware Consciousness	TCI measures of functional processes		
	Agency (SD)	Flexibility (CO)	Understanding (ST)
(1) Intuition	responsible vs controlled	tolerant vs prejudiced	sensible vs repressive
(2) Reasoning	purposeful vs aimless	forgiving vs revengeful	idealistic vs practical
(3) Emotion	accepting vs approval-seeking	empathic vs inconsiderate	transpersonal vs individual
(4) Intention	resourceful vs inept	helpful vs unhelpful	faithful vs sceptical
(5) Action	hopeful sublimation vs compromising deliberation	charitable principles vs self-serving opportunism	spiritual awareness vs local realism

human thought has a 5 × 5 matrix structure that is useful for quantitative measurement. The content of this matrix is summarized in Table 2.4 for dualistic consciousness, which is characteristic of people with personality disorders and the ordinary cognition of most adults. Supporting biopsychosocial data about this way of quantifying thought and its spiral pattern of movement with increasing coherence and social radius in time is presented in detail elsewhere [10].

Sample descriptors of thought are summarized in Figure 2.2. Thoughts in the sexual and material planes (i.e. planes 2 and 3 respectively) are most frequent in individuals with personality disorders that are severe (lacking in basic trust, thought levels from 2.0 to 2.5), moderate (borderline or trusting but lacking in basic confidence, thought levels from 2.6 to 2.7), and mild (narcissistic, i.e. confident but lacking in initiative, thought levels from 2.8 to 3.3), as well as ordinary levels of maturity (thought from 3.4 to 3.9) in the first stage of self-aware consciousness. Note that the average thoughts of

TABLE 2.4   5 × 5 matrix of human thought (dualistic consciousness)

Subplane of thought	Plane 2 (Sexuality)	Plane 3 (Intention)	Plane 4 (Emotion)	Plane 5 (Intellect)	Plane 7 (Spirit)
Spiritual Aspects (7)	{responsible} scorn or exhibition (shy)	{purposeful} power or sarcasm (exploratory)	{self-accepting} contentment or relief of grief (attached)	{resourceful} [self-actualization +oceanic feelings] (perfectionistic)	{coherence} [coherence-seeking]
Intellectual Aspects (5)	{sensible} devaluation or idealization (pessimistic)	{idealistic} pride or inferiority (impulsive)	{transpersonal} tender-minded or tough-minded (sentimental)	{faithful} self-transcendence & patience (eagerness of effort)	{spiritual} [truth-seeking]
Emotional Aspects (4)	Harm Avoidance— worry or denial	Novelty Seeking— anger/envy or stoicism	Reward Dependence— warmth or coldness	Persistence— calmness & conscience	[peace-seeking]
Material Aspects (3)	{tolerant} vulnerability or eroticism (fearful) {prejudiced}	{forgiving} greed/competition or submission (extravagant) {revengeful}	{empathic} sociability or aloofness (aloof) {inconsiderate}	(overachieving) {helpful} cooperativeness or non-prejudice (underachieving) {unhelpful}	{charitable} [merit-seeking]
Sexual Aspects (2)	{victimized} emptiness or lust (fatigable)	{aimless} desire/fight or aversion/flight (disorderly)	{approval-seeking} succorance or rejection (dependent)	(work-hardened) self-directness or irresponsibility (spoiled) {inadequate}	{enlightened} [mastery-seeking]

Experiences that are unlikely to be explicitly clear in the consciousness of most people are labelled in brackets. Adjectives in parentheses indicate the Temperament and Character Inventory (TCI) temperament subscales that provide quantitative measures of the emotional aspects of the conflict within each subplane of thought observed in dualistic consciousness. Adjectives in { } indicate the TCI character subscales that modulate that subplane, except coherence, which is the sum total of all three character scales.

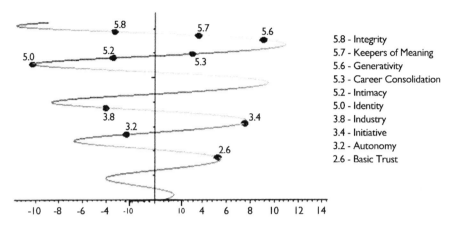

Figure 2.2 Sample descriptors of thought in terms of Erikson's levels of character development as modified by George Vaillant (adapted from Cloninger [10])

individuals described as having a severe personality disorder are lacking in basic trust (which begins at thought level 2.6), so this involves thought in the emotional aspects of sexuality with prominent somatization, or even lower in the material aspects of sexuality with prominent conversion and dissociation. The average thoughts of those with moderate personality disorder involve basic trust but are lacking in confidence, which begins at thought level 2.8 with primary narcissism in the spiritual aspects of sexuality. The average thoughts of individuals with a mild personality disorder involve narcissistic confidence but are lacking in self-awareness, as manifest by initiative and self-efficacy and secondary emotions like empathy. More detailed descriptions are presented elsewhere with examples for the full range of human thought [10].

Notice that typical borderline characteristics occur in plane 2, such as somatization (2.4 to 2.5 in the emotional aspects of sexuality) and splitting (2.7 in the intellectual aspects of sexuality). Primary narcissism is severe at a thought level of 2.8 in the spiritual aspects of sexuality. The fight or flight response occurs at the thought level of 3.0 and oppositional behaviour occurs at 3.1, both in the sexual aspect of the material plane. Guilt and remorse occur at a minimum thought level of 3.2 in those with maximum thoughts at 3.4 or higher. Self-awareness of initiative (i.e. self-efficacy) occurs at level 3.4, which is the beginning of the first stage of self-aware consciousness. Even in the first stage of self-aware consciousness, thought is egocentric and dominated by emotional conflicts. Self-acceptance is the culmination of the first stage of self-awareness at thought level 5.3, which leads to the second stage of self-awareness (i.e. thinking about thinking, metacognition, free association, meditation, or mindfulness) at thought levels 5.4 to 5.7. The third stage of self-awareness is contemplation in which there is a growing awareness of what was previously unconscious, leading to illumination and later wisdom (see [10]).

A person's thought pattern can be described by its average and range (i.e. minimum and maximum). For example, a person with mild ASPD may have an average level of thought at 3.0 (i.e. fight or flight) with a minimum of 2.2 (i.e. hate with dissociative or conversion episodes under stress) and a maximum of 4.0 (i.e. wish for sympathy and emotional support). In other words, a person's level of thought may be elevated under favourable conditions or may regress under stress and function at a lower level of coherence than is usual for him. Such an individual has an immature character in which his primary narcissism (i.e. archaic grandiosity) is associated with a happy mood that is resistant to change because he is not self-aware of reality without distortion. He can lie to others convincingly because he rarely faces reality himself and often believes his own lies. He may be overly familiar, glib, seductive, or superficially charming because his thought is often elevated in the sexual plane. However, when his material wants are frustrated, he is predisposed to react with fighting or flight (i.e. aggression or runaway reactions).

Hence somatization, borderline features like splitting, primary narcissism, and aggression or runaway reactions are nearby in level of coherence of thought. Individuals with thought in this range are lacking in self-awareness, which is associated with inefficiency in activation of brain networks that modulate the branches of mental self-government (i.e. character dimensions). For example, executive functions or TCI self-directedness is highly correlated ($r = 0.75$) with individual differences in the activation of medial prefrontal cortex (Brodmann areas 9/10) [69]. The psychobiological description of ASPD that is needed as a foundation for effective therapy requires a detailed description of the frequency of thought in individuals with and without ASPD throughout its possible range, and a similar description of the human relationships of these same individuals.

MEASUREMENT OF THOUGHT AND HUMAN RELATIONSHIPS IN ASPD

In the course of my clinical work since 1997, I have carried out detailed assessments of the movement of thought in more than 100 adults with ASPD diagnosed according to DSM-IV criteria and more than 2000 individuals representative of the general population of the metropolitan St. Louis, as previously described [40]. The levels of thought were

TABLE 2.5   Diagnosis of the Frequency of Thought (DFT) of people representative of active antisocial personality disorder (ASPD) (above the diagonal) and representative of the general population (GP) (below the diagonal), excluding individuals who have received coherence therapy, with descriptors for group averages in ASPD

| Plane | Group Averages (ASPD/GP)* | | | (Descriptor of ASPD) |
	Mean	Min	Max	
2 (sexuality)	0.4/0.3	0.0/0.0	0.7/0.6	mistrusting
3 (materiality)	0.2/0.3	0.0/0.0	0.5/0.6	greedy
4 (emotion)	0.3/0.3	0.0/0.0	0.4/0.5	unappreciated
5 (intellect)	0.2/0.2	0.0/0.0	0.3/0.4	intolerant
7 (spirituality)	0.0/0.0	0.0/0.0	0.2/0.2	mastery-seeking
Global	3.0/3.2 aggressive	2.2/2.3 hedonistic	4.0/4.3 resentful	

*Expressed in decimal units (0.0 to 0.9) of the possible range of each evolutionary plane of the path of human self-aware consciousness as described in Cloninger C.R. (2004), *Feeling Good: The Science of Well-Being*, Oxford University Press, New York (reprinted by permission of the Center for Well-Being, Washington University).

quantified using my most recent refinements of the method for the detailed Diagnosis of the Frequency of Thought (DFT) [10,40]. Individuals were only excluded if they had previously received treatment according to the principles I have described for coherence therapy, which results in changes in thought and related psychobiological variables [10,40]. The group averages are summarized in Table 2.5 for the mean and range (minimum and maximum values) of thought within each plane of thought. Notice that the verbal descriptors given in Tables 2.5–2.9 are for the group with ASPD, not those of the general population to which they are compared.

The global average of thought in the general population was measured in the material plane at thought level 3.2, which refers to thought at the level Erikson described as "autonomous", which involves competitive conflicts, such as seeking control versus feeling trapped. The average minimum thoughts (i.e. least coherent thoughts) in the general population were in the sexual plane at thought level 2.3, involving a hedonistic sexual conflict leading to condemnation or seduction. The average maximum level of thought in the general population was 4.3, indicating sociability or aloofness related to conflicts about feelings of respect and appreciation for and by others. Sociability versus aloofness is a particular conflict of opposites at the same level of thought, differing primarily in the way temperament biases the response to the social context.

TABLE 2.6   Diagnosis of Human Relationships (DHR) of people representative of active antisocial personality disorder (ASPD) (above the diagonal) and representative of the general population (GP) (below the diagonal), excluding individuals who have received coherence therapy

| Plane | Group Averages (ASPD/GP)* | | | (Descriptor of ASPD) |
	Mean	Min	Max	
2 (sexuality)	0.3/0.3	0.0/0.0	0.5/0.6	exploitative
3 (materiality)	0.2/0.3	0.0/0.0	0.3/0.6	competitive
4 (emotion)	0.2/0.2	0.0/0.0	0.5/0.6	aloof
5 (intellect)	0.1/0.1	0.0/0.0	0.3/0.4	self-serving
7 (spirituality)	0.0/0.0	0.0/0.0	0.0/0.1	heartless
Global	3.0/3.4 aggressive	2.2/2.3 hedonistic	4.2/4.5 vulnerable	

*Expressed in decimal units (0.0 to 0.9) of the possible range of each evolutionary plane of the path of human self-aware consciousness as described in Cloninger C.R. (2004), *Feeling Good: The Science of Well-Being*, Oxford University Press, New York (reprinted by permission of the Center for Well-Being, Washington University).

The averages in the thoughts of people in the ASPD group were lower in ways that are clinically significant, even if the differences appear small numerically. For example, the global average of thought in ASPD was at the bottom of the material plane at 3.0, which indicates frequent unmodulated defence reactions ("fight or flight"), described in Table 2.5 as "aggressive". The average of the minimum thoughts of people with ASPD was low in the material aspects of the sexual plane at 2.2, indicating hedonistic or hateful thoughts. The average of the maximum thoughts in people with ASPD was at the bottom of the emotional plane at 4.0, indicating resentment arising from unmodulated conflicts about the wish to reject others or the unmet need for their sympathy.

The global values are weighted averages of the frequency of thought in each of the five component planes of thought indicated in Table 2.5. The main deviation of individuals with ASPD in the detailed DFT is primarily lower thought in the material plane (i.e. more impulsive–aggressive) and lower maximum thoughts in the other planes.

The diagnosis of human relationships (DHR) of people can be quantified in a similar manner, as in Table 2.6, which is based on measurements related to the thoughts, feelings, and actions evoked by relationship with other people. The DHR method is described in more detail elsewhere with examples illustrating the importance of both sides of a human relationship [10]. The average of the most frequent (i.e. modal) DHR of people in the general population was 3.4 (i.e. showing initiative and self-efficacy to try to cope with conflicts related to aggravation, envy, or jealousy). The averages of the minimum and maximum values ranged from 2.3 (as previously described) to 4.5 (indicating conflicts about emotional security related to high or low reward dependence, which measures the emotional aspects of the plane 4). The human relationships of people with ASPD corresponded to the level of their thoughts with an average of 3.0 ("fight or flight"). The averages of their human relationships ranged from 2.2 to 4.2, indicating some relationships involving emotional attachments in which there was concern about social vulnerability (feeling hurt, wounded, rejected or wanting to be left alone). This showed that individuals with ASPD usually have maximum thoughts and relationships that are self-reflective and amenable to psychotherapy, although their average thoughts and relationships are dominated by defence reactions and are lacking in self-aware emotions like guilt, attachment, or empathy.

MEASUREMENT OF PSYCHOBIOLOGICAL INFLUENCES ON THOUGHT

The differences in personality dimensions, including the level of character development, are strongly associated with individual differences in the activation of specific brain networks that have distinct functions in processing information and emotional cues, as is summarized in detail elsewhere [10]. In brief, the level of maturity of a person depends strongly on differences in brain networks that modulate attention, affect, and character. For example, executive functions, as measured by TCI self-directedness, are correlated strongly ($r = 0.75$) with differences in the efficiency of activation of the medial prefrontal cortex [69]. Legislative functions, as measured by TCI cooperativeness, require self-awareness in an allocentric context, which depends on activation of the inferior parietal region [70]. Judicial functions, as measured by TCI self-transcendence, require orchestration of the entire brain for creative and efficient multi-tasking, which depends on activation of the frontal poles [71] and are strongly correlated (-0.7) with binding of 5HT-1a receptors in the neocortex and other brain regions [72]. The regulation of these three dimensions of character leads to a spiral movement of self-aware consciousness in human beings. In other words, the movement of human thought can spiral up or down and the three dimensions of such spiral movement can be quantified in terms of the elevation of thought (i.e. executive functions, sense of agency, or TCI self-directedness), width of thought (i.e. legislative functions, voluntary social radius, or TCI cooperativeness), and the depth of thought (i.e. judicial functions, depth of understanding, or TCI self-transcendence).

An adequate theory of human personality and self-aware consciousness requires recognition that thought is influenced by both a biological, material aspect (*soma*) and a self-aware, immaterial aspect (*psyche*) [10]. Each person has a rich innate endowment that allows self-organizing development to proceed in creative ways that cannot be fully explained by genetic predisposition or prior environmental conditioning. Extensive empirical data shows that humans have agency and self-efficacy that makes many aspects of personality development to be unpredictable [10,73,74]. For example, variability in human personality is about equally explained by genetic variability and by variability unique to each individual. The functional organization of the soma and the psyche must correspond because psychosomatic coherence of personality is possible, as exemplified in the lives of individuals who are well-integrated and coherent. From this perspective, the treatment of personality disorder may require the development of coherence in the psychobiological influences on human thought. Therefore, treatment of any personality disorder requires an understanding of the detailed structure of thought and human relationships, as well as the underlying psychobiological parameters that modulate them. Description of thought, human relationships, and their psychobiological determinants in terms of categories or traits is not adequate because it reduces a person, who is a self-organizing hierarchy of complex adaptive systems, into something mechanical, lacking in free will and self-awareness, and incapable of radical transformation to a state of well-being because of a perpetual struggle with internal and external conflicts [10]. This is particularly true of deterministic approaches to the description and treatment of ASPD, which usually have assumed that people we do not understand are bad, incorrigible, and untreatable. When a therapist begins with such negative dualistic attitudes toward another person, the negative expectation is a self-fulfilling prophecy because the trust, hope, or compassion that is needed in an effective helping relationship is absent. Therefore, the earlier biomedical and psychosocial observations I have made about ASPD need to be translated into an adequate non-reductive, non-dualistic framework for understanding the dynamics of human thought.

The description of the 5 × 5 matrix structure of human thought (i.e. Table 2.4) provides a suitable framework for a detailed description of the range of thought in each of the five planes, as described in Table 2.5 for ASPD. The psyche influences thought through its three major functions: self-aware memory (i.e. recollection), will, and understanding. Individual differences in recollection can be measured by level of coherence of the intuitive schema that make up a person's world view (i.e. the level of TCI self-

TABLE 2.7   Diagnosis of Freedom of Will (DFW) of people representative of active antisocial personality disorder (ASPD) (shown above the diagonal) and representative of the general population (GP) (shown below the diagonal), excluding individuals who have received coherence therapy, with descriptors of influence on Cooperativeness in ASPD

Plane	Group values (ASPD/GP)*			
	Mean	Min	Max	(Descriptor)
2 (sexuality)	0.2/0.2	0.0/0.0	0.4/0.5	prejudiced
3 (materiality)	0.1/0.2	0.0/0.0	0.3/0.5	revengeful
4 (emotion)	0.1/0.2	0.0/0.0	0.2/0.4	inconsiderate
5 (intellect)	0.1/0.1	0.0/0.0	0.3/0.4	unhelpful
7 (spirituality)	0.0/0.1	0.0/0.0	0.2/0.2	opportunistic
Global	2.7/3.1 sensation-seeking	2.0/2.1 inflexible	3.2/3.8 demanding	

*Expressed in decimal units (0.0 to 0.9) of the possible range of each evolutionary plane of the path of human self-aware consciousness as described in Cloninger C.R. (2004), *Feeling Good: The Science of Well-Being*, Oxford University Press, New York (Center for Well-Being, Washington University).

directedness) and his degree of giftedness in various domains of the mind and spirit. Individual differences in freedom of will influence the degree of a person's cooperativeness in thought. Individual differences in listening to the psyche influence a person's degree of understanding, or TCI self-transcendence. These spiritual parameters are interdependent, so the level of free will and listening to the psyche in each of the planes influences the recollection in those planes and vice versa. For example, there is substantial, but not complete, correspondence between the variability of thought in individuals with ASPD and their variability in the freedom of their will from external conditioning and their frequency of contemplative listening to their psyche (i.e. the degree to which the wisdom of the psyche remains unconscious instead of being awakened).

Variability in free will in each of the five planes of human thought is summarized in Table 2.7 for people with ASPD and the general population. The degree to which a person is cooperative (as measured by the TCI cooperativeness scale) is the mental expression of freedom of will. It is not surprising that individuals with ASPD, who are often highly uncooperative and frequently have substance dependence, are distinguished by lower levels of free will than others, at least in some aspects of their being. Most people have weak flexibility and are dominated by habit in much that they do, but individuals with ASPD are distinguished by marked inflexibility in their maladaptive behaviours. There is a range of flexibility even in ASPD,

TABLE 2.8   Diagnosis of Listening to the Psyche (DLP) of people representative of active antisocial personality disorder (ASPD) (shown above the diagonal) and representative of the general population (GP) (shown below the diagonal), excluding individuals who have received coherence therapy, with descriptions of influence on Self-Transcendence in ASPD

Plane	Group values (ASPD/GP)*			(Descriptor)
	Mean	Min	Max	
2 (sexuality)	0.3/0.3	0.2/0.1	0.5/0.6	repressive somatizing
3 (materiality)	0.0/0.3	0.0/0.1	0.3/0.5	amoral guiltless
4 (emotion)	0.1/0.2	0.0/0.1	0.2/0.4	alienated no empathy
5 (intellect)	0.1/0.2	0.0/0.0	0.3/0.4	sceptical agnostic
7 (spirituality)	0.0/0.1	0.0/0.0	0.2/0.3	irreverent unwise
Global	2.9/3.2 detached	2.1/2.2 empty	3.4/3.8 remorseful	

*Expressed in decimal units (0.0 to 0.9) of the possible range of each evolutionary plane of the path of human self-aware consciousness as described in Cloninger C.R. (2004), *Feeling Good: The Science of Well-Being*, Oxford University Press, New York (Center for Well-Being, Washington University).

nevertheless, so the capacity for positive change is present in this dynamic, changeable aspect of every human being.

Likewise, variability in listening to the psyche in each of the five planes of human thought is summarized in Table 2.8 for individuals with ASPD and for the general population. Human beings have a capacity for intuitive learning by listening to their psyche, which underlies the character trait of TCI self-transcendence. Individuals with ASPD have lower average values in listening to the psyche (i.e. contemplative or transcendent thinking) than the average person in the general population. They are particularly deficient in listening to their psyche in the material and spiritual planes, which is often described as their having a corruptible conscience, ethical unreliability, or lacking in moral ideals [21]. Hence, individuals with ASPD are deficient in their intuitive senses of responsibility, purpose, beauty, truth, or goodness. Their experience is superficial, shallow, or concrete because listening to the psyche is what communicates these qualities to experience. Consequently, they are deficient in self-aware emotions, such as sincere remorse (thought level 3.2), accurate empathy (thought level 4.7), genuine conscientiousness (thought level 5.4), and impartial compassion (thought level 7.5).

Character is developed and thought is elevated by the processes of increasing free will (i.e. decreasing control by habit, conditioning, and other attachments) and by increasing listening to the psyche (i.e. awakening of the intuitive senses). Nearly everyone really wants to be free and awake to the ever-changing wonders of life, including individuals with ASPD. Any treatment that radical transforms a person with personality disorder must target these influences on the dynamics of thought and social development.

Other psychobiological parameters that distinguish individuals with ASPD from the general population are summarized in Table 2.9. These are presented along with the group averages for free will and listening to the psyche to provide an overview of the psychobiological parameters that influence human thought and relationships. Descriptions of these parameters and how to measure them in clinical practice are presented in more detail elsewhere [10]. However, they are mentioned briefly here because two variables are of major clinical importance. The psyche level is reflected in a person's world view, which is not much different in ASPD and the general population, suggesting a good potential for self-efficacy. Following the path of the psyche is reflected in the level of reality testing and self-directedness of an individual; individuals with ASPD are not psychotic but are often maladaptive in their way of living. Low self-directedness and

TABLE 2.9 Overview of psychobiological parameters distinguishing individuals with active antisocial personality disorder (ASPD) from the general population, excluding individuals who have had coherence therapy, with descriptions of influence of fundamental psychobiological parameters on thought and relationships*

Parameter	General average	ASPD average	(Descriptor)
Psyche Level	3.7	3.5	(good potential for self-efficacy)
Following the Path	3.2	2.8	(maladaptive, unwise)
Ego Level	3.9	4.2	(pathological narcissism)
Serenity of Psyche	3.5	2.7	(inappropriate unstable arousal)
Freedom of Will	3.1	2.7	(inflexible, stimulus-bound dependence-prone)
Listening to Psyche	3.2	2.9	(little self-aware emotion like guilt, empathy, conscience)

*Expressed in the evolutionary units of the path of human self-aware consciousness as described by Cloninger C.R. (2004), *Feeling Good: The Science of Well-Being*, Oxford University Press, New York (Center for Well-Being, Washington University).

following of the path of the psyche is typical of personality disorders generally [10,31,38]. Individuals with ASPD are highly narcissistic, as previously described, and this is a mental reflection of the marked inflation of their ego because of their intense and incoherent struggles with themselves, other people, and reality in general. A well-integrated, self-accepting person has an ego level of 3.2 or 3.3, so the average person in the general population is also narcissistic to a lesser degree (average ego level 3.9 in the general population). These struggles create a large gap between the level of the psyche and the usual level of thought and human relationships. The gap between the level of the psyche and the level of individual functioning leads to mental depression and low serenity of the psyche, which are reflected in the mental status by psychomotor arousal, inappropriateness of affect, and lack of equanimity. These parameters help to clarify the psychobiological dynamics that lead to the clinical picture observed in ASPD, and may help to guide us in promising directions for improvement of the treatment of ASPD.

MEASUREMENT OF THE POWER OF THE SOCIAL CONTEXT

The Concept of the Powerful Situation

People with antisocial personality do remit and when they do so they usually attribute their improvement to powerful life-changing situations, such as getting a good job, a good marriage, religious conversion, or an illumination experience [2]. They seldom credit professional treatment in mental health or criminal justice systems for their improvement. To the contrary, many contacts with jails, prisons, and hospitals are recalled unfavourably, consistent with systematic outcome studies that show negative (harmful) effects from certain kinds of treatment. For first offenders, for example, recidivism rates are lower with probation than with imprisonment followed by parole [4].

The situational effects are examples of what is called the effect of "powerful situations" in social psychology [41]. A powerful situation is defined as a situation that alters behaviour in ways that cannot be explained by an individual's personality outside of that situation [75].

The Stanford Prison Experiment is one of a series of experiments in social psychology that have demonstrated the power of social context to transform human behaviour [41,75]. In this experiment, the basement of the psychology building at Stanford University was converted into a simulated prison to study the effect of institutional settings on those who pass through them, including prisoners and their guards. The participants were evaluated in advance to assure that they were psychologically healthy, but their behaviour during the experiment was shocking. Some randomly assigned mock prisoners suffered severely and begged to be released early, whereas others adapted by becoming blindly obedient to the unjust authority of the guards. "Despite the fact that guards and prisoners were essentially free to engage in any form of interaction...the characteristic nature of their encounters tended to be negative, hostile, affrontive and dehumanizing" [68]. Verbal interactions were pervaded by threats, insults, and dehumanizing references that were most commonly directed by guards against prisoners. Prisoners expressed more negative affect than did guards, failed to support one another, and expressed intentions to harm others. Guards more often gave commands and engaged in confrontive or aggressive acts toward prisoners. Several mock guards devised sadistic ways to harass and degrade the prisoners and the others did not try to protect the prisoners from the inappropriate harassment. Most of the worst prisoner treatment came on the night shifts and other occasions when the guards thought they could avoid surveillance and interference of the research team. The planned two-week experiment had to be aborted after only six days because the experience dramatically and painfully transformed most of the participants in ways the experimenters had not anticipated or prepared for. The experimenters themselves felt that their goals and values were being corrupted in ways they had not anticipated. The emotional states and self-concepts of the participants were dramatically changed in ways that could not be predicted by standardized personality tests measured before the experiment or afterwards. "The negative, antisocial reactions observed were not the product of an environment created by combining a collection of deviant personalities, but rather the result of an intrinsically pathological situation which could distort and rechannel the behavior of essentially normal individuals. The abnormality here resided in the psychological nature of the situation and not in those who passed through it" [68].

The Therapeutic Alliance

The psychology of prison settings is the antithesis of the common factors observed in an effective therapeutic alliance. Systematic empirical studies of outcome have failed to demonstrate advantages of different psychotherapy techniques and suggest that treatment outcome is predicted best by the particular relationship formed between the patient and the therapist [76]. Ordinary human relationships can have therapeutic value, but the value depends on particular qualities of the bi-directional human relationship. The common factors that have been most thoroughly documented as beneficial are respect or positive regard (DHR = 4.2), nonpossessive warmth (DHR = 4.3), accurate empathy (DHR = 4.7), and congruence or genuineness (DHR = 5.3) [77]. The first three of these involve relationships in the emotional plane: respect (DHR = 4.2), non-possessive warmth (DHR = 4.3), and accurate empathy (DHR = 4.7), which occur in more elevated relationships of most therapists and some patients with ASPD, as described in the prior section. The effect size of treatment outcome studies indicates that relationships based on strict discipline and power have small positive effects, whereas those based on respect, warmth, and empathy have medium positive effects, as described in next section. Clarkson has also described higher level therapeutic relationships that are transpersonal (i.e. in the second-stage of awareness) or spiritual (i.e. in the third-stage of awareness) [76]. Such higher-level relationships have not been thoroughly studied but may be more likely to facilitate a radical transformation of personality [10].

SYSTEMATIC STUDIES OF TREATMENT OUTCOME

Since at least the 19th century, there have been recurrent cycles of conservative attitudes toward ASPD alternating with liberal attitudes, neither based on sound empirical evidence. The conservative attitude is punitive, emphasizing harsh punishment with long fixed sentences and frequent use of execution, supposedly justified for the security of the general public and possibly deterrence of criminal activity. However, meta-analysis of the effect of increasing the severity and consistency of punitive sanctions show no benefit from more severe community-based sanctions (e.g. longer probation periods) and an increase in criminal recidivism following longer imprisonments [7,78]. In contrast, the liberal attitude is rehabilitative, emphasizing psychosocial treatment, education, skills training, and supportive services, as was advocated in the 60s and early 70s in the United States.

However, even in the fourth (1964) edition of *The Mask of Sanity*, Cleckley noted that "There is, of course, no evidence to demonstrate or to indicate that psychiatry has yet found a therapy that cures or profoundly changes the psychopath." Likewise, Lee Robins found no evidence that any psychiatric treatment had helped to improve the outcome of patients with ASPD in her 30-year follow-up [2]. In 1974 Robert Martinson reviewed treatment programs in correctional settings and concluded that "nothing works", although a more deliberate consideration of available data soon contradicted his earlier impression [4,79]. Martinson's review came at a time of rising crime, growing public fear, and political pressure for more tough-minded approaches, and helped to facilitate the collapse of the liberal rehabilitative ideal in the late 1970s [9,41,80]. "Nothing works" became the conventional wisdom, even though logically the inadequacy of controlled research studies of the treatment of ASPD justified only a conclusion of "not proven" for any psychosocial treatment. The absence of proof is not proof of the absence of a treatment effect; more research was needed using well-defined treatment procedures, randomized assignment of cases, and control groups to evaluate treatments for ASPD before any confident statements could be made about the effectiveness of available treatments, as was acknowledged later by Martinson and others [5,6,81].

Conventional narrative reviews of research on the efficacy of psychological treatments are often unable to reach firm conclusions about the overall effectiveness of treatments, because of variability in the design and outcome of different trials, as shown by divergent results in studies of the treatment of ASPD. Fortunately, meta-analyses have now been carried out to evaluate the effectiveness of treatments to reduce criminal recidivism and other psychosocial aspects of ASPD. These meta-analytic studies had the advantages over earlier narrative reviews that they combine data in a systematic manner from all known treatment studies that included both cases and controls. The effect size of treatments were examined by computing Cohen's d, which is the difference in the means of the treatment and control groups on a specific outcome variable in standard deviation (SD) units. Incidence of crime following treatment is the usual variable for which much data is available and will be used here except when stated otherwise. When pre-treatment and post-treatment functions are compared, an effect size of +1.0 on an outcome criterion indicates that a patient scoring at the mean of the group at admission would be expected to advance 1 SD following treatment, which is an improvement from the 50th percentile to the 84th percentile when the outcome variable is normally distributed. According to traditional terminology, an effect size of 0.2 is weak or small, 0.5 is moderate or medium, and 0.8 or more is strong or large. For example, coronary bypass surgery has a strong effect on relief of angina ($d = 0.80$) but a weak effect on reduction in mortality ($d = 0.15$) [82]. In psychiatry, the use of neuroleptic drugs for reducing agitation in dementia has a moderate effect ($d = 0.37$) whereas use of electroconvulsive therapy for acute relief of major depression has a strong effect ($d = 0.80$). The use of stimulants for behavioural and social outcomes in attention deficit/hyperactivity disorder has moderate to strong effects ($d = 0.47$ to 0.96). Lipsey and Wilson assessed the general efficacy of psychological, educational, and behavioural treatments of a wide range of psychosocial problems in 156 meta-analytic studies in which there were both cases and controls, eliminating studies that exaggerated effect sizes by excluding unpublished studies. These meta-analyses represented approximately 940 individual treatment effectiveness studies and more than one million individual subjects. The grand mean treatment effect was 0.47 standard deviations, or a success rate 62% in treated cases versus a success rate of 38% in controls. 83% of the mean effects sizes were 0.20 or greater, which is a difference of about 10 percentage points between treatment and control success rates (55% versus 45%). An effect size of 0.20 standard deviations also is the mean difference between comparison of treatment to no treatment rather than placebo treatment; that is, 0.20 is approximately the average effect of the psychosocial support derived from placebo treatments for a wide range of problems [82]. In addition, volunteering and persisting in a treatment study is associated with a moderate effect size (about 0.5) when volunteers are compared to those who refuse or drop out of treatment [6].

Meta-analyses of criminal recidivism show that currently available treatments have a positive but weak effect overall and that the best correctional treatments have moderate positive effects in both adolescents and adults [6]. In 443 studies of offenders between 12 and 21 years of age, the mean effect size was $d = 0.17$, with a range from 0.13 to 0.52 [8]. According to Lipsey's meta-analysis, more specific and structured treatments (e.g. skills training) and multimodal treatments were more effective than less structured and less specific treatments (e.g. counselling). Treatment effectiveness was positively related to risk (i.e. individuals at greater risk of recidivism benefited from more intensive intervention), to delivery in the community rather than in institutional settings, and to higher levels of involvement by therapists. In other words, the best outcomes for young offenders observed by Lipsey were obtained in community settings in which there were frequent contacts over a long period of treatment. Such intensive community treatments had moderate effect sizes of 0.4 to 0.5 standard deviations, reducing criminal recidivism by 20% to 40%. Negative effect sizes were obtained for treatment interventions in about one third of studies, confirming that some psychosocial treatments can harm young offenders, and need to be regularly monitored.

Another meta-analytic study included 23 comparisons of adult offenders in addition to 131 comparisons of juvenile offenders [7]. Andrews found a definite but small overall effect of treatment ($d = 0.20$) with no difference in the effectiveness of programs run for adult versus juvenile offenders. The overall estimate of a weak overall effect ($d = 0.21$) is confirmed in another meta-analysis of recidivism in the treatment of adult offenders in Germany [83]. Andrews specified the characteristics of effective correctional service according to three principles, and showed that such appropriate correctional service yielded moderate positive effects, cutting recidivism by more than 50% [7]. The three principles of effective correctional service suggested by Andrews and associates were related to risk of recidivism prior to treatment, targeting criminogenic needs and attitudes, and responsivity. First, only individuals at high risk for criminal recidivism should receive intensive service and low-risk cases should receive minimal intervention. Second, treatment to reduce criminal recidivism must target changeable factors associated with criminal conduct, such as antisocial attitudes, peer associations, chemical dependencies, identification with antisocial models, social skills, and skills in impulse control and mental self-government. Third, social learning is most effective when therapists are "firm but fair" while modelling and rewarding anti-criminal attitudes, feelings, and actions in a structured program. Only a small proportion of highly verbal, self-reflective offenders, who were unlikely to have ASPD, were considered appropriate for non-behavioural, non-directive, emotionally evocative, and unstructured cognitive treatments, such as psychodynamic therapy or therapeutic communities. When programmes followed these principles, treatment effects were larger than otherwise, cutting recidivism moderately [7,8].

Eleven well-controlled trials in adult offenders showed moderate beneficial effects in reducing recidivism in these meta-analyses [7,8], and additional randomized controlled trials have been carried out for ASPD complicated by substance dependence [84–86]. Some of the positive programs relied primarily on cognitive therapy [87,88]. For example, in one Canadian study, adult probationers were randomly assigned to probation officers for individual counselling that focused on modelling problem-solving and anti-criminal attitudes [87]. The counsellors were blindly rated on measures of empathy and socialization, and counselling sessions were recorded, so that researchers could count anti-criminal statements by the officers and the number of times counsellors rewarded anti-criminal statements and disapproved pro-criminal statements by the probationers. Officers high in socialization emitted more of the desirable behaviours. Probationers assigned to officers high in both empathy and socialization had lower recidivism rates during the programme.

Similarly, in another study with positive results from cognitive therapy, probationers were provided social skills training, problem solving, values education, assertion training, negotiation skills training, and social perspective taking by specially trained probation officers [88]. The 80-hour program was taught to small groups of probationers, with random assignment to cognitive training and those assigned to cognitive training, had lower recidivism during the training. However, recidivism after these cognitive treatment programmes was not evaluated, so it is unknown whether the cognitive treatments had a lasting effect on the subjects. Furthermore, criminal recidivism indicates failure of treatment, but its absence does not imply that there has been positive character development. When personality has been directly measured, reductions in criminal activity have been associated with improvements in character, including reductions in psychopathic deviance on the Minnesota Multiphasic Personality Inventory (MMPI), improvements in attitudes toward self and others, and in value orientations. It is important to recognize that such positive character development occurs in community settings and low-security institutions, but not in maximum-security institutions [4].

Other programmes for adult offenders have relied on employment and intensive supportive therapy to reduce criminality and improve socialization. For example, intensive supervision of non-violent offenders in New Jersey was shown to reduce recidivism moderately compared to matched control offenders [89]. The treatment programme required employment, random drug tests, and frequent community contacts with the supervising officer. Treated cases were provided community sponsors who provided help, guidance, anti-criminal modelling and other specialized counselling when needed. The intensely supervised cases had less recidivism, and the programme cost substantially less than the usual programme. Similar results have been obtained in several other studies of intensive supervision, including work showing improvements in aggression, manipulativeness, optimism, and human relations [4].

Multimodal psychiatric treatments have also shown positive outcomes, with results varying from weak to moderate depending on the level of the therapeutic alliances. For example, an intensive long-term milieu therapy programme for adult offenders reduced recidivism slightly more than no treatment [90]. The components of treatment included supportive counselling, individual and group psychotherapy, pharmacological treatments, academic and vocational education, work assignments, and recreation. The programme also involved a graded system of privilege levels, which provided a skillful and fair application of sanction. However, the quality of the therapeutic alliances between therapists and patients and other possible moderators of efficacy were not evaluated. Treatment costs may be large for multimodal therapy programs, so it is important to understand the variables that moderate the effectiveness of treatment in order to evaluate cost-benefit ratios.

A more informative series of randomized controlled trials have been conducted within a well-designed and closely monitored multimodal substance abuse rehabilitation program [84–86]. The studies by Woody and his associates were the first randomized controlled trials of the treatment of ASPD using standard diagnostic criteria and employing psychotherapy that is both manual guided and tape recorded [86]. One hundred and ten nonpsychotic men between 18 and 55 years of age with opiate dependence were randomly assigned to receive paraprofessional drug counselling alone or counselling plus professional psychotherapy. Patients who received supportive-expressive psychotherapy or cognitive-behavioural psychotherapy did better than those who received drug counselling only, and there were no differences in the effectiveness of the two psychotherapy methods. Those who received psychotherapy were subdivided to evaluate the impact of a diagnosis of ASPD on treatment outcome. The sample consisted of 50 men with ASPD, including 30 who were randomly assigned to psychotherapy, compared to 60 other opiate dependent patients, including 32 who were randomly assigned to psychotherapy. Outcome was evaluated using several measures including the Addiction Severity Index (ASI) at the start of treatment and at one-month and seven-month evaluation points. The ASI is an interview that assesses problem severity in several areas of function that are commonly impaired in drug-dependent patients: medical, employment/support, drug abuse, legal, familial/social, and psychological. Independent interviewers who were not aware of the patient's group assignment were used to assess outcome. Patients with ASPD did less well than those without ASPD unless they also had a diagnosis of major depression. The effect sizes of patient improvement on outcome criteria at the seventh month follow-up are summarized in Table 2.10. The global improvement in problem severity was positive for all groups receiving psychotherapy, but drug dependent patients with ASPD and no depression had only small benefits ($d = 0.18$), mostly for reduction in substance abuse. Psychiatric problems actually increased in patients with ASPD without depression, particularly in those who did not form a positive alliance with their therapist ($d = -0.23$). The magnitude of the positive and negative effects of psychotherapy in ASPD is comparable to the overall effects of treatment observed in meta-analyses of adult offenders. However, if patients with ASPD also had a diagnosis of depression, they were better able to form a therapeutic alliance with the psychotherapists and had moderate benefits comparable to patients without ASPD ($d = 0.50$) [86]. Subsequent research showed that the ability to form a trusted helping alliance with the therapist predicted moderate benefits [84]. Treatment outcome in 31 patients with ASPD was correlated more than 0.6 ($p < 0.001$) with both therapist's and patient's assessments of their helping alliance [84]. In addition, the characteristics of patients and counsellors interact, as in any human relationship, so the characteristics of counsellors contribute to outcome as much as the characteristics of the patients [85,91]. There was variability in outcome within the caseloads of the same counsellors, so it is the unique quality of each alliance that determines its effects on treatment outcome. Psychosocial relationships have non-linear dynamics that are not fully determined by past history [10].

Another method of treatment with independent replication of reduced recidivism in a long-term follow-up after treatment has discontinued is transcendental meditation (TM). In a study of ninety prisoners in a maximum security prison who were taught TM, those practising TM for

TABLE 2.10   Effect size (Cohen's d, in standard deviation units) measures of patient improvement on selected outcome criteria (adapted from Woody $et\ al.$ [86])

Outcome variable	ASP+O $(n = 13)$	ASP+O+D $(n = 17)$	O+D $(n = 16)$	O only $(n = 16)$
Medical problems	−0.33	−0.02	0.08	−0.42
Employment problems	0.61	0.91	1.05	1.02
Drug abuse	0.28	0.64	0.64	0.12
Legal problems	0.50	0.97	0.24	0.75
Psychiatric problems	−0.23	0.47	0.58	0.65
Global problem severity (mean effect sizes)	0.18	0.50	0.53	0.40

ASP, antisocial personality disorder; O, opiate dependence; D, depression.

one year had greater improvement in self-awareness and had 30% reduction in criminal recidivism compared to controls in a 3-year follow up [92]. An independent study replicated the reduced recidivism in prisoners practising TM compared with others in a six-year follow-up. Such moderate beneficial effects may be explained at least in part by the volunteer status of those choosing to practise TM.

Pharmacological treatments of ASPD and components of ASPD, such as impulsivity and aggression, have been reviewed in detail elsewhere [5,32,93]. Controlled randomized trials of dopaminergic stimulants to treat ASPD in adults with a childhood history of attention deficit/hyperactivity disorder produced substantial improvements in target symptoms of impulsivity, inattention, hyperactivity, and irritability. About 60% of such patients receiving stimulant medication showed moderate to marked improvement compared with 10% of those receiving placebo [94]. However, the potential for stimulant abuse limits the use of the intervention, and the non-euphoriant stimulant pemoline is no longer approved for use in these patients, despite early favourable results, because of toxicity. A double-blind, placebo-controlled trial of the effect of lithium on aggressive behaviour in men aged 16 to 24 years found moderate reduction in aggressive behaviour, defined as angry threats and actual physical assaults, during the 3 months that lithium was administered in a medium security prison, which has been confirmed in similar studies in children and adults [93,95]. However, compliance with lithium and other mood stabilizers after release from custody is poor in individuals with ASPD, so the intervention is ineffective in the long term. Typical and atypical antipsychotics have been reported to tranquillize the patients and to facilitate compliance with authority [32,93]. Such pharmacological treatment for specifically targeted symptoms can be an important component of the multimodal clinical management of ASPD. However, pharmacological treatment is only one component of a multimodal treatment program designed to facilitate character development [5,32,94,96].

The limited change in personality that results from conventional psychosocial and pharmacological treatments, even when they are intensive, multimodal, and well-matched to the individual needs of the person, underscores the central facts about treatment outcome studies of ASPD. A therapeutic alliance at first-stage (egocentric "adult") or second-stage (allocentric "parent") levels of relatedness in an appropriate treatment program for ASPD still has only moderate benefits (Cohen's d about 0.50), as is true for psychological treatments generally. Many patients with ASPD have a history of abuse and neglect since childhood, and have little trust and hope in mental health professionals. Establishing such confidence takes time and will almost always be tested in ways that can be disturbing and time-consuming for any therapist. Consultation with others may be needed to deal with the strong emotions and counter-transference issues that are often elicited by patients with severe personality disorders [32]. Nevertheless, therapeutic nihilism or blaming of the patient are not justified, because positive and clinically useful results can be obtained even with difficult patients, especially if the psychiatrist is realistically impartial, calm, patiently hopeful and ready to facilitate the small steps involved in the complex process of establishing trust, hope, and self-awareness.

Even when patients are unmotivated to form a trusting therapeutic alliance, a "firm but fair" program structure and behavioural controls combined with a hopeful, kind, and patient attitude with respect for everyone's potential for change has a small benefit (d about 0.2 in SD units), and can be satisfying to both patients and therapists. Sturup, in the Herstedvester Institute for Psychopaths in Denmark, provided treatment for convicted criminals with ASPD [97]. Subjects were placed in a highly structured institutional work program. They were encouraged to express their feelings about their work situation and were closely supervised to detect the emergence of problems. These problems were constructively and reasonably discussed with the patients, so that they could learn to face and understand their problems in the "here and now", thereby providing an opportunity to establish a helping alliance that was directed to something of immediate interest to them. Similarly, when crises arise in individuals with ASPD in the general community, there are often opportunities to engage in constructive work that is of interest to the patient, such as job placement, remedial education, and psychotherapy. Such crisis interventions have produced moderate benefits in randomized controlled trials that are sustained in longitudinal follow-ups for over fifteen years after treatment [8,98].

RADICAL TRANSFORMATION OF ASPD BY COHERENCE THERAPY

What is most needed now in the treatment of ASPD and other personality disorders is a clinical description of how to facilitate radical transformations that improve character. Radical transformations refer to changes in character that are large and stable, indicating a fundamental change in self-understanding, goals, and values. Elsewhere I have described what I suggest are the key elements of treatment that are needed to produce large and sustained character developments in general [10]. Here I will briefly point out promising treatment approaches that merit systematic clinical trials based on my own positive clinical experience and the information previously described.

The narcissism, distrust, aloofness, aggressiveness, and unreliability of patients with ASPD can make the establishment of a trusted helping alliance difficult. Nevertheless, crises and problems do occur for which they have a genuine motivation to obtain help, and they do usually have maximum levels of thought and relationships that are amenable to psychotherapy. Hence the therapist must be patient and ready to provide appropriate service and to thereby establish the beginnings of a working relationship with trust, hope, and compassion. Change in personality is stepwise, and the steps are small and influenced in a non-linear manner by the working alliance and its context. In addition to the principles of effective treatment already described, some additional mental exercises can be helpful in enhancing therapy so that the effect sizes are large rather than small to medium.

First, individuals with ASPD have very shallow thinking, which has been variously described as deficits in superego functions or low levels of the five aspects of self-transcendence shown in Table 2.3. In my experience these deficiencies in self-transcendence can be improved by a simple exercise to awaken their physical and intuitive senses that I call the "Union in Nature" meditation. This is a stepwise awakening of the senses of touch, taste, smell, hearing, and vision. The physical and intuitive senses of people are often partially asleep (i.e. outside of self-aware consciousness) when they are in distress and conflict, which is frequent in individuals with ASPD. For example, individual differences in the sexual aspect of self-transcendence (measured as the tendency toward repression rather than sensory responsivity) are expected to influence sensitivity to touch sensation, as indicated in Table 2.3. In fact, repressive personality style was correlated moderately with the length of sensory stimulation to elicit awareness of touch sensations [99]. In other words, less transcendent individuals take longer to become aware of sensory stimulation. Individuals high in the sexual aspect of self-transcendence recognize the beauty and meaning in sensory experiences intuitively, whereas those who are low in this function are alexithymic. Scores on the Toronto Alexithymia Scale (TAS) were moderately correlated with low scores on all three TCI character scales and the strongest correlation was between the scores on the TCI self-transcendence subscale for sensibility with the TAS subscale for externally oriented thinking ($r = -0.4$, $p < 0.0001$) in a sample of 644 individuals from the general population [10]. These relationships are clinically relevant to people with ASPD, who often have alexithymia and comorbid somatoform disorders.

The Union in Nature exercise is described in depth elsewhere [10]. It takes about a half hour and is enjoyable. It appeals to nearly everyone, including sensation-seeking narcissists who want to be keenly aware of their environment. It should be begun early in therapy, perhaps while working on relapse prevention after detoxification. This meditation is simple to explain and do, but can have profound effects even at an early point in therapy when insight-oriented discussion and reflection are ineffective or even counter-productive.

At this early point it may be useful to combine the regular practice of Union in Nature with the experience of elevated artistic creations. As an example in music, the works of composers like Bach, Mozart, and Schubert often elevate mood, attention, and integrated thinking, regardless of debates about the explanatory mechanisms underlying these effects [100–105]. Benefits can also be obtained from other kinds of artistic creation and from the inspiring writings of highly coherent philosophers listed and described elsewhere [10].

An important clinical caveat should be mentioned about experiencing elevated artistic creations. When people who have been highly repressed (i.e. are poor in listening to their psyche) begin meditation and experiencing elevated creations, they may experience anxiety and other resurgent emotions, as described by the writer Stendhal while viewing inspiring art in Florence. Consequently, patients should be advised simply to interrupt the exercise temporarily if they become disturbed. They should be reassured that their experience is a part of the process of increasing self-awareness. They can be taught simple relaxation exercises, as described next. They can learn to titrate their own reawakening by combining relaxation with meditation. Learning to remain calm and to focus on trying to understand what is happening is an important step in the development of greater self-aware consciousness.

Another specific exercise can be introduced to help the patient to be calm and let go of their struggles with other people or themselves. This exercise is called the "Silence of the Mind" meditation and has three phases that correspond to the three stages of self-aware consciousness: getting calm and accepting, growing in awareness of your subconscious thoughts (i.e. mindfulness or meditation), and contemplation (i.e. listening to the psyche effortlessly). Initially only the first phase is taught as a relaxation technique to be used when someone feels angry, anxious, or has other negative feelings. The full sequence is described elsewhere [10]. The Silence of Mind meditation provides a non-demanding self-paced way by which a person can gradually grow in self-acceptance, self-awareness, and well-being.

Fourth, after patients have begun to be aware of their subconscious conflicts and have an interest in their origins and consequences, further work can be done in a therapeutic alliance to help them become more aware of the degree to which their behaviour is reactive to conditioning and hence not free, flexible, or voluntary. Initiative, self-efficacy, industriousness can be developed by individualized discussion of some of the powerful situations that trigger or maintain the patient's maladaptive behaviours. Simply being aware that such powerful situations exist and that they are not an essential part of one's own lifestyle is a major advance in self-understanding and often reduces the influence of external controls, thereby helping the person become more self-directed.

Fifth, it is important that the patient recognize that the therapist regards him with respect for his human dignity as a free agent in search of understanding. Everyone wants to understand the way to live that satisfies his basic needs for happiness, understanding, and love. Fundamental character change only develops through voluntary self-directed choices in search of a way of living that is satisfying and not self-defeating. Even when dealing with crises, it is useful for the therapist to help the patient recognize general principles of coherent living that recur in many specific guises [10]. Ultimately psychotherapy is a way to well-being, not just a technique for treating disease. A focus on disease or problems obscures the way to radical transformation of character deficits. If you don't want to hit an obstacle on your path, you cannot succeed if you remain preoccupied with not hitting the obstacle. On the other hand, you cannot fail if you focus on where you want to go and what you can do to get there.

SUMMARY

Consistent Evidence

- ASPD is characterized in behavioural terms by childhood or adolescent onset of recurrent antisocial behaviour affecting school, work, family and social life.
- ASPD is also characterized by temperament traits of high novelty seeking (impulsivity), low harm avoidance (risk-taking), low reward dependence (aloofness), low self-directedness, low cooperativeness, and low self-transcendence.

- ASPD occurs in men about four times more often than women, and women with the disorder have a stronger familial loading of ASPD and somatization disorder.
- The risk of ASPD is moderately influenced by genetic factors, weakly by the post-natal rearing environment, and moderately by factors unique to the individual according to twin and adoption studies.
- More than one-third of individuals with ASPD remit or burn-out in adulthood, usually between 30 and 40 years of age.
- Structured behavioural treatments of ASPD in which there is no cooperative therapeutic alliance have a small but positive effect size according to multiple randomized controlled trials (Cohen's d about 0.2).
- Psychotherapy of ASPD in which there is a positive therapeutic alliance has a moderate effect size according to multiple randomized controlled trials (Cohen's d about 0.5).
- Pharmacological treatments of ASPD (lithium for aggressiveness, stimulants for residual ADHD) have a moderate effect size for specific target symptoms but not for character development.
- Therapeutic nihilism about the treatment of ASPD is an invalid but self-fulfilling prophecy that creates a powerful counter-therapeutic situation.

Incomplete Evidence

- ASPD is characterized in psychobiological terms on average by low levels of free will (inflexible, uncooperative), low following of the path of the psyche (maladaptive, unwise), low listening to the psyche (lacking in remorse, empathy, conscience), immaturity of thought and human relationships, inflation of ego (narcissistic), and low serenity (inappropriate arousal). These are expressed mentally as low character development, leading to inflexible maladaptive behaviour with infrequent self-awareness, infrequent self-aware emotions, poor impulse control, inappropriate arousal, and pathological narcissism.
- The maximum levels of thought and human relationships in ASPD are usually in the emotional plane, which is adequate for psychotherapy and the development of a healthy therapeutic alliance.
- Specific mental exercises leading to increased levels of self-aware consciousness activate specific brain networks that are strongly correlated with specific character dimensions and psychobiological functions.

Areas Still Open to Research

- Radical transformation of ASPD and other mental disorders can be facilitated by specific meditative and contemplative exercises designed to increase free will, awaken intuitive senses for listening to the psyche, and reduce pathological narcissism.

• Brain imaging and molecular genetic analyses can provide better characterization of the neurobiological systems involved in regulating human thought, emotion, and behaviour, including ASPD and other mental disorders.

REFERENCES

1. Goodwin D.W., Guze S.B. (1996) *Psychiatric Diagnosis*. Oxford University Press, New York.
2. Robins L.N. (1966) *Deviant Children Grown Up: A Sociological and Psychiatric Study of Sociopathic Personality*. Williams and Wilkins, Baltimore.
3. Robins L.N., Price R.K. (1991) Adult disorders predicted by childhood conduct problems: results from the NIMH Epidemiological Catchment Area Project. *Psychiatry*, **54**: 116–132.
4. Lipton D., Martinson R., Wilks J. (1975) *The Effectiveness of Correctional Treatment: A Survey of Treatment Evaluation Studies*. Praeger, New York.
5. Dolan B., Coid J. (1993) *Psychopathic and Antisocial Personality Disorders: Treatment and Research Issues*. Gaskell, London.
6. Rice M.E., Harris G. (1997) The treatment of adult offenders. In *Handbook of Antisocial Behavior* (Eds D.M. Stoff, J. Breiling, J.D. Maser), pp. 425–435. John Wiley & Sons, New York.
7. Andrews D.A., Zinger I., Hoge R.D., Bontga J., Gendreau P., Cullen F.T. (1990) Does correctional treatment work? A clinically relevant and psychologically informed meta-analysis. *Criminology*, **28**: 369–404.
8. Lipsey M.W. (1992) Juvenile delinquency treatment: a meta-analytic inquiry into the variability of effects. In *Meta-analysis for Explanation* (Eds R.S. Cook, H. Cooper, D.S. Cordray, H. Hartmann, L.V. Hedges, R.J. Light, T.A. Louis, F. Mosteller), pp. 83–125. Russell Sage, New York.
9. Andrews D.A., Bonta J. (1994) *The Psychology of Criminal Conduct*. Anderson, Cincinnati.
10. Cloninger C.R. (2004) *Feeling Good: The Science of Well Being*. Oxford University Press, New York.
11. Pritchard J.C. (1835) *A Treatise on Insanity and Other Disorders Affecting the Mind*. Sherwood, Gilbert, and Piper, London.
12. Rush B. (1962) *Medical Inquiries and Observations upon the Diseases of the Mind*. Hafner, New York.
13. Koch J.L.A. (1889) *Leitfaden der Psychiatrie*, 2nd edn. Dorn, Ravensburg.
14. Kraepelin E. (1909) *Psychiatrie*. Barth, Leipzig.
15. Kahn E. (1931) *Psychopathic Personalities*. Yale University Press, New Haven.
16. Schneider K. (1958) *Psychopathic Personalities*. Cassell, London.
17. Maughs S.B. (1972) Criminal psychopathology. *Progress in Neurology and Psychiatry*, **27**: 275–278.
18. Cleckley H. (1964) *The Mask of Sanity*, 4th edn. Mosby, St. Louis.
19. Hare R.D. (1991) *The Hare Psychopathy Checklist—Revised*. Multi-Health Systems, Toronto.

20. Hart S.D., Hare R.D. (1997) Psychopathy: assessment and association with criminal conduct. In *Handbook of Antisocial Behavior* (Eds D.M. Stoff, J. Breiling, J.D. Maser), pp. 22–35. John Wiley & Sons, New York.

21. Svrakic D.M. (1990) The functional dynamics of the narcissistic personality. *Am. J. Psychother.*, **44**: 189–203.

22. Hart S.D., Hare R.D. (1989) Discriminant validity of the Psychopathy Checklist in a forensic psychiatric population. *Psychol. Assess.*, 211–218.

23. Cloninger C.R., Bayon C., Przybeck T.R. (1997) Epidemiology and Axis I comorbidity of antisocial personality disorder. In *Handbook of Antisocial Behavior* (Eds D.M. Stoff, J. Breiling, J.D. Maser), pp. 12–21. John Wiley & Sons, New York.

24. Zuckerman M., Cloninger C.R. (1996) Relationships between Cloninger's, Zuckerman's, and Eysenck's dimensions of personality. *Person. Indiv. Diff.*, **21**: 283–285.

25. Cloninger C.R., Reich T., Guze S.B. (1975) The multifactorial model of disease transmission: II. Sex differences in the familial transmission of sociopathy (Antisocial Personality). *Br. J. Psychiatry*, **127**: 11–22.

26. Cloninger C.R., Gottesman I.I. (1987) Genetic and environmental factors in antisocial behavior disorders. In *Causes of Crime: New Biological Approaches* (Eds S.A. Mednick, T.E. Moffitt, S.A. Stack), pp. 92–109. Cambridge University Press, Cambridge.

27. Cloninger C.R., Reich T., Guze S.B. (1975) The multifactorial model of disease transmission: III. Familial relationship between sociopathy and hysteria (Briquet's syndrome). *Br. J. Psychiatry*, **127**: 23–32.

28. Robins L.N., Regier D.A. (Eds) (1991) *Psychiatric Disorders in America*. Free Press, New York.

29. Martin R.L., Cloninger C.R., Guze S.B., Clayton P.J. (1985) Mortality in a follow-up of 500 psychiatric out-patients. II. Cause-specific mortality. *Arch. Gen. Psychiatry*, **42**: 58–66.

30. Kessler R.C., McGonagle K.A., Zhao S., Nelson C.B., Hughes M., Eshelman S., Wittchen H.U., Kendler K.S. (1994) Lifetime and 12-month prevalence of DSM-III-R psychiatric disorders in the United States. *Arch. Gen. Psychiatry*, **51**: 8–19.

31. Svrakic D.M., Whitehead C., Przybeck T.R., Cloninger C.R. (1993) Differential diagnosis of personality disorders by the seven factor model of temperament and character. *Arch. Gen. Psychiatry*, **50**: 991–999.

32. Cloninger C.R., Svrakic, D.M. (2000) Personality disorders. In *Comprehensive Textbook of Psychiatry* (Eds B.J. Sadock, V.A. Sadock), pp. 1723–1764. Lippincott Williams & Wilkins, New York.

33. Cloninger C.R., Sigvardsson S., Bohman M. (1988) Childhood personality predicts alcohol abuse in young adults. *Alcoholism: Clinical and Experimental Research*, **12**: 494–505.

34. Cloninger C.R. (1999) Genetics of substance abuse. In *Textbook of Substance Abuse Treatment* (Eds M. Galanter, H.D. Kleber), pp. 59–67. American Psychiatric Press, Washington.

35. Cloninger C.R., Sigvardsson S., Bohman M., von Knorring A.L. (1975) Predisposition to petty criminality in Swedish adoptees. II. Cross-fostering analysis of gene-environment interaction. *Arch. Gen. Psychiatry*, **39**: 1242–1247.

36. Cloninger C.R., Sigvardsson S., von Knorring A.L., Bohman M. (1984) An adoption study of somatoform disorders: II. Identification of two discrete somatoform disorders. *Arch. Gen. Psychiatry*, **41**: 863–871.

37. Cloninger C.R., von Knorring A.L., Sigvardsson S., Bohman M. (1986) Symptom patterns and causes of somatization in men. II. Genetic and environmental independence from somatization in women. *Genet. Epidemiol.*, 3: 171–185.

38. Cloninger C.R., Svrakic D.M., Przybeck T.R. (1993) A psychobiological model of temperament and character. *Arch. Gen. Psychiatry*, 50: 975–990.

39. Gillespie N.A., Cloninger C.R., Heath A.C., Martin N.G. (2003) The genetic and environmental relationship between Cloninger's dimensions of temperament and character. *Person. Indiv. Diff.*, 35: 1931–1946.

40. Cloninger C.R. (2002) Implications of comorbidity for the classification of mental disorders: the need for a psychobiology of coherence. In *Psychiatric Diagnosis and Classification* (Eds M. Maj, W. Gaebel, J.J. Lopez-Ibor, N. Sartorius), pp. 79–106. John Wiley & Sons, Chichester.

41. Haney C., Zimbardo P. (1998) The past and future of U.S. prison policy: twenty-five years after the Stanford Prison experiment. *Am. Psychol.*, 53: 709–727.

42. Svrakic D.M., McCallum K. (1991) Treatment of personality disorders. In *As Varias Faces da Personalidade* (Ed. A. Neto), pp. 369–422. Libru, Belo Horizonte.

43. Crowe R.R. (1974) An adoption study of antisocial personality. *Arch. Gen. Psychiatry*, 31: 785–791.

44. Crowe R.R. (1972) The adopted offspring of women criminal offenders—A study of their arrest records. *Arch. Gen. Psychiatry*, 27: 600–603.

45. Cadoret R.J., O'Gorman T.W., Troughton E., Heywood E. (1985) Alcoholism and antisocial personality—interrelationships, genetics and environmental factors. *Arch. Gen. Psychiatry*, 42: 162–167.

46. Schulsinger F. (1972) Psychopathy, heredity and environment. *Int. J. Ment. Health*, 1: 190–206.

47. Mednick S.A., Gabrielli W.F.J., Hutchings B. (1984) Genetic influences in criminal convictions. Evidence from an adoption cohort. *Science*, 22: 891–894.

48. Sabol S.Z., Nelson M.L., Fisher C., Gunzerath L., Brody C.L., Hu S., Sirota L.A., Marcus S.E., Greenberg B.D., Lucas F.R.T. *et al.* (1999) A genetic association for cigarette smoking behavior. *Health Psychol.*, 18: 7–13.

49. Kotler M., Cohen H., Segman R. (1997) Excess dopamine D4 receptor (D4DR) exon III seven repeat allele in opioid-dependent subjects. *Mol. Psychiatry*, 2: 251–254.

50. Van Gestel S., Forsgren T., Claes S., Del-Favero J., Van Duijn C.M., Sluijs S., Nilsson L.G., Adolfsson R., Van Broeckhoven C. (2002) Epistatic effects of genes from the dopamine and serotonin systems on the temperament traits of novelty seeking and harm avoidance. *Mol. Psychiatry*, 7: 448–450.

51. Benjamin J., Osher Y., Kotler M., Gritsenko I., Nemanov L., Belmaker R.H., Ebstein R.P. (2000) Association of tridimensional personality questionnaire (TPQ) traits and three functional polymorphisms: dopamine receptor D4 (DRD4), serotonin transporter promoter region (5-HTTLPR) and catechol O-methyltransferase (COMT). *Mol. Psychiatry*, 5: 96–100.

52. Strobel A., Lesch K.P., Jatzke S., Paetzold F., Brocke B. (2003) Further evidence for a modulation of Novelty Seeking by DRD4 exon III, 5-HTTLPR, and COMT val/met variants. *Mol. Psychiatry*, 8: 371–372.

53. Ekelund J., Lichtermann D., Jaervelin M.-R., Peltonen L. (1999) Association between novelty seeking and the type 4 dopamine receptor gene in a large Finnish cohort sample. *Am. J. Psychiatry*, 156: 1453–1455.

54. Keltikangas-Jaervinen L., Elovainio M., Kivimaeki M., Lichtermann D., Ekelund J., Peltonen L. (2003) Association between the type 4 dopamine receptor gene polymorphism and Novelty Seeking. *Psychosom. Med.*, **65**: 471–476.

55. Keltikangas-Jaervinen L., Raeikkoenen K., Ekelund J., Peltonen L. (2003) Nature and nurture in novelty seeking. *Mol. Psychiatry*, **8**: 1–4.

56. Ding Y.C., Chi H.C., Grady D.L., Morishima A., Kidd J.R., Kidd K.K., Flodman P., Spence M.A., Schuck S., Swanson J.M. *et al.* (2002) Evidence for positive selection acting at the human dopamine receptor D4 gene locus. *Proc. Natl. Acad. Sci. USA*, **99**: 309–314.

57. Scarr S., McCartney K. (1983) How people make their own environments: a theory of genotype greater than environment effects. *Child Develop.*, **54**: 424–435.

58. Cloninger C.R. (1999) A new conceptual paradigm from genetics and psychobiology for the science of mental health. *Aust. N. Zeal. J. Psychiatry*, **33**: 174–186.

59. Cloninger C.R. (2000) Biology of personality dimensions. *Curr. Opin. Psychiatry*, **13**: 611–616.

60. Sigvardsson S., Bohman M., Cloninger C.R. (1987) Structure and stability of childhood personality: prediction of later social adjustment. *J. Child Psychol. Psychiatry*, **28**: 929–946.

61. Loeber R. (1982) The stability of antisocial and delinquent child behavior: a review. *Child Develop.*, **53**: 1431–1446.

62. Black C.W., Baumgard C.H., Bell S.E. (1995) A 16–45 year follow-up of 71 men with antisocial personality disorder. *Compr. Psychiatry*, **36**: 130–140.

63. Walters G.D. (1990) *The Criminal Lifestyle: Patterns of Serious Criminal Conduct.* Sage Publications, Newbury Park.

64. Cloninger C.R. (1987) A systematic method for clinical description and classification of personality variants: a proposal. *Arch. Gen. Psychiatry*, **44**: 573–587.

65. Cloninger C.R., Przybeck T.R., Svrakic D.M., Wetzel R.D. (1994) *The Temperament and Character Inventory: A Guide to its Development and Use.* Washington University Center for Psychobiology of Personality, St. Louis.

66. Cloninger C.R. (2000) A practical way to diagnose personality disorder: a proposal. *J. Person. Disord.*, **14**: 99–108.

67. Cloninger C.R., Svrakic N.M., Svrakic D.M. (1997) Role of personality self-organization in development of mental order and disorder. *Develop. Psychopathol.*, **9**: 881–906.

68. Haney C., Banks W., Zimbardo P. (1973) Interpersonal dynamics in a simulated prison. *Int. J. Criminol. Penol.*, **1**: 69–97.

69. Gusnard D.A., Ollinger J.M., Shulman, G.L., Cloninger C.R., Price J.L., Van Essen D.C., Raichle M.E. (2003) Persistence and brain circuitry. *Proc. Natl. Acad. Sci. USA*, **100**: 3479–3484.

70. Farrer C., Frith C.D. (2002) Experiencing oneself vs another person as being the cause of an action: the neural correlates of the experience of agency. *Neuroimage*, **15**: 596–603.

71. Burgess P.W., Veitch E., de Lacy Costello A., Shallice T. (2000) The cognitive and neuroanatomical correlates of multitasking. *Neuropsychologia*, **38**: 848–863.

72. Borg J., Andree B., Soderstrom H., Farde L. (2003) The serotonin system and spiritual experiences. *Am. J. Psychiatry*, **160**: 1965–1969.

73. DiClemente C.C., Prochasta J.O., Gibertini M. (1985) Self-efficacy and the stages of self-change of smoking. *Cogn. Ther. Res.*, **9**: 181–200.

74. Kavanagh D.J., Pierce J., Lo S.K., Shelley J. (1993) Self-efficacy and social support as predictors of smoking after a quit attempt. *Psychol. Health*, **8**: 231–242.

75. Ross L., Nisbett R. (1991) *The Person and the Situation: Perspectives of Social Psychology*. McGraw-Hill, New York.

76. Clarkson P., Pokorny M. (Eds) (1994) *The Handbook of Psychotherapy*. Routledge, London.

77. Lambert M.J. (1986) Implications of psychotherapy outcome research for eclectic psychotherapy. In *Handbook of Eclectic Psychotherapy* (Ed. J.C. Norcross), pp. 436–462. Brunner/Mazel, New York.

78. Petersilia J., Turner S., Peterson J. (1986) *Prison Versus Probation in California*. RAND, Santa Monica.

79. Martinson R. (1974) What works? Questions and answers about prison reform. *The Public Interest*, **35**: 22–54.

80. Palmer T. (1992) *The Reemergence of Correctional Intervention*. Sage, Newbury Park.

81. Martinson R. (1979) Symposium on Sentencing: Part II. *Hofstra Law Review*, **7**: 243–358.

82. Lipsey M.W., Wilson D.B. (1993) The efficacy of psychological, educational, and behavioral treatment: confirmation from meta-analysis. *Am. Psychol.*, **48**: 1181–1209.

83. Loesel F., Koferl P. (1989) Evaluation research on correctional treatment in West Germany: a meta-analysis. In *Criminal Behavior and the Justice System: Psychological Perspectives* (Eds H. Wegener, F. Loesel, J. Haisch), pp. 334–355. Springer, New York.

84. Gestley L., McLellan A.T., Alterman A.I., Woody G.E., Luborsky L., Prout M. (1989) Ability to form an alliance with the therapist: a possible marker of prognosis for patients with antisocial personality. *Am. J. Psychiatry*, **146**: 508–512.

85. McLellan A.T., Woody G.E., Luborsky L., Goehl L. (1988) Is the counselor an "active ingredient" in substance abuse rehabilitation? An examination of treatment success among four counselors. *J. Nerv. Ment. Dis.*, **176**: 423–430.

86. Woody G.E., McLellan A.T., Luborsky L., O'Brien C.C. (1985) Sociopathy and psychotherapy outcome. *Arch. Gen. Psychiatry*, **42**: 1081–1086.

87. Andrews D.A. (1980) Some experimental investigations of the principles of differential association through deliberate manipulations of the structure of service systems. *Am. Sociol. Rev.*, **45**: 448–462.

88. Ross R.R., Fabiano E.A., Ewles C.D. (1988) Reasoning and rehabilitation. *Int. J. Offender Ther. Comp. Criminol.*, **32**: 29–35.

89. Pearson F.S. (1988) Evaluation of New Jersey's intensive supervision program. *Crime and Delinquency*, **34**: 437–448.

90. Bloom H.S., Singer N.M. (1979) Determining the cost-effectiveness of correctional programs. In *Evaluation Studies: Review Annual* (Eds L. Sechrest, S.G. West, M.A. Phillips, R. Redner, W. Yeaton), pp. 552–568. Sage, Beverly Hills.

91. Grant J.D., Grant M.Q. (1959) A group dynamics approach to the treatment of non-conformists in the Navy. In *Prevention of Juvenile Delinquency* (Ed. T. Sellin), pp. 126–135. The American Academy of Political and Social Science, Philadelphia.

92. Alexander C.N., Davies J.L., Dixon C.A., Dillbeck M.C., Druker S.M., Oetzel R.M., Muehlman J.M., Orme-Johnson D.W. (1990) Growth of higher stages of consciousness: Maharishi's Vedic psychology of human development. In

Higher Stages of Human Development (Eds C.N. Alexander, E.J. Langer), pp. 286–341. Oxford University Press, New York.

93. Cloninger C.R. (1983) Drug treatment of antisocial behavior. In *Psychopharmacology* (Eds D.G. Grahame-Smith, H. Hippius, G. Winokur), pp. 353–370. Excerpta Medica, Amsterdam.

94. Wender P.H., Wolf L.E., Wasserstein J. (2001) Adults with ADHD: an overview. *Ann. N.Y. Acad. Sci.*, **931**: 1–16.

95. Sheard M.H., Marini J.L., Bridges C.I., Wagner E. (1976) The effect of lithium on impulsive aggressive behavior in man. *Am. J. Psychiatry*, **133**: 1409–1413.

96. Beck A.T., Freeman A. (1990) *Cognitive Therapy of Personality Disorders.* Guilford, New York.

97. Sturup G.K. (1948) Management and treatment of psychopaths in a special institution in Denmark. *Proc. Roy. Soc. Med.*, **41**: 465–768.

98. Shore M.F., Massimo J.L. (1979) Fifteen years after treatment: a follow-up study of comprehensive vocationally-oriented psychotherapy. *Am. J. Orthopsychiatry*, **49**: 240–245.

99. Shevrin H., Ghannam J.H., Libet B. (2002) A neural correlate of consciousness related to repression. *Consciousness and Cognition*, **11**: 334–341.

100. Bodner M., Muftuler L.T., Nalcioglu O., Shaw G.L. (2001) FMRI study relevant to the Mozart effect: brain areas involved in spatial-temporal reasoning. *Neurol. Res.*, **23**: 683–690.

101. Campbell D. (1995) *The Mozart Effect for Children.* William Morrow, New York.

102. Campbell D. (1997) *The Mozart Effect: Tapping the Power of Music to Heal the Body, Strengthen the Mind, and Unlock the Creative Spirit.* Harper Collins, New York.

103. Chabris C.F. (1999) Prelude or requiem for the 'Mozart effect'? *Nature*, **400**: 826–827.

104. Thompson W.F., Schellenberg E.G., Husain G. (2001) Arousal, mood, and the Mozart effect. *Psychol. Sci.*, **12**: 248–251.

105. Twomey A., Esgate A. (2002) The Mozart effect may only be demonstrable in nonmusicians. *Perceptual and Motor Skills*, **95**: 1013–1026.

Commentaries

2.1
Understanding the Antisocial Personality Disorder and Psychopathy Professional Literature

Carl B. Gacono[1]

Before discussing antisocial personality, one must define the disorder. Two issues essential to understanding the plethora of American based literature are: first, that sociopathy, antisocial personality and psychopathy are not the same terms; second, that psychopathy is both a dimensional and categorical construct.

In over 20 years of evaluating and treating antisocial and psychopathic patients in various outpatient, hospital, and correctional settings, and training others to do the same [1,2], the misuse of the terms sociopathy, antisocial personality and psychopathy continues to surprise me. Despite a wealth of published research on psychopathy [3], professionals continue to confuse sociopathy, antisocial personality and psychopathy, inappropriately viewing them as synonymous. Originating along different theoretical lines, these constructs manifest empirically measurable and clinically relevant differences [4].

Sociopathy and antisocial personality disorder (ASPD) are intertwined with the evolution of the DSM. Sociopathy appeared in the DSM-I and included a diverse group of individuals. It was replaced by ASPD in DSM-II. Unlike the traditional definitions of psychopathy, ASPD's mostly behavioural criteria were inspired by a "social deviancy model". Gradually, many of the trait based characteristics associated with psychopathy disappeared from ASPD in subsequent DSMs.

Not linked to the DSM series, the construct of psychopathy contains both trait and behaviourally based criteria [5]. Psychopaths are found in most cultures [6,7]. Murphy [6] notes that in the Inuit (Northwest Alaska) community, the word *kunlangeta* describes "a man who... repeatedly lies and cheats and steals things and does not go hunting and, when the other men are out of the village, takes sexual advantage of many women— someone who does not pay attention to reprimands and who is always

[1] St. Edwards University, P.O. Box 140633, Austin, TX 78714, USA

being brought to the elders for punishment". In the Yorubas community (rural Nigeria), the term *aranakan* describes an individual who "always goes his own way regardless of others, who is uncooperative, full of malice, and bullheaded" [6]. This shared *world view* is held by the majority of NATO countries [7].

As measured by the Psychopathy Checklist—Revised (PCL-R), psycho-pathy includes two factors [3]. Factor 1 contains traits such as glibness, grandiosity, pathological lying, conning and manipulation, lack or remorse and so forth. It is characterized by egocentricity, callousness, and remorse-lessness, and correlates with narcissistic and histrionic personality disorders, low anxiety, low empathy, and self-report measures of Machiavellianism. Factor 2 represents an irresponsible, impulsive, thrill-seeking, unconventional, and antisocial lifestyle and correlates most strongly with criminal behaviours, lower socioeconomic background, lower IQ and less education, self-report measures of antisocial behaviour, and the DSM-IV diagnosis of ASPD [3].

Base rates in forensic settings highlight the differences in the two constructs. Dependent on the security level of the institution, 50% to 75% of the offenders would meet the criteria for ASPD, while only 15% to 25% would be classified as psychopathic. While most criminal psychopaths meet criteria for ASPD, the majority of ASPD patients are not psychopaths.

Psychopaths (PCL-R≥30) comprise a smaller, more *homogenous, violent* group than individuals diagnosed with ASPD; thus, a psychopathy designation carries important implications for both research and clinical usage (prediction and management of behaviour).

Is psychopathy a taxon or a dimensional construct? This is a trick question. Psychopathy is both a categorical designation (taxon; PCL-R≥30) and a dimensional construct, dependent on its application. Dimensional uses are recommended for clinical applications. Clinical usage requires that psychopathy be conceptualized along a continuum of severity, so that individuals who obtain higher PCL-R scores exhibit more serious and pervasive symptoms of psychopathy compared to their lower PCL-R counterparts. Clinically, one is more interested in what ranges of psychopathy are best at predicting behaviour (where specific scores fall within an actuarial based risk prediction instrument) within a specific setting, than whether or not a given individual meets the traditional threshold score for a designation of psychopathy (PCL-R≥30; [2]).

Taxon designations are appropriate and preferred for comparative research, wherein the researcher is concerned with how psychopaths (PCL-R≥30) nomothetically differ from non-psychopaths (PCL-R < 30). Note that statistical approaches that use simple correlational methods to compare categorical variables to the individual PCL-R score (dimensional applica-tion) fail to capture true between-group differences. Identifying whether psychopathy is referenced as a dimensional versus categorical variable is essential to evaluating research findings. Beware of research studies that approach their data in a dimensional fashion and then discuss their findings categorically. Many of these studies have few if any psychopaths in them [8]. Indeed, the resurgence of research on ASPD and psychopathy in the past thirty years require that the consumer has a more sophisticated understanding of these disorders in order to accurately interpret research findings.

REFERENCES

1. Gacono C.B., Meloy J.R. (1994) *The Rorschach Assessment of Aggressive and Psychopathic Personalities.* Erlbaum, Hillsdale.
2. Gacono C.B. (2000) Suggestions for the institutional implementation and use of the Psychopathy Checklists. In *The Clinical and Forensic Assessment of Psychopathy* (Ed. C.B. Gacono), pp. 175–202. Erlbaum, Hillsdale.
3. Hare R.D. (2003) *The Hare Psychopathy Checklist—Revised,* 2nd edn. Multi-Health Systems, Toronto.
4. Gacono C.B., Neiberding R., Owen A., Rubel J., Bodhodt R. (2001) Treating juvenile and adult offenders with conduct-disorder, antisocial, and psychopathic personalities. In *Treating Adult and Juvenile Offenders with Special Needs* (Eds J. Ashford, B. Sales, W. Reid), pp. 99–130. American Psychological Association, Washington.
5. Cleckley H. (1976) *The Mask of Sanity,* 5th edn. Mosby, St. Louis.
6. Murphy J. (1974) Psychiatric labeling in cross-cultural perspective. *Science,* **191:** 1019–1028.
7. Cooke D., Forth A., Hare R. (1998) *Psychopathy: Theory, Research and Implications for Society.* NATO ASI Series, Kluwer, Dordrecht.
8. Gacono C., Loving J., Bodholdt R. (2001) The Rorschach and psychopathy: toward a more accurate understanding of the research findings. *J. Person. Assess.,* **77:** 16–38.

2.2
Developmental Perspectives on Self-Awareness in Antisocial Personality Disorder
Jonathan Hill[1]

Cloninger's chapter highlights, and rises to, many of the challenges posed by the personality disorders. He argues that a personality disorder can be defined as a description of someone whose thoughts and human relationships are usually lacking in self-awareness, defined as awareness of

---

[1] *University Child Mental Health, Mulberry House, Royal Liverpool Children's Hospital, Liverpool L12 2AP, UK*

one's own initiative and self-efficacy. If that is the case, it should be possible to develop ideas regarding the developmental origins of these deficits. Given that the histories of antisocial adults generally go back to early childhood, it is unlikely that they start in a lack of self-awareness, but in its precursors [1].

We find some indicators of where to look in Cloninger's summary of the two factors of the Hare Psychopathy Checklist, the "callous–unemotional" and the "impulsive–emotionally unstable". In terms of self-awareness, the first may be thought of as a failure to be aware of the other in relation to the self, and the second as an excessive awareness of the other. This contrast finds its counterpart in the childhood literature in the contrast between proactive aggression, cold and unprovoked, and reactive aggression, which is angry and occurs in response to perceived or actual aggression from others [2].

According to Stern [3], the development of the self in the young child is underpinned by the experience of emotions and of being the author of one's actions, across situations. In particular, perhaps the experience of effective action is crucial. Certainly self-assertiveness, including aggressive assertion, increases up to around the age of two. In some respects, therefore, the two year old can be seen as having an accumulated knowledge of his own effectiveness, underpinning a robust sense of self. Although many parents experience their two year olds as omnipotent and self-centred, most are not narcissistic psychopaths, because other processes modify their behaviours. These include the interplay between anxiety or fear and interpersonal understanding and problem solving. The interpersonal processes entail the child's capacity to respond to the needs of others, and to look to others to meet his/her needs and help regulate behaviours. The two year old's tendency to behave aggressively towards other children is already influenced by empathy, a complex process involving the recognition of another's distress and the reasons for it, responding to it emotionally, and acting appropriately. The interplay between interpersonal understanding and anxiety or fear seems to be crucial. The awareness of distress in another is likely to generate anxiety, and that anxiety further alerts the person to the distress and the need to do something about it. Empathy in 6 year olds is predicted by high levels of fear in infancy [4], and anxious adults show high empathy [5].

Blair has argued that a failure to respond emotionally to cues for distress in others underpins callous–unemotional traits in children [6]. The experience of anxiety or fear also is central to attachment behaviours. These are generally thought of as occurring in response to threat. However, the infant who does not become anxious in anticipation of, or frightened in response to threat, lacks the motivation to seek comfort. From the parent's perspective this may appear to be a self-contained "good" infant. However, later the dyad may lack the experience of dealing with difficult emotions required to tackle the emerging omnipotence of the two year old [7].

Finally, temperamental models of antisocial behaviours have a central role for anxiety. Harm avoidance (Cloninger) or behavioural inhibition (Gray [8]) is thought to provide the "brakes" for novelty seeking (Cloninger) or behavioural activation (Gray). Thus anxiety has at least three central roles: to drive empathy, to motivate attachment and intimacy, and to inhibit antisocial impulses. Lack of fear or anxiety may be central to processes associated with a limited capacity to reconcile the needs and perspectives of others with an awareness and experience of self-efficacy. In the National Longitudinal Study of Youth (NLSY), high activity level and low fearfulness in infancy was associated subsequently with antisocial behaviours in boys between ages four and eight [9]. In a Canadian general population study, low levels of social anxiety in children who were disruptive when aged 10–12 were predictive of delinquency three years later [10].

The second factor of the Psychopathy Checklist, the impulsive emotionally unstable, finds its counterpart in childhood in reactive and emotionally dysregulated patterns of responding. Here even minor or non-existent provocation appears to trigger extreme angry and aggressive responses. Reactively aggressive children are more likely to attribute hostile intent to others' behaviours and attend to hostile cues in their social environment [11]. The reactively aggressive child seems to view the world as one in which others are effective at his expense. In turn the poorly modulated extreme reactions are generally not effective and so further reduce the experience of initiative and self-efficacy.

Following Stern's idea that repeated effective action experienced across situations underpins a sense of self, the reactively aggressive child is likely to have a fragile sense of self. Intense distress when frustrated appears to be central to this pathway. Stifter *et al.* [12] found that infants who reacted intensely to stress in laboratory tests during the first 18 months were more non-compliant at 30 months. Lack of emotional control during laboratory tests at ages 3 and 5 predicted violent crime at age 18 in the Dunedin Health and Development Study [13]. The parents of infants who show such extreme responses to stress may disengage in an attempt to reduce the distress, hence providing less assistance to the child in managing it [7].

At this stage the idea of two kinds of process in antisocial behaviours, one characterized by a low level of interpersonal awareness and low anxiety, and the other by interpersonal sensitivity and intense emotionality, serves as a useful way of conceptualizing pathways and processes. It is consistent with Cloninger's integration of temperamental concepts and self processes. Future work may clarify whether there are "callous–unemotional/ proactive" and "sensitive–emotional/reactive" individuals, or whether these are contrasting processes commonly found together. Our work using doll play scenarios with young antisocial children suggests that they may work in a potent synergy [14]. We found that, compared to controls, antisocial boys were less likely to tell stories that showed interpersonal awareness in response to a child portrayed as distressed, and more likely to respond with aggressive and violent stories to everyday conflict challenges. This may indicate extreme reactive aggression in response to minor provocation that is unmodified by anxiety or interpersonal awareness at the time or afterwards.

REFERENCES

1. Hill J. (2002) Biological, psychological and social processes in the conduct disorders. *J. Child Psychol. Psychiatry*, **43**: 133–164.
2. Vitaro F., Brendgen M., Tremblay R.E. (2002) Reactively and proactively aggressive children: antecedent and subsequent characteristics. *J. Child Psychol. Psychiatry*, **43**: 495–506.
3. Stern D. (1985) *The Interpersonal World of the Infant*. Basic Books, New York.
4. Rothbart M.K., Posner M.I., Rosicky J. (1994) Orienting in normal and pathological development. *Develop. Psychopathol.*, **6**: 635–652.
5. Dias A., Pickering A.D. (1993) The relationship between Gray's and Eysenck's personality spaces. *Person. Indiv. Diff.*, **15**: 297–306.
6. Blair R.J.R. (1999) Responsiveness to distress cues in the child with psychopathic tendencies. *Person. Indiv. Diff.*, **27**: 135–145.
7. Keenan K., Shaw D.S. (2003) Starting at the beginning: exploring the etiology of antisocial behavior in the first years of life. In *Causes of Conduct Disorder and Juvenile Delinquency* (Eds B.B. Lahey, T.E. Moffitt, A Caspi), pp. 153–181. Guilford, New York.
8. Gray G. (1987) *The Psychology of Fear and Stress*, 2nd edn. McGraw Hill, New York.
9. Colder C., Mott J., Berman A. (2002) The interactive effects of infant activity level and fear on growth trajectories of early childhood behavior problems. *Develop. Psychopathol.*, **14**: 1–23.
10. Kerr M., Tremblay R.E., Pagini L., Vitaro F. (1997) Boys' behavioural inhibition and the risk of later delinquency. *Arch. Gen. Psychiatry*, **54**: 809–816.
11. Dodge K.A., Lochman J.E., Harnish J.D., Bates J.E., Pettit G.S. (1995) Social information-processing patterns partially mediate the effect of early physical abuse on later conduct problems. *J. Abnorm. Psychol.*, **104**, 632–643.
12. Stifter C.A., Spinrad T.L., Braungart-Rieker J.M. (1999) Toward a developmental model of child compliance: the role of emotion regulation in infancy. *Child Develop.*, **70**: 21–32.
13. Henry B., Caspi A., Moffitt T.E., Silva P.A. (1996) Temperamental and familial predictors of violent and non-violent criminal convictions: age three to eighteen. *Develop. Psychol.*, **32**: 614–623.
14. Hill J., Fonagy P., Lancaster G., Broyden N. Social cognition and antisocial behaviour problems in boys: the interplay between aggressive representations and intentionality. Submitted for publication.

2.3
The Complexity of Antisocial Behaviour
John M. Oldham[1]

Building upon his earlier work utilizing the Temperament and Character Inventory (TCI) to assess proposed critical factors delineating varieties of personality functioning, Cloninger applies these constructs to current thinking about antisocial personality disorder (ASPD). His review is clarifying and informative, attempting to disentangle substantial complexities in the ASPD literature. For example, studies reported to be about ASPD are often, instead, studies of criminal behaviour. In turn, studies that exclude institutionalized populations focus, inevitably, on less impaired or disabled individuals of the complete universe of those who would meet either DSM-IV or ICD-10 diagnoses of ASPD. Population ambiguities or inconsistencies of this sort make it difficult to compare discrepant results with respect to issues such as level of disability, longitudinal course, or response to treatment.

Cloninger's subdivision of ASPD into primary psychopaths with prominent narcissistic traits and secondary psychopaths with prominent borderline traits is intriguing but may diverge from the inclusion and exclusion criteria utilized in many published ASPD studies. Further, differentiation of "uncomplicated" ASPD from patients with ASPD complicated by the additional presence of alcohol or drug abuse may lead to different histories regarding criminal behaviour, yet studies of ASPD differ widely with regard to degree of comorbidity.

Cloninger presents excerpts from a complex matrix of development and behavioural analysis that he has been developing, to be presented in more detail in his new book. Seven major steps in human learning ability are delineated, including five of the seven specified to account for individual differences in human thought processes. This system also involves five planes of thought, accompanied by a method to quantify these thought levels. These concepts are extended by a scheme that involves the diagnosis of frequency of thought, and the diagnosis of human relationships, which are described at length as they apply to ASPD. This material serves as an appetizer for Cloninger's book, which provides readers with a more in-depth understanding of these dimensional approaches to human behaviour.

Kagan et al. [1] have described the correlation between conduct disorder in children and ASPD in adults as the most robustly established predictive longitudinal course of psychopathology in the literature, with the identification

_____
[1] Department of Psychiatry and Behavioral Sciences, Medical University of South Carolina, 67 President Street, Charleston, SC 29425, USA

of conduct disorder as a precursor of the adult ASPD condition. The varieties of causality, however, remain multiple. As described by Rutter [2], "twin studies data indicate that genetic factors are probably particularly important in those varieties of antisocial behaviour associated with early-onset, pervasive hyperactivity. Conversely, it is likely that they are least influential in the case of adolescent-onset delinquency that has not been preceded by hyperactivity." Later work reported by Rutter and his group [3] indicated that childhood hyperactivity and conduct disorder showed equally strong prediction of ASPD and criminality in early and mid-adult life, but intermediate life experiences remain important in ultimate outcome and represent an opportunity for intervention.

A major challenge remains regarding ASPD, and that is in this precise area of prevention, intervention, and treatment. Black [4] described a follow-up study of men with ASPD, demonstrating a 24% mortality rate but encouraging outcomes for the survivors, with 58% improved or remitted. These findings contrast with the marked pessimism in the literature about the treatability of this condition. Paris [5], for example, described that "patients with ASPD are famously resistant to therapy, failing to respond to virtually every form of intervention that has been tried....". He cites, nonetheless, exceptions to this rule, and the problem is frequently compounded by the inclusion of prisoners and criminals in reported samples. Motivation for treatment is often negligible, unless comorbidity is present or secondary gain is anticipated.

It is in this respect that Cloninger's review is most encouraging. It may be necessary to prioritize our treatment efforts to the non-institutionalized, less disabled patients with ASPD and to disconnect ourselves from what may be a negative treatment bias at the outset. Cloninger describes strategies called "listening to the psyche", "following the path of the psyche", "union in nature meditation", and "silence of the mind meditation", suggesting that these techniques may be effective with at least selected ASPD populations. These ideas are encouraging and need to be subjected to further research. Recent developments in our understanding of the plasticity of the brain and of the bi-directional nature of the gene–environment interaction [6]—that, as Gabbard [7] puts it, "genetic 'hard-wiring' is a questionable assumption"—help persuade us to challenge old assumptions and explore new methods of intervention and prevention. Cross-fostering studies reinforce our optimism, such as those that clearly demonstrate lifetime behavioural improvements in primates genetically at risk for aggressive behaviour [8]. Similar hopeful signs are emerging as research groups explore family-based interventions with highly dysfunctional families whose youth are already at or beyond the edge of delinquency [9].

REFERENCES

1. Kagan J., Zentner M. (1996) Early childhood predictors of adult psychopathology. *Harv. Rev. Psychiatry*, **3**: 341–350.
2. Rutter M. (1996) Concluding remarks. In *Genetics of Criminal and Antisocial Behavior* (Eds G.R. Bock, J.A. Goode), pp. 265–271. Wiley, Chichester.
3. Simonoff E., Holmshaw J., Pickles A., Murray R., Rutter M. (2004) Predictors of antisocial personality. Continuities from childhood to adult life. *Br. J. Psychiatry*, **184**: 118–127.
4. Black D.W. (1995) A 16- to 45-year follow-up of 71 men with antisocial personality disorder. *Compr. Psychiatry*, **36**: 130–140.
5. Paris J. (2003) *Personality Disorders Over Time: Precursors, Course, and Outcome*, pp. 111–131. American Psychiatric Publishing, Washington.
6. Rutter M. (2002) The interplay of nature, nurture, and developmental influences. *Arch. Gen. Psychiatry*, **59**: 996–1000.
7. Gabbard G.O. (in press) Mind, brain and personality disorders. *Am. J. Psychiatry*.
8. Suomi S.J. (in press) Social and biological mechanisms underlying impulsive aggressiveness in rhesus monkeys. In *Severe Juvenile Delinquency* (Eds B.B.Lahey, T. Moffitt, A. Caspi). Guilford, New York.
9. Henggeler S.W., Sheidow A.J. (2003) Conduct disorder and delinquency. *J. Marital Fam. Ther.*, **29**: 505–522.

2.4
Assessing Research on Antisocial Personality
Lee N. Robins[1]

Any review of research on antisocial personality is hampered by two major problems in the literature: disagreements about the criteria for diagnosis, and use of samples from which milder cases of the disorder are excluded and which consider as "affected" persons who do not actually have the disorder.

While all definitions of the disorder agree that the prototypic case is an adult who shows a variety of antisocial behaviours, the DSM definitions emphasize the history of childhood onset, and Cleckley's [1] and Hare's [2] definitions emphasize the current psychological substrate. We have argued [3] that, since behaviour is always the basis on which we substantiate or disallow the respondent's claim to psychological states incompatible with the disorder (e.g. love, anxiety, and guilt), behaviour is inevitably the ultimate criterion. Cloninger's own contributions to this literature offer a compromise between these two views. His diagnosis uses a psychological

[1] *Department of Psychiatry, Washington University School of Medicine, St. Louis, MO 63110-1093, USA*

substrate similar to Cleckley's, but much elaborated to include temperament and character traits. Recognizing the problem of using current
psychological traits to define a disorder that lasts across the life span, he
reports finding "moderate stability of personality from childhood to
adulthood in most people", and believes these traits are reflected in
biology, and largely genetically determined.

Cloninger found that much of the research relevant to antisocial personality
disorder is based on special samples from which members who do not have
the disorder have not been excluded. Study samples such as former juvenile
delinquents and prisoners do indeed have an elevated rate of antisocial
personality disorder, but its prevalence is nowhere near 100%. Further, such
samples exclude the many persons with antisocial personality disorder who
have not been convicted. Samples of patients with an antisocial personality
diagnosis are very likely to have one or more concurrent disorders as well,
because antisocial personality disorder alone rarely leads to seeking
treatment [4]. The most common associated disorders are substance abuse
and depression.

Cloninger notes the uniform findings from these many studies that
appear despite the variation across studies in diagnostic criteria and type of
sample. Those with antisocial personality disorder characteristically are of
male sex and in childhood had early onset of the disorder and ineffective
and antisocial parents. Early in adulthood, they show irresponsibility and
poor work performance, unstable commitment to partners, illegal behaviour, and substance abuse. These behaviours are generally stable until
middle age, when they often remit partially or completely.

There is no comparable uniformity in the literature with regard to how
treatable antisocial personality disorder is, or what treatment methods are
most effective. Treatment studies in patients with antisocial personality
disorder who have other disorders as well may explain some over-optimism
about antisocial personality disorder's treatability. This will occur when
effective treatment of the co-morbid disorder diminishes symptoms that are
part of the antisocial personality diagnosis. For example, treating depression
or substance abuse may reduce marital breakup and inability to hold a job;
treating substance abuse will reduce theft and violence by reducing the
patient's expenses and his need to participate in illegal transactions.

Cloninger cites epidemiological studies as a prime source of information
about the disorder's diagnostic symptoms and demographic characteristics.
This is justified because, in general population studies, everyone with the
disorder has a known chance of entering the sample. Unfortunately,
epidemiological studies are not very useful for assessing treatment
effectiveness; so small a proportion of those affected come to treatment
[4] that even very large samples do not allow comparing outcomes of
treated and untreated cases.

As a result of these difficulties in assessing treatment effects, there is still little solid information about the treatability of antisocial personality disorder. Future studies could be more useful than those reviewed here if they count among their experimental subjects all those who met the criterion of "intention to treat" rather than only those who completed a course of treatment. Because many antisocial personality patients break off treatment early, the treatment completers are on the whole a more cooperative group than the controls, biasing results in favour of treatment.

Cloninger's review not only summarizes research on antisocial personality disorder, but also provides the author's estimates of proportions of human beings with varying types of thought and the role of temperament and character in psychiatric disorder. It includes his theories about effective treatment styles for all psychiatric disorder, as well as for antisocial personality. I look forward to the publication of Cloninger's new book, which he says contains research evidence supporting his views. If it also evaluates the quality of that research, it will be valuable in discussions of evidence for the biological basis of antisocial personality and of its treatability.

REFERENCES

1. Cleckley H. (1964) *The Mask of Sanity.* Mosby, St. Louis.
2. Hare R.D. (1970) *Psychopathy: Theory and Research.* John Wiley & Sons, New York.
3. Robins L.N. (1978) Aetiological implications in studies of childhood histories relating to antisocial personality. In *Psychopathic Behaviour: Approaches to Research* (Eds R.D. Hare, D. Schalling), pp. 255–271. John Wiley & Sons, New York.
4. Robins L.N., Tipp J., Pryzbeck T. (1991) Antisocial personality. In *Psychiatric Disorders in America* (Eds L.N. Robins, D.A. Regier), pp. 258–290. Free Press, New York.

2.5
Antisocial or Social Adaptation

Janine L. Stevenson[1]

Antisocial personality disorder (ASPD) is a broad concept based on behavioural criteria. Of the 80% of prison inmates who fulfil criteria for ASPD, only a fraction could be said to have the core personality structure of Cleckley's psychopathic personalities [1]. The latter represent only 15 to

[1] *Department of Psychiatry, Westmead Hospital, Westmead, NSW, Australia 2145*

30% of prison inmates. Many people with psychopathic traits are living in the community and not all manifest antisocial behaviours.

The DSM-III and the DSM-III-R define ASPD via behavioural items such as truancy, destroying property, and fighting. This method increases reliability at the expense of validity and is over-inclusive, often applying to the so-called "neurotic psychopath" (borderline personality disorder, BPD in DSM classification, or emotionally unstable in ICD-10). Included here can be the "dyssocial personality" (the member of a socially deviant group), and the "sociopath" whose behaviour resulted from poor parenting.

Hare *et al.* [2] have sought to rectify the problem, revising the original Cleckley descriptors, creating the Psychopathy Check List (PCL and PCL-R). Psychopathy is diagnosed if the score is greater than 30. In the social context, a psychopath is a "non-reciprocator". The high novelty-seeking of which Cloninger speaks and low harm avoidance (impulsivity) make him a risk taker. At the milder end of the continuum these qualities may contribute to success in business. At the severe end are the repeat criminal, arsonist, and serial killer. Persons with a score of less than 30 could be said to show degrees of psychopathy, thus lending some weight to a dimensional approach.

ASPD is a categorical diagnosis. Not all lack remorse and compassion or are committed to a lifelong course of deceiving others. So-called psychopathy on the other hand tends to be stable with age, whereas ASPD declines in the fourth and fifth decades. Research is hampered by the fact that only prison inmates have been studied and the study of subjects in the general population has only occurred to a minor degree. There may be many more successful psychopaths, who are not violent or criminal.

Of all the so-called disorders of personality, ASPD causes the most impact on the population at large. Antisocial personalities are by definition in conflict with society. Paradoxically, the disorder may be encouraged by the very societies in which they live. ASPD is present in many cultures, not only in industrialized countries [3]. For example, the Inuit of Alaska, and the Yorubas of Nigeria recognise the concept and have names for these individuals. However, the level of violence and aggression differs markedly between cultures. In the Yamomamo tribe of the upper Amazon villagers are constantly fighting, within, as well as between, villages. Here, a man's status is determined by his level of aggressiveness. Enculturation and early socialization influence aggression. In collectivistic societies such as China, group loyalties and responsibilities have priority over self-expression. Individualistic societies, such as Australia and the North Americas, may be more likely to produce glibness, grandiosity, multiple marital relationships, and lack of responsibility in relationships. This environment is also heading towards a sociobiological situation characterized by high reproductive effort (promiscuity) and low parenting effort, which encourages "victimful criminal behaviour"[3].

An essential element of psychopathy as defined by Cleckley [1] is a deficit in anxiety or fear. This is not necessarily the case in antisocial subjects, who lack the core affective features. Psychopathy may represent one endpoint along a continuum of responsiveness to punishment cues. Cloninger used his extensive research on temperament and character to explore this in antisocial subjects. Is there an emotional deficiency with a disturbance in affective processing and an inability to experience feelings evoked by reward and punishment [4]? Cloninger found that one prominent feature was a lack of "self-aware consciousness" in people with ASPD. His multidimensional definition allows everyone to be assigned to mutually exclusive groups. He uses a cube to visualize the three temperamental dimensions. The clinical presentation then depends on the level of character development associated with the particular temperament. He goes on to point out that the detailed structure of the person's thought and the level of psychological maturity is a more definitive basis for differential diagnosis than behavioural or checklist criteria. Behaviour in a certain situation is determined by the structure, maturity and coherence of thought processes. Cloninger, using a detailed broad research base, looks at not simply behaviour, but thought processes and maturation. This comprehensive analysis of outcome is much more optimistic than most literature would have us believe.

Biological studies have stressed the complex interaction between biological and environmental or social variables. They have shown that heritable characteristics of adopted children also influence the behaviour of their adoptive parents, leading to negative parenting behaviours. Studies in this area are necessarily complex. Researchers have found abnormalities in the prefrontal cortex, the hippocampus, and right cerebral hemisphere. Frontal lobe injuries can also result in antisocial and aggressive behaviour. Researchers have talked about an emotional deficiency, where affective processing is disturbed. Neuropsychological testing has found deficits in the orbitofrontal and ventromedial area of the brain. Positron emission tomography (PET) and single photon emission computed tomography (SPECT) studies have found abnormalities seeming to suggest that these subjects had deficits in the higher nervous system centres related to moral behaviour [5].

Studies looking at gender postulate that cluster B personality disorders may represent variable expressions of a common diathesis, perhaps influenced by gender. Boys tend to show more aggression and externalizing behaviour patterns and girls show more behavioural inhibition and internalizing problems [6]. As Cloninger points out, "primary psychopaths" are callous, calm, cold-blooded, remorseless, whereas "secondary psychopaths" are anxious and emotionally unstable. The latter nowadays are usually classified as BPD (in DSM-IV) and emotionally unstable disorder (in ICD-10).

Treatment is necessarily complicated by multiple factors: certain antisocial cultural groups see their behaviour as normal, and the wealthy often "buy off" the authorities. The best prognostic factor is actually the absence of psychopathic traits, the absence of predatory narcissism. Meloy [7] offered five contraindications to psychotherapy: sadistic behaviour, absence of remorse, either a very high or very low IQ, absence of attachment and counter-transference fear in the therapist. A multimodal approach addressing cognitive distortions using structured, behavioural, and cognitive behavioural skills-oriented methods in an outpatient rather than most institutional settings is preferred. Cloninger introduces evidence for some meditative approaches, which have promise. He also introduces compelling evidence for an "adventurous" outpatient approach, rather than the structured prison environment.

Is ASPD in an evolutionary adaptation or cultural creation? What is the role of genes/environment? What about degrees of deviance and what does this mean for treatment? What about the neurobiological abnormalities? And why is the incidence so much higher in some societies than others? There are yet many questions to answer, and many routes to those answers.

REFERENCES

1. Cleckley H. (1976) *The Mask of Sanity; An Attempt to Clarify Some Issues about the So-called Psychopathic Personality*, 5th edn. Mosby, St. Louis.
2. Hare, R.D. (1991) *The Hare Psychopathy Checklist—Revised*. Multi-Health Systems, Toronto.
3. Cooke D.J. (1996) Psychopathic personality in different cultures: what do we know? What do we need to find out? *J. Person. Disord.*, **10**: 23–40.
4. Herpetz S.C., Sass H. (2000) Emotional deficiency and psychopathy. *Behav. Sci. Law*, **18**: 567–580.
5. Raine A. (2002) Biosocial studies of antisocial and violent behavior in children and adults. *J. Abnorm. Child Psychol.*, **30**: 311–326.
6. Skodol A.E. (2000) Gender-specific etiologies for antisocial and borderline personality disorders? In *Gender and its Effects on Psychopathology* (Ed. E. Frank), pp. 37–58. American Psychiatric Publishing, Washington.
7. Meloy J.R. (1988) *The Psychopathic Mind*. Northvale, Aronson.

2.6
Antisocial Personality Disorder—The Forgotten Patients of Psychiatry
Donald W. Black[1]

One of the best-validated disorders in the DSM-IV, antisocial personality disorder (ASPD), is rarely diagnosed, researched, or offered treatment [1]. The lack of interest by psychiatrists and researchers is puzzling, because the disorder is of enormous importance. As documented in Cloninger's comprehensive review, ASPD is among the most common psychiatric disorders, and contributes to great suffering by individuals, families, and society at large. ASPD is also associated with increased health care services utilization, early mortality, and poor treatment response in those suffering from major depression or substance use disorders. Direct and indirect costs have never been calculated, yet it must be among the most costly of mental disorders, due primarily to the downstream costs of maintaining the criminal justice and penal systems (because the majority of criminals meet criteria for ASPD).

ASPD is poorly understood in the general population, and even among some psychiatrists and other mental health professionals. Goodwin and Guze [2] have provided one of the best brief definitions. These authors describe ASPD as "a pattern of recurrent, delinquent, or criminal behavior that begins in early childhood or early adolescence and is manifested by disturbances in many areas of life...". The diagnosis relies on the mental health professional's ability to uncover this pattern of misbehaviour and trace it through a patient's life. Isolated misdeeds or those confined to one area of life—work for instance—are not by themselves evidence of ASPD, though they may indicate an underlying pattern of antisocial acts and attitudes. In short, ASPD is a disorder of recurring lifelong misbehaviour.

Cloninger points out that many individuals with ASPD improve by middle age and cites Lee Robins' critical work [3], in which she reported that 12% of 82 subjects followed 30 years into their mid-40s were in remission and an additional 20% had improved. In my own follow-up study, also approximately of 30 years duration, persons were followed into their mid-50s, and rates of remission were slightly higher, suggesting that antisocials continue to improve over time; perhaps an even higher percentage would be in remission if follow-up studies were extended another 10 or 20 years [1]. Both Robins [3] and Black et al. [4] reported that baseline symptom severity was perhaps the most robust predictor of outcome. Cloninger is correct in pointing out that many intelligent and successful individuals are antisocial, though, because of their poor

[1] Psychiatry Research, University of Iowa, Iowa City, IA 52242, USA

educational and occupational achievement, few rise very high on the social ladder. Arguably, one example may be that of the former dictator Sadaam Hussein, who achieved high status prior to his ignominious fall from power. Interestingly, in the Iowa study [5] antisocials fared less well during the follow-up than depressed subjects and normal controls in their marital, occupational, and psychiatric status. They functioned better than schizo-phrenic subjects in their marital status and housing, but not in their occupational status or aggregate psychiatric symptoms.

The cause of ASPD is unknown, though genetic epidemiology—much of it coming from Robert Cloninger—has linked the condition to somatization disorder and substance use disorders. More recently, Krueger *et al.* [6] has written that ASPD, substance use disorders, and disinhibited behaviour are all linked by a latent externalizing factor with high heritability. Exactly what is inherited, and how the disorder is transmitted, is unclear. Other theories that have been pursued posit that ASPD represents the sequelae of a neurodevelopmental insult, and an even older theory posits that chronic autonomic underarousal contributes to the development of ASPD [7]. Neuro-transmitter studies have found that serotonin modulates both impulsivity and aggression, suggesting a tie-in with ASPD [8]. Brain imaging studies of antisocials revealed reduced prefrontal gray matter, an intriguing finding because the prefrontal cortex is well known for helping to regulate mood and behaviour [9]. None of these theories satisfactorily account for the entire antisocial syndrome, and it is likely that ASPD is a multi-determined condition, not unlike schizophrenia.

The treatment of ASPD is vexing and, in fact, few individuals seek psychiatric attention specifically for their condition, although according to the Epidemiologic Catchment Area study nearly one in five antisocials had mental health care within six months of survey participation [10]. One might ask: why antisocials seek psychiatric care? One chart review study indicated that they do so for troublesome problems such as marital discord, alcohol or drug abuse, or suicidal behaviour [11]. Other antisocials may be brought for evaluation by family members or the courts. Because poor insight is a feature of the disorder, antisocials often reject the diagnosis when it is presented to them, or they deny its symptoms.

The diagnosis itself is relatively straightforward when using the DSM-IV criteria. Formal testing, in my opinion, is unnecessary, though may help uncover information in otherwise uncooperative patients. Tests of intelligence and educational achievement may provide useful information about the patient and perhaps in treatment planning. On traditional intelligence tests, antisocials score lower than non-antisocials and are more likely to show evidence of learning disabilities [6].

One of the curious facts about ASPD is that there are no randomized control trials pitting any type of medication or psychotherapy against a control condition. One of the problems in assessing the treatment literature is that we are forced to extrapolate from studies of persons with impulsive personalities, aggressive dementia, mental retardation, or from studies of felons or other offenders, substance abusers, or children and adolescents with conduct disorder. In each case, some of the subjects are arguably antisocial, though in most of the studies the presence or absence of ASPD is not specified [1]. With this in mind, it is hard to conclude that any treatment fully targets the antisocial syndrome. Similarly, the literature on cognitive-behavioural and other psychotherapies is sparse, and mainly limited to case reports or small case series [1]. These reports suggest that, at least in mild cases, cognitive-behavioural approaches may be helpful, but clearly more research is needed to clarify the role of psychotherapy in treating ASPD.

Nonetheless, the view among most practising psychiatrists and mental health professionals is that ASPD is untreatable. In fact, we cannot conclude that it is untreatable, because research is wholly inadequate on this question. If treatments *were* available it is hard to know how many antisocials would benefit. In order to do so, antisocial patients would have to step forward to seek help, comply with treatment recommendations, and follow through. In my view, it is unlikely that more than a handful would ever do so, because antisocials typically lack insight and are unreliable. Additionally, countertransference issues would make it likely that many psychiatrists and therapists would refuse to treat antisocials. Antisocials induce many feelings in psychiatrists and therapists, including fear, rage, or even disgust [12]. Such feelings can interfere with the proper treatment of patients or preclude it altogether. In their book *Psychopathy and Delinquency* [13], sociologists William and Joan McCord describe the challenge of treating antisocials: "The psychopath is like a chow dog who may turn and bite the hand that pets it. The psychopath's hard external shell, his disturbing aggression, and his complete irresponsibility make therapy a thankless task". Their observation was written in 1956 and the situation is not appreciably different in 2004.

REFERENCES

1. Black D.W. (1999) *Bad Boys, Bad Men. Confronting Antisocial Personality Disorder.* Oxford University Press, New York.
2. Goodwin D., Guze S. (1989) *Psychiatric Diagnosis*, 4th edn. Oxford University Press, New York.
3. Robins L. (1966) *Deviant Children Grown Up.* Williams and Wilkins, Baltimore.
4. Black D.W., Monahan P., Baumgard C.H., Bell S.E. (1987) Prediction of long-term outcome in 45 men with antisocial personality disorder. *Ann. Clin. Psychiatry*, 9: 211–213.

5. Black D.W., Baumgard C.H., Bell S.E. (1995) The long-term outcome of antisocial personality disorder compared with depression, schizophrenia, and surgical conditions. *Bull. Am. Acad. Psychiatry Law*, **23**: 43–52.
6. Krueger R.F., Hicks B.M., Patrick C.G., Carlson S.R., Iacono W.G., McGue M. (2002) Etiologic connections among substance dependence, antisocial behavior, and disinhibited personality: modeling the externalizing spectrum. *J. Abnorm. Psychol.*, **111**: 411–424.
7. Hare R.D. (1978) Electrodermal and cardiovascular correlates of psychopathy. In: *Psychopathic Behavior: Approaches to Research* (Eds R.D. Hare, D. Schalling), pp. 107–144. Wiley, New York.
8. Raine A. (1993) *The Psychopathology of Crime*. Academic Press, New York.
9. Raine A., Lencz T., Bihrle S., LaCasse L., Colletti P. (2000) Reduced prefrontal gray matter volume and reduced autonomic activity and antisocial personality disorder. *Arch. Gen. Psychiatry*, **57**: 119–127.
10. Shapiro S., Skinner E.A., Kessler L.G., Von Korff M., German P.S., Tischler G.L., Leaf P.J., Benham L., Cottler L., Regier D.A. (1984) Utilization of health and mental health services. *Arch. Gen. Psychiatry*, **14**: 971–978.
11. Black D.W., Braun D. (1998) Antisocial patients: comparison of persons with and persons without childhood conduct disorder. *Ann. Clin. Psychiatry*, **10**: 53–57.
12. Strasburger L.H. (1986) The treatment of antisocial syndromes: the therapist's feelings. In *Unmasking the Psychopath: Antisocial Personality and Related Syndromes* (Eds W.H. Reid, D. Dorr, J.I. Walker, J.W. Bonner), pp. 191–207. Norton, New York.
13. McCord W., McCord J. (1956) *Psychopathy and Delinquency*. Grune and Stratton, New York.

2.7
A New Conceptualization of Antisocial Personality Disorder
Conor Duggan[1]

Antisocial personality disorder (ASPD) is in many ways both the most important and the most controversial of all personality disorders, because of its high prevalence and negative societal impact. Its Achilles heel, however, lies in its nosological status; specifically, in the overlap between antisocial personality traits and criminal behaviour. The very high prevalence of ASPD found among those in prisons [1] suggests that this overlap is substantial.

As a consequence, psychiatrists are ambivalent when confronted with those with ASPD. For instance, should they function as criminologists and reduce offending behaviour or as mental health professionals and reduce symptomatic distress? Allied to this is their understandable desire to avoid

[1] East Midlands Centre for Forensic Mental Health, Cordelia Close, Leicester LE5 0LE, UK

public ridicule by being seen as a 'soft touch' by those who might use mental disorder as a pretext to avoid responsibility for their behaviour while, at the same time, not wishing to deny interventions to those who legitimately might benefit from them.

One response to these dilemmas is to reduce this overlap by separating antisocial traits from antisocial behaviour [2]. Robert Hare's Psychopathy Checklist (PLC-R) is one of the most widely known instruments that address this task. In his comprehensive review, Robert Cloninger continues this tradition by focusing on the well-known distinction between primary and secondary psychopathy [3]. What is new in this review is Cloninger's attempt to embed this distinction in features of general personality disorder in his Temperament and Character Inventory (TCI) model.

Thus, according to Cloninger's taxonomy, primary psychopathy is associated with impulsivity (high novelty seeking), risk taking and autonomic underarousal (low harm avoidance) and aloofness and social detachment (low reward dependence). Secondary psychopaths, although also impulsive and antisocial, are more affectively labile. In addition to these temperamental difficulties, primary psychopaths display character-ological difficulties, as they are low in TCI self-directedness and cooperativeness. Thus, while a lack of self-reflective capacity underlies all personality disorders, Cloninger argues that it is by attending to the specific combination of TCI defined temperament and character abnormalities in the individual with ASPD that a more advanced and richer ASPD typology will emerge.

Two key underpinnings of primary psychopathy are emotional under-arousal [4] and a lack of empathic awareness. Hence, there is both an input and a processing problem [5]. How does Cloninger's proposal explain these deficits? In response, Cloninger argues that those with ASPD exhibit a primitive form of thought, because of their continued struggles within themselves, and this inability to be self-reflective results in them appearing to be shallow, egocentric and unempathic.

Whether or not one can intervene effectively in those with ASPD is controversial, not least because the purpose the intervention itself is often unclear [6]. Focusing solely on preventing recidivism, current thinking (which is the polar opposite of that which prevailed 20 years ago) is that highly structured programmes that tackle criminogenic needs of high risk offenders show moderate efficacy in reducing recidivism.

An important caveat here is that many such programmes target the behavioural features of secondary psychopathy. It remains to be seen whether they will be as effective for primary psychopaths who, some believe, are made even worse by conventional interventions [7]. Another difficulty that will need to be addressed is Cloninger's proposal of the need to match the 'adventurous' temperament that is a key trait in ASPD by respecting them as free agents. This is not what happens in practice, where treatment, if it is provided at all, is usually only available in very restricted settings (e.g. secure hospitals or prisons) and only very rarely in the community. Finally, as those with ASPD often lack the capacity to engage in a therapeutic relationship, Cloninger recommends a number of meditative and contemplative exercises to promote more reflective thinking. These components, and indeed his coherence therapy more generally, ought to be properly evaluated in this group with the appropriate design. Indeed, it is remarkable how few properly designed randomized treatment trials there have been in this group despite its high prevalence and great societal cost.

In summary, Robert Cloninger, in this thoughtful and challenging review, opens up a vista that allows us to think more constructively about a disorder that has traditionally been shunned by psychiatrists. His proposals, if implemented, would radically change how we manage those with this disorder. Thus, he has set the bar at a high level and it remains to be seen whether mental health workers are equal to the task.

REFERENCES

1. Singleton N., Meltzer H., Gatward R., Coid J., Deasy D. (1998) *Psychiatric Morbidity Among Prisoners in England and Wales*. Stationery Office, London.
2. Lilienfeld S.O. (1994) Conceptual problems in the assessment of psychopathy. *Clin. Psychol. Rev.*, **14**: 17–38.
3. Mealy L. (1995) The sociobiology of sociopathy: an integrated evolutionary model. *Behav. Brain Sci.*, **18**: 523–541.
4. Hare R.D. (1998) Psychopathy, affect and behaviour. In *Psychopathy: Theory, Research and Implications for Society* (Eds D.J. Cooke, A.E. Forth, R.D. Hare), pp. 105–138. Kluwer, Dordrecht.
5. Newman, J.P. (1998) Psychopathic behaviour: an information processing perspective. In *Psychopathy: Theory, Research and Implications for Society* (Eds D.J. Cooke, A.E. Forth, R.D. Hare), pp. 81–104. Kluwer, Dordrecht.
6. Duggan C. (2004) Does personality change and, if so, what changes? *Criminal Behaviour and Mental Health*, **14**: 5–16.
7. D'Silva K., Duggan C., McCarthy L. (in press) Does treatment make psychopaths worse? A review of the evidence. *J. Person. Disord.*

2.8
Cloninger's Theory of Antisocial Personality Disorder
Thomas A. Widiger[1]

Robert Cloninger provides in his review of the antisocial personality disorder (ASPD) a thorough summary of how its diagnosis, aetiology, pathology, and treatment would be understood from the perspective of his temperament and character theory of personality. Perhaps not surprisingly, this is not the only conceptual model of ASPD. Some of the personality disorders have failed to generate much scientific research (e.g. paranoid, schizoid, and obsessive–compulsive). However, this is not true for ASPD. There is a considerable amount of ongoing research devoted to the assessment, diagnosis, aetiology, and pathology of ASPD. Persons interested in learning about other current models and studies of ASPD might find it useful, for example, to consider the seminal texts edited by Stoff *et al.* [1], Cooke *et al.* [2], and Millon *et al.* [3]. A couple of chapters from one of these texts are noted in passing within Cloninger's review, but there is quite a bit of additional material that might also be of interest to persons concerned with ASPD. For example, there is interest among leading investigators of ASPD in the response modulation theory of Newman [4], the low anxiousness, hyporeactivity model of Patrick [5], the interpersonal model of Kosson [6], the social learning model of Dodge [7], the general personality model of Lynam [8], and the affective deficit model of Hare [9]. These alternative models have much to offer in our understanding of the aetiology and pathology of ASPD, and their validity is well supported by a considerable amount of empirical research.

Cloninger's discussion of the treatment of ASPD does cover much of the current literature and research. All of the personality disorders, particularly ASPD, have had the unfortunate perception of being largely untreatable. Personality disorders are among the most difficult of clinical conditions to treat, but there is compelling empirical research to indicate that clinically, personally, and socially meaningful response to treatment does occur. Treatment may not result in a radical change in personality, but even mild to moderate changes in antisocial personality traits can be associated with quite meaningful benefits to the person and to the wider society. As suggested by Cloninger, a nihilistic perspective can in fact be harmful. Therapists should not assume that they have nothing to offer persons seeking treatment for maladaptive personality traits. The potential benefits of treatment for ASPD have also been summarized well in a recent review of this literature by Salekin [10]. I am personally uncertain, however, that

_____
[1] *Department of Psychology, University of Kentucky, Lexington, KY 40506-0044, USA*

Cloninger's Union in Nature and Silence of the Mind meditations, along with an exposure to elevated artistic creations (e.g. classical music), would really be as effective in the treatment of ASPD as he suggests. Cloninger does cite a study to support his approach, but he also acknowledges that the participants in this study probably had a strong a priori interest in and receptivity to meditative self-reflection. To parallel the past hopes of Fox Mulder in his search for extraterrestial life, "I want to believe" in the benefits of an emphasis on self-transcendence rather than succumb to my generally pessimistic expectations, but it is difficult for me to be optimistic in the likelihood of a radical transformation of ASPD through coherence therapy.

REFERENCES

1. Stoff D.M., Breiling J., Maser J.D. (Eds) (1997) *Handbook of Antisocial Behavior.* Wiley, New York.
2. Cooke D.J., Forth A.E., Hare R.D. (Eds) (1998) *Psychopathy: Theory, Research, and Implications for Society.* Kluwer, Dordrecht.
3. Millon T., Simonsen E., Birket-Smith M., Davis R. (Eds) (1998) *Psychopathy. Antisocial, Criminal, and Violent Behavior.* Guilford, New York.
4. Brinkley C.A., Newman J.P., Widiger T.A., Lynam D.R. (in press) Two approaches to parsing the heterogeneity of psychopathy. *Clin. Psychol: Science and Practice.*
5. Patrick C.J. (1994) Emotion and psychopathy: startling new insights. *Psychophysiology,* **31**: 319–330.
6. Kosson D.S., Gacono C.B., Bodholdt R.H. (2000) Assessing psychopathy: Interpersonal aspects and clinical interviewing. In *The Clinical and Forensic Assessment of Psychopathy: A Practitioner's Guide* (Ed. C.B. Gacono), pp. 203–229. Lawrence Erlbaum, Mahway.
7. Dodge, K.A. (2002) Mediation, moderation, and mechanisms in how parenting affects children's aggressive behavior. In *Parenting and the Child's World: Influences on Academic, Intellectual, and Social–Emotional Development* (Eds J.G. Borkowski, S.L. Ramey), pp. 215–229. Lawrence Erlbaum, Mahwah.
8. Lynam D.R. (2002) Psychopathy from the perspective of the five factor model. In *Personality Disorders and the Five Factor Model,* 2nd edn (Eds P.T. Costa, T.A. Widiger), pp. 325–348. American Psychological Association, Washington.
9. Hare R.D. (1996) Psychopathy: a clinical construct whose time has come. *Criminal Justice and Behavior,* **23**: 25–54.
10. Salekin R.T. (2002) Psychopathy and therapeutic pessimism: clinical lore or clinical reality? *Clin. Psychol. Rev.,* **22**: 79–112.

2.9
An Uphill Battle Being Won
Renato D. Alarcón[1]

The discussion of antisocial personality disorder (ASPD) allows a sobering look at the field of clinical psychiatry in general, and its research endeavours in particular.

An extremely important aspect in the overall perception of this disorder is the cultural dimension. The very term "antisocial" reflects the inherence of environmental factors. Cultural relativism plays an important role, particularly in the light of the media and the general public's tendency to easily introduce clinical terms into everyday jargon [1]. Antisocial is a very broad term; antisocial behaviour can be a coping mechanism to deal with an adverse milieu in large cities and small towns alike, in modern Western world metropolis, and in tiny villages in the Sahara desert, the Australian jungles, or Andean communities in Latin American countries [2]. Furthermore, there are the "charming" or "acceptable" psychopaths, many of them living not precisely in the darkness of jails or in the fringes of a society that considers itself "normal".

It is important to realize the enormous influence of social and cultural aspects in what Robert Cloninger calls "self-aware, immaterial aspects of human personality", and subsumes under the concept of psyche. By the same token, it is legitimate to support, as Cloninger does, the notion of different types of antisocial personalities. The hard core criminal may be at one extreme of this true clinical spectrum, and the charming businessman or politician at the other. The severity of levels (and the need to measure them as accurately as possible) are critical factors, with both diagnostic and therapeutic implications.

It is almost paradoxical that some comorbidities make the antisocial personality disordered patient more amenable to therapeutic interventions. This issue is important in that we need to, first, prove whether it is true, and second, what aspects of these interventions may contribute to the relatively better prognosis of multi-morbid ASPD patients. It is logical to speculate that the psychological predispositions (and their neurophysiological underpinnings) of these individuals can make some of them more receptive to reflection, interpersonal transactions, introspection, relearning processes, capacity to self-transcend, and other concepts cogently examined by Cloninger. Yet, the beautiful correlations between temperament, existing diagnostic categories, and factors such as motivation and goal accomplishment, are somewhat blurred when postulating that any of these temperament configurations can occur "in people with either mature or immature

[1] Mayo Psychiatry and Psychology Treatment Center, Rochester, MN, USA

characters". Isn't immaturity a critical feature of personality disorders? If so, isn't it also legitimate to wonder whether we are then talking about ASPD as a diagnosis, or whether the antisocial behaviour is simply a defective (therefore, hopefully correctable) coping mechanism for individuals affectively or emotionally compromised?

The diagnostic placement of ASPD is another controversial matter. While in recent years the efforts of the authors of DSM and ICD have strengthened the descriptive aspect, it is important to keep in mind Jablensky's comment that the clinical use of this label reflects a trend towards "typologizing" conditions that are essentially multidimensional [3]. Even Cloninger's dimensional terms have fallen into the typological, descriptive, categorical usage to which clinical practitioners are so adept. This is not only a reflection of an "occupational deformity" by hurried clinicians, but also the result of the complexity of a disorder that uses descriptive adjectives more generously than any other existing clinical condition. Even Cloninger's terminology abounds in this kind of terms, for both the depiction of ASPD and his novel "coherence therapy" approach. Moreover, to define a personality disorder as a "description of someone whose thoughts and human relationships are usually lacking in self-awareness" may strike some as too broad or simplistic to be of any use in research.

A related question is whether Cluster B is the best niche for ASPD. Answering those who question the very existence of Axis II in any nosological classification, it could be said that ASPD may be one of the strongest reasons to keep it even if, for instance, the connections between ASPD and somatization, or with substance dependence in the patient and his/her relatives, have not been fully explained. On the issue of gender, it has been said that ASPD in men is what histrionic personality is among women [4]. Indeed, ASPD stands alone in its complexity, and the difficulties to be appropriately grasped and tested.

If we are truly faithful to a multidimensional approach in diagnostic parlance, the notion of spectrum may have, in the antisocial personality, one of its most fertile fields of application. Are only criminals to be labelled as ASPDs? I would submit that the spectrum concept would assist in responding to this question. Moreover, the concept of cluster may even be more precise as it may include features such as narcissism and histrionic behaviour, which are part of other personality types, but seem to be also essential components of ASPD. Do the variations in the spiral movement of self-aware consciousness in ASPD imply clinical variations in the spectrum of antisocial behaviours? Taking from Cloninger's approach, the ASPD spectrum would have to include areas beyond the pure phenomenological description, and get into aetiopathogenic, diagnostic and therapeutic grounds. The neurobiological approach would have to produce much more persuasive evidence related to the underlying dysfunction or disruption. Neuroimaging and genetic studies may only contribute to the eventual clarification of the most severe cases within the spectrum, which leaves out a significant number of patients whose ASPD label then may or may not be valid. In this context, the issue of differential diagnosis with other conditions, including bipolar disorder, is extremely pertinent. Clinicians all over the world face the problem of labelling "moodiness", "irritability", and "dysphoria" as mood rather than personality features, and a variant of bipolarity rather than an autonomous Axis II entity.

This is important also for the effort at translating psychophysiological findings into descriptors of symptomatic remission, and consistent responsiveness to therapy, i.e. amenability to Cloninger's "radical transformation of behaviours". The treatment of ASPD is clearly the most challenging and frustrating aspect of this condition. It starts with therapists from different schools, who do not necessarily agree on some of the key descriptive features, such as "lack of empathy", among ASPD patients. How do we explain the fierce loyalty that true antisocials show towards other members of their gangs? Is this a distorted notion of loyalty, or is it loyalty perverted by external pressures and by what are perceived as oppressive realities? Are we talking about antisocials here? Or would reviving the old terms "asocial" or "dissocial" [5] solve these discrepancies? In fact, Gabbard seems to think that these patients profess significant capacity for empathic discernment, even though it is a rather self-serving feature [6]. The "otherness" of the ASPD may have both a psychological and physiological basis, but neither this somewhat abstract concept nor the current neuro- and psychophysiological findings qualify for a "physiological marker" as suggested by some authors. On the other hand, is the grouping in primary and secondary psychopaths just one way to dress up our varying levels of therapeutic expectations and hopes? Furthermore, the verdict is still out regarding the use of well-structured environments and the setting in which they take place (correctional schools, prisons, and the military).

In short, ASPD embodies all the challenges and complexities of a multidimensional entity, and the need to be truly eclectic in studying its many different aspects. Progress has been made, and yet the trite comment that a lot remains to be done has never been truer than at this point in history. The antisocial behaviour is universal, and yet ASPD patients are unique in their biopsychosocial, cultural, and spiritual contexts. This is an uphill battle that, one would like to think, is being won a little step at a time.

REFERENCES

1. Alarcón R.D., Foulks E.F., Vakkur M. (1998) *Personality Disorders and Culture. Clinical and Conceptual Interactions.* Wiley, New York.

2. Reid W.H. (1985) The antisocial personality: a review. *Hosp. Commun. Psychiatry*, **36**: 831–837.
3. Jablensky A. (2002) The classification of personality disorders: critical review and need for rethinking. *Psychopathology*, **35**: 112–116.
4. Nuckolls C.W. (1992) Toward a cultural history of personality disorders. *Soc. Sci. Med.*, **35**: 37–47.
5. American Psychiatric Association (1952) *Diagnostic and Statistical Manual of Mental Disorders*, 1st edn. American Psychiatric Association, Washington.
6. Gabbard G. (1997) Finding the "person" in personality disorders. *Am. J. Psychiatry*, **154**: 891–893.
7. Frank J.D., Frank J.B. (1993) *Persuasion and Healing*. Johns Hopkins University Press, Baltimore.

2.10
Public Health Approaches to Antisocial Personality Disorder

Giovanni de Girolamo and Mariano Bassi[1]

It is very difficult to write a meaningful comment on such a scholarly work as Cloninger's review on antisocial personality disorder (ASPD). His chapter provides a fascinating and comprehensive account of the developmental roots of ASPD and the clinical and treatment issues involving people affected with this disorder. We can only attempt to highlight a few of the public health issues related to ASPD.

One first, crucial point concerns the staggering frequency of ASPD in correctional settings. A systematic review of 62 surveys, conducted over several decades in 12 countries, assessed the prevalence of mental disorders in prisons [1]. The review identified 28 surveys that had investigated the frequency of ASPD with standardized assessment methods in a total of 13 844 prison inmates. Overall, 47% of males and 21% of females were diagnosed with ASPD. If we extrapolate these results to the world prison population, which includes approximately 9 million people worldwide—with 2 million in the USA [2]—it means that millions of people are imprisoned because of their criminal behaviour, which is, however, closely related to their disordered thinking and behaviour.

In public health terms, the most important question then, is the following: how many of these prisoners receive any sort of treatment for their ASPD? Cloninger has convincingly shown that aversive settings such as prisons are unlikely to trigger and foster the personality changes these subjects require. Unfortunately, effective mental health care in prison settings (with appropriate follow-up in the post-release period) has yet to be invented, introduced,

[1] *Department of Mental Health, Local Health Unit, Bologna, Italy*

and tested on a large-scale basis. An additional paradox is that the few mental health teams working in prisons and similar settings are frequently understaffed and do not include the most skilled and expert clinicians available in the field—contrarily to what might logically be expected, since these patients are among the most difficult to engage and maintain in treatment. This occurs for a variety of reasons (e.g. work in these settings is considered poorly rewarding, is poorly paid, is too emotionally demanding, etc....).

The community management of subjects with ASPD requires teamwork. Indeed "the needs of the severely mentally ill can rarely be met by a single individual" [3]. The difficulty of setting up effective mental health teams to treat patients with ASPD is also related to the fact that "adequate service provision requires explanatory models" [4] and that ASPD has long represented "a most elusive category", as Sir Aubrey Lewis noted thirty years ago [5]. This fact can partly explain the absence of ASPD in most mental health worker training curricula. Effective mental health teams capable of managing ASPD patients must be able to deal with two complex (and related) problems: (a) the management of comorbidity, since substance abuse is closely linked to ASPD [6,7], and (b) the assessment, prevention, and treatment of violent behaviour. Disappointingly, in most countries, and in most residency programs, both study areas are missing from mental health worker training curricula. Consequently, mental health workers are generally unprepared to cope with these difficult patients. Indeed, the treatment of comorbidity is often fraught with difficulty and many patients show poor outcomes despite interventions [8,9]. Managing violent patients in the community is equally difficult, as shown by the first randomized trial comparing intensive case management to standard care in patients with psychosis: intensive care was not more effective in reducing violence in these patients [10].

In evaluating treatment effectiveness, we also need to improve treatment evaluation methods as well as methodologies for pooling and assessing results from different trials. For instance, two of the most recent systematic reviews on the topic [11,12] have come to antithetic conclusions about the effectiveness of therapeutic communities in treating offenders, the first review considering therapeutic communities the *least* effective treatment for personality disordered offenders and the second review considering them the *most* effective! Most of these discrepancies can be explained by the different inclusion criteria used in these reviews. Of the 42 studies examined by Salekin [11], only one was included by Warren *et al.* [12] in their own meta-analysis of 117 trials examining personality disordered offenders. This finding clearly points to a persisting lack of clarity in the field, which needs to be urgently addressed. Furthermore, only a very small percentage of the studies evaluated in these two systematic reviews were conducted in prisons and high-security settings, which should actually be a priority target for any type of intervention.

Generally speaking, any comprehensive strategy to tackle ASPD must involve early recognition and intervention during childhood and adolescence [13]. In fact, very well-designed prospective studies have demonstrated that ASPD not preceded by conduct disorders in adolescence is a rare event [14], and this phenomenon may offer prevention opportunities that are generally missed [15]. In this perspective, recognition and treatment of child and adolescent conduct disorders is a paradigmatic example of the "primary prevention of secondary disorders" [16], since conduct disorders precede both ASPD and other disorders (e.g. substance abuse). As Cloninger also underscores, cognitive-behavioural-oriented, multimodal, well-structured, intensive, and long-term programmes are the types of intervention that will most likely have an impact on adolescents with very disturbed or difficult behaviour [17]. Hence, scientifically rigorous evaluations are needed to establish which types of interventions are most effective, under what circumstances, and for whom.

REFERENCES

1. Fazel S., Danesh J. (2003) Serious mental disorder in 23 000 prisoners: a systematic review of 62 surveys. *Lancet*, **359**: 545–550.
2. Walsmey R. (2000) *World Prison Population List*, 2nd edn. Home Office Research, Development and Statistics Directorate, London.
3. Onyett S. (1992) *Case Management in Mental Health*. Chapman & Hall, London.
4. Taylor P.J. (2000) Balancing policy development and research evidence: are we falling short? *Acta Psychiatr. Scand.*, **102**: 1–2.
5. Lewis A. (1974) Psychopathic personality: a most elusive category. *Psychol. Med.*, **4**: 133–140.
6. Brooner R.K., Herbst J.H., Schmidt C.W., Bigelow G.E., Costa P.T. Jr. (1993) Antisocial personality disorder among drug abusers. Relations to other personality diagnoses and the five-factor model of personality. *J. Nerv. Ment. Dis.*, **181**: 313–319.
7. King V.L., Kidorf M.S., Stoller K.B., Carter J.A., Brooner R.K. (2001) Influence of antisocial personality subtypes on drug abuse treatment response. *J. Nerv. Ment. Dis.*, **189**: 593–601.
8. Drake R., Mercer-McFadden C., Mueser K.T. (1998) Review of integrated mental health and substance abuse treatment for patients with dual disorders. *Schizophr. Bull.*, **24**: 589–608.
9. Havassy B.E., Shopshire M.S., Quigley L.A. (2000) Effects of substance dependence on outcomes of patients in a randomised trial of two case management models. *Psychiatr. Serv.*, **51**: 639–644.
10. Walsh E., Gilvarry C., Samele C., Harvey K., Manley C., Tyrer P., Creed F., Murray R., Fahy T. (2001) Reducing violence in severe mental illness: randomised controlled trial of intensive case management compared with standard care. *Br. Med. J.*, **323**: 1093–1096.

11. Salekin R.T. (2002) Psychopathy and therapeutic pessimism. Clinical lore or clinical reality? *Clin. Psychol. Rev.*, **22**: 79–112.
12. Warren F., Preedy-Fayers K., McGauley G., Pickering A., Norton K., Geddes J.R., Dolan B. (2003) *Review of Treatments for Severe Personality Disorders.* Home Office Research, London.
13. Hill J. (2003) Early identification of individuals at risk for antisocial personality disorder. *Br. J. Psychiatry*, **182** (Suppl. 44): S11–14.
14. Loeber R., Burke J.D., Lahey B.B. (2002) What are adolescent antecedents to antisocial personality disorder? *Crim. Behav. Ment. Health*, **12**: 24–36.
15. Stouthamer-Loeber M., Loeber R. (2002) Lost opportunities for intervention: undetected markers for the development of serious juvenile delinquency. *Crim. Behav. Ment. Health*, **12**: 69–82.
16. Kessler R.C., Price R.H. (1993) Primary prevention of secondary disorders: a proposal and agenda. *Am. J. Commun. Psychol.*, **21**: 607–633.
17. Moran P., Hagell A. (2001) *Intervening to Prevent Antisocial Personality Disorder: A Scoping Review.* Home Office Research, Development and Statistics Directorate, London.

2.11
Antisocial Personality Disorder in its Cultural Context

Levent Küey[1] and Ömer Aydemir[2]

Cloninger's review reminds us that multiple genetic and environmental variables interplay in the construct of antisocial behaviour. Keeping the continuity between childhood disruptive behaviour and antisocial personality disorder (ASPD) in mind, research on the developmental model of the origins of early conduct problems help to enlighten this interplay. Child, family, and sociodemographic factors, and specially, the quality of the caregiving environment all play a significant role in the development of early conduct problems [1]. Child rearing practices are strongly shaped by transgenerational transmission of parenthood styles and cultural norms. These cultural norms and expectations determine whether a specific pattern of behaviour will be categorized as psychopathologic or not. Each culture has its own ways of regulating aggressive and sexual drives; culture can be understood as a complex construct of socially transmitted ideas, feelings, and attitudes that shape behaviour, organize perceptions, and label experiences [2].

Epidemiological data underline the fact that male preponderance for antisocial behaviour is universal, but on the other hand, while the

[1] *Psychiatry Department, Beyoglu Training Hospital and Psychology Department, Istanbul Bilgi University, Istanbul, Turkey*
[2] *Department of Psychiatry, Medical School of Celal Bayar University, Manisa, Izmir, Turkey*

prevalence rates of ASPD is stated to increase in the United States, it is unusually low in East Asia [3]. The cross-cultural differences in the prevalence of ASPD seem not to be an artifact of methodological differences in research but a reflection of a real diversity among cultures. Besides the low prevalence rates, the phenomenology of ASPD seems to differ in Eastern or transitional societies. Although criminality is a specific characteristic of ASPD in every culture, the forms, means and the severity of criminal acts may differ. In Turkey, violent, sadistic, or vandalistic crimes seem to be relatively rare among ASPD patients. In a Turkish sample of 140 subjects with a diagnosis of ASPD, while the lifetime prevalence of involvement in street fights is nearly 89% and the frequency of using weapons is 74%, the prevalence of direct physical assault to individuals is 56% and sexual insult is 19% [4]. In this same sample, the high frequency of imprisonment in the past (88%) showed that criminality was high [5], but characterized by low frequency of pre-planned violent and sadistic antisocial behaviours. Lack of the feeling of guilt accompanied by a strong feeling of shame might result in different clinical patterns of ASPD in Eastern or transitional societies.

The low prevalence rates in Eastern societies as well as the different phenomenology may be due to a variety of reasons: an important one is the strong cohesion in families. Traditional Eastern families share some common features protecting from ASPD: fathers are strong and authoritative, expectations from children are high, family and subcommunity loyalty is prized [3]. On the other hand, as in Turkey, these features may mask the antisocial behaviours. A positive and tolerant attitude towards the disobedient behaviours of male adolescents, before their military service at the age of 18–20, especially by their mothers, provide the young men with an environment suitable for externalizing antisocial behaviours. As if he has permission for impulsive acts, he is called "mad blooded" (the Turkish word used to define a male adolescent). The society reinforces this young boy to behave in a so-called masculine manner: impulsive and aggressive behaviours, alcohol over dosage, staying out very late at nights, changing partners frequently, participating in small fights, offensive reactions when even just the words of others are perceived as offensive towards his and his family's or his subcommunity's identity. The cultural legitimatization of delinquency to some extent, in the name of the young boy's process of masculine gender identification, mask many antisocial behaviours of the adolescent. This might have a normalizing effect on aggressive behaviours. A hidden antisocial pattern, a phenomenon sometimes called "latent antisocial structure" may be observed in either upper or lower classes. Here, if the environment fulfills all the needs of the antisocial individual, no decompensation will be expected in the mental organization [6].

In Western societies, contrary to Eastern culture, severe and overt antisocial behaviours are more easily and individually expressed in a milieu of higher psychosocial freedom, and a lesser interdependence in inter-personal relations. As a result of a clear separation and individualization process, typically, children are separated from their families and become the captains of their own lives, by the end of adolescence. These individuals lack the close social control mechanisms on their aggressive power except for their own mental structure [7].

Transitional societies, as in Turkey, carry pre-modern, modern and even post-modern features in socio-cultural norms. While the traditional family and social ties are loosened, new social structures are not yet formed sufficiently enough to provide widely accepted new processes of social control. Subcommunity and local norms frequently challenge the universal constructs for the expression of aggressivity. Frequently, it is observed that the whole group is acting as an antisocial body against the rules; the high prevalence of disobedience to traffic rules is a significant example. Here, disobedience becomes normative and even adjustive.

The sociocultural context affects the developmental psychopathology and the epidemiology and clinical phenomenology of antisocial, delinquent and criminal behaviours. Specially in societies in transition, which encounter paradigm shifts in many facets of life, including their subcultural heritage and norms, the cultural competency of the psychiatrist in his/her daily clinical work and research becomes a more important issue of scientific concern.

REFERENCES

1. Shaw D.S., Bell R.Q., Gilliom M. (2000) A truly early starter model of antisocial behavior revisited. *Clin. Child Fam. Psychol. Rev.*, **3**: 155–172.
2. Lu F.G., Lim R.F., Mezzich J.E. (1995) Issues in the assessment and diagnosis of culturally diverse individuals. In *Review of Psychiatry*, Vol. 14 (Eds. J. Oldham, M. Riba), pp. 842–844. American Psychiatric Press, Washington.
3. Paris J. (1996) Antisocial personality disorder: a biopsychosocial model. *Can. J. Psychiatry*, **41**: 71–80.
4. Turkcapar M.H., Akdemir A., Sayar K., Bahcekapili H. (2000) Sociodemographic features and childhood characteristics of men with antisocial personality disorder: a comparative study. *J. Psychol. Psychiatry Psychopharmacol.*, **8**: 11–16 [in Turkish].
5. Sayar K., Fidan G., Turkcapar M. H., Ceyhun E. (2000) Hopelessness and alexithymia in antisocial personality disorder. *Psychiatry in Turkey*, **1**: 10–20 [in Turkish].
6. Ak I., Sayar K. (2002) Sociobiological factors in antisocial personality disorder. *Bull. Clin. Psychopharmacol.*, **12**: 155–158 [in Turkish].
7. Gabbard G.O. (2000) *Psychodynamic Psychiatry in Clinical Practice*, 3rd edn. American Psychiatric Press, Washington.

3

Borderline and Histrionic Personality Disorders: A Review

Michael H. Stone

Columbia College of Physicians and Surgeons, 225 Central Park West, New York, NY 10024, USA

INTRODUCTION

By the time, a quarter century ago, when the two personality disorders of this chapter—borderline personality disorder (BPD) and histrionic personality disorder (HPD)—were incorporated into the personality disorder section (Axis II) of DSM-III [1], each had undergone a curious evolution, such that they emerged draped in criteria sets that differed importantly from the ways in which "borderline" and "hysteric" (the older term for HPD) had earlier been described. Borderline had been a term of art chiefly in psychoanalytic circles, denoting a group of difficult patients thought to be in the borderland between the healthier "neurotic" patients and psychotic, presumably schizophrenic, patients. But the definition of BPD in DSM-III referred to an unstable condition with strong links to affective disorders, not schizophrenia. Meantime, the millennia-old term *hysteric* was replaced by a term less prejudicial to women: *histrionic*. The old definition (of hysteric character) designated a well-functioning group of patients, "ideal" candidates for psychoanalysis. The criteria for HPD, in contrast, depicted a group of poorly-functioning angry, infantile, over-emotional patients who resembled the hysteric patients only in their emotional excess. In fact, those with HPD now resemble the emotionally unstable, angry BPD patients. On the other hand, many BPD patients are comorbid not only for bipolar II disorder (more than was so of the older, broader definitions of "borderline"), but also for other "dramatic cluster" personality disorders—chiefly HPD. It seems reasonable, therefore, that we discuss BPD and HPD in the same chapter.

Personality Disorders. Edited by Mario Maj, Hagop S. Akiskal, Juan E. Mezzich and Ahmed Okasha.
©2005 John Wiley & Sons Ltd: ISBN 0-470-09036-7

BORDERLINE PERSONALITY DISORDER

There are a number of unusual features about BPD. Although this is only one of ten personality disorders catalogued in the Axis II portion of the DSM-IV [2], it overshadows all the others in relation to the literature devoted to it, to the proportion of time this disorder occupies in the working life of mental health professionals, and to the percentage of personality-disordered patients who appear to exemplify it. In any search of the psychiatric literature, antisocial personality disorder (ASPD) runs a distant second in the number of citations; the others are represented sparsely. Of the 363 conditions listed in DSM-IV, apart from a few eponymous disorders (Asperger's, Rett's, Tourette's), "borderline" is alone in conveying on its surface no hint of what kind of condition it might be. The others, even if their names harken back to old Greek, Latin or Anglo-Saxon roots, announce with some specificity their true nature (anorexia, dementia, reading disorder...). Another peculiarity of BPD resides in its defining features, which now consists of nine "items" in DSM-IV (one more than were noted in the DSM-III of 1980) [1]. If we accept that a personality *trait*, strictly speaking, is an ingrained, habitual way of psychological functioning that emerges during the developmental years [3] and then crystallizes in adult life [4], then we see that, arguably, only three of the BPD items are true personality traits (impulsivity, moodiness, anger), though each of these is carried in BPD to the level of a highly troublesome, symptomatic behaviour. BPD differs in this respect from most of the other criteria for the remaining personality disorders, which are indeed traits in the customary sense (mistrustfulness, aloofness, deceitfulness, shallowness, etc.). One consequence of this reliance on symptom-based, as opposed to trait-based, definitions is that BPD differs more noticeably across cultures than is the case with, for example, schizoid personality disorder. The aloofness that one encounters in schizoid persons is similar the world over. Yet when BPD is diagnosed in Scandinavia or Japan, for example, the typical patients are less angry or tempestuous than their American counterparts; those diagnosed in Japan, though they engage in suicidal behaviours, show most strikingly the traits of dependent personality disorder [5–7].

The term *borderline* represents the interface between traditional psychiatry and psychoanalysis. First used in the late 1800s to denote conditions in the "borderland" between psychosis and the milder "neurotic" conditions [8], borderline was later used in the 1920s, as psychoanalysis was becoming popular, to designate conditions that were not readily amenable to psycho-analytic therapy, yet were not so clearly non-analysable as were the psychoses. In other terms, these conditions were considered borderline with respect to psychosis, especially schizophrenia (which at that time was defined very broadly) [9]. Some of the early descriptors were hypersensitivity to criticism, "masked" depression, ego-weakness, infantile qualities, rage outbursts, and a tendency to externalize blame [10]. One spoke of the borderline *neurosis, state, condition,* or *syndrome* [10–12]. Only with the publication of Kernberg's paper [13] was the term *personality* introduced, within the new phrase: borderline personality organization (BPO). What was meant here was not personality in the usual sense of one's enduring traits, so much as an organization of the whole mind or the Self. Kernberg was making a distinction between a higher (*neurotic*) level of mental organization, where identity-sense and reality testing were both intact, and a lower (*psychotic*) level, where both these functions were grossly impaired. In "borderline" organization, reality testing was preserved (albeit with a tendency to "over-valued ideas" about certain emotion-laden areas), but identity-sense was weakened. The aetiology of BPO remained obscure—an excess of "innate aggression" was suggested—but the concept was now decoupled from that of schizophrenia. *Borderline* was now on its own.

A number of competing usages gained currency: "borderline" as a manifestation of arrested development in the separation-individuation stage [14–16], as a descriptor of the "difficult" patient [17], as a label for four groups of patients (spanning the proximity to psychosis on up to the higher-functioning "anaclitic-depressed" types) [12], as designating a type of narcissistic injury [18], and as a personality disorder defined by criteria that were more easily measured and objectifiable than those of previous definitions [19]. This last concept of a *borderline personality disorder* became one of the two sources (the other being Kernberg's BPO) upon which DSM-III had drawn, when in 1980 BPD was officially included in the "Axis II" section for personality disorders. The strong influence of Kernberg, later of Gunderson, contributed to the retention of the word "personality" in the newly defined *borderline* disorder. This accounts also for BPD being placed in Axis II rather than in Axis I, even though the definition contains more symptoms than traits.

The evolution of the borderline concept as sketched above led to a description of BPD that, besides being distinct from that of schizophrenia, was characterized by a constellation of attributes: a stormy life-style, impulsive behaviour, suicide threats, anger that was easily provoked and excessive in magnitude, lability of mood, and (to a lesser extent) brief psychotic episodes that might have a depressive or paranoid cast, but were not classically schizophrenic [20]. The emerging definition of BPD contributed to another unusual feature of this disorder: by virtue of its dependency on rather non-specific symptoms, with less reliance upon specific traits, BPD is remarkably heterogeneous, and can be found in conjunction with many disorders of Axis I [21] and with almost all of the other Axis II disorders [22,23], though rarely with schizoid personality disorder [7]. Among the Axis I disorders, those commonly encountered include major depression [9], bipolar II disorder [24–30], eating disorders [31], anxiety disorders (such as panic, social anxiety, obsessive-compulsive disorder) [25], substance abuse [27], dissociative disorders [32,33], post-traumatic stress disorder (PTSD) [34], erotomania [35] and other forms of obsessive love [36], and impulsive aggression [37]. Though BPD is encountered mostly in female patients (where overlap with affective disorders of various types is common [25]), male patients exhibiting the condition are apt to show an admixture of antisocial features and a tendency to violence. Violent behaviour is less common in the female patients; when it occurs, it is usually in the context of a failed real or fantasied romance [35,36] or of pathological jealousy [38]. A comprehensive account of symptom pictures that may accompany BPD, including even such rarities as factitious illness, is given by Kernberg *et al.* [39].

The Many Faces of Borderline Personality Disorder

The large number of conditions and other personality configurations that commonly accompany BPD would by itself tend to create considerable variation in the clinical picture of any sample of BPD patients, whether the sample derived from ambulatory or institutional sources. Gender differences have been noted in controlled studies of Axis II comorbidity: male borderlines, for example, were more likely to show antisocial, passive–aggressive, sadistic and narcissistic traits, whereas avoidant and dependent traits were common to both sexes [40,41]. Differences of this kind have led to disagreement among psychiatrists as to the "real" or essential nature of BPD, and to controversy concerning the ideal treatment. Diagnostic labelling can also be affected: clinicians with a primary interest in BPD may see certain patients with strong narcissistic traits as "borderline, with narcissistic features", while another clinician with a primary focus on narcissistic personality disorder may characterize the same patients as "narcissistic, with borderline features".

The multiplicity of aetiological factors is another confounding variable. Genetic, constitutional, and environmental factors have been implicated [7]; many BPD patients show an admixture of several such factors. Many reports on this topic are based on small samples. If an investigator works in a centre where the majority of BPD patients have been incest victims, then the disorder will likely be ascribed to the "trauma factor" [34]. In other samples, bipolar II disorder will appear, correctly, as the chief underlying factor [25]. Cultural differences also have their impact on what is "typical" for BPD in certain locales: the confluence of BPD with dissociative disorders has been noted by a number of investigators in the USA [42,43], but is especially common in Turkey [44]. The interplay of certain traumatic factors and borderline personality that predispose to dissociative phenomena has been documented by Zanarini *et al.* [45], who found four factors associated with later dissociation: inconsistent treatment by a caretaker, sexual abuse by a caretaker, witnessing sexual violence as a child, and adult rape history. There is an interaction between the abuse—especially, the sexual abuse—factor and the gender disparity in BPD. The greater the childhood sexual abuse (especially with penile penetration), the more severe the symptoms experienced by the future BPD (predominantly female) patients [46]. Women appear to have a greater predisposition to affective disorders, constitutionally, but certainly are at greater risk for childhood sexual abuse, intrafamilial as well as extrafamilial. The tendency to a dissociative disorder is probably linked to subtle neurobiological differences—of a sort that render certain persons more vulnerable to dissociative phenomena, given the stress of early traumata, in constrast to other persons who respond to similar traumata with paranoid personality, antisocial behaviours, etc. À propos biological correlates, work has been underway only in the last few years, using positron emission tomography (PET) [47] and functional magnetic resonance imaging (f-MRI) [48] among other techniques, to elucidate the brain differences that may underlie these tendencies. Bremner *et al.* [47], for example, found that women who had experienced both sexual abuse and PTSD showed failure of hippocampal activation and reduced hippocampal volume, when compared with women who had neither abuse nor PTSD. Depression was common in the affected group, as was substance abuse. It is not clear how many would also be considered "borderline", though the early background and symptom picture were similar to many BPD patients. This common symptom-picture of "interpersonal stress, affective instability, impulsivity, and self-injurious behaviour or dissociation" is increasingly understood as stemming from an interaction of genetic and environmental factors that "lead to brain alterations that are the basis for specific presentations of BPD, such as self-injurious and impulsive–aggressive behaviour" [49].

Diagnostic Reliability

After BPD was included as one of the personality disorders of DSM in 1980 (DSM-III), studies of inter-rater reliability were undertaken. Good kappa coefficients of reliability were obtained in a number of such studies [50,51], whether focusing on outpatients or on inpatients. Certain descriptors in DSM-III could be more readily assessed than others: higher reliability attached to items like impulsivity, stormy relationships, and inordinate anger than to more subjective concepts like identity disturbance [20]. A diagnostic schema composed of more easily objectifiable items, developed by Gunderson and his colleagues—the Diagnostic Interview for Borderlines (DIB) [52]—was shown to achieve high reliability by trained judges at other centres, with kappas of 0.80 [53]. This high reliability is maintained also with the revised version (DIB-R) [54].

When clinicians' diagnoses were compared with patients' self-report diagnoses, using the Personality Diagnostic Questionnaire, general lack of agreement was found for the various personality disorders, but the best kappa score (0.46) was for BPD [55]. From the standpoint of face validity, others criticized the DSM set on the grounds that some of the criteria for BPD lacked specificity, and seemed merely to define a nonspecific type of serious character pathology [56]. More recently, several groups of investigators have tested self-report questionnaires designed to be compatible with the DSM criterion set for BPD. One such, the Borderline Personality Inventory (BPI), based on Kernberg's BPO, showed good sensitivity and specificity, and was compatible both with Gunderson's DIB and with the latest DSM, thus emerging as a useful screening instrument for BPD [57]. Similar work has been done with Kernberg's BPO: the Inventory of Personality Organization (IPO) was developed to assess three BPO components: reality testing, primitive defences, and identity diffusion [58]. High scores on these components of the self-report instrument are in turn associated with negative affect, aggressive dyscontrol (akin to impulsivity and inordinate anger) and dysphoria (analogous with lability of mood)— fundamental concepts of "borderline-ness" that link up with BPD (by either the Gunderson's or the DSM definition). Still, BPO represents a much broader domain within the total field of psychopathology, encompassing those of Gunderson and DSM. Approximately four times as many persons would meet BPO criteria in an epidemiological survey than would BPD: some 10% of the community, as opposed to 2.5% for BPD. This is because schizotypal, paranoid, many schizoid, depressive-masochistic, hypomanic, and antisocial persons would also fit under the BPO umbrella.

At first glance there would seem to be a paradox in the situation where BPD shows good reliability and "tightness" as a diagnostic concept, yet can be associated clinically, as we have noted, with a bewildering array of other Axis I and personality disorders, to a far greater extent than any other DSM-defined personality disorder. An analogy with a quite different phenom-enon may make this seeming paradox more understandable. Imagine the "dumpling" section of a Chinese menu. The dumplings may be filled with all manner of ingredients: pork, beef, chicken, mushrooms, shrimp. But from the *outside*, all the dumplings appear nearly identical. This "outside" is BPD. The "inside" is any of the dozen Axis I disorders (depression, cyclothymia, dysthymia, bipolar II disorder, PTSD, premenstrual tension, temporal lobe epilepsy, alcoholism, other substance abuse, anorexia, bulimia . . .), almost any of the other personality disorders, or any combination thereof [59]. A similar comment was made concerning psychodiagnosis in general: "Some psychiatric illnesses may turn out to be clusters of diseases that may have similar symptoms but require different treatments" [60]. Here, the "similar symptoms" are the constellation of descriptors that make up BPD. The "different treatments" are a function of the great diversity of psychiatric conditions that may accompany the BPD, creating the necessity for different therapeutic approaches. These we will examine further on.

The Genetic Component of BPD

Since the reconceptualization of "borderline" by Kernberg in 1967 [13], upon which he expanded in a later book [61], and particularly since BPD was incorporated into DSM, BPD has been an entity apart from schizophrenia. A new definition arose—that of schizotypal personality disorder (SPD)—to occupy the territory immediately surrounding the central concept of schizophrenia, whose descriptors were much nearer to what clinicians meant by an "almost schizophrenic" condition: eccentric thinking, ideas of reference, suspiciousness, constricted affect, and the like. None of these descriptors were a part of the emerging concept of BPD. Evidence that SPD truly belonged, genetically, in the penumbra of schizophrenia came from various family studies, such as that of Baron *et al.* [62]. This still left open the question: was BPD related as a close cousin to the other major psychosis, bipolar disorder? Some of the descriptors had, after all, an affective coloration: mood lability, inordinate anger, suicidal behaviours. The long-term follow-up studies of BPD in the 1980s again argued against the connection to schizophrenia, and suggested at least a partial kinship with affective disorders, given that a proportion of young BPD patients went on, 10 to 25 years later, to develop unmistakable bipolar I or (more often) bipolar II disorders, or else unipolar depression [63,64].

The twin studies did not shed much light on the question: the first one, done twenty years ago, was based on a small sample (10 borderline same-sexed twin probands) and did not show a relationship with affective disorders [65]. A more recent study, however, acknowledges that genetic influences (of some sort) do in all likelihood play a role in the pathogenesis of BPD—as they do in all personality disorders [66]. The evidence suggested high heritability levels, if not for the entire BPD syndrome, at least for some of the key ingredient traits, such as aggressivity and separation anxiety [67].

In a follow-up study that did not address the issue whether BPD was or was not a condition within the affective "spectrum", it was noted that, when BPD and unipolar depression (UNI) occurred together, the risk for certain symptoms was heightened: substance abuse and suicide risk. BPD patients who were not comorbid for UNI had a low suicide rate (2%) [68]. Because depressive symptoms of one kind or another are common in persons with many of the DSM Axis II disorders, some have felt that the relationship between BPD and affective disorder is weak and non-specific [69]. Others, again without commenting on any genetic link between affective disorder and BPD, note that, phenomenologically, adolescents with both major depression and substance abuse (as opposed to those with just one of the two) were more apt to be diagnosed with BPD [70].

When viewed from the perspective of temperament (that is, inborn personality tendencies), research by Cloninger and his colleagues suggests that the temperamental trait called novelty seeking (that may be a function of high brain dopamine levels) is common to most of the "dramatic" Cluster B disorders, including BPD (but not narcissistic personality disorder) [71]. BPD is also characterized in this temperament model by fairly high harm avoidance, but low reward dependence. Their data point to inherited tendencies to certain traits common to BPD (such as intolerance of being alone), though leaving aside the question about any connection to bipolar disorder. Similar to the findings of the Cloninger group, a study from New Zealand showed high novelty seeking in BPD patients, along with high harm avoidance and greater anger than found in other personality disordered patients [72].

A recent controlled family study of outpatients with BPD who happened not to have mood disorder, and who were compared with mood disorder patients, revealed that familial aggregation of psychiatric disorders was similar for both groups; the relatives of the BPD probands had increased rates of mood disorders (as did the relatives of the mood disorder group). This suggested that there may indeed be common aetiological factors between BPD and affective disorder [73], as was proposed earlier in a non-controlled study of BPD patients and their first-degree relatives [74]. The two foregoing studies were based on small samples, a shortcoming that needs to be rectified, as Siever et al. [75] point out, by large-scale family studies with careful diagnostic demarcation and measurement of endo-phenotypes. Still, as of this time, these authors argue that the family, adoptive and twin studies carried out thus far converge to support an underlying genetic component in BPD. But they caution that the genetic basis for the disorder may be stronger for certain dimensions such as impulsivity/aggression and affective instability, rather than for the border-line syndrome as a whole. In line with Cloninger's data, these dimensions may be linked with abnormal levels of key neurotransmitters: impulsive aggression with reduced brain serotonergic activity; affective instability with increased responsivity of cholinergic systems [76].

Follow-up Studies of BPD

The DSM definition of BPD is category-based and polythetic (allowing for over 200 combinations of 5 or more items to fulfil the diagnostic criteria). There are shortcomings in such a model, given the subtleties and complexities one encounters among patients. Viewed dimensionally, for example, some patients *almost* fulfil the DSM criteria, yet seem "borderline" to most clinicians. And we have noted the myriad admixtures of Axis I disorders and other personality profiles that BPD patients routinely present. Even so, the recognition of BPD in DSM-III was a great step forward: it facilitated research into the very validity of the concept itself, into underlying biological and environmental factors, and into the effectiveness of various therapeutic approaches.

There was now vigorous pursuit of follow-up research, thanks to the greater uniformity and reliability of diagnosis, which appreciably reduced the vagueness of the term "borderline" in the years before 1980. A number of studies, all retrospective in design, of formerly hospitalized BPD patients were reported in the late 1980s [64,77–81]. The patients came from all socioeconomic strata, and were mostly in their late teens or early 20s when hospitalized. One of the more robust findings was that about two-thirds of the BPD patients, when evaluated 10 to 25 years later, were functioning at levels compatible with Global Assessment Scores [82] in the mid-60s: "some mild symptoms...but generally functioning pretty well, has some meaningful inter-personal relationships". An equally robust finding, from the other side of the spectrum, was that 3% to 9% of the former patients had committed suicide. The younger the average age of the sample, the higher the rate, since the younger patients had more of the high-risk (3rd decade of life) years to pass through. The larger samples [64,78] yielded large enough subgroups of BPD patients to examine the impact of certain variables. Factors that augured well, prognostically, were high intelligence, self-discipline, artistic talent, attractiveness, and (in the case of borderlines who abused alcohol) ability to commit to Alcoholics Anonymous. Factors associated with poor prognosis (including suicide) included incest by a member of the older generation, parental cruelty, antisocial comorbidity, and chaotic impulsivity (as manifested, for example, by meeting all 8 of the DSM-III criteria). Those who continued to abuse alcohol had a suicide rate of 37%. The suicide rate in BPD was comparable across the studies with that of bipolar disorder or schizophrenia, indicating the seriousness of the condition, despite the majority of the BPD patients outperforming (given a long enough time period) patients with a psychosis. Many patients, as they entered their 30s, began to improve significantly, and no longer met criteria for BPD [83]. 8% or 10% of the adolescents or young adults with BPD went on to develop various forms of affective disorder (bipolar II, or unipolar depression); almost none became schizophrenic.

The results of the long-term studies were encouraging, inasmuch as the impressionistic, short-term studies that preceded them suggested that "borderlines" shared a fate not much different from that of schizophrenics [84]. The same was true of a Danish 20-year follow-up of child and adolescent "borderlines": 40% of 50 adolescents were schizotypal (i.e. "borderline schizophrenics" of the older terminology); 60% had BPD. Many of the schizotypal patients went on to develop schizophrenia, especially those with a childhood onset. By 20 years, the BPD patients had done better than their schizotypal counterparts. The overall suicide rate was 10%, and substance abuse was usually an accompanying factor [85].

Subsequent follow-up work relied more on a prospective design, since the latter promised greater accuracy, and was less at the mercy of the memories, by patients and their relatives, of events from many years earlier.

The recent outcome studies have relied on smaller samples (from 30 to 44 subjects) than the long-term studies of the 1980s (some of which were carried out in 100–200 subjects), and shorter time spans. They have usually been naturalistic and without control groups, though some have compared a particular favoured approach with "treatment as usual" (TAU). A group from Australia [86] found that outpatients with BPD (DSM-III criteria) did well with a 1-year treatment with a Kohutian self-psychological approach: 9 of the 30 no longer met BPD criteria, and the patients as a whole showed less symptom severity, violence, self-harm and hospitalizations than was noted in the pre-treatment phase. Linehan *et al.* [87] carried out a randomized clinical trial with dialectic-behavioural therapy (DBT) versus TAU in the community. Evaluated at 6 months and 1 year into the treatments, the DBT group showed better function and lower rates of suicide gestures and other forms of self-harm ("parasuicidal" behaviours) than the TAU patients; the improvements continued to hold up later on at a 1-year follow-up.

In another naturalistic study, prospective, though without a control group, BPD patients showed a rise in global function from the "poor" (Global Assessment Score, GAS 31–49) to the "fair" (GAS 51–60) level three years after initial evaluation. A few showed decline in function, but erratic (generally uphill, but with brief downturns) improvement was the norm [88]. Less encouraging were the results of a Finnish study in which 42 BPD patients (70% of an original 62) were treated as inpatients for 3 months and then followed for 3 years [89]. At the end of the 3 years, only a third were "continually fit for work", whereas half were "chronically unfit for work". These results resembled those of the short-term (less than 5 years) studies of the 1970s.

In a recent study, mirroring that of Linehan in design, a group of BPD patients in England were treated either with psychoanalytically oriented partial hospitalization (POPH), or with TAU [90]. Here, the POPH patients outperformed the TAU patients, in that, at 18-month follow-up, they showed greater improvement in social and interpersonal functioning, less self-harm, and less need for full inpatient care.

Follow-up study of BPD is beset with some special problems. The great diversity and heterogeneity of the condition requires large sample sizes in order to ensure even approximate similarity across studies from different centres and countries. We now know that many BPD patients do better than was once thought, but the good results are not usually discernible for many years. The studies that have used TAU as a "control" are suspect, because the TAU is much skimpier in what is offered the patients than what is given via the main treatment approach—making it easier for the latter to prove its "superiority". A way around this difficulty is to create a randomized prospective study using several "main" methods (psychodynamic, cognitive-behavioural, supportive), administered by therapists of equal training and experience, who provide their patients equal amounts of therapy-time per week. Such an endeavour would involve about 300 BPD patients, 60 therapists, and the research-team administering standardized questionnaires, plus follow-up of at least 10 years—at a cost in the millions of dollars. Clearly, we will have to learn what we can from much less ambitious projects.

Treatment for Borderline Patients

For many years the mainstay in the treatment of borderline patients, whether in the pre-DSM era or after, was psychoanalytically oriented psychotherapy. There are now so many alternative therapies for BPD, one wonders how this came about. A bit of history will explain. Up till the late 19th century, psychiatry concerned itself mostly with the very ill—those with psychosis—who required institutional care. The less ill, "ambulatory", patients were seen first by the hypnotists, and then, at the turn of the 20th century, by Freud and the pioneering generation of analysts. Their sickest patients—too disturbed for conventional analysis as it was evolving, but not so ill as to need hospitalization—were the in-between cases, the "borderlines". DSM-III made a cleavage between the more *cognitively* disturbed of the "borderlines"—henceforth to be called schizotypal personality, and the more *affectively* disturbed (and incidentally, more reachable psychotherapeutically)—henceforth to be called simply "borderline personality": our BPD.

In lockstep with this change was the development of alternative therapeutic approaches. Currently the approaches most widely employed are the supportive, the cognitive-behavioural, and the psychoanalytically oriented—each with many variations and names. Some who have written extensively on supportive techniques rely on psychoanalytic theory as their explanatory model [91,92]; others rely more on an interpersonal model inspired by Harry Stack Sullivan [93,94]. Cognitive-behavioural therapies (CBT) emphasize working with the patient's faulty assumptions about self and others through the use of reason, as in the therapies of Beck [95] and Ellis [96]. Linehan's DBT [97] represents an adaptation of CBT specifically for BPD patients. The psychoanalytically oriented approaches emphasize work with the transference, but mostly in relation to the "here-and-now", rather than to early childhood (as in classical analysis). In this domain, the guidelines proposed by Kernberg [98] (called "transference-focused therapy" or TFP) and Gunderson (called "exploratory therapy") [99] are currently in wide use. Recently, the American Psychiatric Association published a set of guidelines that embodies elements of all three approaches [100].

Although supportive techniques constitute the foundation for all forms of therapy, there are as yet no controlled studies comparing their effectiveness with dynamic and behavioural methods, though one such is underway [101]. Meanwhile, the effectiveness of supportive psychotherapy has been demonstrated for personality disorders in general (as leading to a seven-fold faster rate of recovery) [102], and has been suggested also for BPD [103,104].

Results from Recent Treatment Studies, including Evidence-based Studies

At 5-year follow-up, female BPD patients treated with multimodal therapy (that might include group, family, as well as individual supportive and exploratory therapies) at McLean Hospital showed a steady decline in suicidal behaviour, but suicidal ideation and (milder forms of) self-harm did not decline notably; in relation to self-harm, most patients showed a fluctuating course and had higher levels of baseline dysphoria [105]. At 6-year follow-up in the larger group ($n = 290$) of borderline inpatients at McLean Hospital, 74% no longer met (full) BPD criteria [106]. In this study, it was noted that impulsive symptoms resolved the most quickly; affective symptoms were the most stubborn.

The effectiveness of analytically oriented therapy, compared with TAU, in the randomized English study [90] has already been mentioned; this method achieved a reduction in suicidal and self-mutilatory acts and an improvement in depressive symptoms—which began at 6 months of treatment, and continued for the 18 months of the study [107].

Comparable results were achieved with TFP, carried out under the auspices of Kernberg's Personality Disorder Institute in New York. BPD outpatients in this program (which emphasizes clarification and transference interpretation, integration of split-off affects and attitudes toward self and others) showed reduced number of suicidal acts and less need for in-patient care, as became demonstrable after 6 to 8 months of twice-weekly therapy (along with whatever medications seemed indicated) [108].

As for Linehan's DBT, the emphasis is on a number of special interventions: validation, skills coaching, acceptance interventions, and suppression of "secondary gain". A patient about to cut herself, for example, may phone her therapist *before* doing so (the ensuing conversation often eliminates the urge to self-harm), but no phone call is permitted if the patient calls *after* having cut herself—a technique designed to extinguish the tendency to self-mutilation or to manipulative suicide gestures [109].

A group in the Netherlands were able to duplicate her findings [110]; namely, that female BPD patients, when treated for a year with either DBT or TAU, showed greater reduction in self-mutilating and self-damaging impulsive behaviours if they had been randomized into DBT. Though DBT was developed for outpatient borderlines, a variant was recently developed that begins with a 3-month period of inpatient care; preliminary results also show a dramatic reduction in parasuicidal acts within several months [111]. This modification will now be adapted for a randomized controlled study. DBT has also been applied to other clinical tasks: the reduction of anger levels [112], and more recently, the treatment of BPD patients with eating disorders [113], substance abuse [114], and opioid dependency [115].

In common with theoreticians of all the dominant schools of therapy, DBT assumes that the emotional dysregulation characteristic of BPD patients is a function not of just environmental/family factors, but of an interaction between these and biological factors. This view underlies the DBT family therapy model currently being developed [116].

Pharmacotherapy

The use of medications in the treatment of BPD is to combat the symptoms which almost invariably accompany the disorder, especially in the initial stages. The main target symptoms are affective, impulsive and (to a lesser extent) cognitive. The medications most favoured currently are the selective serotonin reuptake inhibitors (SSRIs) for depression, and various mood stabilizers for those patients with hypomanic or bipolar II symptoms: lithium, valproic acid [117] or lamotrigine. Valproic acid has also been found to reduce anger and irritability in BPD patients with bipolar II disorder comorbidity [118].The SSRIs have been found useful in alleviating impulsive aggression, as noted in a recent randomized, placebo-controlled, double-blind study [119]. Impulsive aggression is understood in broad terms by some, who consider it a core dimension of BPD, and include within it aggression directed against both *others* (such as domestic violence, property destruction) and self (suicide attempts, self-mutilation, substance abuse). Actually several types of medication have been found useful in minimizing this aspect: SSRIs, atypical antipsychotics such as olanzapine [120], and mood stabilizers [121].

Symptom reduction via medication, while extremely important in the overall treatment of BPD, does little to ameliorate the lingering maladaptive personality traits that typify the disorder (and that long outlive the amelioration of symptoms): clinginess, manipulativeness, vehemence, mercuriality, action-proneness, unruliness, boredom, demandingness, touchiness, etc. For this reason, pharmacotherapy plays a complementary role in the complete approach to the treatment of BPD, alongside psychotherapy in its various forms (including individual, group, family, 12-step, etc., depending on the particularities of each case).

HISTRIONIC PERSONALITY DISORDER

HPD is the term by which DSM-III and IV sought to replace the much older designation: hysterical personality (HyP) [122] or (as the condition was called in the psychoanalytic literature) hysterical character [123]. This taxonomic change was inspired by the desire to avoid further stigmatization of women, given that "hysteria"—stemming from the Greek word for womb—was connected with the notion of behavioural excess and emotional wildness, ascribed since Hippocrates' time to the ill effects of a womb that had somehow travelled to the brain, there to stir up an over-emotionality manifested, so it was believed, only by women [7]. Ironically, HyP was considered by the early generations of psychoanalysts as a healthier condition, nearer to the most mature stage in Freud's developmental schema, than was compulsive character, even though the latter was presumably more common in men. The hallmark of HyP was (in women) coquetry in gait, gaze and speech, paired with apprehensiveness [123], along with suggestibility and quick changes of mood and behaviour. There was a diminished tendency to sublimation. In men one would see softness and over-politeness, feminine facial expression and feminine behaviour. Before HPD was described in DSM, it had already been noted that the clinical picture in some persons with HyP was much sicker. Serious "pre-oedipal" conflicts were present—in what was felt to be prominent "oral", rather than (healthier) genital issues [124]. This observation led to the coining of various labels: hysteroid [125] (meaning like hysteric, only more disturbed); infantile [61] (which amounted to hysteric traits in persons functioning at the borderline level); and hysteroid dysphoric [126] (signifying hysteroid + depressive). Patients so diagnosed presented with the picture of marked impulsivity, open and crude seductiveness, gross attention seeking and florid theatricality, severe separation anxiety defended against by clinginess, and a ragefulness if rejected or disappointed in a love relationship [127]. Whereas those with HyP show a rigid conscience, in HPD one often sees primitivity of defences and an amorality that is reminiscent of antisocial personality [128]. In establishing a criterion set for HPD that answers only to the more disturbed, maladaptive variant (i.e. the hysteroid, or infantile), DSM has in effect rendered HyP a no longer detectable entity (for it is "sub-clinical" with respect to HPD), even though the milder form continues to exist in the community, presumably in greater frequency than HPD.

There is little agreement in the epidemiology literature about the prevalence of HPD: 12% in females and 0% in males, in an Australian study [129]; 1 to 3% of the population in another study [130], albeit 10–15% of patients in clinical settings [131]. Whatever the figures, they are not very meaningful. This is because the essential feature—exaggerated emotionality—exists on a continuum that spans mild "hysteric" traits, to hysteric character, then sub-clinical HPD (e.g. 3 or 4 of the 8 items in DSM, rather than 5 or more), and finally to HPD. Furthermore, as with BPD, HPD almost never occurs in "pure" form, unalloyed with the traits of other DSM disorders. The combination of HPD with BPD is common [132], as is the mixture of HPD with narcissistic personality disorder (one of the DSM items is itself "narcissistic": needing to be the centre of attention). HPD (nearly identical with the extraverted, aggressive hysteroid personality [133]), if mixed with depressive features, is essentially the same as what others have called hysteroid dysphoria. Compared with HyP patients, those with HPD are more likely to abuse alcohol and other substances [134].

The Gender Question

Thorny and politically loaded questions have arisen as to whether HPD is predominantly a condition of women, or whether the descriptions used to define HPD have been "rigged" by men to make it appear so, by way of ensuring that the "weaker" sex remains weaker in appearance (i.e. more suggestible, more vain, less capable of organized thought). The criteria do seem to elicit a feminine stereotype [135]. Of interest, raters asked to react to the criterion sets of HPD (and dependent personality disorder) assume they are associated with "female"; those of compulsive and antisocial personality disorders with "male" [136].

From the viewpoint of evolutionary psychiatry, certain differences between the sexes evolved apparently because of their survival value. Female attractiveness is more important than male attractiveness; male strength and size (in dealing with potential competitors) is more important that female physical strength [137]. Thus the HPD item "uses physical appearance to draw attention to self" may be understood as an exaggeration of a species-relevant need, one that is more relevant to women than to men. In a study of college women with various personality disorders, those with HPD were rated higher in attractiveness than those with other personality disorders [139]. Attractive women had a more varied and supportive social network; those with HPD showed more negative behaviours in close relationships, but were still more accepted as potential mates [64]. Cultural differences may modify this aspect: overt and uninhibited sexuality is more acceptable in Latin than in many Asian cultures [139]. More recent studies suggest that the feminist complaint about HPD as being prejudicial to women was based on inadequate epidemiological data. In young adults, for example, males and females are about *equally* likely to be diagnosed with HPD, but in middle age, HPD is, indeed, seen mostly in women [130]. Males with HPD tended to belong to one of two main groups: (a) passive-feminine men who are either homosexual or, if heterosexual, insecure and inhibited in their sexuality, or (b) heterosexual "Don Juan" types, who used their charm, seductiveness, and flashiness to make one romantic conquest after the other. The Don Juan, with his compulsive sexuality and predatoriness, represents the confluence of HPD with narcissistic and antisocial traits. Some have entertained the idea that HPD and antisocial personality disorder (ASPD) were two sides (the female HPD and male ASPD) of the same coin: namely, the coin of psychopathy [128]. The point here was that both histrionic women and antisocial men utilized psychopathic tactics: exploitativeness, superficial charm, amorality—basically to get something at minimal cost to themselves. In evolutionary terms, both are "free-loaders" who cheat rather than reciprocate [140]. The male deceives the woman about his degree of commitment; the female deceives the male about her faithfulness, lest he worry about his paternity. Some support for this position remains [141,142], but has been challenged by others [143]. The scenario in which psychopathy "causes" both HPD and ASPD is probably more readily explained as a peculiarity of sample variance. That is, some samples of HPD patients may show such a degree of admixture of psychopathic traits and antisocial behaviours as to lend credence to the earlier hypothesis. But there are many other HPD patients who show no such tendencies, apart from the superficial charm and a rather aggressive kind of seductiveness [127].

One might see more of the latter features, and a measure of psychopathic traits, in a sample of HPD patients who had been incest victims [144], when compared with those who had not been.

Clinical Features

When compared with women who had either another, or no, personality disorder, those with HPD show lower sexual assertiveness, more negative attitudes toward sex, greater preoccupation with sex despite lower sexual desire, more orgasmic dysfunction, and greater likelihood to enter into extramarital affairs [145]. Others have emphasized the tendency of those with HPD to seek, with great urgency, protection and affection, rendering them suggestible and overly disposed to adopt the beliefs and attitudes of a lover or mate, in hopes of thus securing that affection [146]. This contributes to the emotional shallowness and lack of authenticity often noted in HPD: a phenomenon akin to the *As-If* personality of the earlier analytic literature [147]. The marked impulsivity of persons with HPD shows its conceptual kinship with BPD, and distinguishes the disorder from the milder HyP [127,148]. HPD patients characteristically show an insecure attachment style [149] and a cognitive style that is global, diffuse, lacking in sharpness [127,150], tending to answer, in response to a question about how life is with their current partner: "Oh, it's great, it's super!" Some have stressed that the intermingling of logical and symbolical thought patterns seen in HPD (and HyP) amount to a kind of dissociation, which in pronounced degree can resemble a formal thought disorder [151,152].

From the perspective of the Five Factor Model of personality [153], HPD is seen as the meeting point of extraversion and (marked) neuroticism [154]. This would accord with the theatricality and emotional dyscontrol in HPD. In contrast to the milder HyP, those with HPD manifest this dyscontrol in more extreme ways: impulsivity with self-destructive overtones (alienating a lover, getting fired from a job), and novelty- or "thrill"-seeking [152]. Characteristics of HPD that are less often mentioned include "secondary gain" from illness, by way of both avoiding difficult situations and gaining sympathy; also, an inability to derive deep satisfaction from any activity or relationship, leading to a pervasive sense of unfulfillment and incompleteness.

Other Perspectives

As there are no long-term follow-up studies devoted exclusively to HPD, we can make only some rough estimates about the fate of persons with this disorder. One study found that Cluster B traits persisted from adolescence to adulthood [155], and predicted an externalizing symptom pattern [156], but did not address treatment issues. Because HPD (as opposed to the milder HyP) is seldom encountered without an admixture of BPD traits, one looks instead to the data on BPD patients who were "co-morbid" for HPD. In one report, there were 49 BPD inpatients (21 with HPD; 28 with the related "infantile" personality) followed for 10 to 25 years [64]. Two-thirds of these were functioning, when traced, at levels consistent with GAS of 61 or more, consistent with good occupational and interpersonal function. Four of the patients (8%) had committed suicide—about average for the borderline patients in that large sample ($n = 206$ with BPD). The "hysterical" (we would call them HPD) patients from the Menninger Study [92] were expected to have the best prognosis (according to the psychoanalytic developmental model) but the few long-term outcomes mentioned fell short of original expectations. Patients with an HPD that is unalloyed with the traits of other Cluster B disorders are exceedingly rare, and there are no evidence-based data, or follow-up results on this small group.

Psychological tests on HPD reveal only what was already expected: the Minnesota Multiphasic Personality Inventory (MMPI) shows predominantly a pattern of high scores on the hysteria and manic scales, and lower score on social introversion (since HPD is associated with extraversion [157]). The Rorschach testing of HPD patients showed higher than average responses involving colour (FC, CF, and C)—considered indices of emotionality [158]. Typical of persons with HPD is a preoccupied attachment style, with some dismissive elements—felt to be consistent with the shallow emotions, yet exaggerated emotionality of this group [159]. Also consistent with the behavioural instability and poor emotional control are the observations on the presumably inborn or temperament parameters of HPD, with high scores on novelty seeking and reward dependence, but low on harm avoidance (the latter correlating with lowered serotonin activity in key brain pathways) [160,161]. Thus there is some evidence for a genetic factor for the temperament aspect of HPD, but not much evidence as to the construct as a whole [162].

As to possible neurophysiological correlates of HPD, one study showed a tendency to cognitive impairment in persons with "dramatic" personalities, especially in tests of planning and sequencing in cognitive functions [163]. The study did not mention which disorders (BPD, HPD or the combined BPD + HPD) showed the greatest abnormalities. Others have suggested that in HPD there may be a hyperresponsiveness of the noradrenergic system, contributing to pronounced emotional reactivity to signs of rejection [164].

Treatment for Histrionic Patients

Because the DSM definition of HPD is no longer applicable to the milder HyP, but describes a more severe disorder, HPD patients are not amenable, as are their "neurotic-level" counterparts, to classical psychoanalysis. And because there are no evidence-based, randomized controlled studies of therapy focusing on HPD, one is left with the consensus of experts. Those who address the topic urge a more active approach to treatment: one where therapists engage the histrionic patient in an empathic and rather more forceful way, and do not behave as an "opaque or rigidly neutral manner" [129]. There are certain psychodynamic issues that surface frequently in therapy with histrionic patients: those that are female had often been raised in homes where maternal nurturance was deficient. This promoted a turning to the father for gratification of dependency needs. Flirtatiousness and exhibitionistic display of emotions would then develop as mechanisms of ensuring father's interest. Idealization of the father is a common consequence. The father may contribute to the overemphasis on seductive-ness through subtle (or not so subtle) indications that he values his daughter to the extent that she is physically attractive, bubbly, sexy—such that her sense of self-worth comes to rely excessively on such attributes [131]. The male histrionic, in parallel fashion, may have become overly attached to the mother, developing along a passive-feminine path [127]. These issues will need attention irrespective whether the therapeutic approach is psychodynamic, cognitive-behavioural, or supportive. We have no reason, in the absence of controlled studies, to assign pride of place to any one of these modalities over the others. The "right" method will have more to do with the original training of the therapist and with the cognitive style of the patient. The style optimal for working with a psychodynamic approach is one in which the capacity for self-reflection (introspectiveness, "mentalization") is adequately developed [165]. But this is what is precisely deficient in most patients with HPD (or BPD as well): they tend to externalize and to act out conflicts rather than deal with them by verbal, introspective means. One sees chaotic impulsivity, and, in the therapy sessions, great difficulty in being able to feel and to think about one's emotion at the same time: HPD (and BPD) patients instead become engulfed in strong emotions which they can scarcely think about, or else will talk in a detached manner about situations laden with affect that they cannot at that moment recognize. As with many BPD patients, those with HPD will often quit treatment precipitously. The hallmark of hysterics in general—the "belle indifference"—is even more prominent in HPD: histrionic patients will often fail to show up for sessions, disappear from therapy for weeks at a time, demonstrating in so doing the noteworthy lack of perseverance and commitment often seen in HPD, which makes such patients much more difficult to treat than compulsive patients. The latter tend to be regular about appointments and, though less in touch with their feelings at first, usually show a better reflective function.

These are some of the main points about HPD that therapists must keep in mind, as they undertake to treat patients with this and related conditions (such as HPD admixed with BPD traits). There will be need for limit-setting (in relation to the acting out), confrontation (about the hidden meanings behind their emotional displays), and emphasis on the need for regularity about appointments. Psychodynamic therapy relies on interpretation of transference and countertransference to accomplish the necessary goals; cognitive therapy relies on working with the irrational schemata encountered in HPD, such as the assumption that "Unless I captivate people, I am nothing". Supportive therapists will utilize such interventions as sympathy, exhortation, education, and advice-giving.

As for the prognosis in HPD, this depends greatly upon the same two considerations that weigh so heavily in the balance for BPD: dimensional aspects and comorbidity. Where is the histrionic patient situated along the continuum between mild hysteric personality and markedly chaotic forms of HPD itself? What are the other personality disorders whose traits accompany the HPD? If narcissistic elements are few and antisocial traits are absent, the prognosis will be good. Pure HPD, as mentioned, is rare, and some BPD traits will usually be present. Here, the prognosis will depend on the intensity and chronicity of anger or ragefulness, and upon how stormy are the close relationships. The more marked these features, the more difficult the task of remediation. The degree to which the therapist can curb the patient's tendency to quit during difficult moments in the treatment, and can help the patient achieve some measure of regularity and reflectiveness (in contrast to impulsivity and acting out) will spell the difference between failure and success.

SUMMARY

Borderline Personality Disorder

Consistent Evidence

- DBT and psychodynamic therapies are both effective in reducing suicidal behaviours within the first year of treatment.
- DBT and psychodynamic therapies are both better than (brief or perfunctory) "treatment as usual", but neither is better, on average, than the other.
- SSRIs are beneficial in reducing levels of impulsivity, anger and depression (and less hazardous than monoamine oxidase inhibitors).
- Despite aetiological heterogeneity, BPD can be reliably diagnosed.
- Given enough time, about two thirds of BPD patients cease meeting DSM criteria, and will function in the GAS 61–70 range.

- The suicide risk in BPD is about equal to that of bipolar disorder and schizophrenia.
- High intelligence is a mitigating factor.
- The Axis I disorders accompanying BPD usually resolve more quickly than the pure personality traits.
- Comorbid personality disorders are mainly of the dramatic cluster type.
- BPD as currently defined has almost no connection to schizophrenia, and has some connection to affective disorders (especially where there is bipolar II disorder comorbidity).

Incomplete Evidence

- There is suggestive evidence that supportive therapy is effective, but there have been no completed controlled studies thus far.
- Low socio-economic status seems to correlate with poor long-term outcome.
- Many cases belong to the affective spectrum as unipolar or bipolar II variants.
- Extreme sexual abuse in childhood can produce a chronic post-traumatic stress syndrome that mimics primary affective disorder, and leads to a type of BPD.
- Antisocial comorbidity is associated with a poor prognosis.
- Similarities of temperament (high novelty seeking, high harm avoidance, etc.) point to genetic underpinnings in BPD.
- 12-step programs are useful in dealing with special "craving disorders" (alcoholism, bulimia, sex addiction).

Areas Still Open to Research

- How does the currently reported suicide rate for BPD compare with that of the earlier long-term follow-up studies?
- How does DBT compare with psychodynamic and supportive therapies in relation to long-term changes in personality, as opposed to short-term benefits in suicidal activity?
- Is BPD more an Axis I disorder than a true personality disorder?
- Will BPD as currently defined be subdivided into different types, after further studies of neurophysiology?
- Adoption studies and larger monozygotic twin studies are needed to map out genetic factors more precisely.
- Cognitive styles of BPD patients make a difference as to which type of therapy will be optimal.

- Whether a dimensional approach to assessing BPD should be added to DSM category-based diagnoses.
- What are the true personality traits that are most often seen in BPD patients?
- In this era of brief hospitalization, are there still any indications for long-term stay?

Histrionic Personality Disorder

Consistent Evidence

- HPD represents the "severe" or "sick" end of the hysteria spectrum (which can only be understood in dimensional rather than in categorical terms).
- Comorbidity with other dramatic ("B") cluster personality configurations is the rule rather than the exception.
- The core features of HPD are exaggerated display of emotion and a need to draw attention to oneself.
- Persons with HPD typically manifest a conflictual attitude toward sex: heightened preoccupation with sex, side by side with negative attitudes about sex.
- Psychological tests reveal tendencies toward global thinking, mild cognitive impairment, and exaggerated emotionality (e.g. on Rorschach responses to colour cards).

Incomplete Evidence

- HPD may be of approximate equal prevalence in young adult men and women, but by middle age there is a female preponderance.
- Long-term follow-up shows favourable responses to therapy, provided that antisocial traits are minimal or absent.
- Attachment style in HPD is predominantly of the "preoccupied" type, with some elements of the "dismissive" type (both representing varieties of insecure attachment).
- The impulsivity and lack of perseverance (one sign of which is a shallowness and lack of commitment to treatment) make HPD patients as challenging to treat as BPD patients.

Areas Still Open to Research

- Further neurophysiological testing is needed to probe whether there are significant neurotransmitter differences that underlie the novelty seeking and reward dependence of HPD patients, and that might help differentiate them from other personality disorders.
- Randomized controlled studies of patients with HPD and related personality disorders are required, using two or more different treatment modalities.
- Further study of attachment patterns, cognitive style, and also of indications for, and response to, mood stabilizers (as a help in curbing chaotic impulsivity) is warranted.
- Further studies of reflectiveness or "mentalization" in HPD and other personality disorders are needed.
- The development of scales to capture the full range of hysteria-related disorders is welcome.

REFERENCES

1. American Psychiatric Association (1994) *Diagnostic and Statistical Manual of Mental Disorders*, 3rd edn. American Psychiatric Press, Washington.
2. American Psychiatric Association (1994) *Diagnostic and Statistical Manual of Mental Disorders*, 4th edn. American Psychiatric Press, Washington.
3. Millon T. (1981) *Disorders of Personality: DSM-III, Axis-II.* Wiley, New York.
4. James W. (1890) *The Principles of Psychology*, Vol. 1. Holt, New York.
5. Aarkrog T. (1981) The borderline concept in childhood, adolescence and adulthood. *Acta Psychiatr. Scand.*, **64** (Suppl. 293).
6. Dahl A.A. (1987) Borderline disorders: a comparative study of hospitalized patients. Thesis, Gaustad Hospitalet, Oslo.
7. Stone M.H. (1993) *Abnormalities of Personality: Within and Beyond the Realm of Treatment.* Norton, New York.
8. Kraepelin E. (1915) *Psychiatrie: Ein Lehrbuch für Studierende und Ärzte*, Vol. 4. Barth, Leipzig.
9. Stone M.H. (1980) *The Borderline Syndromes: Constitution, Personality and Adaptation.* McGraw Hill, New York.
10. Stern A. (1938) Psychoanalytic investigation of and therapy in the borderland group of neuroses. *Psychoanal. Quarterly*, **7**: 467–489.
11. Knight R.P. (1953) Borderline states in psychoanalytic psychiatry and psychology. *Bull. Menninger Clin.*, **17**: 1–12.
12. Grinker R.R. Sr., Werble B., Drye R.C. (1968) *The Borderline Syndrome: A Behavioral Study of Ego-Functions.* Basic Books, New York.
13. Kernberg O.F. (1967) Borderline personality organization. *J. Am. Psychoanal. Assoc.*, **15**: 641–684.
14. Mahler M.S. (1971) A study of the separation-individuation process, and its possible application to borderline phenomena in the psychoanalytic situation. *Psychoanal. Study Child*, **26**: 403–424.

15. Masterson J.F. (1971) Treatment of the adolescent with borderline syndrome. A problem in separation-individuation. *Bull. Menninger Clin.*, **35**: 5–18.
16. Masterson J.F., Rinsley D.B. (1975) The borderline syndrome: the role of the mother in the genesis and psychic structure of the borderline personality. *Int. J. Psychoanal.*, **56**: 163–177.
17. Colson D.B., Allen J.G., Coyne L., Deering D., Jehl N., Kearns W., Spohn H. (1986) Profiles of difficult psychiatric hospital patients. *Hosp. Commun. Psychiatry*, **37**: 720–724.
18. Kohut H. (1971) *The Analysis of the Self*. International University Press, New York.
19. Gunderson J.G., Singer M.T. (1975) Defining borderline patients. *Am. J. Psychiatry*, **132**: 1–10.
20. Tarnopolsky A. (1992) The validity of the borderline personality disorder. In *Handbook of Borderline Disorders* (Eds D. Silver, M. Rosenbluth), pp. 29–52. International University Press, Madison.
21. Skodol A.E., Gunderson J.G., Pfohl B., Widiger T.A., Livesley W.J., Siever L.J. (2002) The borderline diagnosis. I: Psychopathology, comorbidity, and personality structure. *Biol. Psychiatry*, **51**: 936–950.
22. Oldham J.M., Skodol A.E., Kellman H.D., Hyler S.D., Rosnick L., Davies M. (1992) Diagnosis of DSM-III-R personality disorders by two structured interviews: patterns of comorbidity. *Am. J. Psychiatry*, **149**: 213–220.
23. Widiger T.A., Trull T.J. (1989) Prevalence and comorbidity of personality disorders. *Psychiatr. Annals*, **19**: 132–136.
24. Akiskal H.S. (1981) Subaffective disorders: dysthymic, cyclothymic and bipolar-II disorders in the "borderline" realm. *Psychiatr. Clin. North Am.*, **4**: 25–46.
25. Perugi G., Toni C., Travierso M.C., Akiskal H.S. (2003) The role of cyclothymia in atypical depression: toward a data-based reconceptualization of the borderline-bipolar-II connection. *J. Affect. Disord.*, **73**: 87–98.
26. Akiskal H.S., Bougeois M.L., Angst J., Post R., Moller H., Hirschfeld R. (2000) Re-evaluating the prevalence of and diagnostic composition within the broad clinical spectrum of bipolar disorders. *J. Affect. Disord.*, **59** (Suppl. 1), S5–S30.
27. Perugi G., Toni C., Akiskal H.S. (1999) Anxious-bipolar comorbidity. Diagnostic challenges. *Psychiatr. Clin. North Am.*, **22**: 565–583.
28. Pinto O.C., Akiskal H.S. (1998) Lamotrigine as a promising approach to borderline personality: an open case series without concurrent DSM-IV major mood disorder. *J. Affect. Disord.*, **51**: 333–343.
29. Perugi G., Akiskal H.S., Lattanzi L., Cecconi D., Mastrocinque C., Petronelli A., Vignoli S., Bemi E. (1998) High prevalence of "soft" bipolar features in atypical depression. *Compr. Psychiatry*, **39**: 63–71.
30. Akiskal H.S., Judd L.L., Gillin J.C., Lemmi H. (1997) Subthreshold depression: clinical and polysomnographic validation of dysthymic, residual and masked forms. *J. Affect. Disord.*, **45**: 53–63.
31. Root M.P., Fallon P. (1988) The incidence of victimization experiences in a bulimic sample. *J. Interpers. Violence*, **3**: 161–173.
32. Van der Kolk B.A. (1996) The complexity of adaptation to trauma. In *Traumatic Stress: The Effects of Overwhelming Experience on Mind, Body and Self* (Eds B.A. van der Kolk, A.C. McFarlane, L. Weisaeth), pp. 182–213. Guilford, New York.
33. Stone M.H. (1990) Incest in the borderline patient. In *Incest-Related Syndromes of Adult Psychopathology* (Ed. R.P. Kluft), pp. 183–202. American Psychiatric Press, Washington.
34. Kroll J. (1993) *PTSD/Borderlines in Therapy*. Norton, New York.

35. Meloy J.R. (1992) *Violent Attachments*. Aronson, Northvale.
36. Orion D. (1997) *"I Knew You Really Love Me"*: *Stalking and Obsessive Love*. Dell/ Random House, New York.
37. Zanarini M.C. (1993) Borderline personality disorder as an impulse spectrum disorder. In *Borderline Personality Disorder: Etiology and Treatment* (Ed. J. Paris), pp. 67–85. American Psychiatric Press, Washington.
38. White G.L., Mullen P.E. (1989) *Jealousy: Theory, Research, and Clinical Strategies*. Guilford, New York.
39. Kernberg O.F., Dulz B., Sachsse U. (Eds) (2000) *Handbuch der Borderline-Störungen*. Schattauer, Stuttgart.
40. Zanarini M.C., Frankenburg F.R., Dubo E.D., Sickel A.E., Trikha A, Levin A., Reynolds V. (1998) Axis-II comorbidity of borderline personality disorder. *Compr. Psychiatry*, **39**: 296–302.
41. Johnson D.M., Shea M.T., Yen S., Battle C.L., Zlotnick C., Sanislow C.A., Grilo C.M., Skodol A.E., Bender D.S., McGlashan T.H. *et al.* (2003) Gender differences in borderline personality disorder: findings form the collaborative longitudinal personality disorder study. *Compr. Psychiatry*, **44**: 284–292.
42. Fink D. (1991) The comorbidity of multiple personality disorder and DSM-III-R Axis-II disorders. *Psychiatr. Clin. North Am.*, **14**: 547–566.
43. Zanarini M.C., Ruser T., Frankenburg F.R., Hennen J. (2000) The dissociative experiences of borderline patients. *Compr. Psychiatry*, **41**: 223–227.
44. Şar V., Kundakçi Y., Kiziltan E., Yargiç L.I., Tutkun H., Bakim B., Bozkurt O., Özpulat T., Keser V., Özdemir Ö. (1999) Axis-I dissociative disorder comorbidity of borderline personality disorder among psychiatric outpatients. Presented at the 4th Conference of the International Society for the Study of Dissociation, Manchester, May 6.
45. Zanarini M.C., Ruser T., Frankenburg F.R., Hennen J., Gunderson J.G. (2000) Risk factors associated with the dissociative experiences of borderline patients. *J. Nerv. Ment. Dis.*, **188**: 26–30.
46. Zanarini M.C., Yong L., Frankenburg F.R., Hennen J., Reich D.B., Marino M.F., Vujanović A.A. (2002) Severity of reported childhood sexual abuse and its relationship to severity of borderline psychopathology and psychosocial impairment among borderline patients. *J. Nerv. Ment. Dis.*, **190**: 381–387.
47. Bremner J.D., Vythilingam M., Vermetten E., Southwick S.M., McGlashan T., Nazeer A., Khan S., Vaccarino L.V., Soufer R., Garg. P.K. *et al.* (2003) MRI and PET study of deficits in hippocampal structure and function in women with childhood sexual abuse and post-traumatic stress disorder. *Am. J. Psychiatry*, **160**: 924–932.
48. Chabrol B., Decarie J.-C., Fontin G. (1999) The role of cranial MRI in identifying patients suffering from child abuse and presenting with unexplained neurological findings. *Child Abuse Neglect*, **23**: 217–228.
49. Schmahl C.G., McGlashan T.H., Bremner J.D. (2002) Neurobiological correlates of borderline personality disorder. *Psychopharmacol. Bull.*, **36**: 69–87.
50. Tarnopolsky A., Berelowitz M. (1987) Borderline personality: a review of recent research. *Br. J. Psychiatry*, **151**: 724–734.
51. Widiger T.A., Trull T.J., Hurt S.W., Clarkin J., Frances A. (1987) Multidimensional scaling of DSM-III personality disorders. *Arch. Gen. Psychiatry*, **44**: 557–563.
52. Gunderson J.G., Kolb J., Austin V. (1981) The diagnostic interview for borderline patients. *Am. J. Psychiatry*, **138**: 836–903.

53. Armelius B.A., Kullgren G., Renberg E. (1985) Borderline diagnosis from hospital records: reliability and validity of Gunderson's Diagnostic Interview for Borderlines (DIB). *J. Nerv. Ment. Dis.*, **173**: 32–34.
54. Zanarini M.C., Frankenburg F.R., Vujanovič A.A. (2002) Inter-rater and test-retest reliability of the Revised Diagnostic Interview for Borderlines. *J. Person. Disord.*, **16**: 270–276.
55. Hyler S.E., Rieder R.O., Williams J.B., Spitzer R.L., Lyons M., Hendler J. (1989) A comparison of clinical and self-report diagnoses of DSM-III personality disorders in 552 patients. *Compr. Psychiatry*, **30**: 170–178.
56. Zanarini M.C., Gunderson J.G., Frankenburg F.R., Chauncey D.L., Glutting J.H. (1991) The face validity of the DSM-III and DSM-III-R criteria for borderline personality disorder. *Am. J. Psychiatry*, **148**: 870–874.
57. Leichsenring F. (1999) Development and first results of the Borderline Personality Inventory: a self-report instrument for assessing borderline personality organization. *J. Person. Assess.*, **73**: 45–63.
58. Lenzenweger M.F., Clarkin J.F., Kernberg O.F., Foelsch P.A. (2001) The Inventory of Personality Organization: psychometric properties, factorial composition, and criterion relations with affect, aggressive dyscontrol, psychosis proneness, and self-domains in a non-clinical sample. *Psychol. Assess.*, **13**: 577–591.
59. Stone M.H. (1992) The borderline patient: diagnostic concepts and differential diagnosis. In *Handbook of Borderline Disorders* (Eds D. Silver, M. Rosenbluth), pp. 3–27. International University Press, Madison.
60. Hyman S.E. (2003) Diagnosing disorders. *Scientific American*, **289**: 97–103.
61. Kernberg O.F. (1975) *Borderline Conditions and Pathological Narcissism.* Aronson, New York.
62. Baron M., Gruen R., Asnis L., Lord S. (1985) Familial transmission of schizotypal and borderline personality disorders. *Am. J. Psychiatry*, **142**: 927–934.
63. McGlashan T.H. (1983) The borderline syndrome. II: Is it a variant of schizophrenia or affective disorder? *Arch. Gen. Psychiatry*, **40**: 1319–1323.
64. Stone M.H. (1990) *The Fate of Borderlines.* Guilford, New York.
65. Torgersen S. (1984) Genetic and nosological aspects of schizotypal and borderline personality disorders: a twin study. *Arch. Gen. Psychiatry*, **41**: 546–554.
66. Torgersen S. (2000) Genetics of patients with borderline personality disorder. *Psychiatr. Clin. North Am.*, **23**: 1–9.
67. Ruiz-Sancho A., Gunderson J.G. (2000) Familien von Patienten mit Borderline-Persönlichkeitsstörungen: ein Literaturüberblick. In *Handbuch der Borderline-Störungen* (Eds O.F. Kernberg, B. Dulz, U. Sachsse), pp. 771–791. Schattauer, Stuttgart.
68. McGlashan T.H. (1987) Borderline personality disorder and unipolar affective disorder: long-term effects of comorbidity. *J. Nerv. Ment. Dis.*, **175**: 467–473.
69. Gunderson J.G., Phillips K.A. (1991) A current view of the interface between borderline personality disorder and depression. *Am. J. Psychiatry*, **148**: 967–975.
70. Grilo C.M., Walker M.L., Becker D.F., Edell W.S., McGlashan T.H. (1997) Personality disorders in adolescents with major depression, substance use disorders, and coexisting major depression and substance use disorders. *J. Consult. Clin. Psychol.*, **65**: 328–332.
71. Svrakič D.M., Whitehead C., Przybeck T.R., Cloninger C.R. (1993) Differential diagnosis of personality disorders by the seven-factor model of temperament and character. *Arch. Gen. Psychiatry*, **50**: 991–999.

72. Joyce P.R., Mulder R.T., Luty S.E., McKenzie J.M., Sullivan P.S., Cloninger R.C. (2003) Borderline personality disorder in major depression: symptomatology, temperament, character, differential drug response, and 6-month outcome. Compr. Psychiatry, 44: 35–43.
73. Riso L.P., Klein D.N., Anderson R.L., Ouimette P.C. (2000) A family study of outpatients with borderline personality disorder and no history of mood disorder. J. Person. Disord., 14: 208–217.
74. Stone M.H., Kahn E., Flye B. (1981) Psychiatrically ill relatives of borderline patients. Psychiatr. Quarterly, 53: 71–84.
75. Siever L.J., Torgersen S., Gunderson J.G., Livesley W.J., Kendler K.S. (2002) The borderline diagnosis. III: Identifying endophenotypes for genetic studies. Biol. Psychiatry, 51: 964–968.
76. Skodol A.E., Siever L.J., Livesley W.J., Gunderson J.G., Pfohl B., Widiger T.A. (2002) The borderline diagnosis. II: Biology, genetics and clinical course. Biol. Psychiatry, 51: 951–963.
77. Plakun E.M., Burkhardt P.E., Muller J.P. (1985) 14 year follow-up of borderline and schizotypal personality disorders. Compr. Psychiatry, 26: 448–455.
78. McGlashan T.H. (1986) The Chestnut Lodge Follow-Up Study: III. Long-term outcome of borderline personalities. Arch. Gen. Psychiatry, 43: 20–30.
79. Stone M.H., Hurt S.W., Stone D.K. (1987) The P.I.-500: long-term follow-up of borderline in-patients meeting DSM-III criteria. J. Person. Disord., 1: 291–298.
80. Paris J., Brown R., Nowlis D. (1987) Long-term follow-up of borderline patients in a general hospital. Compr. Psychiatry, 28: 530–535.
81. Kroll J.L., Carey K.S., Sines L.K. (1985) Twenty year follow-up of borderline personality disorder: a pilot study. In Proceedings of the 4th World Congress of Biological Psychiatry, Vol. 7 (Ed. C. Shagass), pp. 577–579. Elsevier, New York.
82. Endicott J., Spitzer R.L., Fleiss J.L., Cohen J. (1967) The Global Assessment Scale. Arch. Gen. Psychiatry, 33: 766–771.
83. Paris J. (2002) Implications of long-term outcome research for the management of patients with borderline personality disorder. Harv. Rev. Psychiatry, 10: 315–323.
84. Gunderson J.G., Carpenter W.T. Jr., Strauss J.S. (1975) Borderline and schizophrenic patients. A comparative study. Am. J. Psychiatry, 132: 1257–1264.
85. Aarkrog T. (1994) Borderline Adolescents Twenty Years Later. Schmidt, Copenhagen.
86. Stevenson J., Meares R. (1993) An outcome study of psychotherapy for patients with borderline personality disorder. Am. J. Psychiatry, 150: 847–848.
87. Linehan M.M., Heard H.L., Armstrong H.E. (1993) Naturalistic follow-up of a behavioral treatment for chronically parasuicidal borderline patients. Arch. Gen. Psychiatry, 50: 971–974.
88. Najavits L.M., Gunderson J.G. (1995) Better than expected: improvements in borderline personality disorder in a 3-year prospective outcome study. Compr. Psychiatry, 36: 296–302.
89. Antikainen R., Hintikka J., Koponen H., Arstila A. (1995) A prospective three-year follow-up study of borderline personality disorder patients. Acta Psychiatr. Scand., 92: 327–335.
90. Bateman A., Fonagy P. (2001) Treatment of borderline personality disorder with psychoanalytically oriented partial hospitalization: an 18-month follow-up. Am. J. Psychiatry, 158: 36–42.
91. Rockland L. (1989) Supportive Psychotherapy. Guilford, New York.

92. Wallerstein R.S. (1986) *Forty-Two Lives in Treatment: A Study of Psychoanalysis and Psychotherapy*. Guilford, New York.

93. Searles H.F. (1986) *My Work with Borderline Patients*. Aronson, Northvale.

94. Dawson D., MacMillan H. (1993) *Relationship Management of the Borderline Patient: From Understanding to Treatment*. Brunner/Mazel, New York.

95. Beck A.T., Freeman A. (1990) *Cognitive Therapy of Personality Disorders*. Guilford, New York.

96. Linehan M.M. (1993) *Cognitive Behavioral Treatment of Borderline Personality Disorder*. Guilford, New York.

97. Ellis A. (1963) *Rational-Emotive Therapy*. Institute for Rational-Emotive Therapy, New York.

98. Clarkin J.F., Yeomans F.E., Kernberg O.F. (1999) *Psychotherapy for Borderline Patients*. Wiley, New York.

99. Gunderson J.G. (2001) *Borderline Personality Disorder: A Clinical Guide*. American Psychiatric Press, Washington.

100. Oldham J.M., Phillips K.A., Gabbard G.O., Goin M.K., Gunderson J.G., Soloff P., Spiegel D., Stone M.H. (2001) Practice guidelines for the treatment of patients with borderline personality disorder. *Am. J. Psychiatry*, **158** (Suppl.).

101. Applebaum A., Levy K. (2002) Supportive psychotherapy for borderline patients: a psychoanalytic research perspective. *Am. J. Psychother.*, **62**: 201–202.

102. Perry J.C., Banon E., Ianni F. (1999) Effectiveness of psychotherapy for personality disorders. *Am. J. Psychiatry*, **156**: 1312–1321.

103. Higgitt A., Fonagy P. (1992) Psychotherapy in borderline and narcissistic personality disorder. *Br. J. Psychiatry*, **161**: 23–43.

104. Stone M.H. (1990) Treatment of borderline patients: a pragmatic approach. *Psychiatr. Clin. North Am.*, **13**: 265–285.

105. Sabo A.N., Gunderson J.G., Najavits L.M., Chauncey D., Kisiel C. (1995) Changes in self-destructiveness of borderline patients in psychotherapy. A prospective follow-up. *J. Nerv. Ment. Dis.*, **183**: 370–376.

106. Zanarini M.C., Frankenburg F.R., Hennen J., Silk K.R. (2003) The longitudinal course of borderline psychopathology: 6-year prospective follow-up of the phenomenology of borderline personality disorder. *Am. J. Psychiatry*, **160**: 274–283.

107. Bateman A., Fonagy P. (1999) Effectiveness of partial hospitalization in the treatment of borderline personality disorder: a randomized study. *Am. J. Psychiatry*, **156**: 1563–1569.

108. Clarkin J.F., Foelsch P.A., Levy K.N., Hull J.W., Delaney J.C., Kernberg O.F. (2001) The development of a psychodynamic treatment for patients with borderline personality disorder: a preliminary study of behavioral change. *J. Person. Disord.*, **15**: 487–495.

109. Koerner K., Linehan M.M. (2000) Research on dialectical behavior therapy for patients with borderline personality disorder. *Psychiatr. Clin. North Am.*, **23**: 151–167.

110. Verheul R., van den Bosch L.M., Loeter M.W., De Ridder M.A., Stijnen T., van den Brink W. (2003) Dialectical behavior therapy for women with borderline personality disorder: 12-month, randomized clinical trial in the Netherlands. *Br. J. Psychiatry*, **182**: 135–140.

111. Bohus M., Haaf B., Stiglmayr C., Pohl U., Bohme R., Linehan M.M. (2000) Evaluation of inpatient dialectical-behavior therapy for borderline personality disorder: a prospective study. *Behav. Res. Ther.*, **38**: 875–877.

112. Linehan M.M., Tutek D.A., Heard H.L., Armstrong H.E. (1994) Interpersonal outcome of cognitive behavioral treatment for chronically suicidal borderline patients. *Am. J. Psychiatry*, **151**: 1771–1776.
113. Palmer R.L., Birchall H., Damani S., Gatward N., McGrain L., Parker L. (2003) A dialectical behavior therapy program for people with an eating disorder and borderline personality disorder: description and outcome. *Int. J. Eat. Disord.*, **33**: 281–286.
114. Van den Bosch L.M., Verheul R., Schippers G.M., van den Brink W. (2002) Dialectical behavior therapy of borderline patients with and without substance use problems: implementation and effects. *Addict. Behav.*, **27**: 911–923.
115. Linehan M.M., Dimeff L.A., Reynolds S.K., Comtois K.A., Welch S.S., Haegerty P., Kivlahan D.R. (2002) Dialectical behavior therapy versus comprehensive validation therapy plus 12-step for the treatment of opioid dependent women meeting criteria for borderline personality disorder. *Drug Alcohol Depend.*, **67**: 13–26.
116. Woodberry K.A., Miller A.L., Glinski J., Indik J., Mitchell A.G. (2002) Family therapy and dialectical behavior therapy with adolescents: Part II: a theoretical review. *Am. J. Psychother.*, **56**: 585–602.
117. Hollander E., Allen A., Lopez R.P., Bienstock C.A., Grossman R., Siever L.J., Merkatz L., Stein D. (2001) A preliminary double-blind, placebo-controlled trial of divalproex sodium in borderline personality disorder. *J. Clin. Psychiatry*, **62**: 199–203.
118. Frankenburg F.R., Zanarini M.C. (2002) Divalproex sodium treatment of women with borderline personality disorder and bipolar-II disorder: a double-blind, placebo-controlled study. *J. Clin. Psychiatry*, **63**: 442–446.
119. Rinne T., van den Brink W., Wouters L., van Dyck R. (2002) SSRI treatment of borderline personality disorder: a randomized, placebo-controlled clinical trial for female patients with borderline personality disorder. *Am. J. Psychiatry*, **159**: 2048–2054.
120. Zanarini M.C., Frankenburg F.R. (2001) Olanzapine treatment of female borderline personality disorder patients: a double-blind, placebo-controlled study. *J. Clin. Psychiatry*, **62**: 849–854.
121. Goodman M., New A. (2000) Impulsive aggression in borderline personality disorder. *Curr. Psychiatry Rep.*, **2**: 56–61.
122. Wallerstein R.S. (1980/81) Diagnosis revisited: the case of hysteria and hysterical personality. *Int. J. Psychoanal. Psychother.*, **8**: 533–548.
123. Reich W. (1949) *Character Analysis*, 3rd edn. Farrar, Straus and Giroux, New York.
124. Marmor J. (1953) Orality in the hysterical personality. *J. Am. Psychoanal. Ass.*, **1**: 656–671.
125. Easser R.-R., Lesser S. (1965) Hysterical personality: a re-evaluation. *Psychoanal. Quarterly*, **34**: 390–405.
126. Liebowitz M.R., Klein D.F. (1981) Interrelationship of hysteroid dysphoria and borderline personality disorder. *Psychiatr. Clin. North Am.*, **4**: 67–87.
127. Gabbard G.O. (2000) Cluster B personality disorders. In *Psychodynamic Psychiatry in Clinical Practice*, 3rd edn (Ed. G.O. Gabbard), pp. 517–545. American Psychiatric Press, Washington.
128. Cloninger C.R. (1978) The link between hysteria and sociopathy: an integrative model of pathogenesis based on clinical, genetic, and neurophysiological observations. In *Psychiatric Diagnosis* (Eds H.S. Akiskal, W.L. Webb), pp. 189–218. Spectrum, New York.

230 _____ PERSONALITY DISORDERS

129. Andrews G., Hunt C., Pollack C., Thompson S. (1991) Treatment outlines for borderline, narcissistic and histrionic personality disorders. *Aust. N. Zeal. J. Psychiatry*, **25**: 392–403.
130. Nestadt G., Romanoski A.J., Chahal R., Merchant A., Folstein M.F., Gruenberg E.M., McHugh P.R. (1999) An epidemiological study of histrionic personality disorder. *Psychol. Med.*, **20**: 413–422.
131. Widiger T.A., Bornstein R.F. (2001) Histrionic, narcissistic, and dependent personality disorders. In *Comprehensive Handbook of Psychopathology* (Eds P.B. Sutker, H.E. Adams), pp. 509–531. Kluwer, New York.
132. Ohshima T. (2001) Borderline personality traits in hysterical neurosis. *Psychiatry Clin. Neurosci.*, **55**: 131–136.
133. Sullwold F. (1990) Structure of the hypochondriacal and hysteroid personality. *Zeitschr für Experimentelle und Angewandte Psychologie*, **37**: 642–659.
134. Oldham J.M., Skodol A.E., Kellman H.D., Hyler S.E., Doidge N., Rosnick L., Gallaher P.E. (1995) Comorbidity of Axis I and Axis II disorders. *Am. J. Psychiatry*, **152**: 571–578.
135. Sprock J. (2000) Gender-types behavioral examples of histrionic personality disorder. *J. Psychopathol. Behav. Assess.*, **22**: 107–122.
136. Rienzi B.M., Scrams D.J. (1991) Gender stereotypes for paranoid, antisocial, compulsive, dependent and histrionic personality disorders. *Psychol. Rep.*, **69**: 976–978.
137. Low B.S. (2000) *Why Sex Matters: A Darwinian Look at Human Behavior*. Princeton University Press, Princeton.
138. Bornstein R.F. (1999) Histrionic personality disorder, physical attractiveness, and social adjustment. *J. Psychopathol. Behav. Assess.*, **21**: 79–94.
139. Padilla A.M. (1995) *Hispanic Pathology: Criterial Issues in Theory Research*. Sage, Newbury Park.
140. Stevens A., Price J. (2000) *Evolutionary Psychiatry*, 2nd edn. Routledge, London.
141. Lucchi N., Gaston A. (1990) Cultural relativity of hysteria as a nosographic entity. Hysteria and antisocial behavior. *Minerva Psichiatr.*, **31**: 151–154.
142. Hamburger M.E., Lilienfeld S.O., Hogben M. (1996) Psychopathy, gender and gender roles: implications for antisocial and histrionic personality disorders. *J. Person. Disord.*, **10**: 41–55.
143. Cale E.M., Lilienfeld S.O. (2002) Histrionic personality disorder and antisocial personality disorder: sex-differentiated manifestations of psychopathy? *J. Person. Disord.*, **16**: 52–72.
144. Brunner P., Parzer P., Richert-Appel H., Meyer A.E., Resch F. (1999) Childhood sexual abuse in the history of patients in high-frequency psychoanalytic long-term therapy: prevalence and diagnosis. *Psychotherapie, Psychosomatik, Medizinische Psychologie*, **49**: 178–186.
145. Apt C., Hurlbert D.F. (1994) The sexual attitudes, behavior and relationships of women with histrionic personality disorder. *J. Sex Marital Ther.*, **20**: 125–133.
146. Darcourt G. (1995) Hysterical personality disorder. *Revue du Practicien*, **45**: 2550–2555.
147. Deutsch H. (1942) Some forms of emotional disturbance and their relationship to schizophrenia. *Psychoanal. Quarterly*, **11**: 301–321.
148. Looper K.J., Paris J. (2000) What dimensions underlie Cluster B personality disorders? *Compr. Psychiatry*, **41**: 432–437.
149. Fossati A., Feeney J.A., Donati D., Donini M., Novella L., Bagnato M., Carretta I., Leonardi B., Mirabelli S., Maffei C. (2003) Personality disorders and adult

attachment dimensions in a mixed psychiatric sample: a multivariate study. *J. Nerv. Ment. Dis.*, **191**: 30–37.
150. Shapiro D. (1965) *Neurotic Styles*. Basic Books, New York.
151. Sigmund D. (1994) Die Phänomenologie der hysterischen Persönlichkeitsstörung. *Nervenarzt*, **65**: 18–25.
152. Sigmund D. (1998) The hysterical personality disorder: a phenomenological approach. *Psychopathology*, **6**: 318–330.
153. Costa P.T., Widiger T.A. (Eds) (2002) *Personality Disorders and the Five Factor Model of Person.*, 2nd edn. American Psychological Association, Washington.
154. Trull T.J. (1992) DSM-III-R personality disorders and the Five Factor Model of personality: an empirical comparison. *J. Abnorm. Psychol.*, **101**: 553–560.
155. Crawford T.N., Cohen P., Brook J.S. (2001) Dramatic-erratic personality disorder symptoms: I. Continuity from early adolescence into adulthood. *J. Person. Disord.*, **15**: 319–335.
156. Crawford T.N., Cohen P., Brooks J.S. (2001) Dramatic-erratic personality disorder symptoms: II. Developmental pathways from early adolescence to adulthood. *J. Person. Disord.*, **15**: 336–350.
157. Schotte C., De Doncker D., Maes M., Cluydts R., Cosyns P. (1993) MMPI assessment of the DSM-III-R histrionic personality disorder. *J. Person. Assess.*, **60**: 500–510.
158. Blais M.A., Hilsenroth M.J., Fowler J.C. (1998) Rorschach correlates of the DSM-IV histrionic personality disorder. *J. Person. Assess.*, **70**: 355–364.
159. Bartholomew K., Kwong M.J., Hart S.D. (2001) Attachment. In *Handbook of Personality Disorders: Theory, Research and Treatment* (Ed. W.J. Livesley), pp. 196–230. Guilford, New York.
160. Cloninger R.C., Przybeck T.R., Svrakič D., Wetzel R.D. (1994) *Temperament and Character Inventory (TCI): A Guide to its Development and Use*. Washington University Center for Psychobiology of Personality, St. Louis.
161. DePue R.A., Lenzenweger M.F. (2001) A neurobehavioral dimensional model. In *Handbook of Personality Disorders: Theory, Research and Treatment* (Ed. W.J. Livesley), pp. 136–176, Guilford, New York.
162. Niggs J.T., Goldsmith H.H. (1994) Genetics of personality disorders: perspectives form personality and psychopathology research. *Psychol. Bull.*, **115**: 346–380.
163. Burgess J.W. (1992) Neurocognitive impairment in dramatic personalities: histrionic, narcissistic, borderline and antisocial. *Psychiatry Res.*, **42**: 283–290.
164. Klein D.F. (1999) Harmful dysfunction, disorder, disease, and evolution. *J. Abnorm. Psychol.*, **108**: 421–429.
165. Fonagy P., Target M. (1997) Attachment and self-reflection: their role in self-organization. *Develop. Psychopathol.*, **9**: 679–700.

Commentaries

3.1
From Shifting Diagnoses to Empirically-based Diagnostic Constructs

W. John Livesley[1]

The scholarly account of borderline and histrionic personality disorders by Michael Stone beautifully illustrates the problem with current classifications of personality disorder and the challenges faced in developing more valid diagnostic concepts. The very meaning of diagnostic concepts shifts over time, not so much in response to new empirical findings but more in response to changing opinions and even fashions. With borderline personality, these changes created a diagnosis beset by multiple problems. The underlying conceptualization of the disorder is confusing, ranging from an assumed personality structure through problems with emotional regulation to impulsivity and aggression. The diagnosis overlaps to an unacceptable degree with other diagnoses. The criteria set is a combination of traits and symptoms that is inconsistent with how other personality diagnoses are represented, adds to diagnostic instability, and creates confusing overlap with various Axis I disorders. Histrionic personality disorder suffers from similar problems. Although originally formulated as an extreme personality pattern in psychoanalytic theory, its meaning has changed so that now it seems little more than a milder variant of borderline personality.

Given this confusion, it is reasonable to ask where we go from here and how the core ideas captured by these shifting conceptions can be translated into the kind of diagnoses one would expect of a scientific classification. Perhaps the time has come to relinquish efforts to refine current diagnostic concepts based as they are on a mish-mash of clinical observation and speculative theories and replace them with an empirical nosology. Current conceptions of borderline and histrionic personality disorders do not match the way personality disorder is organized at either phenotypic or genetic levels. There is little evidence to suggest that such discrete categories exist. There is, however, overwhelming evidence that the features of personality

[1] *Department of Psychiatry, University of British Columbia, 2255 Wesbrook Mall, Vancouver, BC V6T 2A1, Canada*

disorder merge with normal variation and with each other. There is also substantial evidence that a handful of broad dimensions underlie personality disorder diagnoses [1] and that these dimensions reflect the genetic architecture of personality [2].

What we refer to as borderline personality disorder seems to represent the extreme of a dimension variously labelled asthenia [1] and emotional dysregulation [2,3] that is continuous with the normal personality dimension of neuroticism [4]. Such a formulation captures the pervasiveness of this form of psychopathology more effectively than current categorical concepts. Persons who attract the diagnosis of borderline personality disorder show a wide range of features, several of which are not included in the DSM-IV criteria set. They also exhibit multiple Axis I symptoms that originally prompted suggestions of a relationship with schizophrenia and more recently with mood disorders.

Formulating borderline as the extreme of emotional dysregulation or neuroticism clarifies these relationships: neuroticism appears to predispose to both personality disorder and a wide range of Axis I disorders, including mood disorder [5]. It also clarifies the extensive patterns of co-occurrence with other personality disorders: neuroticism and emotional dysregulation are associated with multiple personality disorder diagnoses [6,7]. The pervasiveness of the clinical picture is also illuminated by empirical analyses of the structure of emotional dysregulation. This broad pattern is made up of a larger number of basic traits such as anxiousness, affective lability, submissiveness, insecure attachment, cognitive dysregulation, and social apprehensiveness [2]. These traits are not simply components of emotional dysregulation. Instead, they are separate entities with a distinct genetic aetiology [8]. They form an important second tier to a dimensional model of personality disorder. The range of features encompassed by emotional dysregulation seems to reflect the clinical picture presented by patients with this diagnosis better than the more circumscribed criteria set of DSM-IV, which omits important features such as anxiousness, a key component of neuroticism and a characteristic of most patients that increases distress and dysphoria at times of crisis. This omission was part of an unsuccessful attempt to differentiate the diagnosis from other disorders, especially cluster C disorders. But the system cannot be shorn up in this artificial way.

If diagnoses are to be useful, they need to reflect natural patterns of personality and psychopathology and aetiological differences. Attempts to establish a more valid representation of the disorder need to incorporate an explicit understanding of the core features of the disorder. Is borderline a form of personality organization, a problem with impulse regulation, or primarily a problem with emotional regulation that leads to impulsive behaviour? Multivariate studies of the phenotypic and genetic structure of borderline [2] and some treatment approaches such as dialectical behavioural therapy [9] suggest the latter. Whichever conception is adopted, it needs to be stated explicitly and be consistent with empirical findings.

Having argued for a dimensional model of borderline pathology, it is appropriate to ask how histrionic personality disorder would fit into such a system. The important issue is whether a diagnosis of histrionic personality disorder is needed. The concept does not seem distinct from borderline. As a mild variant of this condition, histrionic is probably redundant. However, the older concept of hysterical personality may contain features that have clinical relevance. These are probably best represented using the lower order or basic traits that form the second tier of the classification.

Problems with diagnosis and classification inevitably create problems for treatment studies. Fortunately the concept and criteria set for borderline personality disorder contains reliable variance (even though current concepts are not optimal) that make outcome studies feasible. Here the results are encouraging. A meta-analysis of outcome studies reveals that both psycho-dynamic and cognitive-behavioural therapies are effective [10]. This is an important finding that should correct specious claims that some approaches are more effective than others—they may be, but current evidence does not support this contention. Unlike Michael Stone, however, I do not think that there is much to learn from studies that compare the outcome of different treatments. No single approach stands out as more effective than the others and no current therapy is sufficiently comprehensive to treat all forms of the disorder or all aspects of the psychopathology of personality. Under these circumstances we need to pursue an integrated and eclectic approach in which interventions are selected on the basis of what works for a given problem or dimension of psychopathology rather than on the basis of unsubstantiated theories of psychopathology or therapy [11].

It is clear from Stone's review that we are far from constructing valid diagnostic constructs to represent the psychopathology encompassed by borderline and histrionic personality disorders. It is also clear that the current approach with ever changing conceptions and criteria sets based on artificial categories cannot form the foundation for a scientific classification. This is not to say that these diagnoses do not capture important clinical insights—they do. The problem is how to represent these insights using reliable and valid constructs that reflect the etiological structure of personality disorder.

REFERENCES

1. Mulder R.T., Joyce P.R. (1997) Temperament and the structure of personality disorder symptoms. *Psychol. Med.*, **27**: 1315–1325.

2. Livesley W.J., Jang K.L., Vernon P.A. (1998) The phenotypic and genetic architecture of traits delineating personality disorder. *Arch. Gen. Psychiatry*, **55**: 941–948.
3. Livesley W.J. (2002) Diagnostic dilemmas in the classification of personality disorder. In *Advancing DSM: Dilemmas in Psychiatric Diagnosis* (Eds K. Phillips, M. First, H.A. Pincus), pp. 153–189. American Psychiatric Press, Washington.
4. Taylor S. (1995) Commentary on borderline personality disorder. In *Handbook of Personality Disorders* (Ed. W.J. Livesley), pp. 165–172. Guilford, New York.
5. Clark L.A., Watson D., Mineka S. (1994) Temperament, personality and the mood and anxiety disorders. *J. Abnorm. Psychol.*, **103**: 103–116.
6. Costa P.T., Widiger T.A. (Eds) (2002) *Personality Disorders and the Five Factor Model of Personality*, 2nd edn. American Psychological Association, Washington.
7. Bagge C.L., Trull T.J. (2003) DAPP-BQ: factor structure and relations to personality disorder symptoms in a non-clinical sample. *J. Person. Disord.*, **17**: 19–32.
8. Jang K.L., McCrae R.R., Angleitner A., Riemann R., Livesley W.J. (1998) Heritability of facet-level traits in a cross-cultural twin study: support for a hierarchical model of personality. *J. Person. Soc. Psychol.*, **74**: 1556–1565.
9. Linehan M.M. (1993) *Cognitive-behavioural Treatment of Borderline Personality Disorder*. Guilford, New York.
10. Leichsenring F., Leibing E. (2003) The effectiveness of psychodynamic therapy and cognitive therapy in the treatment of personality disorders: a meta-analysis. *Am. J. Psychiatry*, **160**: 1223–1232.
11. Livesley W.J. (2003) *Practical Management of Personality Disorder*. Guilford, New York.

3.2
What is a Personality Disorder, a Set of Traits or Symptoms?

Allan Tasman[1]

Michael Stone's scholarly review highlights the critically important factors in present day understanding of both histrionic and borderline personality disorders from the perspective of diagnosis, aetiology, and treatment. One of the most intriguing aspects of his discussion occurs early in his chapter, where he highlights the concern in descriptive diagnosis of personality disorders relating to the issue of personality traits versus symptoms. At a time when the international community is struggling with the need to better refine our approach to psychiatric diagnosis, this point is worth emphasis.

The major diagnostic systems in use in psychiatry around the world, the DSM from the American Psychiatric Association and the ICD from the World Health Organization, still use a symptom cluster approach to psychiatric diagnosis. This approach has led to greater uniformity and greater inter-rater

[1] Department of Psychiatry, University of Louisville School of Medicine, Louisville, KY 40292, USA

reliability in diagnosis. The impact of these systems on the research advances in psychiatry has been dramatically positive. Understandably, however, we are still a long way from the implementation of an aetiologically based system of diagnosis. In this vacuum, to be filled in as our understanding of psychiatric pathophysiology increases, clinicians and researchers struggle to find common diagnostic ground. The area of personality diagnosis is no exception.

One of the critical baseline issues in personality disorder diagnosis involves agreement on the nature of personality per se. While categorical approaches to diagnosis of pathology are useful, many patients are seen to have substantial overlap of personality diagnosis when, for example, the DSM is used [1]. The evolution of a more dimensional approach seems to provide the opportunity to approach diagnosis of a personality disorder from the perspective of an agreement on the basic nature of personality itself. Work by Cloninger [2], Costa and McCrae [3], and Widiger [4] have contributed to the scientific advancement of this approach.

For example, Cloninger's work is based on the idea that there are four temperaments of reward dependence, harm avoidance, novelty seeking, and persistence [2]. Costa and McCrae's work suggests five dimensions: neuroticism versus emotional stability, introversion versus undependability, antagonism versus agreeableness, and closedness versus openness to experience [3]. Only when our understanding of the nature of personality reaches maturity will our ability to clearly define personality disorders become much more reliable and valid. This is particularly true regarding borderline personality disorder.

Stone clearly reviews the shifting and evolving understanding of borderline personality disorder and the changes in diagnostic criteria of this disorder over the decades of the twentieth century. I have been in practice long enough to have lived through changes in thinking regarding borderline personality, which encompassed its relationship to schizophrenia, mood disorders, traumatic abuse, and developmental arrest. With such aetiological lack of clarity, and in a group of very troubled and troubling patients, it is no surprise that our treatment interventions have fallen short of our and our patients' hope for effectiveness. And, our effectiveness with patients with histrionic personality seems little better.

Kernberg's work, as Stone notes, transformed the discourse about borderline personality, and led to a treatment approach which was based on the aetiology of the illness as it related to the basic, flawed organization of the personality in this group of individuals. And, the treatments which have followed have maintained the focus on the need to change broad individual cognitive, affective, and behavioural responses in a wide range of situations. Such approaches seem appropriate, and even necessary, for this group, or for that matter, any group of individuals diagnosed with a personality disorder.

But, Kernberg's model is rooted in a psychoanalytic theoretical base, especially influenced by the work of Melanie Klein and several generations of advances in understanding the "object relations" approach to normal and pathological development. In spite of the tremendous clinical utility of this model, there is little agreement in the field at large on its validity. Further, the impact of developmental differences across cultures is not addressed in Kernberg's model. Such differences likely account for the lack of uniformity of clinical characteristics and outcomes of patients diagnosed and studied in various countries, as highlighted in Stone's review.

Perhaps the most important day to day issue for clinicians related to treatment of personality disorders has to do with understanding the course of the illness, and treatment selection and duration. We are all aware that, in most parts of the world, there are extreme shortages of mental health clinicians and resources for treatment. Given such a situation, such resources often are targeted to treatment of psychotic and mood disorders. Personality disorders, even those as disruptive as borderline and histrionic, are not seen as treatment priorities.

Stone importantly points out that, in an era of emphasis on pharmacotherapy and brief psychotherapeutic interventions, the successful treatment of borderline and histrionic disorders requires a long term commitment of time and clinical resources. And, he demonstrates, there is little literature supporting the role of pharmacotherapy as a primary modality in these patients. With the long standing nature of personality disorders, and the severe disruption of adaptive capacities they entail, it is unlikely that the modern emphasis on crisis intervention approaches will be effective. And, many clinicians know from personal clinical experience that long term treatment commitments, often lasting years, can produce substantial positive clinical change.

Finding the resources to support such treatment interventions remains an important challenge for governments around the world. Given the social costs of borderline disorders, and the risk for self harm and comorbid substance abuse problems in this group, it is to be hoped that solutions to make treatment more available will be found in the not too distant future.

REFERENCES

1. Widiger T.A., Trull T.J. (1998) Performance characteristics of the DSM-III-R personality disorder criteria sets. In *DSM-IV Sourcebook*, Vol. 4 (Eds T.A. Widiger, A.J. Frances, H.A. Pincus), pp. 357–373. American Psychiatric Association, Washington.
2. Cloninger C.R. (2000) A practical way to diagnosis of personality disorders: a proposal. *J. Person. Disord.*, **14**, 99–108.

3. Costa P.T., McCrae R.R. (1992) *Revised NEO Personality Inventory (NEO PI-R) and NEO Five-Factor Inventory (NEO-FFI) Professional Manual.* Psychological Assessment Resources, Odessa.
4. Widiger T.A., Trull T.J., Clarkin J.F. (2002) A description of the DSM-IV personality disorders with the five-factor model of personality. In *Personality Disorders and the Five-Factor Model of Personality*, 2nd edn (Eds P.T. Costa, T.A. Widiger), pp. 89–99. American Psychological Association, Washington.

3.3
Mentalization and Borderline Personality Disorder

Anthony W. Bateman[1]

The concept of borderline personality disorder (BPD) and histrionic personality disorder (HPD) has inspired some of the most stimulating debates in contemporary psychiatry and this is reflected in the review by Michael Stone. In essence the disorder has become a focus of diagnostic debate and a challenge to biological, psychological and sociological understanding both from an aetiological viewpoint and from a treatment perspective. The diagnosis of HPD is likely to be evicted from the next DSM classification and so in this brief commentary I intend to focus on BPD. I will emphasise a few aspects that are hinted at but remain undeveloped in Stone's review. First is the question of aetiology of BPD and second is the impact that this understanding has on treatment.

There is increasing evidence that BPD results from a complex interplay between genetic and environmental factors, but that it is the environment that determines the phenotypic expression of an underlying genetic vulnerability. Environmental risk factors include childhood neglect, sexual abuse and physical violence, although these are not reported in all patients [1]. But these events take place in the context of attachment relationships and it is the quality of those relationships, which may determine the effect of trauma and childhood experience on personality development.

Although attachment theory is about proximity and the evocation of an experience of safety, it is also about the consequential development of robust, flexible, psychological processes that protect the individual from the stresses of human interaction and everyday life. From an attachment perspective, borderline patients are conceived of as failing to develop a stable sense of self, because of disturbance in early attachment relationships. Different attachment styles in children are apparent and these have

[1] *Royal Free and University College Medical Schools, Halliwick Unit, St. Ann's Hospital, St. Ann's Road, London N15 3TH, UK*

been linked to BPD. A study comparing patients with BPD with those with either antisocial personality disorder or bipolar II disorder [2] found greater separation–abandonment complex and greater conflict about the expression of emotional need and anger in borderline patients. Reliance on transitional objects is suggested to reflect BPD patients failed early attachment experiences [3] which have been suggested to be of the anxious–ambivalent subtype [4,5]. There are at least seven studies which have demonstrated extremely insecure attachments in patients with BPD, characterized by alternating fear of involvement and intense neediness [6]. Variables most strongly related to BPD features are lack of expressed care and over-protection by mother and an anxious and ambivalent attachment pattern.

The experience of safety within the context of a close emotional relationship is essential for the development of an autonomous sense of self and anything that undermines the emergent self leads to anxiety and potentially an angry response as the child attempts to stabilize himself [7]. Under conditions of chronic neglect and insensitivity, instability of the self results first in anger and then aggression, which is evoked so frequently because of repeated parental neglect that it becomes incorporated into the self-structure, with the result that self-assertion, demand, wishes, needs have to be accompanied by aggression if the self is to remain intact and stable. Such distortions to the self are not irreversible. The acquisition of the capacity to create a "narrative" of one's thoughts and feelings, to mentalize, can overcome flaws in the organization of the self that can flow from the disorganization of early attachment. Thus the robustness of the self-structure is dependent on the capacity to mentalize.

Mentalizing depends substantially on optimal functioning of prefrontal cortex [8], a brain structure which has been linked to the regulation of interpersonal relationships, social co-operativity, moral behaviour and social aggression [9]. The most favourable functioning of the prefrontal cortex in turn depends on optimal arousal, and Arnsten [10] and Mayes [11] have argued that when arousal exceeds a certain threshold, it is as if a neurochemical switch is thrown. This switch shifts us out of the executive mode of flexible reflective responding into the fight-or-flight mode of action-centred responding. Those with insecure or disorganized attachment relationships are sensitized during development to intimate interpersonal encounters, experience higher arousal, and the relative level of arousal in the frontal or posterior part of the cortex overwhelms their executive functions more easily than individuals who have experienced a secure attachment relationship. Thus in BPD we have potentially interlocking vicious developmental circles in which attachment disturbance leads to affective hyperarousal, which in turn results in a failure of mentalization; all are intertwined. This has gained further credence from the work of Rinne *et al.* [12,13], who found that in BPD severe and sustained traumatic stress in childhood affects the serotonin (5-HT) system and especially 5-HT1A receptors. This appears to be independent of the BPD diagnosis but dependent on the presence of severe trauma, the severity of which may account for the heterogeneity of patients with BPD in terms of symptomatology, pathogenesis, and type of co-morbidity, with less overt trauma having less effect on receptors and threshold levels of arousal. Hence not all patients with BPD report neglect and abuse, but those that do show the most severe symptoms [14].

This biopsychosocial model has important consequence for treatment. Impulsivity, outwardly directed aggression, and auto-aggression may be helped with medication [15], but mentalization can only develop using psychological techniques. Whilst Michael Stone discusses evidence for outcome of treatment, the question remains about why very different treatments, for example dialectical behavioural therapy and psychoanalytic therapy, seem to "work". According to the aetiological stance discussed earlier, if robust psychological change is to take place, the focus of treatment needs to be on improving mentalization rather than developing skills to control affective disturbance and dysfunctional behaviour. The greater emphasis on mentalization in the psychoanalytic treatment [16] may explain why the follow-up of patients was possibly better for psychoanalytic therapy than behaviour therapy [17]. Yet both approaches give some lasting improvement. However, I would argue that all effective treatments are actually operating though improvements in mentalization and that mentalization is a common theme of all psychotherapies for BPD.

What, then, are the arguments in favour of mentalization as the common pathway for effective treatments for BPD? Firstly, the foundation of any therapeutic work must by definition be implicit mentalization. Without social engagement there can be no psychological therapy, and without mentalization there can be no social engagement. Secondly, psychotherapy invariably activates the attachment system and as a component generates secure base experience. The experience of being understood generates an experience of security, which in turn facilitates "mental exploration", the exploration of the mind of the other to find oneself therein. Thirdly, the therapists of all patients, but particularly of borderline patients, whose experience of their mental world is diffused and confusing, will continually construct and reconstruct in their own mind an image of the patient's mind. They label feelings, they explain cognitions, they spell out implicit beliefs. Fourthly, mentalizing in psychological therapies is prototypically a process of shared, joint attention, where it is the mental state of the patient which forms the area of interest for both patient and therapist. The shared attentional processes entailed by all psychological therapies serve to strengthen the interpersonal integrative function made up of affect regulation, effortful control by attentional mechanisms and mentalization

[18]. Fifthly, the explicit content of the therapist's intervention will be mentalistic regardless of orientation, whether the therapist is principally concerned with transference reactions, automatic negative thoughts, dialectics, reciprocal roles or linear thinking. These approaches all entail explicit mentalization in so far that they succeed in enhancing coherent representations of desires and beliefs. Finally, the dyadic nature of therapy inherently fosters the patient's capacity to generate multiple perspectives.

All these features of psychotherapy require an appropriately arranged treatment context which itself must facilitate the development of mentalization. Part of the benefit which severely personality disordered individuals derive from treatment comes through their experience of being involved in a well-constructed, well-structured and coherent interpersonal endeavour. What may be helpful is the internalization of a thoughtfully constructed structure, the understanding of the interrelationship of different reliably identifiable components, the causal interdependence of specific ideas and actions, the constructive interactions of professionals, and above all the experience of being the subject of reliable, coherent and rational thinking. Social experiences such as these are not specific to any treatment modality, but rather are correlates of the level of seriousness and the degree of commitment with which teams of professionals approach the problem of caring for this group, who may be argued on empirical grounds to have been deprived of exactly such consideration and commitment during their early development and quite frequently throughout their later life. While this suggestion is speculative, it may also be helpful in distinguishing successful from unsuccessful interventions and pointing the way to the creation of even more efficacious protocols in the future.

REFERENCES

1. Salzman J., Salzman C., Wolfson A., Albanese A., Looper J., Ostacher M., Schwartz J., Chinman G., Land W., Miyawaki E. (1993) Association between borderline personality structure and history of childhood abuse in adult volunteers. *Compr. Psychiatry*, **34**: 254–257.
2. Perry J.C., Cooper S.H. (1986) A preliminary report on defenses and conflicts associated with borderline personality disorder. *J. Am. Psychoanal. Assoc.*, **34**: 863–893.
3. Modell A. (1963) Primitive object relationships and the predisposition to schizophrenia. *Int. J. Psycho-Anal.*, **44**: 282–292.
4. Fonagy P., Leigh T., Kennedy R., Mattoon G., Steele H., Target M., Steele M., Higgitt A. (1995) Attachment, borderline states and the representation of emotions and cognitions in self and other. In *Rochester Symposium on Developmental Psychopathology: Cognition and Emotion* (Eds D. Cicchetti, S.S. Toth), pp. 371–414. University of Rochester Press, Rochester.

5. Gunderson J.G. (1996) The borderline patient's intolerance of aloneness: insecure attachments and therapist availability. *Am. J. Psychiatry*, **153**: 752–758.
6. Dozier M., Stovall K., Albus K. (1999) Attachment and psychopathology in adulthood. In *Handbook of Attachment: Theory, Research and Clinical Applications* (Eds J. Cassidy, P. Haver), pp. 497–519. Guilford, New York.
7. Sroufe L.A. (1996) *Emotional Development: The Organization of Emotional Life in the Early Years*. Cambridge University Press, New York.
8. Siegal M., Varley R. (2002) Neural systems involved in "theory of mind". *Nat. Rev. Neurosci.*, **3**: 463–471.
9. Kelley W.M., Macrae C.N., Wyland C.L., Caglar S., Inati S., Heatherton T.F. (2002) Finding the self? An event-related fMRI study. *J. Cogn. Neurosci.*, **14**: 785–794.
10. Arnsten A.F. (1998) The biology of being frazzled. *Science*, **280**: 1711–1712.
11. Mayes L.C. (2000) A developmental perspective on the regulation of arousal states. *Semin. Perinatol.*, **24**: 267–279.
12. Rinne T., Westenberg H.G., den Boer J.A., van den Brink W. (2000) Serotonergic blunting to meta-chlorophenylpiperazine (m-CPP) highly correlates with sustained childhood abuse in impulsive and autoaggressive female borderline patients. *Biol. Psychiatry*, **47**: 548–556.
13. Rinne T., de Kloet E.R., Wouters L., Goekoop J.G., DeRijk R.H., van den Brink W. (2002) Hyperresponsiveness of hypothalamic-pituitary-adrenal axis to combined dexamethasone/corticotropin-releasing hormone challenge in female borderline personality disorder subjects with a history of sustained childhood abuse. *Biol. Psychiatry*, **52**: 1102–1112.
14. Zanarini M.C., Yong L., Frankenburg F.R., Hennen J., Reich D.B., Marino M.F., Vujanovic A.A. (2002) Severity of reported childhood sexual abuse and its relationship to severity of borderline psychopathology and psychosocial impairment among borderline inpatients. *J. Nerv. Ment. Dis.*, **190**: 381–387.
15. Coccaro E.F., Kavoussi R.J. (1997) Fluoxetine and impulsive aggressive behaviour in personality disordered subjects. *Arch. Gen. Psychiatry*, **54**: 1081–1088.
16. Bateman A., Fonagy P. (in press) *Psychotherapy for Borderline Personality Disorder: Mentalisation Based Treatment*. Oxford University Press, Oxford.
17. Bateman A., Fonagy P. (2001) Treatment of borderline personality disorder with psychoanalytically oriented partial hospitalisation: an 18-month follow-up. *Am. J. Psychiatry*, **158**: 36–42.
18. Fonagy P., Target M., Gergely G., Allen J., Bateman A. (2003) The developmental roots of borderline personality disorder in early attachment relationships: a theory and some evidence. *Psychoanal. Inquiry*, **23**: 412–458.

3.4
Complex and Diverse, Yet Similar?
Sigmund Karterud, Theresa Wilberg and Øyvind Urnes[1]

Michael Stone's vivid description of the complexities of the borderline and the histrionic disorders demonstrates to the reader why these dramatic disorders fascinate us so much. Sometimes perhaps at the expense of the less extroverted [1], the shy and inhibited relative, the avoidant personality disorder, which in fact is far more prevalent in the population [2] and even in clinical settings [3]. Given a set of diagnostic criteria, there should be no surprise that the condition defined as borderline personality disorder (BPD) can be reliably assessed, as Stone documents. However, in light of the complexities, it is worth noting that the BPD construct also has a high construct and prototype validity [4]. BPD contains both diversity and unity. Altogether there are 256 ways of fulfilling the criteria for the BPD diagnosis. In a recent study of 252 BPD patients, we found that 136 of these theoretically possible ways were represented in our material. Yet the criteria exhibited good psychometric qualities and indicated a unitary theoretical construct [4]. Concerning the pragmatics of the diagnosis, we only suggested that the diagnostic efficiency ranking of the criteria in the DSM-IV manual should be revised, and that the emptiness criterion should be more properly defined.

The upcoming revision of the DSM system has stirred a discussion of the validity of the current personality disorders. A high construct (or prototype) validity (as demonstrated for BPD) does not necessarily imply a high genetic or neurobiological validity. The principal question is: should one go for "conceptual kinds" or "natural kinds"? Livesley has argued in favour of "natural kinds" and suggested that current clinical and genetic data indicates four broad dimensions of personality dysfunction, e.g. emotional dysregulation, dissocial behaviour, inhibitedness and compulsivity [5]. The current BPD would certainly load high on emotional dysregulation, as would histrionic personality disorder (HPD), probably in combination with low inhibitedness.

In his review Stone argues that the histrionic criteria being implemented in 1980 covered a more severe disorder than the antecedent hysterical personality. Even so, Norwegian epidemiological data indicate that the current HPD is amongst the least severe personality disorders [6]. Our clinical data can be interpreted the same way. Amongst 861 patients with personality disorder from eight different day treatment programmes in Norway, there were only seven patients with the diagnosis of HPD, and for most of them HPD was one of several co-occurring personality disorder

[1] Department for Personality Psychiatry, Ullevål University Hospital, 0407 Oslo, Norway

diagnoses [7]. The general opinion in this Norwegian Network of Psycho-therapeutic Day Hospitals has been that histrionic patients seldom reach the level of severity (Global Assessment of Functioning, GAF score in the lower 40s) that is necessary for referral to partial hospitalization in Norway. And when they do, our data indicate that it is the co-occurrence of other personality disorder traits that contributes to the impaired level of functioning. In contrast, borderline personality traits, in our material, turned out to be among the most severe in areas such as global functioning, symptomatic and interpersonal distress, self-destructive as well as outwardly directed aggressive and antisocial behaviour, and need for psychiatric hospitalization [7].

At the end of his review Stone suggests that attachment issues and mentalization are important problem areas for histrionic patients. We would like to add that these problem areas are even more documented for borderline patients, indicating a dominance of the insecure preoccupied attachment pattern [8]. There is a challenge to find more differentiated models than the traditional broad attachment patterns. Accordingly we are now studying borderline patients with Crittenden's dynamic maturational system, which contains interpersonal strategies around use of falsified enhanced affect in combination with restricted cognition [9]. However, the broad attachment pattern categories have demonstrated significant predictive validity. Several studies have found that disorganized attachment is a risk factor for later development of serious personality pathology [10]. According to Fonagy et al. [10], the end result is malfunctioning interpersonal interpretive mechanisms, involving deficient mentalizing capabilities. It is promising that this theory can be linked to treatment strategies for borderline patients [11] that have been proved effective [12].

REFERENCES

1. Wilberg T., Urnes Ø., Friis S., Pedersen G., Karterud S. (1999) Borderline and avoidant personality disorders and the five-factor model of personality: a comparison of DSM-IV diagnoses and NEO-PI-R. *J. Person. Disord.*, **13**: 226–240.
2. Torgersen S., Kringlen E., Cramer V. (2001) The prevalence of personality disorders in a community sample. *Arch. Gen. Psychiatry*, **58**: 590–596.
3. Karterud S., Pedersen G., Bjordal E., Brabrand J., Friis S., Haaseth Ø., Haavaldsen G., Irion T., Leirvåg H., Tørum E. *et al.* (2003) Day hospital treatment of patients with personality disorders. Experiences from a Norwegian treatment research network. *J. Person. Disord.*, **17**: 243–262.
4. Johansen M., Karterud S., Pedersen G., Gude T., Falkum E. (in press) An investigation of the prototype validity of the borderline DSM-IV criteria. *Acta Psychiatr. Scand.*
5. Livesley J.W., Jang K.L. (2000) Toward an empirically based classification of personality disorder. *J. Person. Disord.*, **14**: 137–151.

6.   Torgersen S. (2002) Epidemiology of personality disorders. Presented at the 5th ISSPD European Congress on Personality Disorders, Munich, July 5.
7.   Wilberg T., Karterud S., Pedersen G., Urnes Ø. Functional impairment and symptomatic distress in patients with paranoid, borderline, avoidant, dependent, obsessive-compulsive or unspecified personality disorders. Manuscript in preparation.
8.   Dozier M., Stovall K.C., Albus K.E. (1999) Attachment and psychopathology in adulthood. In *Handbook of Attachment* (Eds J. Cassidy, P.R. Shaver), pp. 497–519. Guilford, New York.
9.   Crittenden P.M. (2000) *The Organization of Attachment Relationships: Maturation, Culture, and Context. A Dynamic-Maturational Approach to Continuity and Change in Pattern of Attachment.* Cambridge University Press, New York.
10. Fonagy P., Gergely G., Jurist E.L., Target M. (2002) *Affect Regulation, Mentalization, and the Development of the Self.* Other Press, New York.
11. Bateman A., Fonagy P. (in press) *Psychotherapy for Borderline Personality Disorder: Mentalisation Based Treatment.* Oxford University Press, Oxford.
12. Bateman A., Fonagy P. (2001) Treatment of borderline personality disorder with psychoanalytically oriented partial hospitalization: an 18-month follow-up. *Am. J. Psychiatry*, **158**: 36–42.

3.5
The Need for New Paradigms in the Research Approaches to Borderline Personality Disorder

Larry J. Siever[1]

Michael Stone brings a breadth of clinical wisdom as well as a scholarly review of the evidence with regard to borderline and histrionic personality disorders. Yet, it is clear in reading this review that much of what we "know" about the personality disorders rests on clinical anecdote and experience rather than a solid empirical base of research. Part of the reason for the relative dearth of evidence in these disorders can be attributed to several issues or questions, which Stone raises in his article. Are the personality disorders really medical disorders such as diabetes or hypertension, as has been increasingly acknowledged for the major Axis I disorders such as schizophrenia or major mood disorders? What are the aetiologic factors contributing to the personality disorders, including both genetic susceptibilities and environmental factors such as abuse? How do we understand the considerable comorbidity with Axis I disorders that is to be found in the personality disorders? How can we interpret the gender

[1] *Department of Psychiatry, Mount Sinai School of Medicine, One Gustave L. Levy Place, New York, NY 10029, USA*

differences in these disorders? What are the implications of these issues for treatment of personality disorders?

Personality disorders represent an extreme on a continuum of individual differences in personality and temperament that fall within the range of normality to clearly symptomatic disorders that may have considerable morbidity, as, for example, in the self-injurious behaviour and suicide attempts of borderline personality disorder (BPD). Because we can all recognize individual differences in personality, research in this area has been considered somewhat "soft" and the serious morbidity associated with them often underestimated. A more parsimonious model which is consistent with most medical disorders is that these variations exist on a continuum conceptualized in terms of dimensional traits with prominent temperamental underpinnings such as impulsivity or affective instability. Like hypertension, there may be a continuous distribution between normal and pathologic blood pressures, with genetic and environmental contributors to these dimensions. We may use the extremes of these dimensions as exhibited in the personality disorders as a means to more easily identify underlying genetic susceptibilities or environmental determinants. This approach has proved useful in the studies of impulsive aggression, affective instability, cognitive disorganization, and pain sensitivity in BPD. The identification of intermediate phenotypes may inform a search for candidate genes as well as indicate how genetic susceptibilities interact with environmental stressors. For example, polymorphisms related to the serotonin transporter promoter site, the 5-HT$_{2a}$ receptor, 5-HT$_{1b}$ receptor, and the MAO-A gene have associated with impulsive behaviour. The MAO-A genotype may only be expressed as impulsivity if occurring after a developmental history of abuse [1]. This trauma may need to interact with a vulnerable genetic substrate in order to yield the behavioural phenotype. Trauma may have a number of other effects in altering hypothalamic–pituitary–adrenal (HPA) axis activity [2]. Such a vulnerability model, with genetic and environmental factors interacting to determine the degree of personality pathology, may thus accommodate observations of individual differences in personality as well as the more severe personality disorders, but what is now required is a better understanding of the underlying genetic, developmental, and stress related aspects of this aetiology. A related question is that of comorbidity between Axis I and Axis II disorders. Michael Stone points out that BPD can be analogized to the "outside" of a Chinese dumpling while the "inside" consists of any of a dozen or more Axis I disorders, including mood, anxiety, and substance abuse disorders. This model might suggest that the traits of BPD are really only a superficial manifestation of underlying aetiological disorders such as the major mood or anxiety disorders. However, an examination of comorbidity of personality disorders and Axis I disorders such as that of depression and

BPD suggest the traits of BPD may be better predictors of external validating factors including biology, treatment, and outcome than the comorbid Axis I disorder. A more likely model may be that multiple genetic vulnerability factors and environmental precipitants may yield the phenotype of BPD, some of which are shared with Axis I disorders such as the affective or anxiety disorders [3–5].

In this context, the meaning of gender differences in prevalence of these disorders may be explored. Differences in prevalence across gender might reflect biologic differences in the brain issuing from genetic or hormonal distinctions between the sexes to differences in culturally sanctioned behaviours, as Stone alludes to. Again, without some idea of susceptibility mechanisms for the disorders, these gender differences become difficult to investigate.

Finally, the treatment interventions can be targeted to specific vulner-abilities such as impulsivity or affective dysregulation. Thus, dialectical behavioural therapy employs strategies that encourage reflection prior to action and avoid rewarding impulsive and self-destructive behaviours [6]. Medications which were initially targeted to comorbid conditions such as depression or anxiety are now being studied in relation to dimensions of vulnerability such as impulsivity and affective instability [7]. For both psychopharmacologic and psychosocial interventions, however, there needs to be a clearer appreciation of the specific vulnerabilities and strengths an individual patient presents, so that the treatment, as Stone suggests, can be tailored for them. Thus, our work is cut out for us in terms of advancing knowledge in this area to arrive at a truly evidence based treatment, but new paradigms in investigative approaches may bring us towards these goals more expeditiously.

REFERENCES

1. Caspi A., McClay J., Moffitt T.E., Mill J., Martin J. Craig I.W., Taylor A., Poulton R. (2002) Role of genotype in the cycle of violence in maltreated children. *Science*, **297**: 851–854.
2. Grossman R., Yehuda R., Santamaria N., Silverman J., Lee R., Siever L.J. (in press) Hypothalamic–pituitary–adrenal axis activity in personality disordered subjects: associations with major depression, psychological trauma, and post-traumatic stress disorder. *Am. J. Psychiatry*.
3. Siever L.J., Davis K.L. (1991) A psychobiologic perspective on the personality disorders. *Am. J. Psychiatry*, **148**: 1647–1658.
4. Gunderson J.G., Phillips K.A. (1991) A current view of the interface between borderline personality disorder and depression. *Am. J. Psychiatry*, **148**: 967–975.
5. Koenigsberg H.W., Anwunah I., New A.S., Mitropoulou V., Schopick F., Siever L.J. (1999) Relationship between depression and borderline personality disorder. *Depress. Anxiety*, **10**: 158–167.

6. Shearin E.N., Linehan M.M. (1994) Dialectical behavior therapy for borderline personality disorder: theoretical and empirical foundations. *Acta Psychiatr. Scand.*, **89** (Suppl. 379): 61–68.
7. Koenigsberg H.W., Woo-Ming A.M., Siever L.J. (2002) Pharmacological treatment for personality disorders. In *A Guide to Treatments That Work*, 2nd edn. (Eds P.E. Nathan, J.M. Gorman), pp. 625–641. Oxford University Press, New York.

3.6
Borderline Personality Disorder: From Clinical Heterogeneity to Diagnostic Coherence

Cesare Maffei[1]

It is well known that the term "borderline" has always been controversial, because it contains many sources of heterogeneity: pathogenetic, diagnostic, therapeutic. However, recent empirical research seems to shed light on sources of coherence. In this comment some recent data will be presented and commented.

Pathogenesis: traumatic factors. Borderline personality disorder (BPD) probably derives from the interaction of multiple pathogenetic factors, both biological and enviromental, differently combined in different subgroups of subjects. In the 1990s, many clinicians and researchers emphasized the role of childhood traumatic experiences, especially sexual abuse. However, results in this field should be considered cautiously. Available research data derive from very heterogeneous studies: sampling strategies, abuse definitions, source of information (mainly patients, without any external additional information) and methodology used to obtain information are problematic areas. A meta-analytic study [1] of the published literature, performed to evaluate the common effect size of the association between childhood sexual abuse and BPD, showed a moderate pooled r (0.279). The results of this study did not support the hypothesis that childhood sexual abuse is a major risk factor or a causal antecedent of BPD, while suggesting that it should be related to specific psychopathological features (e.g. stress-related dissociative symptoms) present in some, but not all, borderline patients.

Pathogenesis: biological components. The identification of significant temperamental characteristics, that is the genetically based component of personality, could give an important contribution to the search for specific "core dimensions" of BPD. In Cloninger's model, the role of high levels of novelty

---

[1] *Vita-Salute San Raffaele University, Via Stamira d'Ancona 20, 20127 Milan, Italy*

seeking has been considered: research data [2] showed that this temperamental dimension significantly differentiates borderline patients from patients with other Cluster B personality disorders, but also from patients with Cluster A and Cluster C diagnoses, and from mixed psychiatric patients. These differences remained significant when controlling for the effect of attachment variables and suggested that insecure attachment could be an unspecific characteristic of patients with personality disorder, more than a "marker" of BPD. Indeed, a subsequent study [3] showed a relationship between attachment patterns and personality disorders organized along two dimensions, avoidant and anxious. This relationship, however, seemed to be selective for some personality characteristics and not for the whole disorders. The specific role played by novelty seeking in BPD could contribute to confirm that impulsivity really represents a core construct of this disorder, as hypothesized by many researchers. Impulsivity can be considered as a component of novelty seeking, or, using different terms, of impulsive unsocialized sensation seeking [4]. Moreover, since impulsivity is a multidimensional construct, the different importance of its dimensions should be identified. Few data are available: a preliminary study in nonclinical subjects [5] showed that the dimension called motor impulsivity, or "acting without thinking" significantly predicted both borderline and antisocial characteristics. However, dimensions of aggressiveness were differently associated with borderline and antisocial personality disorder features: the former were associated with irritability, resentment and guilt, while the latter were associated with physical aggression, indirect aggression and negativism. A second study in patients [6] confirmed these findings.

Diagnostic validity. Even if the clinical features of BPD could seem very heterogeneous, and its categorial model questionable, the few available empirical studies [7–9] on factor analytical structure obtained partially comparable results, showing the presence of two or three factors. These factors were mainly related to identity and interpersonal problems, affective dysregulation, impulse/behaviour dysregulation. One study [10] showed a unidimensional construct of BPD and a different efficiency of the various diagnostic criteria. The rank order obtained suggested that identity problems, interpersonal difficulties and impulsivity could be the most typical features of BPD. Moreover, exploratory latent class analysis gave some evidence of a categorial structure. These results are not in contrast with those previously quoted, because all the studies show that the BPD diagnosis is not a hotchpotch of heterogeneous clinical phenomena. On the contrary, BPD seems to show some structural validity, and characteristic "core dimensions" are identifiable. However, this does not mean that borderline patients are a homogeneous group of patients. Sources of heterogeneity should be better understood, but the present results give some useful indications for treatment plans.

REFERENCES

1. Fossati A., Madeddu F., Maffei C. (1999) Borderline personality disorder and childhood sexual abuse: a meta-analytic study. *J. Person. Disord.*, **13**: 268–280.
2. Fossati A., Donati D., Donini M., Novella L., Bagnato M., Maffei C. (2001) Temperament, character and attachment patterns in borderline personality disorder. *J. Person. Disord.*, **15**: 390–402.
3. Fossati A., Feeney J.A., Donati D., Donini M., Novella L., Bagnato M., Carretta I., Leonardi B., Mirabelli S., Maffei C. (2003) Personality disorders and adult attachment dimensions in a mixed psychiatric sample: a multivariate study. *J. Nerv. Ment. Dis.*, **191**: 30–37.
4. Zuckerman M. (1993) Sensation seeking and impulsivity: a marriage of traits made in biology? In *The Impulsive Client. Theory, Research and Treatment* (Eds W.G. McCown, J.L. Johnson, M.B. Shure), pp. 71–91. American Psychological Association, Washington.
5. Fossati A., Barratt E.S., Carretta I., Leonardi B., Maffei C. (in press) Predicting borderline and antisocial personality disorder features in nonclinical subjects using measures of impulsivity and aggressiveness. *Psychiatry Res.*
6. Fossati A., Barratt E.S., Carretta I., Leonardi B., Maffei C. Unfolding the latent connections between impulsivity, aggression, and DSM-IV personality disorders: a factor analytic study in an outpatient sample. Submitted for publication.
7. Rosenberger P.H., Miller G.A. (1983) Comparing borderline definitions: DSM-III borderline and schizotypal personality disorders. *J. Abnorm. Psychol.*, **98**: 161–169.
8. Clarkin J.F., Hull J.W., Hurt S.W. (1993) Factor structure of borderline personality disorders criteria. *J. Person. Disord.*, **7**: 137–143.
9. Sanislow C.A., Grilo C.M., McGlashan T.H. (2000) Factor analysis of the DSM-III-R borderline personality disorder criteria in psychiatric inpatients. *Am. J. Psychiatry*, **157**: 1629–1633.
10. Fossati A., Maffei C., Bagnato M., Donati D., Namia C., Novella L. (1999) Latent structure analysis of DSM-IV borderline personality disorder criteria. *Compr. Psychiatry*, **40**: 72–79.

3.7
Borderline Personality Disorder: Problems of Definition and Complex Aetiology

Jiri Modestin[1]

Borderline personality disorder (BPD) is the most discussed while clinically the most relevant and challenging personality disorder (PD). It is a "young" disorder, absent in its present form in the older PD surveys and not introduced in the official classifications until 1980. As Stone rightly stresses, only a minority (3/9) of the defining items are true personality traits, the remaining items representing symptoms or behavioural patterns. It is just

[1] *Psychiatric Hospital Burghölzli, Lenggstrasse 31, CH-8029 Zurich, Switzerland*

the non-trait criterion of interpersonal relationships that has a special diagnostic weight, due to its high positive predictive power, age-independence and sufficient sensitivity [1,2].

Stone credits Kernberg [3] with the attribution of the borderline pathology to the personality domain; indeed, the conception of borderline personality organization (BPO) represents one of the roots of the DSM BPD definition. One of the DSM BPD items, identity disturbance—incidently, more clearly and reliably defined by DSM-III-R and less so by DSM-IV—represents in its uniqueness as an inferential criterion a direct heritage of Kernberg's BPO, where it is viewed as a core characteristic. Theoretically, the Kernberg's conception of BPO is much broader than the DSM conception of BPD; actually, the majority of the DSM PD types have been claimed to have BPO [4]. However, the overlap between BPO and the whole PD category is far from being perfect: admittedly, identity disturbance, one of the basic defining features of BPO, can be encountered in all PD types; however, it was absent in about a half of all patients with PD diagnosis including a proportion of patients with BPD [5]. Due to its large overlap with other PDs, "BPD appears to constitute a broad, heterogeneous category with unclear boundaries that embraces a general PD concept" [6]—just as BPO does. In any case, there is a considerable variation in the clinical picture of any sample of BPD patients. This is due to the comorbidity with Axis I and II, but also to the DSM BPD definition itself. If five of nine criteria are necessary for the diagnosis, then two patients may share only one single criterion.

PD scores tend to diminish with age. This negative correlation is strongest with the four PDs in Cluster B including BPD [7]. Along with the criterion of physically self-damaging acts, it is the criterion of identity disturbance which is significantly less frequently met in older BPD patients: it was found in 55% of patients aged <35, but in 27% of older patients [8]. Some patients will achieve their identity with a delay due to a later maturation, maybe helped by psychotherapy; some others develop their identity later on in accordance with their social role: role identity would transform into personal identity. Identification or even overidentification with a patient role may help some BPD patients to cope with the stigma of mental disorder [9] and/or to stabilize their own identity [10].

Stone rightly points to the complex aetiology of BPD; on the one hand, there is probably a genetic basis for some BPD dimensions such as impulsivity and affective instability. On the other hand, a correlation between a history of traumatic experiences (sexual abuse) and borderline pathology has repeatedly been found in many samples [11–13]. Trauma experiences of different kind could contribute to BPD characteristics such as identity disturbance, unstable interpersonal relationships and self-damaging behaviour. Different borderline domains, having different aetiolological

252 _____ PERSONALITY DISORDERS

roots and pathogenetic pathways, could be amenable to different therapeutic approaches. We can hardly treat impulsivity and identity problems in the same way. Beyond that, negative environmental factors— along with the initial severity of the disorder—seem to be associated with a poor prognosis. The long-term BPD prognosis itself is, however, obviously better than previously thought. The majority of patients maintain some of their symptoms but, generally, are functioning pretty well; we are not sure whether this outcome reflects the impact of treatment or the natural course of the disorder.

REFERENCES

1. Clarkin J.F., Widiger T.A., Frances A., Hurt S.W., Gilmore M. (1983) Prototypic typology and the borderline personality disorder. *J. Abnorm. Psychol.*, **92**: 236–275.
2. Dahl A.A. (1986) Some aspects of the DSM-III personality disorder illustrated by a consecutive sample of hospitalized patients. *Acta Psychiatr. Scand.*, **73** (Suppl. 328): 61–67.
3. Kernberg O.F. (1967) Borderline personality organization. *J. Am. Psychoanal. Assoc.*, **15**: 641–684.
4. Kernberg O.F. (1975) *Borderline Conditions and Pathological Narcissism*, pp. 33–47. Aronson, New York.
5. Modestin J., Oberson B., Erni T. (1998) Identity disturbance in personality disorders. *Compr. Psychiatry*, **39**: 352–357.
6. Nurnberg H.G., Raskin M., Levine P.E., Pollack S., Siegel O., Prince R. (1991) The comorbidity of borderline personality disorder and other DSM-III-R axis II personality disorders. *Am. J. Psychiatry*, **148**: 1371–1377.
7. Zimmerman M., Coryell W.H. (1990) DSM-III personality disorder dimensions. *J. Nerv. Ment. Dis.*, **178**: 686–692.
8. Modestin J. (1987) Quality of interpersonal relationships: the most characteristic DSM-III BPD criterion. *Compr. Psychiatry*, **28**: 397–402.
9. Goffman E. (1963) *Stigma: Notes on the Management of Spoiled Identity*. Prentice-Hall, Englewood Cliffs.
10. Dreitzel H.P. (1972) *Die Gesellschaftlichen Leiden und das Leiden an der Gesellschaft*. Enke, Stuttgart.
11. Herman J.L., Perry J.C., van der Kolk B.A. (1989) Childhood trauma in borderline personality disorder. *Am. J. Psychiatry*, **146**: 490–495.
12. Paris J., Zweig-Frank H., Guzder J. (1994) Psychological risk factors for borderline personality disorder in female patients. *Compr. Psychiatry*, **35**: 301–305.
13. Zanarini M.C., Williams A.A., Lewis R.E., Reich R.B., Vera S.C., Marino M.F., Levin A., Yong L., Frankenburg F.R. (1997) Reported pathological childhood experiences associated with the development of borderline personality disorder. *Am. J. Psychiatry*, **154**: 1101–1106.

3.8
Some Problems in the Current Conceptualization of Borderline and Histrionic Personality Disorders

Enrique Baca Baldomero[1]

At present, there are still several conceptual problems concerning personality disorders (PDs), which can be summarized as follows [1]: (a) the concept of PDs as a collection of *dimensions* which can be identified by using factor analysis techniques, versus the idea of *specific structures* which determine distinct and specific nosologic categories; (b) a genetic basis for these dimensions or structures, versus an origin based on early-life subject-environment interactions; (c) a dimensional continuity between normal personalities and PDs, versus the existence of *qualitative* differences which neatly separate pathology from normality; (d) a unitarian concept of PD versus the typification of different entities; (e) the conceptualization of PDs as diseases within a strictly medical model, versus their conceptualization as social deviations or abnormal variations in Kurt Schneider's use of the term.

All these matters have been debated at some point in the recent history of psychiatry. They need to be resolved to allow a satisfactory development in the research and understanding of PDs. In the last years there has been an accumulation of data, but research has been neglected on these conceptual aspects.

PDs can be understood as an alteration of two levels of personality construction: biological modulation, in terms of "styles of brain functioning", which conditions the aspects called "temperamental" after the works of Kretschmer and Cloninger, and the values acquired during the development period, which are operative in adult life and condition the aspects subsumed under the term "character". It is quite possible that the proportion in which temperamental and characterial aspects are involved determines conceptually different PDs: the psychopathic disorders would result from a greater alteration of temperamental aspects, while the abnormal personality developments, whose pathogenesis and dynamic are close to neurotic mechanisms, would be caused by a specific alteration of characterial structures. This distinction may help clarify the obscure aspects which are nowadays common in many PDs described in international classifications, among them borderline personality disorder (BPD) and histrionic personality disorder (HPD).

Two problems can be found in the current conceptualization of BPD: (a) its inclusion among PDs without taking into consideration that the term

[1] *Department of Psychiatry, Autonomous University of Madrid, Spain*

BPD comprises both symptoms which should belong to Axis I, and personality alterations which should be classified in Axis II (this means that BPD is in fact a complex group of disorders, which have been wrongly "concentrated" under a confusing term); (b) the lack of a basic structure which would give a unified meaning to the symptomatic variations which are observed, and could explain the different evolutive forms of the disorder and the lack of uniformity in treatment response. There is dire need of a proposal which can address these two questions, in order to give a proper explanation to all the problems which are detected daily in clinical practice, in which the fulfilment of the established diagnostic criteria does not allow to establish homogeneous intervention plans with a good chance of obtaining an adequate response. The high comorbidity rates which are found in BPD seem to support the idea of a clinical and conceptual heterogeneity of the disorder, rather than explaining the extreme variation in the course and therapeutic response. In the field of psychiatry, comorbidity is often an indicator of weakness of a diagnostic construct.

The situation concerning HPD is somewhat different. European psychiatry kept the concept of hysterical neurosis until the implementation of DSM classifications. This was understood as a stable structure in which traits of intolerance to frustration, inability to build solid and well founded relationships, and a tendency to manipulation, appear together with affective immaturity, tendency to the utilisation of others, constant search of attention, and egocentric behaviour, all of it presided by the theatricality of emotional expressions, in contrast to the affective isolation and the lack of syntony with the usual feelings of other people. Thus this disorder, unlike BPD, shows an adequate internal consistency and cohesion among traits and symptoms. This allows the distinction between two types of comorbidity, depending on whether the personality problem is primary or secondary (e.g. a patient with HPD may suffer from anxiety or depression, but, if the personality problem is primary, the Axis I disorder will be completely modulated and determined by the underlying personality structure).

The co-existence or relatedness of BPD and HPD may probably be explained by the above mentioned inconsistency and mediocre validity of the construct of BPD, which is frequently used as an inappropriate diagnosis in severe cases of HPD, especially in those in which the disruptive aspects of behaviour predominate in the clinical picture.

REFERENCE

1. Baca E., Roca M. (2004) Personalidad y trastorno de la personalidad: historia y evolución de los conceptos. In Trastornos de Personalidad (Ed. M. Roca), pp. 3–31. Ars Médica, Madrid.

3.9
Borderline (and Histrionic) Personality Disorders: Boundaries, Epidemiology, Genetics and Treatment

Svenn Torgersen[1]

Michael Stone presents a very comprehensive overview of what we know today about borderline personality disorder (BPD). He feels also compelled to include histrionic personality disorder (HPD), as this is necessary to clarify the status of BPD. In my opinion, he raises the following questions: (a) the appropriateness of the criteria for BPD in DSM-IV and the delineation to HPD; (b) the relationship between BPD and major depression; (c) the prevalence of BPD; (d) the causes of BPD, especially the genetic ones; (e) the treatment of choice for BPD; (f) the question of continuity of BPD and HPD traits, from normality to severe disorder. I am going to address in this commentary these six topics.

It is true that the conceptual status of the DSM-IV criteria for personality disoders is somewhat muddy, with some being personality traits, other single behaviours (what Stone calls "symptoms"). However, this is even more the case for antisocial personality disorder and also, among others, schizotypal personality disorder. DSM-IV is pragmatic: as long as they correlate, items are put together. ICD-10 is even worse. The criteria for obsessive (anancastic) and avoidant (anxious) personality disorders are partly obsessive and anxiety symptoms.

As to HPD, Stone states the same as Kernberg [1]: that HPD defines a severe hysterical personality type. I am afraid I do not agree. Those with HPD are functioning very well, just as those with obsessive personality disorder. They are quite happy, have a relatively high level of self-realization, a relatively low level of dysfunction and are well integrated socially [2]. Their only problem is a high tendency to break relationships. They fall in love and change partners.

As Stone maintains, it is assumed that there exists a relationship between BPD and major depression. However, the data are equivocal. A large study of psychiatric outpatients did not disclose such a relationship [3]. A study of co-twins and first-degree relatives of patients with major depression did not observe a high frequency of BPD [4]. On the other hand, BPD predicts relapses and chronicity in major depression [5].

Stone states that the prevalence of BPD is 2%. This percentage is a little too high. Eleven epidemiological studies display a prevalence between 0 and 3.2%. Only three studies showed a prevalence of 2% or higher. The median prevalence of these studies was 1.1% and the pooled prevalence

---

[1] Oslo University, P.O. Box 1094, Blindern, N-0317 Oslo, Norway

was 1.04% [6–16]. On the other hand, the prevalence of HPD is higher: it was between 0.3 and 4.5% in the eleven studies, with a median of 2.1 and a pooled prevalence of 2.19% [6–16]. The reason why the prevalence of BPD appears so high is that no other personality disorder implies such a strong tendency to seek treatment [2].

The study of dysfunctional personality traits among twins shows that genetic factors are important, both for traits similar to BPD and for those similar to HPD, while shared environment is of no importance [17]. A twin study of BPD and HPD displays that genetic factors are very important in their development [18], and that shared environment could not be excluded for these disorders.

No doubt the best studies of treatment effects are related to Linehan's dialectical behaviour therapy. Too many studies, unfortunately, are naturalistic without adequate control. When different theory related treatment methods are investigated, the effects appear to be the same irrespective of the specific type of psychotherapeutic treatment. What counts is the therapist's warmth, optimism, ability to create bonds to the patient [19].

When we look at published studies of the relationship between BPD and the five factor model of personality, we find that individuals with BPD are characterized by high neuroticism and relatively low agreeableness and conscientiousness, irrespective of whether BPD is assessed by interview or questionnaire [20–22]. Extraversion is not related to BPD.

As to the question of continuity from normality to severe disorder, studies of quality of life and dysfunction show that there is a linear relationship between number of criteria fulfilled for BPD (and HPD) and quality of life and dysfunction [2]. There is no natural cutting point for disorder/not disorder, and even one criteria of BPD fulfilled implies more dysfunction than zero criteria.

REFERENCES

1. Kernberg O. (1984). *Severe Personality Disorders*. Yale University Press, New Haven.
2. Cramer V., Torgersen S., Kringlen E. (2003) Personality disorders: prevalence, socio-demographic correlations, quality of life, dysfunction, and the question of continuity. *Persønlichkeitstørungen*, 7: 189–198.
3. Alnæs R., Torgersen S. (1988) The relationship between DSM-III symptom disorders (Axis I) and personality disorders (Axis II) in an outpatient population. *Acta Psychiatr. Scand.*, 78: 485–492.
4. Torgersen S., Onstad S., Skre I., Edvardsen J., Kringlen E. (1993) "True" schizotypal personality disorder: a study of co-twins and relatives of schizophrenic probands. *Am. J. Psychiatry*, 150: 1661–1667.

5. Alnæs, R., Torgersen, S. (1997) Personality and personality disorders predict the development and relapses of major depression. *Acta Psychiatr. Scand.*, **95**: 336–342.
6. Drake R.E., Adler D.A., Vaillant G.E. (1988) Antecedents of personality disorders in a community sample of men. *J. Person. Disord.*, **2**: 60–68.
7. Zimmerman M., Coryell W. (1989) DSM-III personality disorder diagnoses in a nonpatient sample. Demographic correlates and comorbidity. *Arch. Gen. Psychiatry*, **46**: 682–689.
8. Reich J., Yates W., Nduaguba M. (1989) Prevalences of DSM-III personality disorders in the community. *Soc. Psychiatr. Epidemiol.*, **24**: 12–16.
9. Black D.W., Noyes Jr. R., Pfohl B., Goldstein R.B., Blum N. (1993). Personality disorders in obsessive-compulsive volunteers, well comparison subjects, and their first-degree relatives. *Am. J. Psychiatry*, **150**: 1226–1232.
10. Maier W., Lichtermann D., Klingler T., Heun R., Hallmayer J. (1992) Prevalences of personality disorders (DSM-III-R) in the community. *J. Person. Disord.*, **6**: 187–196.
11. Bodlund O., Ekselius L., Lindström E. (1993) Personality traits and disorders among psychiatric outpatients and normal subjects on the basis of the SCID screen questionnaire. *Nordic J. Psychiatry*, **47**: 425–433.
12. Samuels J.F., Nestadt G., Romanoski A.J., Folstein M.F., McHugh P.R. (1994) DSM-III personality disorders in the community. *Am. J. Psychiatry*, **151**: 1055–1062.
13. Moldin S.O., Rice J.P., Erlenmeyer-Kimling L., Squires-Wheeler E. (1994) Latent structure of DSM-III-R Axis II psychopathology in a normal sample. *J. Abnorm. Psychol.*, **103**: 259–266.
14. Klein D.N., Riso L.P., Donaldson S.K., Schwartz J.E., Anderson R.L., Oiumette P.C., Lizardi H., Aronson T.A. (1995) Family study of early-onset dysthymia: mood and personality disorders in relatives of outpatients with dysthymia and episodic major depressive and normal controls. *Arch. Gen. Psychiatry*, **52**: 487–496.
15. Lenzenweger M.F., Loranger A.W., Korfine L., Neff C. (1997) Detecting personality disorders in a nonclinical population: application of a 2-stage procedure for case identification. *Arch. Gen. Psychiatry*, **54**: 345–351.
16. Torgersen S., Kringlen E., Cramer V. (2001) The prevalence of personality disorders in a community sample. *Arch. Gen. Psychiatry*, **58**: 590–596.
17. Jang K.L., Livesley W.J., Vernon P.A., Jackson D.N. (1996) Heritability of personality disorder traits: a twin study. *Acta Psychiatr. Scand.*, **94**: 438–444.
18. Torgersen S., Lygren S., Øien P.A., Skre I., Onstad S., Edvardsen J., Tambs K., Kringlen E. (2000) A twin study of personality disorders. *Compr. Psychiatry*, **41**: 416–425.
19. Orlinsky D.E., Grawe K., Parks B.K. (1994) Process and outcome in psychotherapy. In *Handbook of Psychotherapy and Behavioral Change* (Eds A.E. Bergin, S.L. Garfield), pp. 270–376. Wiley, New York.
20. Costa P.T. Jr., McCrae R.R. (1990) Personality disorders and the five factor model of personality. *J. Person. Dis.*, **4**: 362–371.
21. Trull T.J. (1992) DSM-III-R personality disorders and the five-factor model of personality: an empirical comparison. *J. Abnorm. Psychol.*, **101**: 553–560.
22. Soldz S., Budman S., Demby A., Merry J. (1993) Representation of personality disorders in circumplex and five-factor space: exploration with a clinical sample. *Psychol. Assess.*, **5**: 41–52.

3.10
Categorical Conundrums
John F. Clarkin[1]

The diagnostic system currently applied to personality disorders has been in existence since the introduction of DSM-III in 1980, long enough to expose both its advantages and disadvantages. The strength of the review by Michael Stone is to remind us of the history of conceptualization of character pathology, personality organization, and the articulation of the personality disorders in the DSM-III system and its successors. His paper highlights some of the difficulties with the current diagnostic approach: (a) the unfortunate combination of traits, behaviours, and symptoms used unevenly as criteria for the various disorders; (b) the rampant co-morbidity among personality disordered patients with this diagnostic scheme; (c) the historical context in which DSM, with its emphasis on phenomenology and reliable assessment, has changed the underlying conception of clinical syndromes of borderline and hysterical character pathology; (d) following DSM, the collection of data, most benefical to our field, but based on the criteria that mix symptoms and traits. Stone is masterful in making sense of the historical progression, and in attempting to understand the complexity of the patients that present in our offices.

The clear differences between the clinical tradition prior to DSM and that which flows from the DSM, that Stone articulates so clearly, continue to this day. DSM guides much of the empirical research work that Stone refers to, but at the same time clinicians do not use the specific criteria to guide their assessment and treatment planning [1]. Instead of using the symptom and trait criteria, clinicians pursue the patients' patterns of relating inter-personally, and how they interact in the therapeutic relationship.

The review of current empirical work on the phenomenology and treatment of borderline personality disorder is thorough. One could only wish that Stone would suggest what to make of the effectiveness of the various treatments for this disorder, which treatments to use for what types of patients (granted, there are no data on this), and where the research might go in the future. In regards to most recent longitudinal studies of borderline personality disorder, a large multi-site study (not mentioned by Stone) seems to suggest that the patients are characterized by instability in DSM criteria but stability in poor work and social functioning [2]. To this writer, the implication is that the status of work and relationships is more important than many of

[1] New York Presbyterian Hospital, Cornell Medical Center, 21 Bloomingdale Road, White Plains, New York, NY 10605, USA

the criteria in the DSM criteria set. This has implications for the future of Axis II.

By having the same author review both borderline and histrionic personality disorder, the discrepancy in available information on the two disorders is striking. With borderline personality disorder, there is phenomenological, longitudinal, and treatment data. In sharp contrast there are no longitudinal nor treatment data on histrionic personality disorder, so Stone is reduced to making suggestions for treatment based on clinical hunches and speculation. This is not to criticize what he says, but is rather reflective of the state of our field. It raises an interesting question as to why some personality disorders gather so much attention, and others so little.

In summary, the field is faced with a conundrum: (a) the DSM categorical diagnostic system for personality disorders uses criteria that focus unevenly upon symptoms, behaviours, and traits (which of course, contributes to the confusion between Axis II personality disorders and Axis I symptom disorders); (b) some disorders as currently defined (e.g. borderline personality disorder) attract much research attention and others (e.g. histrionic personality disorder) attract virtually none, and (c) there is a large discrepancy between practices in clinical evaluation of personality disorders and the criteria set of DSM.

REFERENCES

1. Westen D. (1997) Divergences between clinical and research methods for assessing personality disorders: implications for research and the evolution of Axis II. *Am. J. Psychiatry*, **154**: 895–903.
2. Skodol A., Gunderson J.G., McGlashan T., Dyck I., Stout R., Bender D., Grilo C., Shea M.T., Zanarini M., Morey L. *et al.* (2002) Functional impairment in patients with schizotypal, borderline, avoidant, or obsessive-compulsive personality disorder. *Am. J. Psychiatry*, **159**: 276–283.

3.11
Are Cyclothymic Temperament and Borderline and Histrionic Personality Related Concepts?

Giulio Perugi[1]

As Michel Stone clearly states in his excellent review, the definition of borderline and histrionic personality disorders in the DSM-III and DSM-IV refers to conditions characterized by persistent "emotional instability" and excessive "mood reactivity", with strong links to affective disorders, in particular bipolar II and related cyclothymic depressions. In this comment, we further develop the view that cyclothymic temperament and DSM-IV borderline and histrionic personality disorders may describe largely overlapping clinical pictures from different perspectives.

The concept of "affective temperament" derives from Greco-Roman and continental European psychiatry and refers to specific constitutionally-based affective dispositions, i.e. the melancholic-dysthymic, choleric-irritable, sanguine-hyperthymic and cyclothymic. It is a dimensional construct, which only in its extremes may be considered abnormal in a statistical, and perhaps clinical, sense. Kraepelin [1] described the cyclothymic disposition as one of the constitutional substrates from which manic-depressive illness arose. Kretschmer [2] went one step further and proposed that this constitution represented the core characteristic of the illness.

The criteria found in modern psychiatric literature for cyclothymic temperament, operationalized by Akiskal [3], are characterized, throughout much of the patient's lifetime, by rapid alternation of opposite moods or conditions, such as hypersomnia and a decreased need for sleep; introverted self-absorption and uninhibited people-seeking; taciturnity and talkativeness; unexplained tearfulness and buoyant jocularity; psychomotor inertia and a restless pursuit of activity; lethargy or somatic discomfort and a sense of energetic well being; dulled senses and keen perception; slow-wittedness and alert, clear thinking; low self-confidence and overconfidence; pessimistic brooding and carefree optimism.

Cyclothymic temperament is characterized by extreme lability and, as a result, distinct hypomanic episodes are not easily discernible as part of the baseline of this temperament. The bipolar nature of cyclothymic temperament is confirmed by the propensity of a patient to switch to hypomania and/or mania when treated with antidepressants, as well as by a family history of bipolar disorders [4,5]. When affective oscillations become extreme and associated with very significant disruption and interpersonal

---

[1] *Department of Psychiatry, University of Pisa, and Institute of Behavioural Science G. De Lisio, Pisa-Carrara, Italy*

conflict, many cyclothymic individuals also meet criteria for so-called "borderline" and other erratic personality disorders. Studies focused on borderline personality cohorts have also reported high rates of cyclothymia [6] and/or soft bipolar spectrum diagnoses [7]. In a German study [8], which rigorously rated "sub-affective personality disorders", borderline and irritable-cyclothymic conditions overlapped considerably. Furthermore, as expected, borderline personality has been found to be a predictor of pharmacological hypomania [9].

In patients with cyclothymic temperament and bipolar II disorder, lifetime co-morbidity with anxiety disorders (in particular panic disorder-agoraphobia), bulimia nervosa, body dysmorphic disorder, alcohol and substance abuse disorder and both Cluster C (anxious) and Cluster B (dramatic) personality disorders, is the rule rather than the exception [10]. A large proportion of these patients meets DSM-IV criteria for borderline personality disorder [11,12]. Cyclothymic-bipolar II-borderline patients display a long-lasting "stable" hyper-reactivity to many psychological (i.e. rejection, separation) and physical (i.e. food, light, drugs) stimuli. This marked reactivity of mood could also explain the frequent concomitance of impulse control disorder and substance and alcohol abuse. The presence of a long-lasting cyclothymic-anxious-sensitive disposition seems to constitute a common background to the complex syndromic pattern of anxiety, mood and impulsive disorders which patients in this realm display during their adolescence and young adulthood [12]. We are aware that prominent investigators with a long record of experience in this field [13] downplay the affective component in bipolar personality disorder and argue instead that the extreme emotionality and behavioural dyscontrol of these patients reflects a childhood legacy of emotional and physical abuse. Obviously, both nature and nurture contribute to this process, in varying degrees, and opposing viewpoints in this realm could reflect the difference between those who give precedence to innate temperamental factors (affective traits) and those who attribute characterological (borderline) pathology to a developmental origin.

Recently, we attempted to provide an empirically-based response to the problem of separating the shifting affective symptomatology of bipolar II patients with atypical depression from their long-term temperamental and characterologic attributes. The study [14] revealed that the presence of cyclothymic temperament explains much of the relationship between bipolar II disorder and borderline personality disorder. The diagnosis of borderline personality disorder in these patients was favoured by the co-existence of an affective cyclothymic temperamental dysregulation with anxious-dependent traits. We find no reason to separate bipolar II with cyclothymic instability from the persistent instability of the borderline type [15], since mood lability is a common characteristic of both sets of disorders. Furthermore, correlational analyses [16] indicate that, in bipolar II atypical depressives, mood reactivity and interpersonal sensitivity traits might be related constructs with a cyclothymic temperamental matrix. Interpersonal sensitivity and usual mood reactivity seem to represent two strongly related temperamental features, representing different aspects (cognitive and affective) of the same psycho(patho)logical dimension. On the other hand, the presence of cyclothymic traits also appears to be related to interpersonal sensitivity and extreme mood reactivity, suggesting a common temperamental background between these constructs.

The overlap of the first two axes of the DSM system suggests that to take into account systematically combined trait and state features may be useful in order to increase the validity of current diagnostic categories. This is particularly true for affective disorders, which usually undergo a complex development during a patient's entire lifetime, influencing cognitive, emotional, and behavioural functioning even during relatively "asymptomatic" phases. Inadequate attention to this trait-state relationship represents one of the major limitations of the current diagnostic systems. The introduction of a separate Axis II for personality disorders, based on the assumption of a relative independence between mental disorders and personality traits, cannot resolve this problem. It actually appears to have broadened the gulf between affective and personality disorders (and their respective researchers!).

REFERENCES

1. Kraepelin E. (1921) *Manic-depressive Insanity and Paranoia*. Livingstone, Edinburgh.
2. Kretschmer E. (1936) *Physique and Character*. Kegan, Paul, Trench, Trubner and Co., London.
3. Akiskal H.S., Khani M.K., Scott-Strauss A. (1979) Cyclothymic temperamental disorders. *Psychiatr. Clin. North Am.*, **2**: 527–554.
4. Akiskal H.S., Djenderedjian A.M., Rosenthal R.H., Khani M.K. (1977) Cyclothymic disorder: validating criteria for inclusion in the bipolar affective group. *Am. J. Psychiatry*, **134**: 1227–1233.
5. Klein D.N., Depue R.A., Slater J.F. (1986) Inventory identification of cyclothymia. IX. Validation in offspring of bipolar I patients. *Arch. Gen. Psychiatry*, **43**: 441–445.
6. Levitt A.J., Joffe R.T., Ennis J., MacDonald C., Kutcher S.P. (1990) The prevalence of cyclothymia in borderline personality disorder. *J. Clin. Psychiatry*, **51**: 335–339.
7. Deltito J., Martin L., Riefkohl J., Austria B., Kissilenko A., Corless P. (2001) Do patients with borderline personality disorder belong to the bipolar spectrum? *J. Affect. Disord.*, **67**: 221–228.
8. Sab H., Herpertz S., Steinmeyer E.M. (1993) Subaffective personality disorders. *Int. Clin. Psychopharmacol.*, **1** (Suppl. 1): 39–46.
9. Levy D., Kimhi R., Barak Y., Viv A., Elizur A. (1998) Antidepressant-associated mania: a study of anxiety disorders patients. *Psychopharmacology*, **136**: 243–246.

BORDERLINE/HISTRIONIC PERSONALITY DISORDERS: COMMENTARIES ___ 263

10. Perugi G., Akiskal H.S. (2002) The soft bipolar spectrum redefined: focus on the cyclothymic-anxious-sensitive, impulse-dyscontrol, and binge-eating connection in bipolar II and related conditions. *Psychiatr. Clin. North Am.*, **25**: 713–737.
11. Soloff P.H., George A., Nathan R.S., Schulz P.M. (1987) Characterizing depression in borderline patients. *J. Clin. Psychiatry*, **48**: 155–157.
12. Perugi G., Akiskal H.S., Lattanzi L., Cecconi D., Mastrocinque C., Patronelli A., Vignoli S., Bemi E. (1998) The high prevalence of soft bipolar (II) features in atypical depression. *Compr. Psychiatry*, **39**: 1–9.
13. Gunderson J.G., Phillips K.A. (1991) A current view of the interface between borderline personality disorder and depression. *Am. J. Psychiatry*, **148**: 967–975.
14. Perugi G., Akiskal H.S. (in press) Are bipolar II, atypical depression and borderline personality overlapping manifestations of a common cyclothymic-sensitive diathesis? *J. Clin. Psychiatry*.
15. Henry C., Mitropoulou V., New A., Koenigsber H., Silverman J., Siever L. (2001) Affective instability and impulsivity in borderline personality and bipolar II disorders: similarities and differences. *J. Psychiatr. Res.*, **35**: 307–312.
16. Perugi G., Toni C., Travierso M.C., Akiskal H.S. (2003) The role of cyclothymia in atypical depression: toward a data-based reconceptualization of the borderline-bipolar II connection. *J. Affect. Disord.*, **73**: 87–98.

3.12
Borderline and Histrionic Personality Disorders: Implications for Health Services

Brian Martindale[1]

This WPA volume on personality disorders will have been most worthwhile if it makes a contribution to overcoming the common finding that "Many clinicians and mental health practitioners are reluctant to work with people with personality disorder because they believe that they have neither the skills, training or resources to provide an adequate service, and because many believe there is nothing that mental health services can offer" [1].

Michael Stone's review achieves the important tasks of delineating the phenomena encountered within contemporary definitions of borderline and hysteroid personality disorders and gives grounds for cautious optimism about treatment possibilities. However, in Western societies, it is a sad but realistic fact that we will only see greater investment on behalf of these troubled persons when there is much harder evidence of financial costs to the community when untreated and financial benefits from therapeutic interventions. The societal, psychological and practical problems that will be encountered in achieving this necessary research are considerable.

[1] *Psychotherapy Department, West London Mental Health Trust, Uxbridge Road, Southall, Middlesex UB1 3EU, UK*

Amongst many factors, major obstacles include the professional and social stigma against this clinical population, the predominant medical model in psychiatry that focuses on symptoms and current state disorders rather than underlying traits and developmental issues (with the excessive dependence on the pharmaceutical industry for research money), and not least the problematic fact that any worthwhile research needs to be long term when we are talking about personality disorders.

There is one essential point that follows from Stone's description of these two personality disturbances that is in keeping with everyday clinical experience. All persons who engage over time with these persons will inevitably be subject to stress and distress, because these particular personality disturbances manifest themselves in disturbing relations with others, and clinicians are not spared this consequence. This 'clinical' fact is probably the main underlying reason for the frequent rejection of these persons from services other than emergency care. The rejection often only leads to more frequent, often escalating, contact across a spectrum of services including mental health, social services, general practitioners and the criminal justice system. On the other hand, it is this same effect on others that is the source of the cautious optimism expressed by those whose training equips them to engage with the patient and with those same interpersonal stress and distress, and to manage it in a therapeutic manner, whatever the theoretical model being used.

It is therefore not surprising that there is an emerging consensus about the conditions that allow for a degree of success in treatment. For example, Bateman and Fonagy [2], when discussing day treatment services in their review of the effectiveness of psychotherapeutic treatment of personality disorder, state: "There are no data to suggest that the mere inclusion of psychotherapy within a day hospital is sufficient to ensure good outcome. All studies use an integrated and organised treatment programme within a singular, coherent (and to the patients understandable) system. Only such integrated programmes, with clinicians with various tasks and functions working to the same strategic goals, permit patients with severe problems in understanding human motives to feel sufficiently safe to engage effectively with the treatment".

In 2003, the UK National Health Service (through the new National Institute for Mental Health in England) gave its first ever formal policy implementation guidelines for personality disorders [1]. These guidelines involved careful consultation with patients who had personality disorder and experience of UK mental health services. The guidelines include a long list of factors experienced as helpful and unhelpful aspects of services. The guidelines stress the need for therapy to be relatively long term and to involve a clear treatment alliance between therapist and patient. It will be interesting to see if other national bodies and professional mental health organizations provide personality disorder treatment guidelines and give expectations of service provision. This could be another route by which the treatment culture changes, as surely such guidelines will lead to patient expectations and patient groups challenging health services perhaps even through the courts when such services fail to be provided to recommended standards.

Although there are different approaches to the treatment of borderline and histrionic personality disorders, the advances in recent decades in psychoanalytic understandings of the more "primitive" mental mechanisms used by such patients should not be underestimated. The realization of the extent to which splitting, projection and projective identification mechanisms are central mental phenomena in these disorders has very considerable therapeutic implications. The understanding has the potential to be of considerable assistance when attending to the various feelings of other family members, and of health and mental health staff. Although great care has to be taken in disentangling the psychology of the recipient from that of the person with the personality disordered person, borderline and histrionic personality disorder patients are capable of arousing extremes of feelings in others and between others. Utilization of these feelings as sources of information (countertransference) has led to considerable changes in technique and practice of psychoanalytically informed clinicians compared with those of the classical analysts, who often worked within a "one mind" psychology and were discomfited by powerful feelings stirred up by patients.

REFERENCES

1. National Institute for Mental Health in England (2003) Personality disorder: no longer a diagnosis of exclusion. www.doh.gov.uk/mentalhealth/personalitydisorder.pdf
2. Bateman A., Fonagy P. (2000) Effectiveness of psychotherapeutic treatment of personality disorder. *Br. J. Psychiatry*, **177**: 138–143.

3.13
Psychotherapy for Borderline Personality Disorder: Some Tentative Interpretations of the Available Empirical Findings

Roel Verheul[1]

In this commentary on Michael Stone's excellent review, I will primarily discuss some issues surrounding the available empirical evidence for the effectiveness of psychotherapeutic treatments for borderline personality disorder (BPD). In my opinion, it is possible to conclude more from the available studies than Stone actually does.

First of all, Stone does not compare the outcome results of the treatment models of Linehan (i.e. dialectical behaviour therapy, DBT) and Bateman/ Fonagy (i.e. mentalization based treatment, MBT). The most important trials for DBT include Linehan et al.'s original study with a separate one-year post-treatment follow-up and a replication of the pre-post part by Verheul et al. [1]. The 6-month post-treatment follow-up of this replication study is still under way. A randomised evaluation of 18 months of MBT with a 18-month post-treatment follow-up has been published by Bateman and Fonagy. In summary, both treatments show similar effects on suicidal and self-mutilatory acts, but MBT is superior to DBT in terms of the reduction of anxiety and depressive symptoms. Furthermore, the data seem to indicate that the benefits are better maintained in MBT as compared to DBT. Thus I think that it is fair to state that, although the effectiveness of DBT has been documented in more studies than the effectiveness of MBT, the clinical results from the first trial on MBT are more impressive than those published for DBT. What does this mean? As far as I can see, there are three competing explanations: the differential results can result from theoretical and technical differences, or from dosage differences, or from a combination thereof. DBT is 12 months of outpatient treatment without aftercare, whereas MBT is 18 months of day treatment with aftercare. Thus, the treatments that have been studied differ not only in terms of the treatment model (i.e. theory and techniques) but also in terms of dosage (i.e. setting, duration, and aftercare). To establish whether model or dosage is the decisive factor, one would have to conduct a randomized controlled trial (RCT) with 2×2 arms defined by model × dosage.

Second, the available evidence does not seem to support DBT as a treatment of choice for BPD per se. Based upon multiple effectiveness studies, it is now well established that DBT is an efficacious treatment of high-risk behaviours among patients with BPD. This is probably due to

[1] Center of Psychotherapy De Viersprong, University of Amsterdam, Post Box 7, 4660 AA Halsteren, The Netherlands

some of DBT's distinguishing features: (a) routine monitoring of the risk for these behaviours throughout the treatment program; (b) an explicit focus on the modification of these behaviours in the first stage of treatment; (c) encouragement of patients to consult with therapists by phone preceding these behaviours; and (d) prevention of therapist's burnout through frequent supervision and consultation group meetings. Across studies, however, DBT has not shown effectiveness in terms of a reduction of depression, hopelessness, and improvements in survival and coping beliefs or overall life satisfaction [2]. In addition, Verheul *et al.* [1] showed that DBT was differentially effective in reducing self-harm in chronically parasuicidal borderline patients, whereas the impact of DBT in low-severity patients was similar to treatment as usual. Together, these findings suggest that DBT should—consistent with its original aims [3]—only be a treatment of choice for chronically parasuicidal borderline patients, and should perhaps be extended or followed by another treatment, focusing on other components of BPD, as soon as the high-risk behaviours are sufficiently reduced. Alternatively, it can be hypothesized that DBT is a treatment of choice for patients with severe, life-threatening impulse control disorders rather than for BPD per se, implying that also some patients with other severe impulse regulation disorders (e.g. substance use disorders or eating disorders) might benefit from it. The latter interpretation is consistent with the development of modified versions of DBT for the treatment of BPD patients with a comorbid diagnosis of drug dependence [4] or patients with a binge-eating disorder [5].

Third, many authors tend to limit discussions about effective treatments for BPD to those treatments that have been investigated in RCTs, i.e. MBT and DBT. Three issues should be taken into account: (a) the limitations of the RCT research model (e.g. limited external validity or generalizability, cross-overs, care consumption during follow-up, etc.) and the advantages of nonrandomized studies (e.g. better external validity, larger samples, more representative clinical conditions, etc.) are often not recognized; (b) treatments without empirical evidence supportive of their effectiveness are still possibly evidence-based treatments; (c) randomized trials of long-term and inpatient treatments are more difficult to get financed, ethically approved and conducted.

Given the fact that there are virtually no direct comparisons between treatment models, it is perhaps wise to point to the essential characteristics of effective treatments rather than to attempt to identify a treatment of first choice for BPD. In a recent review of psychotherapeutic treatment of personality disorder, Bateman and Fonagy [6] conclude that treatments shown to be moderately effective have certain common features. They tend: (a) to be well structured; (b) to devote considerable effort to enhancing compliance; (c) to have a clear focus, whether that focus is a problem behaviour such as self-harm or an aspect of interpersonal relationship patterns; (d) to be theoretically highly coherent to both therapist and patient, sometimes deliberately omitting information incompatible with the theory; (e) to be relatively long term; (f) to encourage a powerful attachment relationship between therapist and patient, enabling the therapist to adopt a relatively active rather than a passive stand, and (g) to be well integrated with other services available to the patient. It is the overall integration that is crucial. I would personally add that there is increasing clinical consensus that day treatment, or partial hospitalization, has unique advantages for the treatment of BPD. Such treatment may offer patients the optimal level of intensiveness and containment, resulting in less regressive dependency and acting-out behaviour [7]. It is less restrictive than inpatient treatment, but provides more sustained and intensive support than outpatient treatment. It is not unlikely that partial hospitalization followed by outpatient psychotherapy followed by less intensive aftercare is the best combination treatment. Future research should focus on the optimal duration of those components.

REFERENCES

1. Verheul R., Bosch L.M.C., van den Koeter M.W.J., van den Brink W., Stijnen T., de Ridder M. (2003) Efficacy of dialectical behaviour therapy: a Dutch randomized controlled trial. *Br. J. Psychiatry*, **182**: 135–140.
2. Scheel K.R. (2000) The empirical basis of dialectical behavior therapy: summary, critique, and implications. *Clin. Psychol. Sci. Pract.*, **7**: 68–86.
3. Linehan M.M. (1987) Dialectical behavior therapy: a cognitive behavioral approach to parasuicide. *J. Person. Disord.*, **1**: 328–333.
4. Linehan M.M., Schmidt H.I., Dimeff L.A., Craft J.C., Kanter J., Comtois K.A. (1999) Dialectical behavior therapy for patients with borderline personality disorder and drug dependence. *Am. J. Addict.*, **8**: 279–292.
5. Wiser S., Telch C.F. (1999) Dialectical behavior therapy for binge-eating disorder. *J. Clin. Psychol.*, **55**: 755–768.
6. Bateman A.W., Fonagy P. (2000) Effectiveness of psychotherapeutic treatment of personality disorder. *Br. J. Psychiatry*, **177**: 138–143.
7. Miller B.C. (1995) Characteristics of effective day treatment programming for persons with borderline personality disorder. *Psychiatr. Serv.*, **46**: 605–608.

3.14
How to Cope with the Burden of Trying to Help a Borderline Patient?

Vera Lemgruber[1]

Michael Stone's paper reviews the outcome of a work that culminated in 1980, with the publication of the DSM-III, and continued to the DSM-IV in the 1990s. This work was performed for the American Psychiatric Association by a group of researchers, who did an excellent job in reducing the vagueness of the terms to be used by clinicians not only in the caring of their patients but also in filling the papers for health bureaucracy, insurance companies or health maintenance organizations (HMOs), where categories need to be specified.

Medical doctors who want to keep in touch with the extremely rapid and significant progress of research surely must rely on data based on evidence. Nevertheless, in everyday practice, facing each patient, with his own idiosyncrasies and behavioural problems with possible serious social implications, as it is sometimes the case for the patient with borderline personality disorder (BPD), the clinician is urged to follow his/her own experience and feeling.

BPD patients, with their stormy life-style, impulsive behaviour, suicide threats, easily triggered excessive anger, lability of mood, may understandably represent a burden to the psychiatrists and easily frustrate their efforts in treating them. Maybe this is why, in order to alleviate and soften a problem for which we still do not have a solution, we tend to make jokes about them. In a book called "Oral Sadism and the Vegetarian Personality", written in 1984 as a parody of traditional scientific papers, a very sarcastic article called "Thanatotherapy: A One-Session Approach to Brief Psychology" [1] identified BPD patients as the ones indicated for that kind of "radical" therapy, and depicted them as "patients notorious for late night irrelevant 'emergency' phone-calls, no common sense, no redeeming qualities, no income and no health insurance".

"The stability of instability" could be a good definition for BPD and could also be applied to histrionic personality disorder (HPD), bipolar II disorder and also some cases of post-traumatic stress disorder (PTSD), especially those with sexual/aggressive family abuse factors. A tentative proposal could be to encompass these category-based diagnostics into a dimensional spectrum, including different grades of specific traits like negative affect, lability of mood, impulsivity, aggression. This proposal could be added to

_____

[1] _WHO Collaborating Center for Research and Training in Psychotherapy, Santa Casa General Hospital, Rio de Janeiro, Brazil_

the list presented by Michael Stone in the final section of his review. Really this is an area still open to research and needing much study!

The improvement of the reliability of the various diagnoses has already helped to emphasize the necessity of different therapeutic approaches to different problems, which also included the overcoming of the ancient notion that psychoanalysis was a kind of "panacea" for all mental problems.

In the case of BPD, medication, while extremely important in reducing several symptoms, does little to ameliorate the lingering maladaptive personality traits that typify the disorder, like clinginess, manipulative attitude, vehemence, action-proneness, unruliness, touchiness etc. For this reason, pharmacotherapy plays an ancillary role in the complete approach to the treatment of BPD.

Progress of neuroscience will probably in the future help us to sharpen our medical procedures, providing us with evidence about the neurophysiological pathways underlying our current category-based diagnoses. Until then, we must rely on our clinical expertise and on what we can identify by our clinical examination through the signs and symptoms presented by the patient, and, above all, try to develop a strong therapeutic alliance.

REFERENCE

1. McDonald K.M., Wampold B.E. (1984) Thanatotherapy: a one-session approach to brief psychotherapy. In *Oral Sadism and the Vegetarian Personality* (Ed. G. Ellenbogemk), pp. 45–50. Brunner-Mazel, New York.

3.15
Borderline Personality Disorder: A Complex Disorder, but not just Complex Post-traumatic Stress Disorder

Christian Schmahl[1]

The turn towards borderline personality disorder (BPD) in psychiatry constitutes a fascinating phenomenon. Twenty years ago the disorder's complexity, about which there is no doubt among clinicians and researchers, scared off most people involved ("no borderline patient on my unit nor in my lab"). In contrast, nowadays these patients are among the most searched for, and the disorder has become a major focus of interest in psychiatric

[1] *Department of Psychosomatic Medicine and Psychotherapy, Central Institute of Mental Health, J 5, D-68159 Mannheim, Germany*

research. There appear to be several possible explanations for this phenomenon. One is that the economic burden of patients with BPD, a frequent and often difficult to treat disorder, has become a major problem in our general health systems. In this context the growing interest of the pharmaceutical industry and of public and private funding sources appears to be of special importance and has definitely contributed to the preoccupation with the disorder.

Another possibility for this growing interest is that the complexity does no longer scare off but in contrast attracts researchers. In fact, the advantage of complex disorders with open boundaries towards other diagnostic entities is that research approaches can be transferred from these overlapping conditions. Thus, during the last two decades, research in BPD has been stimulated by the neighbourhood of schizophrenia and then of the affective disorders. Later the boundaries towards the impulsive and also the dissociative disorders spectrum has become the most relevant areas of research. In the realm of interpretation, the inclusion into a neighboured diagnostic entity can be speculated to be an attempt to get rid of an unloved diagnosis.

One of the latest debates in this context is whether BPD constitutes a form of complex post-traumatic stress disorder (PTSD) [1]. There is a large overlap between PTSD and BPD regarding aetiology as well as clinical presentation. Prevalence of childhood physical and sexual abuse is high in both of them (between 29 and 71%) and about 50% of patients with BPD fulfil the diagnostic criteria for PTSD. Two findings from neuroimaging studies may add to the discussion of this problem. A major neurobiological finding of the last decade is a reduction in hippocampal volume as assessed by magnetic resonance-based volumetry in combat-related as well as abuse-related PTSD. There is an ongoing debate as to whether this volume reduction is due to an elevated activity of stress-associated neurobiological systems such as the hypothalamic-pituitary-adrenal axis or is genetically determined. On the other hand, all studies investigating amygdala volumes in patients with PTSD did not find any significant difference compared to controls. In contrast to this, several studies, including our own [2] revealed about 10–20% volume reductions of hippocampus and even more pronounced of amygdala volumes in patients with BPD. These findings suggest that, in contrast to PTSD, not only hippocampus but also amygdala volumes seem to be reduced in patients with BPD.

A second line of research is the investigation of memories of stressful life events in patients with PTSD and BPD. We studied neural responses to scripts depicting autobiographical situations of sexual or physical abuse as well as abandonment situations in patients with BPD during positron emission tomography (PET) imaging. Similar studies of traumatic reminders in PTSD have revealed prefrontal cortex dysfunction with a failure of anterior cingulated activation. In our studies, memories of trauma were associated with increases in blood flow in right dorsolateral prefrontal cortex as well as decreased blood flow in left dorsolateral prefrontal cortex in traumatized women without BPD. There was also increased blood flow in right anterior cingulate and left orbitofrontal cortex in women without BPD. Women with BPD failed to activate anterior cingulate gyrus as well as orbitofrontal cortex during memories of trauma. Also, no blood flow differences were seen in dorsolateral prefrontal gyrus in women with BPD [3]. In comparison, during abandonment memories there was a more pronounced pattern of prefrontal dysfunction with marked deactivation in anterior cingulate and activation in dorsolateral prefrontal cortex [4]. It can be concluded that traumatic memories involve similar circuits in both disorders and that traumatic stress is an important factor in the development of BPD, but that other types of interpersonal stress, e.g. situations of abandonment, may be of similar or even greater importance for the development of BPD. To test this hypothesis directly, a comparison study of the two diagnostic groups using different types of stress-related scripts would be necessary.

Taken together, these neuroimaging findings underline common features of both PTSD and BPD, but also differences in brain structure and function in these disorders. In my opinion, another fruitful approach in neurobiological research in BPD is the investigation of the underlying biology of clinical features that appear to be relatively distinct for BPD, such as self-injurious behaviour and pain dysregulation.

REFERENCES

1. Driessen M., Beblo T., Reddemann L., Rau H., Lange W., Silva A., Berea R.C., Wulff H., Ratzka (2002) Is the borderline personality disorder a complex post-traumatic stress disorder—The state of research. *Nervenarzt*, **73**: 820–829.
2. Schmahl C.G., Vermetten E., Elzinga B.M., Bremner J.D. (2003) Magnetic resonance imaging of hippocampal and amygdala volume in women with childhood abuse and borderline personality disorder. *Psychiatry Res.: Neuroimaging*, **122**: 109–115.
3. Schmahl C.G., Vermetten E., Elzinga B.M., Bremner J.D. (in press) A PET study of memories of childhood abuse in borderline personality disorder. *Biol. Psychiatry*.
4. Schmahl C.G., Elzinga B.M., Vermetten E., Sanislow C., McGlashan T.H., Bremner J.D. (2003) Neural correlates of memories of abandonment in women with and without borderline personality disorder. *Biol. Psychiatry*, **54**: 142–151.

3.16
Borderline Personality Disorder between Axis I and Axis II Diagnosis
Tarek A. Okasha[1]

Michael Stone's seminal paper reviews the controversial subject of borderline personality disorder and histrionic personality disorder. It is worth mentioning that nearly 1000 years before Hippocrates used the term hysteria, ancient Egyptians, in the Kahun Papyrus (a papyrus for uterine diseases) described a series of morbid states, all attributed to the displacement of the uterus. They ascribed these morbid states to the "starvation" of the uterus by its upward displacement with a consequent crowding of other organs. As treatment, the genitalia were fumigated with precious and sweet smelling substances to attract the womb, or evil tasting and foul smelling substances were injected or inhaled to repel the organ and drive it away from the upper part of the body where it was thought to have wandered. Most of these diseases are defined clearly enough to be recognizable today as hysterical disorders [1].

An Egyptian study comparing the diagnosis of 1000 patients presenting to an outpatient university clinic in 1967 and in 1990 showed a two fold increase in the diagnosis of personality disorder, mainly due to the addition of the term borderline personality disorder (BPD), where previously they would be diagnosed as hysterical or psychopaths [2].

In another study carried out in Egypt, an all night polysomnographic assessment was made for 20 ICD-10 borderline patients (without comorbid depression), 20 patients with major depression and 20 healthy controls. The study showed a high similarity in EEG sleep profile in the borderline and depressed groups, including significantly increased sleep latency, increased rapid eye movement (REM) percentage and density as well as increased first REM period, though the changes in the depressed group were more robust. This study was a step in line with the hypothesis of affective dysregulation in borderline personality at the neurophysiological level [3].

A number of investigations point to similarity in pathophysiology between borderline personality disorders and depression. Neuroendocrine abnormalities—dexamethasone suppression test (DST) and thyrotropin-releasing hormone (TRH) test—were found in a total of 75% of borderline women, independent of whether or not they met DSM-III criteria for major depressive disorder [4]. These findings suggest that some patients with borderline personality disorder share a neuroendocrine abnormality with some affective disorder patients [5]. However, other studies [6] showed no

[1] Institute of Psychiatry, Ain Shams University, 3 Shawarby Street, Kasr El Nil, Cairo, Egypt

evidence of an endocrine biological link between BPD and major depression.

Recently, Akiskal [7] argued that the affective dysregulation of patients given borderline diagnosis can be more precisely delineated in terms of atypical, dysthymic, cyclothymic and bipolar II disorders, and that understanding the temperamental underpinning of these disorders has important therapeutic implications. As the diagnosis of schizotypal disorder falls within the category of the psychotic spectrum in the ICD-10, and remains as a personality disorder in the DSM-IV, it is believed that BPD should be included within the spectrum of affective disorders, either as an atypical form of affective disorders [8] or as a "soft" bipolar disorder [9]. The fact that there is a high comorbidity with Axis I diagnoses—including mood disorders, eating disorders and substance abuse—sheds some doubt on the validity and reliability of the diagnosis of BPD. Sometimes the symptoms are discussed as a trait, sometimes as a state, which is more confusing than clarifying. Further research is required to delineate the diagnosis of BPD as being related more to Axis I or whether it is actually related to the emotionally erratic and dramatic cluster of Axis II.

REFERENCES

1. Okasha A., Okasha T. (2000) Notes on mental disorders in pharaonic Egypt. *History of Psychiatry*, **11**: 413–424.
2. Okasha A., Sief El Dawla A., Asaad T. (1993) Presentation of hysteria in a sample of Egyptian patients—an update. *Neurol. Psychiatry Brain Res.*, **1**: 155–159.
3. Asaad T., Okasha T., Okasha A. (2002) Sleep EEG findings in ICD-10 borderline personality disorder in Egypt. *J. Affect. Disord.*, **71**: 11–18.
4. Sternbach H.A., Fleming J., Extein I., Pottash A.L., Gold M.S. (1983) The dexamethasone suppression and thyrotropin-releasing hormone tests in depressed borderline patients. *Psychoneuroendocrinology*, **8**: 459–462.
5. Garbutt J.C., Loosen P.T., Tipermas A., Prange A.J. Jr. (1983) The TRH test in patients with borderline personality disorder. *Psychiatry Res.*, **9**: 107–113.
6. De la Fuente J.M., Mendlewicz J. (1996) TRH stimulation and dexamethasone suppression in borderline personality disorder. *Biol. Psychiatry*, **40**: 412–418.
7. Akiskal H.S. (2000) Die borderline-personlichkeit: Affektive grundlagen symptome und syndrome In *Handbuch der Borderline-storungen* (Eds O.F. Kernberg, B. Dulz, U. Sachsse), pp. 259–270. Schattaur, Stuttgart.
8. Akiskal H.S. (1981) Subaffective disorders: dysthymic, cyclothymic and bipolar-II disorders in the "borderline" realm. *Psychiatr. Clin. North Am.*, **4**: 25–46.
9. Perugi G., Akiskal H.S., Lattanzi L., Cecconi D., Mastrocinque C., Petronelli A., Vignoli S., Bemi E. (1998) High prevalence of "soft" bipolar features in atypical depression. *Compr. Psychiatry*, **39**: 63–71.

3.17
Histrionic and Borderline Personality Disorders: A View from Latin America

Néstor M.S. Koldobsky[1]

Very significant advances in the study of personality disorders have taken place recently, but this development has been unequal. Not all disorders have received the same interest. Borderline personality disorder (BPD) has attracted the most significant attention and research grants, in relationship to its severity and social implications. Other personality disorders, like histrionic personality disorder (HPD), have been understudied in the post-DSM-III era. The concepts of hysteria and HPD have been criticized, in particular by the feminist movement, because of their pejorative and stigmatizing implications, which has probably somewhat influenced the scientific attitude.

The term histrionic refers to a very dramatic style of self-presentation, when this style becomes excessive and maladaptive. Many social traits (friendly, expressive, sociable, warm, lively, dramatic, energizing, seductive) are normal to some extent, but sometimes they become a source of suffering and maladaptation. In Argentina, we studied the prevalence of HPD in two samples. The former was a group of 46 severe male offenders (mean age 28.38 years, range 18–48 years) studied at the Neuropsychiatry Institute of Security, Penitentiary Division of the Buenos Aires Province, La Plata, Argentina. We used the DSM-IV and the Millon Clinical Multiaxial Inventory (MCMI III), validated in Argentina by M. Casullo. We found a prevalence of 3.85% [1]. The latter was a sample of 1032 academic graduates (both sexes, age from 35 to 55 years) applying for a job in the Department of Justice of the Buenos Aires Province, all evaluated by the DSM-IV criteria and the MCMI III [2]. We found a prevalence of 9.88% in males and 13.56% in females. HPD was the most frequent personality disorder among females.

The presence of BPD in different cultures is currently a subject of debate. In the above-mentioned study of 46 severe male offenders evaluated by the MCMI III, we found a prevalence of this disorder of 7.69% [1]. In the above-mentioned sample of academic graduates, the prevalence of BPD was 8.13% in men and 6.20% in females [2]. In a sample of outpatients with a diagnosis of substance use disorder, the prevalence was 7.98% in males and 0.63% in females. These results confirm that BPD, as defined by the DSM-IV, is not a rare condition in Latin America. This was also the conclusion of a survey of Latin American experts which I coordinated recently in my quality of

[1] La Plata National Medicine School, La Plata, Argentina

President of the Personality Section of the Latin American Psychiatric Association. The hope is that the definition of this disorder will be further refined, so that this category stops to be, as it is in some clinical contexts, a mere label to diagnose difficult cases, which cannot be placed in any other diagnostic category.

REFERENCES

1. Koldobsky N.M.S., Astorga C., Ranze S. (1997) Antisocial personality disorders or psychopathic personality: subtypologies. Presented at the 5th International Congress on the Disorders of Personality, Vancouver, June 1.
2. Koldobsky N.M.S., Casullo M.M., Astorga C., Ibarbide P. (1999) Use of MCMI III in a sample of 1032 individuals. Presented at the 6th International Congress on the Disorders of Personality. Geneva, September 15.

Narcissistic Personality Disorder: A Review

Elsa Ronningstam

*McLean Hospital, Harvard Medical School,
Belmont, Massachusetts, USA*

INTRODUCTION

Our knowledge on narcissism and narcissistic personality disorder (NPD), accumulated during the past century, stems mostly from three major areas of inquiry: individual case studies of treatment of narcissistic people in psychoanalysis and dynamic psychotherapy; empirical studies using structured and semi-structured diagnostic instruments for evaluating narcissistic characteristics and NPD in patients in psychiatric settings; and studies in the field of academic social psychology using laboratory experiments and inventories for exploring specific narcissistic traits and behaviours. This paper reviews both clinical and psychoanalytic, and empirical psychiatric and psychological evidence based studies of pathological narcissism and NPD. It includes an outline of a diagnostic formulation and criteria for NPD that integrate present observations on self-esteem dysregulation, affect dysregulation and specific behaviours and dysregulations in interpersonal relationships. Three types of NPD are discussed as well as some of the most important differences vis-à-vis near neighbour Axis I and Axis II disorders.

THE SCOPE OF NPD

Definitions of Pathological Narcissism and NPD

The terms "pathological narcissism", "narcissistic disorder" and "narcissistic personality disorder" have been used interchangeably in the clinical

Personality Disorders. Edited by Mario Maj, Hagop S. Akiskal, Juan E. Mezzich and Ahmed Okasha.
©2005 John Wiley & Sons Ltd: ISBN 0-470-09036-7

literature. For the purposes of clarification, the following definitions of pathological narcissism, narcissistic traits/features/characteristics, and NPD will be used throughout this paper.

Narcissism refers to a dimension ranging from healthy, to pathological, to the enduring NPD, and identified by degree of severity, dominance of aggression versus shame, and by the extent to which its manifestations are overt or internally hidden. Pathological narcissism differs from healthy or normal narcissism since the self-esteem regulation is dysfunctional, serving to protect and support a grandiose but fragile self. Affect regulation is compromised by difficulties to process and modulate feelings, specifically anger, shame and envy. Interpersonal relationships are also affected as they are used primarily to protect or enhance the self-esteem and other self-regulatory functions at the expense of mutual relativeness and intimacy.

Pathological narcissism can be more or less obtrusive on an individual's sustained personality functioning. When the level of pathological narcissism is less severe, temporary, situational or limited to a set of specific character features that interfere to a lesser degree with regular personal, interpersonal and/or vocational functioning, it is referred to as narcissistic disturbance or narcissistic traits. The diagnostic term NPD refers to a stable long-term characterological functioning that meets the DSM-IV criteria for NPD or any other comprehensive diagnostic description [1–8]. NPD refers to specific deformations in the personality structure that involve a pathological grandiose self, impaired affect regulation, unintegrated object relations, and inconsistent and/or overly harsh superego functioning. The self-esteem is inconsistent and fragile and maintained by pathologically defensive, expressive and supportive regulatory processes. Affect regulation is influenced by feelings of rage, shame and envy, and the capacity for empathy and interpersonal commitment is impaired.

In addition, in a recently proposed diagnostic term, "trauma-associated narcissistic symptoms" (TANS) [9], the stress associated with an external traumatic experience overwhelms the self and triggers symptoms such as shame, humiliation and rage. Although underlying vulnerability to such stress can stem from the presence of pathological narcissism or NPD, even people with relatively healthy self-esteem can develop narcissistic symptoms after experiencing a more or less severe narcissistic humiliation.

These definitions indicate the complexity of pathological narcissism, i.e. that there are context-dependent, reactive types of pathological narcissism with changeability and fluctuations between healthy and pathological functioning, as well as more enduring, stable forms of NPD with clearly identifiable character pathology and a long-term course [9,10]. These definitions also suggest that pathological narcissism encompasses different levels of functioning or degrees of severity [11–13]. They can range from extraordinarily high levels of functioning combined with exceptional capabilities, to context-determined narcissistic reactions, to a personality disorder with mild to severe symptoms that limit functioning in the interpersonal and vocational areas, to malignant forms of narcissism and to antisocial or psychopathic behaviour found in severe criminals. Pathological narcissism can, independent of level of severity, range from being overt, striking and obtrusive to being internally concealed and unnoticeable [14]. Furthermore, pathological narcissism can also co-occur with other forms of character pathology or major mental disorders and interact with other significant personality characteristics or symptomatology such as: psychopathy [15], borderline personality disorder [6,12], the bipolar spectrum disorders [16], eating disorders [17,18] and substance abuse disorders [19]. Vicissitudes between healthy and more or less severe pathological narcissism are constantly present, and the coexistence of and intertwined interaction between healthy and pathological aspects of narcissistic functioning can make it specifically challenging to identify and understand the NPD [20–22].

Clinical Presentation

Differences in cultural expressions, overtly predominant core character features and level of functioning in people with NPD contribute to significant variability in clinical presentation. Some people with NPD present themselves as obliviously confident and arrogant, boastful, attention-seeking and entitled, and they bluntly and even proudly verify their narcissistic characteristics [6,16]. While in some cultures or social contexts individual assertiveness and arrogance are more accepted or even promoted, in others this behaviour may cause strong social disapproval or condemnation. Other narcissistic people may pride themselves on being modest and consciously hide their narcissistic strivings, or they may, due to shame and insecurity, deny any tendencies of feeling special or superior [3,14]. In some cultures, such as the North American, modesty and self-effacing behaviour can be both socially and professionally handicapping, while in other cultures they are considered a virtue and hence highly socially valued. Since such narcissistic people appear sensitive, compliant, timid and inferior, it may take an extended psycho-diagnostic evaluation or a longer period of psychotherapy until a correct diagnosis can be established. Still other narcissistic people, closer to the psychopathy range, are ruthlessly insensitive and entitled to be exploitative, charming and cunning with manipulative and sadistic behaviour [13,23]. Of diagnostic and clinical importance, is the additional fact that people who initially may present with strikingly overt narcissistic features can para-doxically have less severe narcissistic pathology and be capable of both empathy and interpersonal commitments. Others who appear concerned and interpersonally "tuned in" can have a much more severe hidden underlying narcissistic pathology, being cunning, envious, spiteful, contemptuous, revengeful and incapable of mutual interpersonal relationships. None of the present diagnostic descriptions or instruments takes into account these variations.

Heritability and Early Origins

Two studies have suggested a genetic influence on the development of personality disorders, including the narcissistic. Jang and colleagues [24] found an average of 45% heritability for the dimension of narcissism, including "need for adulation", "attention seeking" and "grandiosity" as main facets. Torgersen *et al.* [25] showed that nearly 80% of the variation in the trait of DSM-III-R NPD could be explained by genes. While the meaning and consequences of these findings still await future research, there are indications that of specific importance for the development of narcissistic personality disorder are inherited variations in hypersensitivity, strong aggressive drive, low anxiety or frustration tolerance, and defects in affect regulation. Schore [26] suggested that of relevance for the development of NPD are the specific early vicissitudes of hyperactivation and affect under-regulation in the interaction between caregiver and child, later resulting in overt grandiosity, entitlement, and aggressive reactions to others. Early infant observations suggest that the child is intensively attended to, and specially valued as a regulator of the parent's self-esteem, but the child is not valued and seen in his/her own right [27]. Nevertheless, the childhood family environment for NPD patients may be ostensibly structured and even admiring, but parents are generally unempathic, emotionally unavailable and unable to attune to the child's emotional personal or age appropriate needs and reactions. P. Kernberg [27] identified a specific risk factor for development of NPD, i.e. when parents give their children roles or functions beyond or inconsistent with the child's normal developmental tasks.

Prevalence

Although there is a general opinion that narcissistic disorders are becoming more common in Western society, the prevalence rate of NPD in the general population is still very low (0–0.4%) [28,29], suggesting that NPD is among the least common personality disorders [30]. Others report consistent low to moderate prevalence rates, less than 1% in the general population [25,31]. A few studies found somewhat higher rates of NPD (3.9–5.3%) [32,33] using non-clinical control samples. Studies also indicate that NPD is more frequently found among people in higher education or special professional groups. In a study of personality maladjustment among first-year medical students, 17% met criteria for NPD [34]. Narcissistic personality traits or disorder were the most commonly occurring Axis II diagnosis (20%) in a military clinical outpatient sample [35,36]. Johnson [37] suggested that military service may appeal to narcissistic people because of the focus on appearance, rewards and public displays of reinforcement.

The use of the NPD diagnosis is probably more common in some clinical settings such as forensic psychiatric clinics and private hospitals or in the private practices of psychoanalysts, psychotherapists and marriage counsellors. In the adult clinical population, rates between 1% and 16% have been found [19,38], and high rates of NPD were identified in the personality disorder population (22%) [39] as well as in specific clinical samples. A study of cocaine abusers reported 32% comorbid diagnosis of NPD [40]. In an Australian study on bipolar patients, 47% met criteria for NPD [41]. In a Japanese study on personality disorders in depressed patients [42], 21% met the DSM-III-R diagnostic criteria for NPD. In a post-mortem study conducted in Israel, Apter *et al.* [43] found that, among young males in the army who had committed suicide, as many as 23.3% had a diagnosis of NPD. However, studies of prevalence in clinical populations do not reflect clinicians' usage of the NPD diagnosis, and the DSM criteria often fail to identify patients whom clinicians consider having NPD. Only 10 of 24 patients clinically diagnosed as NPD met the threshold for the DSM-III-R NPD diagnosis [38].

Gender and Age Differences

Research reports disagree on the gender distribution of NPD. Some studies support the idea that NPD is more common in males than in females [6,25,44], while others believe NPD is equally prevalent in both sexes [45]. The DSM-IV claims that 50% to 75% of those diagnosed with NPD are male. Ninety-five percent of patients diagnosed as narcissistic (with traits or personality disorder) in a military sample were male, indicating a professionally related gender difference [35].

Narcissistic disturbances are frequent among people in their late teens and early twenties, due to the specific developmental challenges in the transition from adolescence to adulthood. Such disturbances are usually corrected through developmental life experiences and normally do not develop into adult NPD [10]. However, the presence of NPD in both children and adolescence has been empirically verified [46,47]. Unlike other dramatic cluster disorders, NPD does not necessarily remit with advanced age. In fact, middle age is an especially critical period for the development or worsening of NPD, with chronic denial, emptiness, devaluation, guilt and cynicism [48]. Significant narcissistic pathology and personality disorder have also been found in elderly people [49,50].

International Conceptualizations of Narcissism and NPD

Narcissism and NPD have been considered phenomena of the Western world. Studies of narcissism originated in Europe (Austria, England, Hungary) and continue to progress in the United States. The emphasis on inner separateness and autonomous self-motivation, assertiveness and mobility in the Western societies would urge narcissistic functioning and lay the ground for the development of pathological narcissism [51–53]. The international controversy about the existence of NPD and the fact that NPD is still not included in the ICD-10 probably underscores such an impression.

Contrary to this view is the fact that pathological narcissism and NPD by now are studied worldwide. The international usage of the DSM Axis II and structured diagnostic instruments have encouraged studies of personality disorders including NPD. Although most of these studies also have faced the limitations of small samples of NPD, studies of co-occurring pathological narcissism and NPD in other psychiatric conditions have added valuable knowledge. Those include: substance abuse in Norway [19], psychopathy in Canada [15], suicidality in Germany and Israel [43,54,61], social anxiety/anthropophobia in Japan [55,56], mood disorders in Australia [41], factitious illness in Germany [57], hypochondriasis in former Yugoslavia [58]. The Quality Assurance Project for psychiatric practice in Australia and New Zealand [59] was the first in the world to include NPD in treatment guidelines for cluster B personality disorders.

The introduction of the "shy" narcissistic personality [3,4,7,8,14,60] and the new understanding of the complex, less overt or intrapsychic narcissistic functioning made the identification of pathological narcissism less dependent on cultural contexts. Warren and Capponi [53] suggested that the exhibitionistic form of NPD which so far has been considered more prevalent in the United States has counterparts in the shy narcissism in Japan and Denmark. Moreover, the connection between narcissism and shame [62,63] has stimulated discussions on narcissism in more shame-dominated cultures, especially Japan [64]. The Western-defined narcissism concept was applied to a specific Japanese clinical problem, *taijin kyofu* or anthropophobia, i.e. intense self-consciousness in close social circles, and strong needs to preserve a grandiose self-image and to be perceived as unique and visible, suggesting a link to narcissism and insecure self-esteem [55].

HISTORICAL DEVELOPMENT

Early Psychoanalytic Contributions

The phenomenon of narcissism was introduced to psychiatry by H. Ellis [65] in a psychological study of autoeroticism in which he described the "Narcissus-like" tendency to absorb sexual feelings into self-admiration. The following year P. Näcke [66] was first to use the term "narcissism" in a study of sexual perversions. Freud first mentioned narcissism in a footnote added in 1910 to "Three essays on the theory of sexuality" [67] as a phase in the development of male homosexuality. In his paper "On narcissism" [68] and in his later comments on the subject [69,70], Freud outlined definitions of primary and secondary narcissism, identified narcissistic object-choice, and connected narcissism to the development of the ego-ideal and to self-preservation and self-regard as the "libidinal complement of egoism". Of much relevance for the contemporary discussion of narcissism, was the relationship between narcissism and inferiority. Freud suggested that the impoverishment of the ego due to the withdrawal of libidinal cathexes contributed to feelings of inferiority.

In a remarkable thoughtful and still most relevant and timely report, Jones [71] described the character traits of people with a "God Complex". He suggested that the excessive narcissism and exhibitionism involved in such fantasy of being God or godlike and the accompanying admiration of one's own power and qualities were manifested in a range of character traits. Contrary to later accounts of narcissistic personalities, Jones highlighted self-modesty, self-effacement, aloofness and inaccessibility as the main features of this narcissistic personality. The person is surrounded by a cloud of mystery, unsociable and protective of his privacy. Jones distinguished between two major types: those whose qualities indeed are valuable, adaptable and truly God like, and those whose unrealistic self-evaluation and difficulties to adjust to social life leave them dissatisfied and outside.

In another early account, Waelder [72] discussed the intellectual functioning of the "narcissistic scientist", a person with a superior attitude who, although fully able to understand others intellectually, was indifferent to them and pursued "to create a world for oneself". Waelder also outlined the difference between narcissism and psychosis, an essential distinction, as psychoanalysts by then had acknowledged that the transference technique was not applicable either for narcissistic fixations or psychosis.

After these earliest thoughtful and nuanced accounts, the descriptions of narcissistic personalities became more influenced by the connection between narcissism and aggression. This trend has been most influential in outlining the present arrogant type of NPD. In 1931, Freud [73] introduced the "narcissistic libidinal type": "The main interest is focused on self-preservation; the type is independent and not easily overawed. The ego has a considerable amount of aggression available, one manifestation of this being a proneness to activity". People of this type impress others as being "personalities" and "they readily assume the role of leader". Following Freud, W. Reich [74] proposed the phallic-narcissistic character: self-confident, arrogant, vigorous and impressive individuals, who are haughty, cold, reserved or aggressive with disguised sadistic traits in relation to others. They resent subordination and readily achieve leading positions. When hurt, they react with cold reserve, deep depression or intense aggression. Their narcissism is expressed in an exaggerated display of self-confidence, dignity and superiority. They are often considered highly desirable as sexual partners because of their masculine traits, despite the fact that they usually show contempt for the female sex. Sexuality serves less as a vehicle of love than as one of aggression and conquest. Less frequent in women, Reich believed that the phallic-narcissistic character could develop either into a "creative genius or into a large scale criminal". He also noted that these characters can have the opposite, passive tendencies of daydreaming and addiction.

The connection between narcissism and self-esteem regulation, first alluded to by Freud [68] in his discussion of self-regard and the development of the ego-ideal, was discussed further by Horney [75], who differentiated healthy self-esteem from pathological unrealistic self-inflation, a substitute for an undermined self-esteem. A. Reich [76] added substantially to the understanding of pathological self-esteem regulation which serves to maintain grandiosity and undo feelings of inadequacy and insufficiency. She described the strategy of compensatory narcissistic self-inflation, which fails and results in hypochondriac anxiety and depression. Excessive inner aggression and inordinate self-consciousness leading to dependency on outside approval, contribute to these regulation failures. Kohut [77] identified defects in self-esteem regulation as one of the core disturbances in NPD, and Goldberg [78] proposed a separate diagnostic category of acute narcissistic injury to one's self-esteem that may manifest itself as depression, but should be differentiated and treated differently from general depressive reactions or disorder.

Narcissistic Personality Disorder

The origin of NPD as a diagnostic category is more difficult to establish. Terms like narcissistic neurosis, schizophrenia and psychosis have often been used interchangeably, reflecting the initial close interrelation between narcissism and these illnesses. In his theory of narcissistic and autoerotic regression, Freud [68,79] explained schizophrenic symptoms as a libidinal withdrawal from the object world and regression to a narcissistic stage. In addition, the observation that the capacity to develop classical transference during psychoanalysis was absent in patients diagnosed with narcissistic neurosis [68] further connected narcissism to psychosis and schizophrenia. In addition, narcissism was associated with paranoia and suicide. Not until the late 1960s were the terms narcissistic personality structure, introduced by Kernberg [51], and narcissistic personality disorder, proposed by Kohut [80], used to describe a long-term organized characterological functioning defined as a personality disorder. Based on radical reformulations of psychoanalytic theory and technique, both Kohut and Kernberg defined NPD in terms of a pathological self-structure, atypical transference development and strategies for psychoanalytic treatment.

Kernberg and the Egopsychological Object Relational Perspective

Inspired by Rosenberg, Kernberg [12,51] outlined the narcissistic personality structure as having a pathological grandiose self characterized by aggression, excessive self-absorption and superior sense of grandiosity and uniqueness. This narcissistic person has serious problems in interpersonal relations, with superficial but also smooth and effective social adaptation, entitlement, and lack of empathy. Kernberg's [1,2] narcissistic personality shows devaluation, contempt and depreciation of others, is extremely envious and unable to receive from others, and has severe mood swings. Kernberg also highlighted the presence of superego pathology in people with this diagnosis, a less severe level with lack of integrated sense of values, and a more severe with malignant narcissism—antisocial features, ego-synthonic aggression and sadism and a general paranoid orientation. Narcissistic pathology can be found in political leaders, selfless ideologists and social redeemers [81]. However, Kernberg also recognized some atypical features found in patients with NPD: they can be anxious and tense, timid and insecure, have grandiose fantasies and daydreams, be sexually inhibited, and have a lack of ambition.

Kohut and the Self-Psychological Perspective

Kohut included NPD in his diagnostic spectrum of primary self-disorders. He differentiated between NPD, with hypochondria, depression, hypersensitivity and lack of enthusiasm/zest, and narcissistic behaviour disorder, which, in addition, displays perverse, delinquent and/or addictive behaviour that can expose the individual to physical or social danger [21,82]. Kohut also introduced the concept of the "Tragic Man" [21], a type of narcissistic personality suffering from repressed grandiosity and guiltless despair. This person knows and understands that his ambitions have not been realized and that his self-realization has not occurred. He has failed to attain his goals for self-expression and creativity. Morrison [83] stated that the major distinguishing affective experience of the Tragic Man is shame, caused by "the failure to realize ambitions, to gain response from others, and the absence of ideals". Kohut also described the individual with the "the depleted self", suffering from empty depression due to "unmirrored ambitions" and the absence of ideals [21]. Kohut's NPD subjects have repressed grandiosity, low self-esteem and hypocondriacal preoccupation and are prone to shame and embarrassment about needs to display themselves and their needs for other people.

Both Kernberg's and Kohut's contributions introduced an enormously productive epoch in the debate on narcissism and studies of narcissistic disorders all over the world. Especially the radical change in the understanding of treatability spurred both clinical and empirical interest in narcissistic patients. The introduction of NPD in DSM-III [84] and the proposition of a discrete set of diagnostic criteria led to its inclusion in official diagnostic instruments and in empirical studies of the Axis II personality disorders. These studies have helped to refine the criteria set for NPD and differentiate NPD from other mental disorders. It also began to encourage international exchange and communication on narcissistic disorders, especially in the clinical and psychodynamic/psychoanalytic field.

Empirical Research on Narcissism and NPD

Despite this, it has been challenging to establish an empirical base for defining NPD [38]. The complex nature of this disorder, i.e. high level of functioning, lack of symptoms or consistent behavioural signifiers, hidden or denied intrapsychic problems (even when severe), and lack of motivation to seek psychiatric treatment out of shame, pride, or self aggrandizing denial, have made it difficult to identify people in general psychiatric settings who meet the official criteria for NPD. Consequently, funding for psychiatric research on NPD has been less publicly urgent, especially in comparison to antisocial personality disorder (ASPD) and borderline personality disorder (BPD), for which more obvious human suffering, and extensive social and mental health costs, have impelled research on aetiology, course and treatment.

Nevertheless, two series of studies of clinically well defined narcissistic patients were conducted at Austen Riggs Center and McLean Hospital. Using data from a long-term follow-up study including medical records and self questionnaires from people who had been in long-term treatment at the Austen Riggs Center, Plakun [45,85–87] confirmed the validity of the NPD diagnosis vis-à-vis BPD, schizophrenia and major affective disorder. He also identified a group of patients with unusually severe NPD, with history of long inpatient treatment and several re-hospitalizations. Compared to BPD, this group of severe narcissistic patients had lower social and global functioning at follow-up, more re-hospitalizations, lower level of subjective satisfaction and less capacity for recovery in mid-life. He also found that self-destructive behaviour in NPD was associated with poor social functioning at follow-up.

In the other series of studies at McLean Hospital, Ronningstam, in collaboration with John Gunderson and colleagues, developed the first semi-structured diagnostic interview, the Diagnostic Interview for Narcissism (DIN) [5] (Table 4.1), specifically designed for studying pathological narcissism in psychiatric patients. People in inpatient or outpatient treatment with clinically well established diagnosis of pathological narcissism and NPD were interviewed and compared to others with a broad range of related psychiatric disorders (BPD, ASPD, bipolar disorder, anorexia nervosa, and others) [16,18,88–90]. These studies contributed to a delineation of pathological narcissism and helped identify diagnostic criteria for NPD that proved useful for the development of the DSM-IV criteria [38,91]. The DIN has later been adapted for both adolescents [47] and pre-adolescents. In a first prospective follow-up study, we found that narcissistic patients changed over time and that corrective life events, achievements, new durable relationships, and disillusionments, contributed to such changes. We also identified characteristics that indicated long-term stable and enduring narcissistic pathology [10]. Notable is that, in both these studies, the participating narcissistic patients had clinically well identified diagnoses of NPD and pathological narcissism from multiple diagnostic sources over an extended work-up period.

Parallel efforts to study narcissism were using self-reports, the Millon Clinical Multiaxial Inventory [92] for Axis II personality disorders, and the Narcissistic Personality Inventory (NPI) [93,94] to examine narcissistic personality styles and behaviour. Both these methods proved sensitive to identify certain aspects of narcissistic character function and have generated a substantial amount of valuable research results. Millon's inventory was adjusted to the changes in DSM-III-R and DSM-IV, and evaluates the egotistical, self-confident, superior, disdainful and exploitive behaviour of narcissistic people in clinical samples. It has been translated to nearly 20 languages and is used widely in clinical personality disorder studies. The NPI is a 40-item self-questionnaire which intends to measure narcissism identified in terms of leadership/authority, superiority/arrogance, self-absorption/self-admiration, and vulnerability/sensitivity [95] and captures

TABLE 4.1   Diagnostic Interview for Narcissism (DIN) [5,89]

Grandiosity (3-years framework)

1. The person exaggerates talents, capacity and achievements in an unrealistic way.
2. The person believes in his/her invulnerability or does not recognize his/her limitations.
3. The person has grandiose fantasies.
4. The person believes that he/she does not need other people.
5. The person regards himself/herself as unique or special compared with other people.
6. The person regards himself/herself as generally superior to other people.
7. The person behaves self-centredly and/or self-referentially.
8. The person appears or behaves in a boastful or pretentious way.

Interpersonal relations (3-years framework)

9. The person has a strong need for admiring attention.
10. The person unrealistically idealized other people.
11. The person devalues other people including feelings of contempt.
12. The person has recurrent and/or deep feelings of envy toward other people.
13. The person reports or behaves entitled, i.e. has unreasonable expectations of favours or other special treatment.
14. The person appears or behaves in condescending, arrogant, or haughty ways.
15. The person is exploitative, i.e. takes advantage of or uses other people.
16. The person lacks empathy (is unable both to understand and to feel for other people's experiences).
17. The person has been unable to make close, lasting emotional commitments to others.

Reactiveness (3-years framework)

18. The person is hypersensitive.
19. The person has had unusually intense feelings in response to criticism or defeat.
20. The person has behaved or felt suicidal or self-destructive in response to criticisms or defeat.
21. The person has reacted with inappropriate anger in response to criticism or defeat.
22. The person has hostile, suspicious reactions in response to the perception of others' envy.

Affects and mood states (1-year framework)

23. The person has deep, sustained feelings of hollowness.
24. The person has deep, sustained feelings of boredom.
25. The person has deep, sustained feelings of meaninglessness.
26. The person has deep, sustained feelings of futility.
27. The person has deep, sustained feelings of badness.

Social and moral adaptation (5-years framework)

28. The person has been capable of high school/work achievement (academic, employment, creative)
29. The person has superficial and changing values and interests.
30. The person shows a disregard for usual/conventional values or rules of society.
31. The person has broken laws one or a few times under circumstance of being enraged or as a means to avoid defeat.
32. The person has recurrent antisocial behaviour.
33. The person's sexual behaviour includes perversions, promiscuity, and/or a lack of inhibitions.

both healthy and maladaptive aspects of narcissism [96]. Despite that research with NPI was conducted on non-clinical samples, the results, especially with regard to self-esteem and affect regulation, have proved increasingly relevant and applicable to pathological narcissism. These efforts have been integrated into a dynamic self-regulatory processing model for narcissistic functioning by Morf and Rhodewalt [97].

Publications

There are by now several important publications updating clinical and empirical progress on narcissism. A special issue of Psychiatric Clinics of North America in 1989, guest edited by O. Kernberg, was the first major effort to integrate clinical, psychoanalytic and psychiatric research contributions to the field. In 1990, Plakun [87] published an anthology which also covered both psychoanalytic conceptualization and case discussions, as well as empirical research on narcissistic patients. Several psychoanalytic volumes specifically addressed identification and treatment of narcissistic patients [60,62, 98–104]. The author edited the volume "Disorders of Narcissism— Diagnostic, Clinical, and Empirical Implications" [105], now translated into both Japanese and Italian. It includes new discussions of theoretical perspectives and treatment efforts, as well as an overview of the accumulating empirical research. In addition, several practical handbooks on dealing with narcissistic individuals and problems in the corporate workplace [106,107], and in couples and families [108–110] have added to a broader interest in understanding narcissistic behaviour and interpersonal relativeness. In addition, a practical semi-autobiographical handbook with accompanying websites was written by a layperson, Sam Vaknin [111].

CONTEMPORARY PERSPECTIVES AND CONTROVERSIES

DSM-IV

The present official guideline for diagnosing NPD is the set of nine criteria and the diagnostic description found in DSM-IV [112] (Table 4.2). Narcissistic personalities are usually identified by overt and striking grandiose sense of self-importance, i.e. a tendency to exaggerate talents or achievement and expectations to be recognized as superior. Grandiose fantasies of unlimited success, power, brilliance etc. serve to expand their sense of themselves. They believe they are special and unique and can only be understood by, or

TABLE 4.2 DSM-IV diagnostic criteria for narcissistic personality disorder

A pervasive pattern of grandiosity (in fantasy or behaviour), need for admiration and lack of empathy, beginning in early adulthood and present in a variety of contexts, as indicated by five (or more) of the following:

1. Has a grandiose sense of self-importance (e.g. exaggerates achievement and talents, expects to be recognized as superior without commensurate achievements)
2. Is preoccupied with fantasies of unlimited success, power, brilliance, beauty, or ideal love
3. Believes that he or she is "special" and unique and can only be understood by, or should be associated with, other special or high-status people (or institutions)
4. Requires excessive admiration
5. Has a sense of entitlement, i.e. unreasonable expectations of especially favourable treatment or automatic compliance with his or her expectations
6. Is interpersonally exploitive, i.e. takes advantage of others to achieve his or her own ends
7. Lacks empathy; is unwilling to recognize or identify with the feelings and needs of others
8. Is often envious of others or believes that others are envious of him or her
9. Shows arrogant, haughty behaviours or attitudes

should associate with, other special or high status people. Entitlement (unreasonable expectations of especially favourable treatment), need for excessive admiration, and arrogant and haughty behaviour characterize their interactions with other people. In addition, envy of others or the belief that others envy them, as well as unempathic and exploitive attitudes and behaviour towards other people or society, are additional character traits that impair the narcissistic individual's capacity for interpersonal functioning and long-term commitments.

Revisions of the DSM Axis II have over the years significantly improved the criteria set for NPD, and although some of the criteria still fail in specificity, i.e. grandiose fantasies and entitlement, the NPD criteria seem to adequately capture the central features of pathological narcissism. Empirical studies render support for the content validity and discriminating capacity of these criteria. Blais *et al.* [113] found in their factor analytic study that grandiosity is a core feature for NPD and that three domains underlie pathological narcissism: grandiosity in fantasy and behaviour, need for admiration, and lack of empathy. When compared to the near neighbours ASPD and BPD, the unique criteria for NPD were: grandiosity, belief in being special and unique, needing admiration, entitlement, and arrogant and haughty behaviour [114]. DSM-IV NPD criteria appear more distinct from BPD while both the above studies indicate a relationship between

NPD and ASPD or sociopathy. Interpersonally exploitive behaviour, lack of empathy and envy were shared with ASPD in the latter study, while the former identified a sociopathic component consisting of lack of empathy, exploitation, envy, and grandiosity. Ronningstam [88] found high discriminating ability for five DSM-III-R/DSM-IV criteria: exaggeration of talents, uniqueness, grandiose fantasies, entitlement, and needs admiration. Morey [115], on the other hand, was more critical and concerned about the low internal consistency, empirical incoherence and high diagnostic overlap in the DSM criteria. He argued for radical changes adding reactions to threats to self-esteem, need for interpersonal control, interpersonal hostility and lack of self-destructive tendencies to the future list of criteria.

A major problem, i.e. the general limitations of DSM-IV Axis II to capture the full range of personality pathology and the failure of the system to identify patients whom clinicians consider having personality disorders diagnosis [38,115,116], is particularly consequential for NPD. People with traits of pathological narcissism that range beyond the DSM-IV criteria set, or people who have less severe and overt narcissistic pathology and for various reasons do not meet the DSM-IV criteria for NPD, will consequentially not be correctly identified. In addition, the conceptual meaning and dynamic expressions of several of the concepts—such as entitlement, empathy and exploitiveness—are unclear and poorly defined, and the interaction between interpersonal interactions, self-esteem fluctuations and affect dysregulation remains unclear.

The specific nature of pathological narcissism, with grandiosity and sensitivity to threats to self-esteem, reduces the reliability of self-assessment and one-time diagnostic evaluations with direct inquiries in structured interviews [96,117]. Questions on narcissistic themes may evoke defensive reactions [5], as narcissistic people make more or less conscious efforts to present themselves in an optimal and favourable way in the service of self-esteem regulation. The nature of some specific narcissistic characteristics, such as self-conscious emotions of shame and envy, which are often hidden or bypassed [118] and therefore inaccessible to immediate diagnostic evaluation, adds further difficulties in empirical evaluations. In addition, the origin and range of impairments in empathic processing as a personality disorder characteristic, one of the core narcissistic interpersonal features, has so far been insufficiently empirically explored to warrant accurate diagnostic assessment.

Similar problems with assessment using structured methods and self-reports have been observed in the research on people with psychopathy [15]. Hart noticed that self-report measures of psychopathy proved to be more useful and reliable in studies of "normal" non-patient populations. This has also been the case for social psychological studies of narcissism in non-clinical samples using the NPI [93,94] and observations of narcissistic functioning of normal adults in laboratory settings. Of interest for future assessment of pathological narcissism is a progressive effort to revise Axis II and develop clinically useful assessment methods. Westen and Shedler [119,120] propose a dimensional system for diagnosing personality disorders, and diagnostic criteria that actually "describe personality dynamics underlying manifest symptoms...e.g. the function of psychological symptoms, the processes that maintain them, the accompanying affect, the manner of regulating distress".

Beyond DSM-IV

Presently there are both clinical and empirical support for identifying the core of narcissistic pathology as centering on three major areas of functioning: self-esteem dysregulation, affect dysregulation and dysfunctions in interpersonal relationships. The following is an outline of clinical and empirical evidence for a set of diagnostic criteria that takes into consideration both the dimensional quality of pathological narcissism and the relationship between the arrogant, the shy and the psychopathic type of NPD.

THE ARROGANT NPD

Self-esteem Dysregulation

Narcissism has historically been associated with self-esteem, and defects in self-esteem regulation, usually described in terms of inflated or vulnerable self-esteem, is one of the core disturbances in narcissistic disorder [12,76–78,81,121]. Recent research [122] has found that people with unstable self-esteem have more fluctuations in self-evaluation and place greater importance on such self-evaluations for determining their overall self-worth. Rhodewalt *et al.* [123,124] concluded that narcissistic people have greater self-esteem instability and mood variability, are more sensitive to ego threats which lower their self-esteem, and tend to react with anger and hostility to such threats. Rhodewalt *et al.* also suggested that self-aggrandizing and self-attributions used for protection of the grandiose self cause hypersensitivity to criticism and more extreme reactions to both success and failure. Narcissistic people externalize failure and attribute success to their own ability—a strategy that sets the stage for narcissistic rage reactions.

Grandiosity

In clinical settings, characteristics describing grandiosity differentiate narcissistic patients from all other psychiatric patients [6]. Grandiosity refers to an unrealistic sense of superiority, a sustained view of oneself as better than others that causes the narcissistic person to view others with disdain, or as different or inferior. It also refers to a sense of uniqueness and specialness, the belief that few others have much in common with oneself and that one can only be understood by a few or very special people. Additional attitudes and behaviours that serve to support and enhance the inflated self-esteem include: admiring attention-seeking, boastful and pretentious attitudes, and unrestrained self-centred and self-referential behaviour [6]. Grandiose fantasies serve to protect, complement or expand the grandiose self-experience. Narcissistic fantasies stem from a need to change the self to overcompensate for experienced defects.

Grandiosity has been considered the core trait of NPD and its most distinguishing characteristic [6,113,123]. Nevertheless, grandiosity is also reactive and state-dependent [10]. For instance, it can be influenced by brief depressive reactions or depressive disorder causing a more self-critical and humble attitude, or by moving from late adolescence to adulthood with experiences of more realistic achievements and interpersonal experiences that stabilize the self-esteem. It can also be influenced by corrective life events, such as achievements and disillusionments that contribute to a more realistic alignment of the self-esteem and evaluation of one's own capacity and potential. In addition, sudden threats to the self-esteem can temporarily increase expressions of a defensive grandiose self-experience [9] or lower grandiosity [97]. Differentiating between state-dependent signs or temporary increase of grandiosity and stable symptoms of grandiose self-experience may require specific diagnostic attention. This changeability in grandiosity suggests that the diagnosis of NPD should not depend as heavily on grandiosity as has been suggested in the empirical and clinical literature [10].

Real or Exaggerated Achievements

Closely related to grandiosity is the narcissistic individuals' tendency to make self-aggrandizing attributions to enhance self-esteem [123] and exaggerate their talents and achievements [6]. Many narcissistic people are indeed very capable and do have sustained periods of successful academic, professional or creative accomplishments [6]. The combination of exceptional talents or intellectual giftedness, grandiose fantasies, and strong self-investment can, in certain cases, lead to extraordinary intellectual, creative or innovative contributions or unusual ability for leadership. Such a capacity may compensate for or counterbalance other interpersonal or emotional difficulties that the narcissistic person experiences in other areas in life. Although high achievements and professional success are not considered diagnostic criteria, their presence distinguishes people with NPD from those with most other personality disorders [6]. The capacity for high achievement is frequently a source or justification of a sense of superiority—a reason for the importance of doing a thorough evaluation of both unrealistic and realistic aspects of actual capability, high self-esteem and superiority. It is specifically important to differentiate realistic competence and high self-esteem in a person coming across as haughty and superior from defensive unrealistic exaggerations and bragging, as well as from actual potentials and capabilities hidden behind grandiose fantasies and self-effacing or arrogantly disdainful attitude.

Reactions to Criticism

Low capacity to discriminate NPD and high presence in other personality disorders prompted the decision to exclude reactions to criticism as a criteria for NPD in DSM-IV [38]. However, recent research on self-esteem regulation [97,124–126] has helped to identify specific patterns that discriminate narcissistic reactivity. In general, ego threats disrupt self-regulatory effectiveness in people with high self-esteem. Narcissistic people tend to interpret tasks and events as opportunities to show off, to demonstrate their superiority and to compete with others. When criticized, they ward off intolerable criticism or threats by overestimating their own contributions, ignoring or devaluing the critique or the person who criticizes, or by aggressively counter-arguing or defending themselves; they also use self-aggrandizing strategies and self-illusion to boost positive feedback, commit to unrealistic goals and take exaggerated credit for a success. Several studies [123,127–129] support the observation that people with high narcissism tend to have strong aggressive and violent reactions to threats to their sense of superiority or self-esteem. Aggressive reactions to criticism may be more or less controlled and obvious—ranging from cognitive reconstructions of events and subtle, well hidden feelings of disdain or contempt, to intense aggressive argumentativeness, criticism and rage outbursts, to more or less controlled aggressive and violent behaviour. Intense emotional reactions such as rage and shame reflect both shifting levels of self-esteem and affect dysregulation [124] (see below). Such reactions also differentiate NPD from antisocial and hypomanic people who are less prone to reactions and affectively more stable [115].

TABLE 4.3   Self-esteem dysregulation in the arrogant narcissistic personality disorder

- Sense of superiority and uniqueness[1]
- Exaggeration of talents and achievements[1, 2]
- Grandiose fantasies[1]
- Self-centred and self-referential behaviour[1]
- Boastful and pretentious attitude[1]
- Need for admiring attention[1]
- Strong reactions to criticism and defeat[2,3]

1. Ronningstam and Gunderson [6]
2. Rhodewalt and Morf [123]
3. Morey and Jones [115]

Summary

The main overt characteristics of narcissistic people's self-esteem regulation centre around grandiosity, which is expressed in an inner sense of superiority and uniqueness, and in grandiose fantasies of being best, powerful, attractive, admired etc. (see Table 4.3). The most noticeable manifest behavioural signs of grandiosity are self-centred and self-referential behaviour and a boastful or pretentious attitude. Admiring attention from others serves to protect and enhance the grandiose self-experience, and narcissistic people make various more or less oblivious or obvious efforts to gain such supportive attention. The most important sign of narcissistic self-esteem dysregulation is the various strong reactions to criticism, defeats or other threats to the self-esteem. Manifestations of such reactions can range from subtle internal re-evaluations, to active self-aggrandizing and self-protecting behaviour, and to intense feelings of rage and shame.

Affect Dysregulation

People with narcissistic personality disorder are challenged both by the presence of strong affects, especially rage, shame and envy [8], and by the low tolerance of the nature and intensity of such feelings. This is especially evident in their difficulties in modulating affects, and their proneness to self-criticism and sensitivity to experiencing failures in maintaining inner control. Excessive, uncontrollable rage outbursts or proneness to self-shaming and extreme reactions to both success and humiliation are signs of such affect dysregulation. In addition, certain aspects of narcissistic people's affect regulation and reactivity actually reflect shifts in self-esteem [115]. Narcissistic people are hypersensitive and prone to rapidly interpreting situations as narcissistically threatening or humiliating [130]. However, there are notable differences in expressions of such hypersensitivity. While some people may appear stoic, cold and unemotional, obsessionally preoccupied with details, or detached and avoidant, others come across as emotionally lively, reactive and intensive, and even erratic or dramatic. An inability to acknowledge and communicate feelings is a common sign of affect dysregulation, especially among ambitious, intelligent narcissistic people. The term alexithymia, i.e. having no words for emotions, has been used to capture this inability to use affects for information processing [131–133]. While empirical studies on narcissistic anger and rage, and on shame unrelated to narcissism, have been most valuable in outlining narcissistic affect dysregulation, studies of envy are still missing.

Anger and Rage

As mentioned above, studies have verified the connection between narcissism and emotional reactivity and the fact that narcissistic people indeed have intense hostile reactions to threats to their egos and self-esteem [123,126]. Kohut [134] described narcissistic rage, a specific form of rage that is triggered in a narcissistically shame-prone or vulnerable individual in response to a narcissistic injury. This rage, which can range from a deep chronic grudge to an archaic violent fury, is related to the need for absolute control of the environment, to righting something wrong, or to undo hurt, for the main purpose of maintaining self-esteem. It is based on a desire to turn a passive experience of victimization into an active act of inflicting injury onto others. As such, it can also be motivated by a need for revenge. Narcissistic rage is archaic in nature, and characterized by relentlessness, sharp reasoning, lack of empathy, and unforgivingness. However, narcissistic rage can also involve self-protection [135] and serve to restore a sense of internal power and safety. As such, it is associated to self-preservation and entitlement and to the urge to destroy any interference to such rights [136]. Turned towards the self, this type of rage can lead to suicidal ideations and behaviour.

Shame

Feelings of shame have been strongly associated with narcissism [62], and specifically with self-evaluation and self-esteem regulation. Tangney and colleagues [118,137,138] have in their extensive empirical studies on shame identified several significant characteristics: shame is a debilitating emotion that often serves to paralyse the self. It can be overwhelming and devastatingly painful and involve the entire self, leading, at least temporarily, to a crippling of adaptive self-functions. Shame involves a significant shift in self-perception, accompanied by a sense of exposure, a sense of shrinking, and feelings of worthlessness and powerlessness. In other words, both the feeling of shame in itself and the perception of one's own feelings of shame tend to lower an individual's self-esteem.

Since shame has been strongly associated with the urge to hide, the impact of shame in interpersonal relationships has usually been overlooked. On the other hand, the pain of shame can motivate anger, hostility and humiliated fury [139,140], which usually cause severe difficulties in interpersonal relationships. It can lead to irrational and aggressive shame-blame cycles with subsequent rejections from the targeted or blamed person [141]. As the distress and pain associated to shame tend to shift the person's attention inward, shame feelings also tend to have a negative impairing effect on the capacity for empathy and for concern and connection to other people [118]. As shame can remain hidden and be effectively rationalized or defended against, feelings of shame have usually been associated with the shy narcissistic personality (see below). However, the connection between shame and anger, hostility and blaming makes the presence of shame more manifest and a central feeling in the arrogant narcissistic personality as well.

Envy

Envy is considered one of the most essential features of pathological narcissism and NPD [12,81] and Rosenfeldt [142] even suggested that the narcissistic character structure is a defence against envy and dependency. Nevertheless, the connection between narcissism and envy has been especially difficult to clarify, as awareness of one's own feelings of envy, in and by itself, tends to lower self-esteem and evoke feelings of shame [143]. In other words, a strong internal readiness to deny feelings of envy, usually accompanied by social reinforcements of such denial, makes envy a vexatious inquiry. In psychoanalytic studies, envy is considered to be rooted in constitutional aggression and defined as hatred directed towards good objects. Compared to "regular" hatred, when the good object is protected and the bad object is attacked, in hatred with primitive envy the other person's goodness is experienced as a threat to the person's own grandiosity or idealized self-experience and the goodness is destroyed [144].

Barth [143] suggested a relationship between narcissistic injury and envious feelings, such that envy can be both a stimulus for and a result of self-esteem dysregulation. Envy may represent both an attempt to avoid painful injury to one's self-esteem, and an effort to maintain a positive self-esteem. In a cycle of self-esteem dysregulation, feelings of inadequacy and/or inferiority and envious rage—which includes a wish to destroy either the possessor or that which is possessed—are followed by self-criticism and shame for such hateful, hostile, and greedy feelings. In this process "the ability to value oneself and one's possession (including personal characteristics, feelings of being loved, personal and professional achievement and so on) is often destroyed" [143]. In other words, "envy not only makes it difficult for the individual to appreciate (take in) what the envied person offers, but it also interferes with the individual's ability to appreciate what he or she already has" [143]. Rage and greed that accompany envy can represent attempts to restore or protect self-esteem. "The rage may be empowering, may help to compensate for feelings of inadequacy which trigger the envy in the first place" [143]. However, Barth also noted that feelings of rage paradoxically also may increase the feelings of shame. Envy is always disguised and it hardly ever appears in a straightforward manner [145]. The expressions of envy in social and interpersonal contexts can be extremely subtle and undermining, ranging from discrete spoiling behaviour and withholding a person's needs such as praise, empathy, warmth, attention, admiration, support or comfort, to actively spoiling or destroying the object [146].

While narcissistic people readily deny feelings of envy towards others, they often report intense reactions to the perception of others' envy [6]. In other words, the belief that other people envy them because of their special talents or unique qualities is associated with suspicious and hostile reactions. Such reactions may remain hidden or be overtly expressed, depending upon the nature and level of the individual's narcissistic functioning. On the one hand, while the preoccupation with others' envy may represent a projection of one's own intolerable envy onto other people, it may also be a sign of hypersensitivity and a perception of other people's envy as a threat to one's own self-esteem and grandiose self-experience. On the other hand, the sensitivity to others' envy can also be associated with a particular superior awareness of others' attention, self-righteous anger and even a sadistic satisfaction in causing a sense of inferiority and painful feelings in others.

Mood and Hypochondria

Mood swings in narcissistic patients, i.e. irritability, cynicism or brief reactive depression, or excitement, optimism and confidence, reflect shifting levels of self-esteem and are highly dependent on external support of the self-esteem or on perceived threats to the grandiose self . Sharp mood variations in response to such threats can also include states of elevated mood or sudden explosive rage [8].

Summary

The most significant characteristic of narcissistic affect dysregulation is the predominance of feelings of anger, shame and envy and the individual's

TABLE 4.4   Affect dysregulation in the arrogant narcissistic
personality disorder

• Strong feelings of shame and envy[1,2] • Intense aggressive reactions to threats to self-esteem[3,4] • Sharp mood variations[1] • Intense reactions to the perception of others' envy[5]

1. Cooper and Ronningstam [7]; Cooper [8]
2. Kernberg [81]
3. Morey and Jones [115]
4. Rhodewalt and Morf [123]
5. Ronningstam and Gunderson [6]

strong proneness to react intensively with such feelings to perceived humiliations and threats to self-esteem (see Table 4.4). While anger reactions, ranging from silent contempt to overt hostility and explosive rage outbursts, are usually noticeable and obvious, the feelings of shame and envy may be more hidden or indirectly expressed, such as in the tendency to blame or in reactions to the perception of others' envy. Mood variations including depression, irritability, elation or hypomania reflect shifting levels of self-esteem.

Interpersonal Relations

Interpersonal relations represent the most consequential area of functioning for people with NPD. Not only are they sensitive to and reliant upon support and feedback from others for their self-knowledge and self-esteem regulation, but they also actively use the social environment and other people to get admiring attention from others, and to protect and enhance their self-esteem [6,124]. On the other hand, other people also represent a constant threat to the narcissistic individual's self-experience and in as much as others can make a narcissist feel superior, entitled and confident, they can also contribute to his/her feeling extremely ashamed, inferior, worthless, irritable and enraged. Problems with commitment, difficulties to take on others' perspective and to interpret other people and to understand and tolerate others' feelings, combined with entitlement and unrealistic expectations of others, often lead to severe interpersonal failures and to potential isolation. Such problems are also the most serious obstacle to engaging in and benefiting from treatment. Although there is a general consensus on several of the characteristics for narcissistic interpersonal functioning, i.e. entitlement, empathy and exploitiveness, the lack of empirical and clinical agreement on their expression in narcissistic patients has made assessment difficult.

Entitlement

Despite being one of the most significant criteria for NPD, entitlement is not among the strongest discriminators [6]. The complex clinical and dynamic expressions and its close relationship to exploitive behaviour contribute. Entitlement may stem either from a sense of grandiose self-righteousness or function as a defence against feelings of envy, guilt, shame, depression or the threat of closeness [147]. Expressions of entitlement can range from infuriated reactions (irritability, hostile rejecting or vindictive behaviour) to feeling surprised, hurt, unappreciated, unfairly treated or even exploited. Entitlement is closely related to a passive attitude and lack of self-initiative [148], and to an experience of not getting as much as one deserves [149]. It can also be associated with expectations or hopes for reparation of past damages or correction of injustices [147]. An expectation that things should come easily and be provided by others often comes with negative or even shameful feeling towards the requirement of one's own efforts. Further explorations of people's feelings of entitlement may reveal a striking contrast between inner experiences of defectiveness, undesirability or worthlessness, and an overt special entitled attitude of unrealistic rights, expectations and exemptions [150]. Entitlement in such dynamic context may have its roots in unmodulated aggression and harsh judgmental self-criticism. Paradoxically, and despite strong feelings of entitlement, narcissistic people may also feel ambivalent and suffer from an inability to feel that they fully deserve what seems to be the basic rights and conditions in the lives of other people.

Empathy

Although lack of empathy has, besides grandiosity, been considered one of the main characteristics of NPD, there have nevertheless been substantial difficulties making valid assessments of this capacity [6]. Empathy refers to the ability to feel and perceive the inner psychological state, and identify the feelings and needs of other people. It also requires the ability to tolerate, feel and identify one's own emotions [151]. As narcissistic people often come across as unsympathetic to and ignorant of other people's feelings, it has readily been assumed that they also lack empathy. This general notion, also held by DSM-IV, seems to neglect cognitive, emotional and interpersonal variations in empathic processing. However, so far no studies have focused specifically on the relationship between self-esteem and affect dysregulation and narcissistic interpersonal functioning to empathic processing.

Of relevance for narcissistic empathic dysfunction is the impaired capacity for understanding our own emotions and reactions. In addition, impairment or disconnection in interpersonal interpretive functioning also contributes to low empathy. "The individual might experience affect in relation to other's distress but this is inappropriately or inadequately linked to a representation of the belief and intentional state of that person" [152]. In other words, this corresponds to the narcissistic individual's tendencies to misinterpret states and emotions in others and to a disconnection between cognitive and emotional interpretative processes.

Low affect tolerance is incompatible with empathic processing [26]. The perception of the other person's emotional state may evoke both intolerable feelings in the narcissistic person and a sense of incompetence and helplessness which seriously interferes with empathy. Proneness to shame tends to impair the capacity for other-oriented empathic concern [117], and both feelings of shame and envy are accompanied by the urge to withdraw which hinders active interpersonal processing of empathy. Biased self-perception, egocentricity and self-preoccupation interfere with the ability for perspective taking and emotional resonance. By nature, entitlement and the readiness for self-serving expectations on others are incompatible with empathy. In addition, self-enhancement and other strategies to protect and increase self-esteem are also incompatible with interpersonal orientation and empathy [153].

The clinical presentation of impaired empathic capacity in narcissistic people may range from tuned in unassuming interest, subtle inattention or inability to listen, to superior intellectual demonstrations of capability to identify mental states and feelings in others, to complete insensitive obliviousness. In addition, empathic dysfunctions may be expressed as efforts to control others' inner states, or as overtly disdainful or critical reactions towards others' feelings and distress, or, in more severe forms of pathological narcissism, as attempts to con, manipulate or emotionally exploit others based on identification of those others' inner state and distress. In the diagnostic evaluation and treatment planning with narcissistic people, it is of crucial importance to differentiate between emotional and cognitive origins of empathic dysfunction, as well as to identify the specific developmental origin and the pattern of attachment and attunement that could have contributed to empathic impairment.

Arrogance, Control and Hostility

Some narcissistic people present themselves as strikingly arrogant and haughty [6], others might initially appear more timid but gradually present more hidden and specific areas of disdainful or pejorative attitude. Morey [115] identified expressions of active or passive interpersonal hostility. The degree and type of hostility can vary from less obvious passive-aggressive behaviour to overtly belittling, exploitive, or sadistic behaviour, especially towards subordinates. The need for interpersonal control [114] or dominance [156] represent an unempathic, detached involvement with self-serving purposes or a strategy to manage hostility and regulate self-esteem.

Interpersonal Commitment

The inability to engage in long-term commitments has primarily been associated with the lack of tolerance for the challenge to self-esteem and the intensity of affects involved in a deep long-term mutual relationship. Cooper [8] noted a relational pattern of early enthusiasm that is followed by disappointment. Lack of commitment is an indicator of more long-term, enduring forms of NPD [10] and is associated with poor prognosis and absence of change. Lack of commitment can also be an expression of a more severe narcissistic disturbance in the context of irresponsible, actively exploitive, or even corruptive interpersonal behaviour. On the other hand, a capacity for long-term commitment to others, even in the presence of other severe signs of narcissistic pathology, points towards changeability and better prognosis, as it enables the person to commit to tasks, family and treatment team.

Exploitiveness

Exploitiveness, a feature associated with pathological narcissism and NPD and traditionally focused on privileges, material or monetary gain, or personal or professional resources of others, did not distinguish narcissistic people in our studies [6,89,90]. Neither did exploitive behaviour differentiate NPD in relation to BPD and ASPD in Holwick et al.'s study [114]. It seems that exploitiveness in narcissistic people is closely linked with grandiosity and entitlement and border to psychopathy. Consequently it is important to differentiate between the more active and consciously exploitive behaviour found in antisocial and psychopathic individuals and the need-fulfilling exploitive behaviour found in borderline patients, from the more passive, manipulative, and entitled, emotionally focused exploitive behaviour that serve to support or enhance self-esteem in narcissistic individuals. It is also important to differentiate exploitive behaviour from aggressive entitlement, i.e. the sense of right to pick on, blame, and misuse others, and revengeful or malignant entitlement [155], i.e. the right to retaliate, parasite on, or violate others. The dynamics behind such entitlement is different from the one leading to exploitive behaviour.

Summary

Narcissistic individuals are usually identified by their specific interpersonal pattern, with a more or less overtly arrogant and haughty attitude, and entitled and controlling behaviour (see Table 4.5). Hostility can range from subtle passive aggressive behaviour to sadistic or explosive behaviour. Inability to commit to others is the sign of a long-term, enduring narcissistic personality disorder. Specific attention should be paid to the range of empathic dysfunctions and varieties in expressions of impaired empathic processing that can be found in narcissistic individuals.

THE SHY NPD

The "shy narcissist" is now a common label for people with a different clinical presentation of pathological narcissism, and several reports have outlined the features and diagnostic criteria for this type of NPD [3,4,7,8,14,60]. Although these specific expressions of narcissistic disorder are not yet included in the official DSM-IV criteria set, they are nevertheless acknowledged as associated features. They include: vulnerable self-esteem, feelings of shame, sensitivity and intense reactions of humiliation, emptiness or disdain in response to criticism or defeat, and vocational irregularities due to difficulties tolerating criticism or competition [111]. The identification of this group of narcissistic personality disorder, also called the "hypervigilant" [4], "diffident" [156], "closet narcissist" [60] or "covert" [8] stems from the recognition of the fragile, vulnerable self-structure in some narcissistic people and the role of shame in the development of pathological narcissism [157]. This type of narcissistic individual appears quite different compared to those captured in the regular NPD criteria set: hypersensitive

TABLE 4.5 Abnormal interpersonal relations in the arrogant narcissistic personality disorder

- Arrogant and haughty behaviour[1]
- Entitlement[1,2]
- Impaired empathic capacity[2]
- Interpersonal control and hostility[3]
- Lack of sustained commitment to others[2,4]

1. Ronningstam and Gunderson [6]
2. Cooper and Ronningstam [7]; Cooper [8]
3. Morey and Jones [115]
4. Ronningstam et al. [10]

and self-effacing [4]; inhibited and unassuming [7]; modest, humble, and seemingly uninterested in social success [3] with a mentality of the loser escaping to grandiose fantasies [156].

While clinical descriptions formed the foundation of this type, two studies confirm two facets in pathological narcissism. In one study [130], narcissism divided into two factors, one implying grandiosity-exhibitionism and another vulnerability-sensitivity. Both were associated with conceit, self-indulgence, and disregard for others, but the vulnerability factor also captured anxiety and pessimism, introversion, defensiveness, anxiety and vulnerability to life trauma. Another study [63] showed that narcissism consists of two different styles, a "phallic" grandiose style and a vulnerable style. Shame contributed to the major differences between these styles, correlating negatively with the grandiose style and positively with the more vulnerable style.

Grandiosity

The shy narcissistic personalities usually hide their grandiosity. Grandiose desires are not expressed and acted upon, and narcissistic pursuits are often performed on a fantasy level [3,7]. In fact, their grandiose fantasies may be excessively compensatory, replacing actual achievements and interactions, and compensating for inhibitions and the inability to expose and realize inner wishes and motivations. Gabbard suggested that "at the core of their inner world is a deep sense of shame related to their secret wish to exhibit themselves in a grandiose manner" [4]. Both such feelings of excessive shame, and the presence of a strict conscience [3] and harsh self-criticism tend to seriously inhibit the shy narcissistic individual, impair executive functioning and force him/her to hide both grandiose strivings and actual ambitions, competence and achievements. In addition, avoiding ambitions and exposure to competitive and challenging situations is an important part of the shy narcissist's self-esteem dysregulation [4]. This is in sharp contrast to the arrogant narcissist, who seeks out opportunities for self-exposure and competition, and often comes across as self-assured, knowledgeable and competent. A specific diagnostic challenge with these types of patients involve differentiating unrealistic grandiosity and grandiose fantasies, from hidden ambitions, realistic capabilities and pursuits, and from inhibitions due to shame or excessive self-criticism.

Affect Regulation

The shy narcissist is highly sensitive, has easily hurt feelings and is prone to feeling ashamed, embarrassed and humiliated, especially when confronted with the recognitions of unsatisfied need or deficiencies in his/her capacities [4,8]. The exceptional sensitivity to exposure and attention and accompanying overwhelming feelings of shame and anxiety is one of the more specific features of this narcissistic type [3,4]. Hypochondria, a sign of affect regression and expression of affects as somatic symptoms, serves defensive purposes to cover grandiosity, omnipotence and masochism [3,8]. Unhappiness, pessimism and sense of lack of fulfilment, inner yearning, and waiting and hoping for recognition and changes to come are major characteristics of the inner affect state of this narcissism [3,130,156].

Interpersonal Relativeness

The shy narcissists are extremely attentive to others. They are hypersensitive and tend to pay specific attention to others' reactions to them, especially slights and criticism [4]. Their capacity for empathy is compromised due to their envy, self-denigration and extreme self-preoccupation. Shy narcissistic people often come across as empathic and sensitive and they can appear interested in, and even "tuned in" to other people. Some may even be capable of identifying feelings and inner experiences in others, i.e. capable of empathic registration. Their unassuming shyness and wish to be noticed may mistakenly be perceived as a genuine interest in and capacity to care for others. However, they are equally unable to genuinely respond to others' needs and to involve in enduring mutual personal relationships as their arrogant counterpart [7]. They may also be ambivalent towards their sense of entitlement, struggling with feelings of not deserving what they actually are entitled to, or they may suppress exaggerated entitlement together with self-righteousness, aggression and grandiosity behind a façade of shyness and aloofness [147].

Superego Functioning

Contrary to the arrogant type, shy narcissistic individuals are able to feel remorse for their incapacity to empathize with others [3] and guilt caused by awareness of their shallowness and lack of concern for others [7]. Akhtar [3] also noticed that shy narcissists have a stricter conscience and hold high moral standards with less tendencies to inconsistency and compromises of ethical values and rules. On the other hand, this strictness also makes the individual hide and suppress grandiosity and ambitions.

Summary

Unlike the arrogant type, who is more openly aggressive, vocationally involved, and actively seeking narcissistic gratification and self-enhancement in his life, the shy narcissist is constricted both interpersonally and vocationally. The self-esteem regulation in shy narcissistic people is much more influenced by shaming, which inhibits not only the expressions of grandiosity but also the individual's pursuits of actual capabilities and opportunities in his real life. The hypersensitivity and attentive readiness for slights and criticism from others calls for an extreme vulnerability. In addition, the intense feelings of shame increase interpersonal detachment and hiding which contribute to feelings of unhappiness, isolation and inner yearning. Although the shy narcissist, because of his/her timid, kind, helpful and unassuming presentation, may be less involved in aggressive conflicts with others, his/her shallowness, envy and inability to genuinely and consistently care for others cause other types of interpersonal conflicts and rejections. Since their presentation is not easily recognizable, correct diagnosis usually requires several sessions or a longer period of assessment (see Table 4.6).

SUPEREGO REGULATION AND RELATION TO PSYCHOPATHY AND ASPD

An additional dimension of diagnostic importance for evaluating NPD, especially in relation to psychopathy and ASPD, concerns moral and ethical values and functioning. Narcissistic individuals can be found among those who openly take pride in their high moral standards, and who can criticize and devalue people with different and "lower" sets of rules and values. In more extreme cases, the narcissistic person may even show intolerance and condemnation of others to highlight the virtue of his/her own superior ethics. Nevertheless, in most narcissistic individuals, moral and value systems can be more consistently relativistic or corrupt [8,14,158]. They show disregard for conventional values and society's rules through deceitful and dishonest behaviour. Akhtar [3] specifically noted the tendencies to shift values and to lie. Other behaviours range from seductive, Don-Juan-like recurrent efforts to conquer or passively exploit others emotionally or financially to conscious efforts to do the "perfect crime", or to actual crimes of revenge or to protect self-esteem or status. However, narcissistic people who can present a variety of antisocial behaviour are usually aware of moral norms and standards and able to feel guilt and concern, but lack the capacity for deep commitment [159]. A more severe level of superego dysfunction has been captured by the term "malignant narcissism" [13,160], characterized by antisocial behaviour, ego-syntonic sadism or characterological aggression, and paranoid orientation.

NPD and ASPD

The relationship between NPD and ASPD and psychopathy has been noted by several researchers [161–163]. Harpur *et al.* [23] suggested that

TABLE 4.6   The shy narcissistic personality disorder

Features shared with the arrogant narcissistic type
• Sense of superiority and uniqueness
• Lack of sustained commitment to others
• Impaired capacity for empathy
• Strong feelings of envy

Features exclusive for the shy narcissistic type
• Compensatory grandiose fantasies[1]
• Shame for ambition and grandiosity[1,2,3]
• Shuns being the centre of attention[2]
• Hypersensitive to slights, humiliation and criticism[2]
• Harsh self-criticism[1]
• Proneness to intense shame reactions[1,2]
• Interpersonal and vocational inhibitions[1,2]
• Modest, humble and unassuming[3]
• Hypochondria[1,3]
• Dysphoric affect state with unhappiness, pessimism, lack of fulfillment, yearning, and waiting[3,4]

1. Cooper and Ronningstam [7]; Cooper [8]
2. Gabbard [4]
3. Akhtar [3,14]
4. Wink [130]

psychopathic symptomatology should be divided into two facets. One is related to narcissism and called "selfish, callous and remorseless use of others", and includes interpersonal and affective characteristics, such as egocentricity, superficiality, deceitfulness, callousness, and lack of remorse, empathy and anxiety. The other represents more prototypic psychopathy with socially deviant behaviour. Kernberg [13] suggested a spectrum of narcissistic pathology, with antisocial behaviour ranging from narcissistic personality, to the syndrome of malignant narcissism, to antisocial personality, representing the most severe form of pathological narcissism. The antisocial person's more severe superego contrasts to the dynamics of the narcissistic individuals, which involves defences against unconscious envy with capacity to recognize good aspects in others, and their antisocial behaviour stem more from ego-syntonic entitlement and greed. The relatively high diagnostic overlap between ASPD and NPD (25%) [90] supports the view that ASPD may be conceptualized as laying along a continuum of narcissistic personality and pathological narcissism. Holdwick *et al.* [117] found that NPD and ASPD share interpersonal exploitiveness, lack of empathy and envy, and Blais [115] identified a sociopathic factor in NPD lack of empathy, exploitation, envy, and grandiose sense of self-importance.

One study [90] confirms intrapsychic and interpersonal similarities between people with NPD and ASPD: both have grandiose fantasies and believe in their invulnerability; both are in need of admiring attention and are entitled, envious and have strong reactions to criticism. The major *differences* found in this study relate to narcissists being more grandiose—exaggerating their talents and feeling unique and superior—while people with ASPD are more actively exploitive and feel more empty. Both narcissistic and antisocial people are *unempathic* and *exploitive*. However, while antisocial people lack motivation for identifying the needs and feelings of others, narcissistic people's empathic failures are due to an emotional or cognitive inability to identify with and feel for other people. Exploitiveness in antisocial patients is more likely to be consciously and actively related to materialistic or sexual gain, while exploitive behaviour in narcissistic patients is more passive, or unwitting. More specifically, in people with NPD, exploitive behaviour may be unconsciously motivated, a result of feeling superior or entitled, and serving to enhance self-image by gaining attention, admiration and status. Exploitiveness can also stem from the narcissistic person being unempathic and unable to identify the boundaries and feelings of others [36,90]. In addition, interpersonal manifestations and affective reactivity, especially rage reactions in response to criticism, are much more evident in NPD, while antisocial people show more acting out, particularly with drug and alcohol abuse, chronic unstable antisocial and criminal life style, impulsivity, and sensation seeking [15,90,117]. NPD patients normally do not display recurrent antisocial behaviour (except for those with advanced drug abuse who finance their addiction through regular criminal behaviour), but they can occasionally commit criminal acts if enraged or as a means of avoiding defeat [6]. The question whether some narcissistic personalities may represent a "white collar", entrepreneurial type of ASPD has also been raised. Studies of violence in social psychological and clinical studies provide another connection between antisocial and narcissistic disorders. Threats towards superior self-regard predicted aggressive and violent behaviour [127] and NPD symptoms correlated with violence in adolescence and young adults [164]. Nestor [165] suggested that narcissistic personality traits are a clinical risk factor for violence. Narcissistic injury constitutes a specific pathway, as it increases the risk for violent reactions especially in psychopaths and people with antisocial conditions.

Summary

Obviously psychopathic behaviour also serves to protect or enhance the inflated self experience, and the sense of grandiosity is strongly related to feeling envious and entitled to exploit others. Lack of empathy, and aggressive, sadistic, revengeful behaviours are more pronounced, and the specific superego pathology with lying, deceitful behaviour (see Table 4.7).

TABLE 4.7   The psychopathic narcissistic personality
disorder

- Lack of empathy[1]
- Entitled exploitativeness[2]
- Irritability and raging reactions[3]
- Violent behaviour[4]
- Interpersonal sadism[5]
- One or a few crimes[2]
- Deceitfulness[6]
- Cunning/manipulative[6]
- Lack of remorse or guilt[6]

1. Holdwick et al. [114]
2. Gunderson and Ronningstam [90]
3. Morey and Jones [115]
4. Baumeister et al. [127]
5. Kernberg [13]
6. Harpur et al. [23]

DIFFERENTIATING NPD FROM OTHER DISORDERS

NPD and BPD

Studies have previously reported on extensive overlap between these
disorders [39,89]. Similarities between NPD and BPD include sensitivity to
criticism, ragefulness and entitlement [89,166]. Entitled rage can be found in
both NPD and BPD, but while this rage in narcissistic people is triggered by
threats to their superiority and to their sense of deserving special or
inordinate rights, privileges, status and security, the entitled rage in
borderlines is triggered by their needs not being met and feelings of
entitlement because of their suffering or victimization. It is very important
to identify this type of rage as, when ignored, it tends to cause unproductive
thriving on the patient's identification as a victim and prevent progress in
treatment. Holdwick et al. [116] found that NPD shares with BPD affect
dysregulation, impulsivity and unstable relationships. However, efforts to
find a conceptual relativeness between NPD and BPD have actually
resulted in both empirical and clinical evidence supporting their separateness. The most important discriminator is the inflated self-concept of NPD
and its various manifestations of grandiosity, including exaggeration of
talent, grandiose fantasies, sense of uniqueness [83,89,116,117].

Akhtar [169] identified the following structural and functional differences. While NPD has a more cohesive self, with fewer tendencies to
regressive fragmentation, BPD has a more poorly integrated self, with risk
for the occurrence of psychotic-like states. Identity diffusion is manifest in
BPD, but masked in NPD. Due to the higher level of self-cohesiveness, NPD

is associated with greater tolerance for aloneness, and better work record, impulse control and anxiety tolerance, while BPD patients, due to their lower level of cohesiveness, show more of self-mutilation and persistent rage. People with NPD are covertly shame-ridden and insecure, and BPD patients have sustained identity diffusion and inferiority feelings. While narcissistic patients are less overtly self-destructive and less preoccupied with dependency and abandonment concerns [114,117], they show more passive-aggressive features [117] and greater arrogance and haughtiness. However, in response to severe humiliation, criticism and defeat, people with NPD may react self-destructively, with a controlled and calculated intention to kill themselves [168]. This contrasts with BPD patients, whose self-destructive behaviour is more impulsive and aimed at regaining caring attention [166]. Both groups regard attention as important, but while borderlines seek nurturing attention because they need it, narcissists feel they deserve admiring attention because they consider themselves superior or exceptional [89].

Recent extensive research efforts on identifying distinctive traits for borderline patients have improved discriminability of the BPD category in relation to other Axis II disorders, especially NPD. Zanarini et al. [169] found the following features to be specific for BPD: quasi-psychotic thoughts, self-mutilation, manipulative suicide efforts, abandonment/engulfment/annihilation concerns, demandingness/entitlement, treatment regression and countertransference difficulties. Gunderson [166] suggested an integrated clinical synthesis for borderline patients, consisting of intolerance of aloneness with impulsive behaviour and lapses in reality testing as major reactions to separateness or abandonment. The corresponding traits for narcissistic patients would probably be intolerance of threats to the grandiose self-image, and intense reactions, including protective cognitive and interpersonal manoeuvres and feelings of rage and shame, in response to such threats. However, while borderlines' reactivity is more consistently manifest, the narcissistic people's reactions may be expressed as overt anger, insecurity or self-aggrandizing behaviour, but may also remain hidden and not involve overt behaviours or emotional reactions. In addition, studies of the pathogenesis of BPD have identified parental separations and losses, and experiences of sexual abuse as significant for the development of borderline pathology [170]. These features together clearly demarcate BPD from NPD.

NPD and the Bipolar Spectrum Disorder

Several accounts in the clinical literature have outlined narcissistic characteristics in bipolar patients, and both Kohut [77] and Morrison [62] described manic/hypomanic states that occurred in narcissistic patients. DSM-IV identifies grandiosity and inflated self-esteem as the most distinct feature both in NPD and in bipolar manic or hypomanic episodes. NPD is one of the most commonly occurring personality disorders among bipolar patients, and bipolar disorder is the third most common Axis I disorder found in narcissistic patients (5–11%) [171].

Two major attempts to conceptualize this overlap have been made by Akiskal [172,173] from the bipolar spectrum perspective, introducing the hyperthymic temperament, and by Akhtar [174] from a psychoanalytic perspective, suggesting a hypomanic personality disorder. People with hyper-thymia bear several similarities with the narcissistic personality, i.e. being ambitious, high achieving, grandiose, boastful, exuberant, overoptimistic, self-assertive and overconfident. They usually deny psychiatric symptoms, but can have histories of brief episodes of depression, and they have been considered belonging to the bipolar spectrum mainly because of their strong family history of bipolar disorder. The hypomanic personality disorder shares grandiosity, self-absorption, social ease, articulateness, seductiveness, and moral, aesthetic and vocational enthusiasm with narcis-sistic personalities. However, contrary to people with NPD, the hyperthymics are warm, people seeking and meddlesome, and the hypomanics do not have the devaluating, secretly envious attitude of the narcissists nor their seething vindictiveness, and dedicated steadfast pursuit for perfectionism [175].

Our study [16] found noteworthy similarities between the experiential, affective and behavioural manifestations in both disorders, in that bipolar patients in a hypomanic and acute manic phase actually exhibit most of the core characteristics for NPD, i.e. overt grandiosity, self-centredness, entitle-ment, lack of empathy, arrogance and boastful/pretentious behaviour. Notable differences between narcissistic and bipolar disorders included the active search for admiring attention, devaluation of others and secret profound envy of others in narcissistic patients, which are not found in patients with bipolar mania. However, we found no evidence of a narcissistic character structure or consistent features of pathological narcissism in bipolar patients when euthymic.

It is reasonable to conclude that hyperthymia/hypomania and patholo-gical narcissism are conceptually and phenomenologically different. It also seems appropriate to propose an interactive model for co-occurring pathological narcissism/NPD and the bipolar spectrum disorders in that narcissistic personality related events and experiences can evoke and influence mood swings, and mood swings can have a major impact on narcissistic self-esteem and affect dysregulation. In a similar sense, in the relationship between NPD and substance abuse and addiction, Vaglum [19] concluded that, although narcissistic traits and NPD seem unrelated to the further course of addiction, NPD may increase the risk of becoming an addict and may contribute to medical disorders and death among addicts. Of interest is what factors make some but not all NPD patients become bipolar or, vice versa, what make some bipolar patients maintain enduring pathological narcissism. Notable is the bipolar NPD patients' appreciation for mood elevation and capability to integrate high energy and activity level into periods of successful personality functioning, and even highly valuable professional or creative achievements. In other words, in these patients we find a strong positive co-variation between both healthy and pathological aspects of narcissism and bipolarity. The presence of genetic or biological communalities awaits further research.

NPD and Depressive Disorder/Dysthymia

Acute depression as a reaction to severe narcissistic injuries, failures, or losses, often in combination with suicidal ideations, can force the normally symptom free narcissistic patient to psychiatric treatment. Depression in such patients usually occurs in the context of a failure in the self-regulatory processes that support the pathological grandiose self. In other words, depression can be seen as an effect of decreased self-esteem, and a consequence of the depleted or depreciated self in narcissistic patient [12,21]. Major depression and dysthymia are the most common concomitant Axis I disorders in patients with NPD (42–50%). Studies of the opposite interrelation, i.e. the presence of NPD in major depression, have earlier shown much lower prevalence rates (0% to 5%) [171]. However, more recent empirical studies of major depression in personality disorders by Fava et al. [175,176] reported higher prevalence rates for NPD (8.1%–16.4%). They found NPD and several other personality disorders to be more common in depression with anger attacks than without such attacks and significantly more common in early-onset major depression [174]. They also found instability in personality disorder diagnosis. Following an eight-week fluoxetine treatment, there was a significant reduction both in the number of patients meeting criteria for NPD (and eight other personality disorders) and in the mean number of NPD criteria met among the narcissistic patients. Decrease in the number of criteria met for NPD was significantly related to improvement in depressive symptoms [177]. These results are interesting and notable, as they contradict some of the previous clinical observations on depression in narcissistic patients, i.e. of a temporary decrease in major narcissistic traits, such as grandiosity, in acutely depressed narcissistic patients [10] and increased NPD rates in patients with remitted depression [178]. In addition, the previously noted treatment resistant depression in NPD patients was also challenged by Fava's studies. These different observations indicate a complexity of co-occurring pathological narcissism and depression and point to an important avenue for further empirical and clinical explorations of the role of personality functioning in treatment of major mental syndromes.

TREATMENT

Psychoanalysis and psychoanalytically oriented psychotherapy have been considered the treatment of choice for patients with NPD. However, recently new treatment strategies for narcissistic disorders outside the psychoanalytic realm have been developed, i.e. cognitive [179,180], short-term [181], group [182], couples and family [183–185], and therapeutic milieu [186]. These strategies have been initiated in part as a result of the increasing recognition of narcissistic patients by clinicians outside private practices or psychiatric outpatient clinics. In addition, treatment of narcissistic patients in programmes and modalities focusing on other major symptoms, such as addiction or affective disorders, have also been reported on [19,174]. Psychopharmacological treatment is often challenging, due to the narcissistic patients' reluctance to subordinate themselves to instructions, and their hypersensitivity to side effects, especially those affecting sexual and intellectual functioning.

The often symptom-free narcissistic individuals usually seek treatment for three reasons: due to acute crises caused by vocational or personal failures or losses; in response to requests or ultimata from family, employer, or court; or due to an increasing sense of dissatisfaction or meaninglessness in their life. The level of motivation varies greatly depending upon such factors as the patient's experiences of urgency and ultimateness, and the absence or availability of outside sources of narcissistic gratification that support a continuation of the patient's narcissistic views and lifestyle. Narcissistic people who suffer from disorders such as substance use, impulsivity or affective disorder are often forced to seek treatment due to consequences of their symptoms. Other motivating factors relate to the degree that narcissistic character patterns are ego-syntonic, i.e. that reasons for failures or problems can be considered related to oneself. The patient's general psychological mindedness, curiosity, and comfort in interpersonal relations can facilitate motivation, whereas rigidity, suspiciousness and high anxiety level can prevent motivation. A helpful motivating factor is the availability of family members, or a network of relatives or friends that are willing to support or even participate in the treatment [187].

For the purpose of diagnostic and clinical assessment, a thorough evaluation of both healthy and well as pathological aspects of the patient's narcissistic functioning is essential, in addition to significant experiences of stressors, failures and losses, that might have seriously challenged the narcissistic patient's self-esteem and usual self-experience. The presence of acute or chronic suicidal ideation, or chronic preoccupation with the meaning of life, has to be evaluated with particular care, especially if the patient has experienced serious failures or losses.

The initial phase in treatment of narcissistic patients is usually characterized by the resistance to get involved in a mutually collaborative therapeutic alliance, and by the establishment of an alternative alliance of self-object type, i.e. the patient places the therapist in a position that serves to support his/her own grandiose self-experience and protect him/her from feelings of inferiority and shame. The therapist can be seen as a naive but appreciative listener, as well as a potential intruder whom the patient has to control or constrain. This can be noticed in the patient's unwillingness to listen to the therapist's comments, in avoidance of eye contact, or in a suspicious attitude. Tendencies to feel misunderstood, or humiliated by the therapist, or a general argumentative behaviour are common, as well as an overly critical, devaluating attitude, or a cheerful, talkative, bragging and dominant behaviour with tendencies to show off. Some patients can devote themselves to ideological or technical expositions, or detailed descriptions of their life, vocational development, or childhood experiences for a long period of time.

The therapist is challenged by the difficulty of establishing an alliance and by the particular transference-countertransference enactments that can develop. Gabbard [190] conceptualized countertransference as providing useful information not only about the therapist's own conflicts but also about the patient's internal world and conflicts. The therapist is treated as an extension of the patient him/herself. Following this view, the different countertransference issues that emerge can be instrumental in the process of understanding the narcissistic patient and delineating the treatment strategy. Such countertransference feelings as emptiness, rage and contempt, or sustained periods of feeling idealized, controlled, or bored can be useful for the therapist in understanding and formulating the dynamics of the patient's internal world. Comments like "It seems as if you feel a need to keep me under control", or "Can it be so that you don't want to be aware of and feel the feelings you might possibly have?" or " I wonder if you are concerned that I might misunderstand you", can be useful. However, a well established therapeutic alliance has to exist before such comments and interpretations can be useful for the patient.

Two psychoanalytic strategies have proved effective. One, suggested by Kernberg [12,156], relies heavily on reality testing and confrontation and interpretation of the pathological grandiose self and the negative transference. The other approach, developed by Kohut [20,21,77,80], focuses on empathic observations and the development and working through of three types of transference—mirroring, idealizing and twinship or alter ego transference [189]—as a way of correcting the structural deficits that characterize narcissistic disorders. A third less well-known strategy [101, 190] uses a method of active interpersonal co-participant psychoanalytic inquiry, which alternates between confrontational and empathic exploration of the narcissistic transference-countertransference matrix. This strategy focuses on the patient's difficulties in tolerating challenges to subjective perspectives and self-esteem, while actively engaging the patient in an exploration of interpersonal interactions.

Explorations and a new understanding of psychic change [191] have had specific relevance for the treatment of narcissistic disorders. Relevant for NPD is new understanding of transference and countertransference development and of projective identification and enactment [192,193], combined with a broadened scope of therapeutic interventions [194]. Several recent clinical reports have documented advances in the treatment of narcissistic disorders as the therapist/analyst acknowledged enactment and counter-transference [195–199].

Short-term treatment of narcissistic patients has become more common, primarily called for by changes in the health care system and by requirements of cost-effectiveness. However, in short-term modalities the therapist and the patient can set up limited goals, and the partially or moderately motivated narcissistic patient can engage in a treatment that focuses on changes in clearly well defined areas of functioning [183]. Replacing narcissistically ingrained interpersonal behaviour, or pointing out and discussing alternatives to grandiose beliefs and self-experience, or high-lighting how symptomatic behaviour ineffectively protects fragile self-esteem, are beneficial strategies that can diminish the narcissistic patient problems with the environment at work or home. Such modalities may also be more appealing and less threatening to the narcissistic person's self-esteem as experiences of changes and positive feedback increase a sense of competence.

Based on cognitive strategies, the schema-focused therapy [180] identifies narcissistic states or behaviours, called schema moods, that are modified during the treatment. Focus is on the patient's close relations, on the vulnerable mood that include defectiveness and emotional deprivation schemas, and the special self-experience that include entitlement, super-iority and approval seeking. The therapist uses the therapeutic relationship to promote change by helping the patient to contain and tolerate strong feelings and prevent the patient's shift between different narcissistic moods and schemas.

Comorbid NPD can have serious implications in the treatment of patients with some Axis I disorders. Clinical observations suggest that the presence of pathological narcissism is associated with low treatment compliance in Axis I disorders [200,201]. Paradoxically, symptom reduction might not be of primary interest for the narcissistic patients if the symptomatology coincides with or accentuates grandiose self-experience or narcissistic pursuits. Axis I symptomatology, such as substance abuse and hypomania or mania, can be specifically agreeable for the narcissistic patient as they lead to an increase in the sense of grandiosity, mastery and control, self-sufficiency and limitlessness [201–203].

SUMMARY

Summarizing the evidence on pathological narcissism indicates that, although DSM-IV adequately captures some of the major features of NPD, the range of level of functioning and clinical variations and the specific challenges involved in diagnosing some characteristics of pathological narcissism have not been adequately addressed. The evidence also indicates the international studies and usage of NPD and pathological narcissism and call for its inclusion in the ICD system as well.

Consistent Evidence

- *Grandiosity*, an inner sense of superiority and uniqueness, and grandiose fantasies of being successful, powerful, attractive, brilliant, etc. Admiring attention from others serves to protect and enhance the grandiose self-experience. The more noticeable manifest behavioural signs of grandiosity are self-centred and self-referential behaviour and a boastful or pretentious attitude.
- *Reactions to criticism* is the most important sign of narcissistic self-esteem dysregulation and consequential to the grandiose self-experience. Reactions include various strategies for self-aggrandizing and self-attributions used for protection of the grandiose self, as well as aggressive reactions to threats to their sense of superiority or self-esteem.
- *Shame.* Clinical and empirical studies have independently rendered support for this very important characteristic of pathological narcissism. Both the feeling of shame in itself and the perception of one's own feelings of shame tend to lower an individual's self-esteem, and the pain of shame can motivate anger, hostility and humiliated fury.
- *Arrogant, haughty behaviour, interpersonal control and hostility, and aggressive reactions.* Expressions of aggression in narcissistic people may range from subtle cognitive reappraisal and silent contempt, to overt hostility and explosive rage outbursts, and even sadistic and violent behaviour.

Incomplete Evidence

- *Envy* is among the most essential features of narcissistic affect dysregulation, although the connection between narcissism and envy has been especially difficult to clarify. Awareness of one's own feelings of envy, in and by itself, tends to lower self-esteem and evoke feelings of shame. Reactions to the perception of others' envy need further empirical studies.
- *Impaired empathic capacity* is one of the least empirically explored characteristics for NPD. Despite its central role in narcissistic character functioning, the relatively narrow definition fails to identify cognitive, emotional and interpersonal variations in empathic processing, and specifically the relationship between self-esteem and affect dysregulation and narcissistic interpersonal functioning to empathic processing.
- *Lack of sustained commitments to others.* This criterion is imprecise and does not differentiate between various reasons for and types of inabilities to commit, underlying dynamics, attachment problems, intolerance of affects or self-esteem.
- *Entitlement.* Entitlement may stem either from a sense of grandiose self-righteousness or function as a defence against feelings of envy, guilt, shame, depression or the threat of closeness. Expressions of entitlement can range from infuriated reactions (irritability, hostile rejecting or vindictive behaviour) to feeling surprised, hurt, unappreciated, unfairly treated or even exploited. This needs much further clarification.
- *The psychopathic NPD.* This interface is specifically complicated by the fact that both problems with self-esteem regulation and with moral values and consciousness co-exist.

Areas Still Open for Research

- *The interface between bipolar spectrum disorders and pathological narcissism/ NPD.* This is a very complex area of study that requires careful and long-term assessment of co-variation. Family studies and studies of early aetiological origins would help further differentiation. The differences between mood variability as reactions to self-esteem fluctuations and bipolar mood variations, as well as their co-occurrence, have high priority.
- *The shy narcissistic personality.* No research studies identifying patients with shy NPD have so far been conducted. The proposed criteria, such as predominance of shyness, shame, and inhibitions with a hidden inner narcissistic self-esteem dysregulation need further research on their assessment and validation.

REFERENCES

1. Kernberg O.F. (1983) Clinical aspects of narcissism. Presented at the Grand Rounds, Cornell University Medical Center, Westchester Division, September 9.
2. Kernberg O.F. (1985) Clinical diagnosis and treatment of narcissistic personality disorder. Presented at the Meeting of the Swedish Association for Mental Health, Stockholm, August 28.
3. Akhtar S. (1997) The shy narcissist. Paper presented at the 150th American Psychiatric Association Meeting, San Diego, May 19.
4. Gabbard G.O. (1989) Two subtypes of narcissistic personality disorder. *Bull. Menninger Clin.*, **53**: 527–532.
5. Gunderson J., Ronningstam E., Bodkin A. (1990) The diagnostic interview for narcissistic patients. *Arch. Gen. Psychiatry*, **47**: 676–680.
6. Ronningstam E., Gunderson J. (1990) Identifying criteria for narcissistic personality disorder. *Am. J. Psychiatry*, **147**: 918–922.
7. Cooper A.M., Ronningstam E. (1992) Narcissistic personality disorder. In *American Psychiatric Press Review of Psychiatry*, Vol. 1 (Eds A. Tasman, M. Riba), pp. 80–97. American Psychiatric Press, Washington.
8. Cooper A.M. (1998) Further developments of the diagnosis of narcissistic personality disorder. In *Disorders of Narcissism: Diagnostic, Clinical, and Empirical Implications* (Ed. E. Ronningstam), pp. 53–74. American Psychiatric Press, Washington.
9. Simon R.I. (2001) Distinguishing trauma-associated narcissistic symptoms from posttraumatic stress disorder: a diagnostic challenge. *Harv. Rev. Psychiatry*, **10**: 28–36.
10. Ronningstam E., Gunderson J., Lyons M. (1995) Changes in pathological narcissism. *Am. J. Psychiatry*, **152**: 253–257.
11. Groopman L.C., Cooper A.M. (1995) Narcissistic personality disorder. In *Treatments of Psychiatric Disorders*, 2nd edn (Ed. G.O. Gabbard), pp. 2327–2343. American Psychiatric Press, Washington.
12. Kernberg O.F. (1975) *Borderline Conditions and Pathological Narcissism*. Aronson, New York.
13. Kernberg O.F. (1998) The psychotherapeutic management of psychopathic, narcissistic and paranoid transference. In *Psychopathy. Antisocial, Violent and Criminal Behavior* (Eds T. Millon, E. Simonsen, M. Birket-Smith, R.D. Davis), pp. 372–392. Guilford, New York.
14. Akhtar S. (1989) Narcissistic personality disorder: descriptive features and differential diagnosis. *Psychiatr. Clin. North Am.*, **2**: 505–530.
15. Hart S.D., Hare R.D. (1998) The association between psychopathy and narcissism—Theoretical views and empirical evidence. In *Disorders of Narcissism—Diagnostic, Clinical and Empirical Implications* (Ed. E. Ronningstam), pp. 415–436. American Psychiatric Press, Washington.
16. Stormberg D., Ronningstam E., Gunderson J., Tohen M. (1998) Pathological narcissism in bipolar patients. *J. Person. Disord.*, **12**: 179–185.
17. Steiger H., Jabalpurwala S., Champagne J., Stotland S. (1997) A controlled study of trait narcissism in anorexia and bulimia nervosa. *Int. J. Eat. Disord.*, **22**: 173–178.
18. Ronningstam E. (1992) Pathological narcissism in anorexic subjects. Presented at the American Psychiatric Association 145th Meeting, Washington, May 7.

19. Vaglum P. (1999) The narcissistic personality disorder and addiction. In *Treatment of Personality Disorders* (Eds J. Derksen, C. Maffei, H. Groen), pp. 241–253. Kluwer/Plenum, New York.

20. Kohut H. (1966) Forms and transformations of narcissism. *Am. J. Psychother.*, **14**: 243–271.

21. Kohut H. (1977) *The Restoration of the Self*. International University Press, New York.

22. Watson P.J., Biderman M.D. (1993) Narcissistic personality inventory factors, splitting and self-consciousness. *J. Person. Assess.*, **61**: 41–57.

23. Harpur T.J., Hare R.D., Hakstian A.R. (1989) A two-factor conceptualization of psychopathy: construct validity and implications for assessment. *J. Consult. Clin. Psychol.*, **1**: 6–17.

24. Jang K.L., Livesley W.J., Vernon P.A., Jackson D.N. (1996) Heritability of personality disorder traits: a twin study. *Acta Psychiatr. Scand.*, **94**: 438–444.

25. Torgersen S., Lygren S., Oien P.A., Skre I., Onstad S., Edvardson E., Tambs K., Kringeln E. (2000) A twin study of personality disorders. *Compr. Psychiatry*, **41**: 416–425.

26. Schore A. (1994) *Affect Regulation and the Origin of the Self*. Erlbaum, Hillsdale.

27. Kernberg P. (1989) Narcissistic personality disorder in childhood. *Psychiatr. Clin. North Am.*, **12**: 671–694.

28. Coryell W.H., Zimmerman M. (1989) Personality disorders in the families of depressed, schizophrenic, and never ill probands. *Am. J. Psychiatry*, **146**: 496–502.

29. Reich J., Yates W., Nduaguba M. (1989) Prevalence of DSM-III personality disorders in the community. *Soc. Psychiatry Psychiatr. Epidemiol.*, **24**: 12–16.

30. Mattia J.I., Zimmerman M. (2001) Epidemiology. In *Handbook of Personality Disorders* (Ed. W.J. Livesley), pp. 107–123. Guilford, New York.

31. Reich J., Yates W., Ndvaguba M. (1989) Prevalence of DSM-III personality disorders in the community. *Soc. Psychiatry Psychiatr. Epidemiol.*, **24**: 12–16.

32. Bodlund O., Ekselius L., Lindström E. (1993) Personality traits and disorders among psychiatric outpatients and normal subjects on the basis of the SCID screen questionnaire. *Nordisk Psychiatrisk Tidskrift*, **47**: 425–433.

33. Klein D.N., Riso L.P., Donaldson S.K., Schwartz J.E., Anderson R.L., Oiumette P.C., Lizardi H., Aronson T.A. (1995) Family study of early-onset dysthymia: mood and personality disorders in relatives of outpatients with dysthymia and episodic major depressive and normal controls. *Arch. Gen. Psychiatry*, **52**: 487–496.

34. Maffei C., Fossati A., Lingiardi V., Madeddu F., Borellini C., Petrachi M. (1995) Personality maladjustment, defenses and psychopathological symptoms in non-clinical subjects. *J. Person. Disord.*, **9**: 330–345.

35. Crosby R.M., Hall M.J. (1992) Psychiatric evaluation of self-referred and non-self-referred active duty military members. *Military Med.*, **157**: 224–229.

36. Bourgeois J.A., Crosby R.M., Hall M.J., Drexler K.G. (1993) An examination of narcissistic personality traits as seen in a military population. *Military Med.*, **158**: 170–174.

37. Johnson W. (1995) Narcissistic personality as a mediating variable in manifestations of post-traumatic stress disorder. *Military Med.*, **160**: 40–41.

38. Gunderson J., Ronningstam E., Smith L. (1991) Narcissistic personality disorder: a review of data on DSM-III-R descriptions. *J. Person. Disord.*, **5**: 167–177.

39. Morey L.C. (1988) Personality disorders in DSM-III and DSM-III-R: an examination of convergence, coverage, and internal consistency. *Am. J. Psychiatry*, **145**: 573–577.

40. Yates W., Fulton A.I., Gabel J.M., Brass C.T. (1989) Personality risk factors for cocaine abuse. *Am. J. Publ. Health*, **79**: 891–892.

41. Turely B., Bates G., Edwards J., Jackson H. (1992) MCMI-II personality disorders in recent-onset bipolar disorders. *J. Clin. Psychol.*, **48**: 320–329.

42. Sato T., Sakado K., Uehara T., Sato S., Nishioka K., Kasahara Y. (1997) Personality disorders using DSM-III-R in a Japanese clinical sample with major depression. *Acta Psychiatr. Scand.*, **95**: 451–453.

43. Apter A., Bleich A., King R., Kron S., Fluch A., Kotler M., Cohen D. (1993) Death without warning?—A clinical postmortem study of suicide in 43 Israeli adolescent males. *Arch. Gen. Psychiatry*, **50**: 138–142.

44. Golomb M., Fava M., Abraham M., Rosenbaum J.F. (1995) Gender differences in personality disorders. *Am. J. Psychiatry*, **154**: 579–582.

45. Plakun E.M. (1990) Empirical overview of narcissistic personality disorder. In *New Perspectives on Narcissism* (Ed. E.M. Plakun), pp. 101–149. American Psychiatric Press, Washington.

46. Abrams D.M. (1993) Pathological narcissism in a eight year old boy: an example of Bellak's T.A.T. and C.A.T. diagnostic system. *Psychoanalytic Psychology*, **10**: 473–591.

47. Kernberg P., Hajal F., Normandin L. (1998) Narcissistic personality disorder in adolescent inpatients—A retrospective record review study of descriptive characteristics. In *Disorders of Narcissism: Diagnostic, Clinical and Empirical Implications* (Ed. E. Ronningstam), pp. 437–456. American Psychiatric Press, Washington.

48. Kernberg O.F. (1980) *Internal World and External Reality*. Aronson, New York.

49. Berezin M.A. (1977) Normal psychology of the aging process, revisited-II. *J. Geriatric Psychiatry*, **10**: 9–26.

50. Kernberg O.F. (1977) Normal psychology of the aging process, revisited II. Discussion. *J. Geriatric Psychiatry*, **10**: 27–45.

51. Kernberg O.F. (1967) Borderline personality organization. *J. Am. Psychoanal. Ass.*, **15**: 641–685.

52. Lash C. (1979) *The Culture of Narcissism*. Norton, New York.

53. Warren M.P., Capponi A. (1995–1996) The place of culture in the etiology of the narcissistic personality disorder: comparing the United States, Japan and Denmark. *Int. J. Comm. Psychoanal. Psychother.*, **11**: 11–16.

54. Henseler H. (1991) Narcissism as a form of relationship. In *Freud's "On Narcissism: An Introduction"* (Eds J. Sandler, E.S. Person, P. Fonagy), pp. 195–215. Yale University Press, New Haven.

55. Tatara M.P. (1993) Patterns of narcissism in Japan. In *Narcissism and the Interpersonal Self* (Eds J. Fiscalini, A. Grey), pp. 223–237. Columbia University Press, New York.

56. Shimizu K., Kaizuka T. (2002) Anthropophobic tendency and narcissistic personality in adults. *Jap. J. Education. Psychol.*, **50**: 54–64.

57. Ehlers W., Plassman R. (1994) Diagnosis of narcissistic self-esteem regulation in patients with factitious illness (Munchausen Syndrome). *Psychother. Psychosom.*, **62**: 69–77.

58. Starcevic V. (1989) Contrasting patterns in the relationship between hypochondriasis and narcissism. *Br. J. Med. Psychol.*, **62**: 311–323.

59. The Quality Assurance Project (1991) Treatment outlines for borderline, narcissistic and histrionic personality disorders. *Aust. N. Zeal. J. Psychiatry*, **25**: 392–403.

60. Masterson J. (1993) *The Emerging Self—A Developmental, Self, and Object Relations Approach to the Treatment of the Closet Narcissistic Disorder of the Self.* Brunner/Mazel, New York.

61. Etzersdorfer E. (2001) The psychoanalytical positions on suicidality in German speaking regions. Presented at the International Congress on Suicidality and Psychoanalysis, Hamburg, August 31.

62. Morrison A.P. (1989) *Shame, the Underside of Narcissism.* Analytic Press, Hillsdale.

63. Hibbard S. (1992) Narcissism, shame, masochism, and object relations: an exploratory correlational study. *Psychoanal. Psychol.*, **9**: 489–508.

64. Ronningstam E. (2001) Foreword. In *Disorders of Narcissism—Diagnostic, Clinical and Empirical Implications* (Japanese Edition). Tokyo.

65. Ellis H. (1898) Auto-erotism: a psychological study. *Alienist and Neurologist*, **19**: 260–299.

66. Näcke P. (1899) Die sexuellen perversitäten in der irrenanstalt. *Psychiatriche en Neurologische Bladen*, **3**.

67. Freud S. (1910) Three essays on the theory of sexuality. In *The Standard Edition of the Complete Psychological Works of Sigmund Freud, Vol. 7* (Ed. J. Strachey) (1957), pp. 125–243. Hogarth, London.

68. Freud S. (1914) On narcissism. In *The Standard Edition of the Complete Psychological Works of Sigmund Freud, Vol. 14* (Ed. J. Strachey) (1957), pp. 66–102. Hogarth, London.

69. Freud S. (1915) Instincts and their vicissitudes. In *The Standard Edition of the Complete Psychological Works of Sigmund Freud, Vol. 14* (Ed. J. Strachey) (1957), pp. 109–140. Hogarth, London.

70. Freud S. (1917) Metapsychological supplement to the theory of dreams. In *The Standard Edition of the Complete Psychological Works of Sigmund Freud, Vol. 14* (Ed. J. Strachey) (1957), pp. 217–235. Hogarth, London.

71. Jones E. (1913) The God Complex. In *Essays in applied psychoanalysis, Vol. 2* (Ed. E. Jones) (1951), pp. 244–265. Hogarth, London.

72. Waelder R. (1925) The psychoses: their mechanisms and accessibility to influence. *Int. J. Psychoanal.*, **6**, 259–281.

73. Freud S. (1931) Libidinal types. In *The Standard Edition of the Complete Psychological Works of Sigmund Freud, Vol. 21* (Ed. J. Strachey) (1957), pp. 217–220. Hogarth, London.

74. Reich W. (1933) (1972) *Character Analysis*, 3rd edn. Farrar, Strauss & Giroux, New York.

75. Horney K. (1939) *New Ways in Psychoanalysis*. Norton, New York.

76. Reich A. (1960) Pathological forms of self-esteem regulation. *Psychoanal. Study Child.*, **15**: 215–232.

77. Kohut H. (1971) *The Analysis of the Self*. International Universities Press, New York.

78. Goldberg A. (1973) Psychotherapy of narcissistic injuries. *Arch. Gen. Psychiatry*, **28**: 722–726.

79. Freud S. (1911) Psychoanalytic notes on an autobiographical account of a case of paranoia. In *The Standard Edition of the Complete Psychological Works of Sigmund Freud, Vol. 12* (Ed. J. Strachey) (1957), pp. 9–82. Hogarth, London.

80. Kohut H. (1968) The psychoanalytic treatment of narcissistic personality disorder. *Psychoanal. Study Child.*, **23**: 86–113.
81. Kernberg O.F. (1998) Pathological narcissism and narcissistic personality disorder. Theoretical background and diagnostic classifications. In *Disorders of Narcissism—Diagnostic, Clinical and Empirical Implications* (Ed. E. Ronningstam), pp. 29–51. American Psychiatric Press, Washington.
82. Kohut H., Wolf E. (1978) The disorders of the self and their treatment: an outline. *Int. J. Psychoanal.*, **59**: 413–425.
83. Morrison A.P. (1986) Shame, ideal self and narcissism. In *Essential Papers on Narcissism* (Ed. A.P. Morrison), pp. 348–371. New York Universities Press, New York.
84. American Psychiatric Association (1980) *Diagnostic and Statistical Manual of Mental Disorders*, 3rd edn. American Psychiatric Association, Washington.
85. Plakun E.M. (1987) Distinguishing narcissistic and borderline personality disorder. *Compr. Psychiatry*, **26**: 448–455.
86. Plakun E.M. (1989) Narcissistic personality disorder: a validity study and comparison to borderline personality disorder. *Psychiatr. Clin. North Am.*, **12**: 653–671.
87. Plakun E.M. (Ed.) (1990) *New Perspectives on Narcissism*. American Psychiatric Press, Washington.
88. Ronningstam E., Gunderson J. (1989) Descriptive studies on narcissistic personality disorder. *Psychiatr. Clin. North Am.*, **12**: 585–601.
89. Ronningstam E., Gunderson J. (1991) Differentiating borderline personality disorder from narcissistic personality disorder. *J. Person. Disord.*, **5**: 225–232.
90. Gunderson J., Ronningstam E. (2001) Differentiating antisocial and narcissistic personality disorder. *J. Person. Disord.*, **15**: 103–109.
91. Gunderson J., Ronningstam E., Smith L. (1996) Narcissistic personality disorder. In *DSM-IV Sourcebook, Vol. 2*, pp. 745–756. American Psychiatric Association, Washington.
92. Millon T., Davis R.D., Millon C. (1996) Millon Clinical Multiaxial Inventory—III, Manual. National Computer System, Minnetonka.
93. Raskin R.N., Hall C.S. (1979) A narcissistic personality inventory. *Psychol. Rep.*, **45**: 590.
94. Raskin R.N., Terry H. (1988) A principal-component analysis of the narcissistic personality inventory and further evidence of its construct validity. *J. Person. Soc. Psychol.*, **54**: 890–902.
95. Emmons R.A. (1984) Factor analysis and construct validation of the narcissistic personality inventory. *J. Person. Assess.*, **48**: 291–300.
96. Rhodewalt F., Morf C.C. (1995) Self and interpersonal correlates of the narcissistic personality inventory: a review and new findings. *J. Res. Person.*, **29**: 1–12.
97. Morf C.C., Rhodewalt F. (2001) Unraveling the paradoxes of narcissism: a dynamic self-regulatory processing model. *Psychol. Inquiry*, **12**: 177–196.
98. Grundberger B. (1971) *Narcissism: Psychoanalytic Essays*. International Universities Press, New York.
99. Rothstein A. (1980) *The Narcissistic Pursuit for Perfection*. International Universities Press, New York.
100. Bach S. (1985) *Narcissistic States and the Therapeutic Process*. Aronson, New York.
101. Fiscalini J., Grey A.L. (1993) *Narcissism and the Interpersonal Self*. Columbia University Press, New York.

102. Sigrell B. (1994) *Narcissism—Ett Psykodynamiskt Perspectiv [Narcissism—A Psychodynamic Perspective]*. Natur och Kultur, Stockholm.
103. Sandler J., Person E.S., Fonagy P. (Eds) (1991) *Freud's "On Narcissism: An Introduction"*. Yale University Press, New Haven.
104. Giovaccini P. (2000) *Impact of Narcissism*. Aronson, Northvale.
105. Ronningstam E. (Ed.) (1998) *Disorders of Narcissism—Diagnostic, Clinical and Empirical Implications*. American Psychiatric Press, Washington.
106. Maccoby M. (2002) *The Productive Narcissist*. Reed Business Information, New York.
107. Brown N.W. (2002) *Working with the Self-Absorbed*. New Harbinger Publications, Oakland.
108. Solomon M.F. (1989) *Narcissism and Intimacy. Love and Marriage in an Age of Confusion*. Norton, New York.
109. Donaldson-Pressman S., Pressman R.M. (1994) *The Narcissistic Family—Diagnosis and Treatment*. Jossey–Bass, San Francisco.
110. Brown N.W. (2001) *Children of the Self-Absorbed*. New Harbinger Publications, Oakland.
111. Vaknin S. (1999) *Malignant Self Love—Narcissism Revisited*. Narcissus Publication, Prague.
112. American Psychiatric Association (1994) *Diagnostic and Statistical Manual of Mental Disorders*, 4th edn. American Psychiatric Association, Washington.
113. Blais M.A., Hilsenroth M.J., Castelbury F.D. (1997) Content validity of the DSM-IV borderline and narcissistic personality disorder criteria sets. *Compr. Psychiatry*, **38**: 31–37.
114. Holdwick D.J., Hilsenroth M.J., Castlebury F.D., Blais M.A. (1998) Identifying the unique and common characteristics among the DSM-IV antisocial, borderline and narcissistic personality disorder. *Compr. Psychiatry*, **39**: 277–286.
115. Morey L.C., Jones J.K. (1998) Empirical studies of the construct validity of narcissistic personality disorder. In *Disorders of Narcissism: Diagnostic, Clinical and Empirical Implications* (Ed. E. Ronningstam), pp. 351–373. American Psychiatric Press, Washington.
116. Westen D., Arkowitz-Westen L. (1998) Limitations of Axis II in diagnosing personality pathology in clinical practice. *Am. J. Psychiatry*, **155**: 1767–1771.
117. Hilsenroth M.J., Handler L., Blais M.A. (1996) Assessment of narcissistic personality disorder: a multi-method review. *Clin. Psychol. Rev.*, **16**: 655–693.
118. Tangney J.P. (1995) Shame and guilt in interpersonal relations. In *Self-Conscious Emotions. The Psychology of Shame, Guilt, Embarrassment and Pride* (Eds J.P. Tangney, K.W. Fischer), pp. 114–139. Guilford, New York.
119. Westen D., Shedler J. (1999) Revising and assessing Axis II, Part I: developing a clinically and empirically valid assessment method. *Am. J. Psychiatry*, **156**: 258–272.
120. Westen D., Shedler J. (1999) Revising and assessing Axis II, Part II: Toward an empirically based and clinically useful classification of personality disorders. *Am. J. Psychiatry*, **156**: 273–285.
121. Perry J.D., Perry J.C. (1996) Reliability and convergence of three concepts of narcissistic personality. *Psychiatry*, **59**: 4–19.
122. Kernis M.H., Cornell D.P., Sun C.-R., Berry A., Harlow T. (1993) There's more to self-esteem than whether it is high or low: the importance of stability of self-esteem. *J. Person. Soc. Psychol.*, **65**: 1190–1204.

123. Rhodewalt F., Morf C.C. (1998) On self-aggrandizement and anger: a temporal analysis of narcissism and affective reactions to success and failure. *J. Person. Soc. Psychol.*, **74**: 672–685.

124. Rhodewalt F., Madrian J.C., Cheney S. (1998) Narcissism, self-knowledge organization, and emotional reactivity: the effect of daily experiences on self-esteem and affect. *Person. Soc. Psychol. Bull.*, **24**: 75–87.

125. Baumeister R.F., Heatheron T.F., Tice D.M. (1993) When ego threats lead to self-regulation failure: negative consequences of high self-esteem. *J. Person. Soc. Psychol.*, **64**: 141–156.

126. Smalley R.L., Stake J.E. (1996) Evaluation sources of ego-threatening feedback: self-esteem and narcissistic effects. *J. Res. Person.*, **30**: 483–495.

127. Baumeister R.F., Smart L., Boden J.M. (1996) Relation of threatened egotism to violence and aggression: the dark side of high self-esteem. *Psychol. Rev.*, **103**: 5–33.

128. Papps B.P., O'Carrol R.E. (1998) Extremes of self-esteem and narcissism and the experience and expression of anger and aggression. *Aggress. Behav.*, **24**: 421–438.

129. Bushman B.J., Baumeister R.F. (1998) Threatened egotism, narcissism, self-esteem, and direct and displaced aggression: do self-love or self-hate lead to violence? *J. Person. Soc. Psychol.*, **75**: 219–229.

130. Wink P. (1991) Two faces of narcissism. *J. Person. Soc. Psychol.*, **61**: 590–597.

131. Krystal H. (1998) Affect regulation and narcissism: trauma, alexithymia and psychosomatic illness in narcissistic patients. In *Disorders of Narcissism: Diagnostic, Clinical and Empirical Implications* (Ed. E. Ronningstam), pp. 299–325. American Psychiatric Press, Washington.

132. Nemiah J.C., Sifneos P.E. (1970) Affect and fantasy in patients with psychosomatic disorder. In *Modern Trends in Psychosomatic Medicine—2* (Ed. O.W. Hill), pp. 26–34. Butterworth, London.

133. McDougall J. (1985) *Theaters of the Mind*. Basic Books, New York.

134. Kohut H. (1972) Thoughts on narcissism and narcissistic rage. *Psychoanal. Study Child.*, **27**: 360–400.

135. Dodes L.M. (1990) Addiction, helplessness and narcissistic rage. *Psychoanal. Quart.*, **59**: 398–419.

136. Murray J.M. (1964) Narcissism and the ego ideal. *J. Am. Psychoanal. Assoc.*, **12**: 477–511.

137. Tangney J.P. (1991) Moral affect: the good, the bad, the ugly. *J. Person. Soc. Psychol.*, **61**: 598–607.

138. Tangney J.P., Wagner P., Gramzow R. (1992) Proneness to shame, proneness to guilt and psychopathology. *J. Abnorm. Psychol.*, **101**: 469–478.

139. Tangney J.P., Wagner P., Fletcher C., Gramzow R. (1992) Shamed into anger? The relation of shame and guilt to anger and self-reported aggression. *J. Person. Soc. Psychol.*, **62**: 669–675.

140. Tangney J.P., Wagner P., Hill-Barlow D., Marschall D.E., Gramzow R. (1996) Relation of shame and guilt to constructive versus destructive responses to anger across the lifespan. *J. Person. Soc. Psychol.*, **70**: 797–809.

141. Lewis H.B. (1971) *Shame and Guilt in Neurosis*. International Universities Press, New York.

142. Rosenfeldt H. (1987) *Impasses and Interpretations*. Tavistock Publications, London.

143. Barth F.D. (1988) The role of self-esteem in the experience of envy. *Am. J. Psychoanal.*, **48**: 198–210.

144. Klein M. (1957) Envy and gratitude. In *Envy and Gratitude and Other Works 1946–1953* (Ed. M. Klein). Macmillan, New York.
145. Etchegoyen H.R., Benito M.L., Rabih M. (1987) On envy and how to interpret it. *Int. J. Psychoanal.*, **68**: 49–61.
146. Schwartz-Salant N. (1982) *Narcissism and Character Transformation. The Psychology of Narcissistic Character Disorder*. Inner City Books, Toronto.
147. Moses R., Moses-Hrushovski R. (1990) Reflections on the sense of entitlement. *Psychoanal. Study Child.*, **45**: 61–78.
148. Kerr N.J. (1985) Behavioral manifestations of misguided entitlement. *Perspect. Psychiatr. Care*, **23**: 5–15.
149. Havens L. (1993) The concept of narcissistic interactions. In *Narcissism and the Interpersonal Self* (Eds J. Fiscalini, A. Grey), pp. 189–199. Columbia University Press, New York.
150. Cohen S.J. (1988). Superego aspects of entitlement (in rigid characters). *J. Am. Psychoanal. Assoc.*, **36**: 409–426.
151. Feshbach N.D. (1975) Empathy in children: some theoretical and empirical considerations. *Counsel. Psychol.*, **5**: 25–30.
152. Fonagy P., Gergely G., Jurist E.L., Target M. (2003) *Affect Regulation, Mentalization, and the Development of the Self*. Other Press, New York.
153. Campbell W.K., Reeder G.D., Sedikides C., Elliot A.J. (2000) Narcissism and comparative self-enhancement strategies. *J. Res. Person.*, **34**: 329–347.
154. Raskin R., Novacek J., Hogan R. (1991) Narcissism, self-esteem, and defensive self-enhancement. *J. Person.*, **59**: 19–38.
155. Kernberg O.F. (1984) *Severe Personality Disorders*. Yale University Press, New Haven.
156. Hunt W. (1995) The diffident narcissist: a character-type illustrated in The Beast in the Jungle by Henry James. *Int. J. Psychoanal.*, **76**: 1257–1267.
157. Broucek F.J. (1982) Shame and its relationship to early narcissistic developments. *Int. J. Psychoanal.*, **65**, 369–378.
158. Millon T. (1998) DSM narcissistic personality disorder. Historical reflections and future directions. In *Disorders of Narcissism: Diagnostic, Clinical and Empirical Implications* (Ed. E.F. Ronningstam), pp. 75–101. American Psychiatric Press, Washington.
159. Kernberg O.F. (1989) The narcissistic personality disorder and the differential diagnosis of antisocial behavior. *Psychiatr. Clin. North Am.*, **12**: 553–570.
160. Kernberg O.F. (1992) *Aggression in Personality Disorders and Perversions*. Yale University Press, New Haven.
161. Gunderson J. (1984) *Borderline Personality Disorder*. American Psychiatric Press, Washington.
162. Stone M. (1993) *Abnormalities of Personality: Within and Beyond the Realm of Treatment*. Norton, New York.
163. Livesley W.J., Jackson D.N., Schroeder M. (1992) Factorial structure of traits delineating personality disorders in clinical and general population samples. *J. Abnorm. Psychol.*, **101**: 432–440.
164. Johnson J.G., Cohen P., Smailes E., Kasen S., Oldham J.M., Skodol A.E., Brooks J.S. (2000) Adolescent personality disorders associated with violence and criminal behavior during adolescence and early adulthood. *Am. J. Psychiatry*, **157**: 1406–1412.
165. Nestor P. (2002) Mental disorders and violence: personality dimensions and clinical features. *Am. J. Psychiatry*, **159**: 1973–1978.

166. Gunderson J.G. (2001) *Borderline Personality Disorder. A Clinical Guide.* American Psychiatric Publishing, Washington.
167. Akhtar S. (1992) *Broken Structures: Severe Personality Disorders and Their Treatment.* Aronson, Northvale.
168. Ronningstam E., Maltsberger J. (1998) Pathological narcissism and sudden suicide-related collapse. *Suicide and Life-Threatening Behaviour*, **28**: 261–271.
169. Zanarini M.C., Gunderson J.G., Frankenburg F.R., Chaunccey D.L. (1990) Discriminating borderline personality disorder from other Axis I disorders. *Am. J. Psychiatry*, **147**: 161–167.
170. Zanarini M.C. (2000) Childhood experiences associated with the development of borderline personality disorder. *Psychiatr. Clin. North Am.*, **23**: 89.
171. Ronningstam E. (1996) Pathological narcissism and narcissistic personality disorder in Axis I disorders. *Harv. Rev. Psychiatry*, **3**: 326–340.
172. Akiskal H.S., Mallya G. (1987) Criteria for the "soft" bipolar spectrum: treatment implications. *Psychopharmacol. Bull.*, **23**: 68–73.
173. Akiskal H.S. (1992) Delineating irritable and hyperthymic variants of the cyclothymic temperament. *J. Person. Disord.*, **6**: 326–342.
174. Akhtar S. (1988) Hypomanic personality disorder. *Integr. Psychiatry*, **6**: 37–52.
175. Fava M., Rosenbaum J.F. (1998) Anger attacks in depression. *Depress. Anxiety*, **8** (Suppl. 1): 59–63
176. Fava M., Alpert J.E., Borus J.S., Nierenberg A.A., Pava J.A., Rosenbaum J.F. (1996) Patterns of personality disorder comorbidity in early-onset versus late-onset major depression. *Am. J. Psychiatry*, **153**: 1308–1312.
177. Fava M., Farabaugh A.H., Sickinger A.H., Wright E., Alpert J.E., Sonawalla S., Nierenberg A.A., Worthington J.J. (2002) Personality disorders and depression. *Psychol. Med.*, **32**: 1049–1057.
178. Joffe R., Regan J. (1988) Personality and depression. *J. Psychiatr. Res.*, **22**: 279–286.
179. Beck A., Freeman A. (1990) *Cognitive Therapy of Personality Disorders.* Guilford, New York.
180. Young J., Flanagan C. (1998) Schema-focused therapy for narcissistic patients. In *Disorders of Narcissism: Diagnostic, Clinical, and Empirical Implications* (Ed. E. Ronningstam), pp. 239–267. American Psychiatric Press, Washington.
181. Oldham J. (1988) Brief treatment of narcissistic personality disorder. *J. Person. Disord.*, **2**: 88–90.
182. Roth B. (1998) The narcissistic patient in group psychotherapy – containing affects in the early group. In *Disorders of Narcissism: Diagnostic, Clinical, and Empirical Implications* (Ed. E. Ronningstam), pp. 221–237. American Psychiatric Press, Washington.
183. Solomon M. (1998) Manifestations and treatment of narcissistic disorders in couples therapy. In *Disorders of Narcissism: Diagnostic, Clinical, and Empirical Implications* (Ed. E. Ronningstam), pp. 269–293. American Psychiatric Press, Washington.
184. Kirshner L.A. (2001) Narcissistic couples. *Psychoanal. Quarterly*, **70**: 789–806.
185. Lansky M.R. (1985) Masks of the narcissistically vulnerable marriage. In *Family Approaches to Major Psychiatric Disorders* (Ed. M.R. Lansky), pp. 1–12. American Psychiatric Press, Washington.
186. Beaumont R. (1998) Treatment of narcissistic disorders in the intensive psychiatric milieu. In *Disorders of Narcissism: Diagnostic, Clinical, and Empirical Implications* (Ed. E. Ronningstam), pp. 195–219. American Psychiatric Press, Washington.

187. Ronningstam E., Gunderson J. (1997) Working with narcissistic personalities. In *Directions in Clinical and Counseling Psychology, Vol. 7, Lesson 9*, pp. 1–16. Hatherleigh, New York.

188. Gabbard G.O. (1998) Transference and countertransference in the treatment of narcissistic patients. In *Disorders of Narcissism: Diagnostic, Clinical, and Empirical Implications* (Ed. E. Ronningstam), pp. 125–145. American Psychiatric Press, Washington.

189. Ornstein P. (1998) Psychoanalysis of patients with primary self-disorder. In *Disorders of Narcissism: Diagnostic, Clinical, and Empirical Implications* (Ed. E. Ronningstam), pp. 147–169. American Psychiatric Press, Washington.

190. Fiscalini J. (1994) Narcissism and coparticipant inquiry—explorations in contemporary interpersonal psychoanalysis. *Contemporary Psychoanalysis*, **30**: 747–776.

191. Horowitz M.J., Kernberg O.F., Weinshel E.M. (Eds) (1993) *Psychic Structure and Psychic Change. Essays in Honor of Robert S. Wallerstein*. International Universities Press, Madison.

192. Renik O. (1993) Countertransference enactment and the psychoanalytic process. In *Psychic Structure and Psychic Change. Essays in Honor of Robert S. Wallerstein* (Eds M.J. Horowitz, O.F. Kernberg, E.M. Weinshel), pp. 135–158. International Universities Press, Inc., Madison.

193. Renik O. (1998) The Role of countertransference enactment in a successful clinical psychoanalysis In *Enactment—Towards a New Approach to the Therapeutic Relationship* (Eds S. Ellman, M. Moskowitz), pp. 111–128. Aronson, Northvale.

194. Stewart H. (1990) Interpretation and other agents for psychic change. *Int. Rev. Psycho-Anal.*, **17**: 61–69.

195. Jorstad J. (2001) Avoiding unbearable pain. Resistance and defense in the psychoanalysis of a man with a narcissistic personality disorder. *Scand. Psychoanal. Rev.*, **24**: 34–45.

196. Kernberg O.F. (1999) A severe sexual inhibition in the course of the psychoanalytic treatment of a patient with a narcissistic personality disorder. *Int. J. Psycho-Anal.*, **80**: 899–908.

197. Bateman A. (1998) Thick- and thin-skinned organizations and enactment in borderline and narcissistic disorders. *Int. J. Psycho-Anal.*, **79**: 13–25.

198. Ivey G. (1999) Transference-countertransference constellations and enactments in the psychotherapy of destructive narcissism. *Br. J. Med. Psychol.*, **72**: 63–74.

199. Glasser M. (1992) Problems in the psychoanalysis of certain narcissistic disorders. *Int. J. Psycho-Anal.*, **73**: 493–503.

200. Smith T.E., Deutsch A., Schwartz F., Terkelsen K. (1993) The role of personality in the treatment of schizophrenic and schizoaffective disorder patients: a pilot study. *Bull. Menninger Clin.*, **57**: 88–99.

201. Jamison K.R., Akiskal S. (1983) Medication compliance in patients with bipolar disorder. *Psychiatr. Clin. North Am.*, **6**: 175–192.

202. Jamison K.R., Gerner R.H., Hammen C., Padesky C. (1980) Clouds and silver linings: Positive experiences associated with primary affective disorders. *Am. J. Psychiatry*, **137**: 198–202.

203. Wurmser L. (1974) Psychoanalytic considerations of the etiology of compulsive drug use. *J. Am. Psychoanal. Assoc.*, **22**: 820–843.

Commentaries

Personality Pathology as Pathological Narcissism

Leslie C. Morey[1]

Elsa Ronningstam has provided a comprehensive and insightful discussion of the history, controversies, and variants of the concept of narcissistic personality. Her contribution is valuable in that it highlights how much the field has learned about this construct, but it also underscores how much remains to be learned. In my commentary, I will attempt to elaborate on some of the points that she references with respect to the boundaries and core of the narcissism construct.

In reading Ronningstam's description of the different theoretical views of narcissistic personality as they have evolved over time, one is struck by the diversity of personality adjectives applied to individuals with these conditions. For example, the following are only a sample of the adjectives presented in her review: arrogant, self-effacing, attention-seeking, shameful, entitled, insecure, exploitative, charming, cunning, spiteful, contemptuous, revengeful, boastful, embarrassed, grandiose, self-modest, aloof, inaccessible, intellectually understanding, indifferent, anxious, haughty, cold, reserved, aggressive, daydreaming, timid, sexually inhibited, and unambitious. The complexity of this list and its apparent inconsistencies illustrate the challenges to the field posed by this construct. One must then wonder how I, as noted by Ronningstam, could advocate broadening [1] the construct in any way, given the wide range of phenomena already subsumed across various theorists. I will try to offer some insight into this view.

One of the most striking and consistent findings among the personality disorders is that of comorbidity; it is far more common for individuals to have co-occurring than single personality disorder diagnoses. This result has often been cited as an important weakness of the DSM manual, and a potential reason to move toward a dimensional system for describing personality disorder [2]. However, it is interesting to note that individuals with personality disorders tend to lie within similar "regions" of the space defined by these dimensional systems, even across different dimensional

[1] Texas A&M University, College Station, TX, USA

approaches [3,4]. For example, within the Five-Factor personality trait model [5], virtually all the personality disorders appear to present with high neuroticism, low agreeableness, and low conscientiousness scores [3]. As with the DSM, it is possible to view such results as indicating potential problems with the discriminant validity of the system. However, I believe that it is important to also consider these results as compelling evidence that there are essential similarities among these disorders; similarities that are not adequately captured by the DSM system.

To illustrate, I present information from three different data sets, each of which included information about every DSM-defined personality disorder criterion. These data sets included a sample of 291 patients described via clinician checklist [6], 95 college students assessed by a self-report questionnaire [7], and 668 patients evaluated using a semi-structured diagnostic interview for personality disorders [8]. To examine the notion that some essential dimension was foundational to the entire collection of criteria, I calculated coefficient alpha [9] as an indication of the internal consistency of a scale formed by simply summing the count of all personality disorder criteria present in a particular client. In these three data sets, the coefficient alpha values were 0.81, 0.96, and 0.94, respectively. Such results suggest that the problematic behaviours and characteristics listed in the criteria for the various DSM personality disorders, which importantly include most of the adjectives cited above, form an internally consistent dimension that cuts across virtually all of the disorders.

In order to provide more information about the nature of this global dimension, the criteria demonstrating the largest correlations with the total number of features were identified, using the data from Morey [6]. These criteria are listed in Table 4.1.1. To further articulate the continuum, a Rasch scaling (e.g. [10]) of these criteria was performed to determine which criteria were informative at the higher end of the continuum and which at the lower end. The values in Table 4.1.1 represent the threshold parameter for these criteria, with larger numbers indicating that the criterion is representative of the more severe end of the continuum. Two aspects of Table 4.1.1 are particularly interesting: first, while criteria from many personality disorders are represented, narcissistic features are represented across the full spectrum; and second, the "anchor point" for the extreme of this global continuum is the core narcissistic feature, "lack of empathy". All of the features listed bear a strong relationship to Ronningstam's observation that a lack of empathy contributes to "the narcissistic individual's tendencies to misinterpret states and emotions in others and to a disconnection between cognitive and emotional interpretative processes". The finding that this empathic failure reflects the core of this global dimension suggests that, at the heart of personality pathology, lies pathological narcissism.

TABLE 4.1.1   Rasch scaling of DSM personality disorder criteria highly associated with global personality pathology

Criterion (disorder)	Threshold Parameter
Hypersensitivity to criticism (schizotypal)	−0.453
Reacts to criticism with rage, shame (narcissistic)	−0.311
Hypersensitive to rejection (avoidant)	−0.103
Easily slighted, quick to take offence (paranoid)	0.042
Overreaction to minor events (histrionic)	0.257
Carries grudges, unforgiving of insults (paranoid)	0.435
Chronic emptiness, boredom (borderline)	0.439
Uniqueness of one's problems (narcissistic)	0.516
Intense searching for confirmation of bias (paranoid)	0.828
Exaggeration of difficulties (paranoid)	0.885
Expects exploitation by others (paranoid)	0.963
Reads hidden threats (paranoid)	1.011
Protests demands of others (passive-aggressive)	1.583
Critical and scornful of authority (passive-aggressive)	1.779
Lack of empathy (narcissistic)	2.351

Approaching personality pathology from this perspective casts many of the conclusions drawn by Ronningstam in an interesting light. First, the notion of narcissism as a dimension is foundational, and it may be hypothesized that the continuum reflects various degrees of failure in a natural development process of the type described by various theorists (e.g. [11]). Second, the low diagnostic prevalence of narcissistic personality disorder relative to other personality disorders may reflect the fact that the criteria tend to focus upon the most severe (and hence less common) presentation of features that underlie most or all personality disorders. The diversity of the presentation of the variants of narcissistic disorders described by Ronningstam (for example, the arrogant vs. the shy narcissist) may be understood as an interaction between narcissistic pathology (which may be developmental in origin) and trait temperament (which may be largely heritable and account for the described heritability estimates). For example, while the arrogant and shy narcissists may share core empathic failures, they represent different temperamental forms of presentation of these failures, with the arrogant variant perhaps demonstrating an extroverted form that manifests features in an active, outwardly directed manner; and the shy variant being temperamentally introverted with empathic failures most notably prominent in internal processes such as fantasy or appraisal.

In conclusion, Ronningstam has provided an excellent overview of a construct that is both ambiguous and at the same time foundational to an understanding of personality pathology. Ideally, future developments will help disentangle core elements of the construct from other aspects that may moderate its presentation.

REFERENCES

1. Morey L.C., Jones J.K. (1998) Empirical studies of the construct validity of narcissistic personality disorder. In *Disorders of Narcissism: Theoretical, Empirical, and Clinical Implications* (Ed. E. Ronningstam), pp. 351–373. American Psychiatric Press, Washington.
2. Clark L.A., Livesley W.J., Morey L.C. (1997) Personality disorder assessment: The challenge of construct validity. *J. Person. Disord.*, **11**, 205–231.
3. Morey L.C., Gunderson J.G., Quigley B.D., Shea M.T., Skodol A.E., McGlashan T.H., Stout R.L., Zanarini M.C. (2002) The representation of borderline, avoidant, obsessive-compulsive and schizotypal personality disorders by the five-factor model. *J. Person. Disord.*, **16**, 215–234.
4. Morey L.C., Warner M.B., Shea T.M., Gunderson J.G., Sanislow C.A., Grilo C.M., McGlashan T.H. (2003) The SNAP dimensional representations of four personality disorders. *Psychol. Assess.*, **15**, 326–332.
5. Costa P.T., Widiger T.A. (2000) *Personality Disorders and the Five-Factor Model of Personality*, 2nd edn. American Psychological Association, Washington.
6. Morey L.C. (1988) Personality disorders under DSM-III and DSM-III-R: an examination of convergence, coverage, and internal consistency. *Am. J. Psychiatry*, **145**, 573–577.
7. Morey L.C., Warner M.B., Boggs C. (2002) Gender bias in the personality disorders criteria: an investigation of the five bias indicators. *J. Psychopathol. Behav. Assess.*, **24**, 55–65.
8. Gunderson J.G., Shea M.T., Skodol A.E., McGlashan T.H., Morey L.C., Stout R.L., Zanarini M.C., Grilo C.M., Oldham J.M., Keller M. (2000) The Collaborative Longitudinal Personality Disorders Study. I: Development, aims, design, and sample characteristics. *J. Person. Disord.*, **14**, 300–315.
9. Cronbach L.J. (1951) Coefficient alpha and the internal structure of tests. *Psychometrika*, **16**, 297–334.
10. Wright B.D. (1977) Solving measurement problems with the Rasch model. *J. Educational Measurement*, **14**, 97–116.
11. Kernberg O.F. (1986) *Severe Personality Disorders: Psychotherapeutic Strategies*. Yale University Press, New Haven.

4.2
Narcissism within Psychiatry: Past and Future Perspectives
Eric M. Plakun[1]

Elsa Ronningstam provides a comprehensive review of narcissistic personality disorder (NPD). As she notes, NPD is a disorder with a relatively low prevalence. It has, however, attracted considerable interest within psychoanalysis, where study of pathological narcissism has contributed greatly to the understanding of severe personality disorders, stimulating a debate about treatment technique and about the role of the self in psychoanalytic theory.

Within the domain of empirical psychiatry, investigation of NPD has tended to demonstrate its validity and its value as a diagnostic concept, despite its relative infrequency in most samples. My own empirical research into NPD followed the initial introduction of the disorder in DSM-III in 1980. Although our sample was relatively small and unusual, coming from a specialized long-term treatment centre for previously treatment refractory patients, it offered early contributions to the study of the validity of the disorder, assessed the utility of the DSM-III criteria in differentiating between NPD and borderline personality disorder (BPD), compared NPD and BPD in terms of demographic and clinical variables, and studied predictors of outcome in NPD [1].

In our Austen Riggs Center sample, NPD and BPD were best distinguished with a five-variable model that included four DSM-III NPD criteria (grandiosity, entitlement, fantasies of success, and exhibitionism) and one BPD criterion (inappropriate intense anger). This list of core NPD criteria has substantial overlap with those reported by several researchers, as summarized by Ronningstam.

In order to address the questions about validity, longitudinal course and outcome that were of interest at that time, I selected for study patients with relatively pure diagnoses of NPD and BPD. Patients who had a significant mood disorder or who met criteria for both NPD and BPD, or those with BPD or NPD who met four instead of five criteria for the reciprocal disorder, were eliminated from the sample. This excluded from scrutiny a severely disturbed group of patients with comorbid NPD and BPD, who had among the most complex and difficult treatment courses of any patients in our sample. In retrospect I realize that many of these patients with comorbid BPD and NPD, but also other of the so-called "pure NPD" patients, were probably patients presenting with Kernberg's syndrome of malignant narcissism, with prominent antisocial features, ego-syntonic

[1] Austen Riggs Center, 25 Main Street, Stockbridge, MA 01262-0962, USA

aggression and sadism, severe suicide risk, and a general paranoid orientation. Patients in our sample who met the schizotypal criterion for ideas of reference had worse outcomes than other NPD patients. Perhaps this criterion was a marker for the general paranoid orientation of malignant narcissism.

A provocative finding in our sample of NPD patients can be framed by paraphrasing an old saw; that is, in our NPD sample the rich got richer, while the poor got better. There was a correlation between good outcome and middle class versus upper class socioeconomic status and between good outcome and shorter length of index treatment (though the mean length of the index treatment was over a year). A review of cases suggested that those NPD patients whose financial circumstances led to the experience of having to face the reality (and the metaphor it offered for the psychotherapy) that their resources for treatment and in life were, in fact, not endless, were able to use this to advantage in treatment, perhaps contributing to better outcomes. An approach to the use of resource limitation as a metaphor in treatment is described more fully elsewhere [2,3].

In collaboration with J. Christopher Perry we are currently conducting a prospective, longitudinal study of 226 patients who were in treatment at Riggs. We are assessing both symptom and psychodynamic measures of change, including reliably measured defences and conflicts. To date we have reliably diagnosed 171 patients. Among them, 9% or 15 patients clearly meet DSM-IV criteria for NPD and 20% (34 patients) have significant NPD traits. This compares with 49% [83] with BPD and 37% [64] with BPD traits. When data collection and analysis is complete, we will offer data about longitudinal course and outcome, about the conflicts and the defences deployed by patients who meet criteria for NPD or BPD, and about how conflicts and defences change over time in these disorders.

REFERENCES

1. Plakun E.M. (1990) Empirical overview of narcissistic personality disorder. In *New Perspectives on Narcissism* (Ed. E.M. Plakun), pp. 103–149. American Psychiatric Press, Washington.
2. Plakun E.M. (1996) Economic grand rounds: treatment of personality disorders in an era of resource limitation. *Psychiatr. Serv.*, **47**: 128–130.
3. Plakun E.M. (2002) Jihad, McWorld and enactment in the post-modern mental health world. *J. Am. Acad. Psychoanal.*, **30**: 341–353.

4.3
Some Psychodynamics of Narcissistic Pathology
Arnold M. Cooper[1]

Elsa Ronningstam has provided a superb review of the current status of narcissistic personality disorder (NPD), a topic of increasing importance in psychiatry during the past quarter century. I shall attempt to add some clinical insights to her largely empirical presentation.

More perhaps than most psychiatric disorders, NPD cries out for a dimensional rather than categorical classification, since narcissistic qualities appear along the full spectrum from health to disorder, and it is not always easy to distinguish appropriately high self-confidence from grandiosity. Kohut [1], in distinguishing "Tragic Man" from "Guilty Man", emphasized the role of idealization and ambition in the development of the "normal" self and the tragedy inherent in the fact that infantile goals always exceed realistic grasp and leave us with a residue of awareness of our puniness in the universe. Psychoanalysts and infant researchers [2] agree that the development of a satisfactory sense of self requires the early experience of empathic care—"the good enough mother" [3]—who is able to respond to the infant's cues, mirror the infant's affective state, and provide necessary feelings of efficacy and satisfaction. This early mothering experience, essential for the development of a sturdy self concept as well as for the development of the capacity to understand the minds of others, is later supplemented by the psychosocial support derived from the creation of what Kohut termed "self-objects". Self-objects are those close relationships in which one carries a sense of the other in one's mind and derives increased strength and confidence from that enduring relationship which no longer requires the actual presence of another person. When these intrapsychic and developmental support systems fail to develop, defects of the self, the superego and affect regulation will develop, often in the form of what is overtly NPD.

An account of narcissistic pathology should include the concept of the mind in conflict. In clinical work with pathological narcissism one observes sets of underlying fantasies and defences of which the overt behaviour is an outcome. Grandiosity, for example, is regularly found to be a compensatory behaviour for inner feelings of rageful inadequacy, often not revealed until a collapse of the narcissistic structure into depression with harsh superego reproaches of inadequacy, failure and fraudulence. The pathologically narcissistic individual attempts an artificial inflation of the self in order to undo the injury of early non-responsive, unempathic care.

_____

[1] *Weill-Cornell Medical College, New York, USA*

The treatment of patients with NPD is made immensely difficult by their apparent lack of emotional connectedness and contempt for all other living creatures including, of course, the therapist. It was Kohut who recognized that what seemed to be an absence of transference, thus paralysing the therapist, was in fact the special form of transference occurring in narcissistic patients. They are unable to view another as a full human being, but attempt to use the other either to fill in missing parts of themselves, or to reassure their shaky self-esteem by contempt and murderous rage for the other. Therapy requires some degree of empathic immersion in the patient's primitive inner world, as well as the ability to interpret the anger the patient experiences at every attempt to understand or assist him. The recognition that the apparent lack of empathy and emotional aloofness has defensive qualities, protecting the self from disappointment and humiliation, enables the therapist to begin to have a sense of emotional contact with the patient and to institute a treatment process. Bitter rage is an unavoidable aspect of therapy of NPD and represents, in part, a defensive consequence of the patient's beginning recognition of his own self-hatred projected outward.

The fragility of narcissistic grandiosity is also illustrated by the inability of patients with NPD to experience solid attachment, either to their work or their relationships. In the face of constant inner superego attack on themselves, the maintenance of their self-esteem requires endless outer trappings of praise, money, status, adornment, etc. These patients are unable to get secure and lasting satisfaction from their own often very notable achievements, and lapse into denigrating depression when outer reinforcement is not available. Similarly their attachments to people—their capacity to love—is severely damaged, providing little genuine satisfaction or security. The love of others is valued only as a marker for their grandiosity and not emotionally internalized.

An aspect of narcissistic pathology that has particularly interested me is its close tie to masochistic behaviours, and I have urged that we consider a category of narcissistic-masochistic character [4]. These are patients who, rather predictably, manage to snatch defeat from the jaws of victory. Individuals with great business acumen engage in petty thievery which destroys their achievement, their reputation and their lives. A man who had finally won the love of a woman he had ardently pursued managed to kill the romance with a series of minor humiliations capped by being caught in sexual liaison with another woman. A highly successful business executive turns over a critical negotiation to an assistant whom he had never trusted who bungled the deal, with dire consequences. These narcissistic-masochistic characters are frequently observed and difficult to understand. I have suggested that one aspect of pathological narcissism is a carryover of childhood intolerance of frustrations which were dealt with by attempting to make unavoidable frustrations—narcissistic humiliations, in effect—into narcissistically acceptable events by the intrapsychic mechanism of attempting to take credit for the frustrations. No one hurt me against my will—I commanded them to do so. These individuals get a curious sense of satisfaction out of the frustrations they unconsciously organize, although consciously they respond with fury and depression. The self-defeating behaviours of many or most individuals with NPD is an important aspect of their pathology that often comes to the fore in the course of psychoanalytic treatment.

We owe a debt of thanks to Elsa Ronningstam for her comprehensive update of NPD.

REFERENCES

1. Kohut H. (1977) *The Restoration of the Self*. International Universities Press, New York.
2. Stern D. (1985) *The Interpersonal World of the Infant*. Basic Books, New York.
3. Winnicott D.W. (1971) *Playing and Reality*. Basic Books, New York.
4. Cooper A. (1988) The narcissistic-masochistic character. In *Masochism: Current Psychoanalytic Perspectives* (Eds R.A. Glick, D.I. Meyers). The Analytic Press, Hillsdale.

4.4
Complexity of Narcissism and a Continuum of Self-Esteem Regulation
Paul J. Watson[1]

As Ronningstam's review makes clear, pathological narcissism is a complex phenomenon even at the most basic definitional level. Complexity is obvious not only in clinical interactions with individuals who receive the diagnosis of narcissistic personality disorder (NPD), but also in personality research in which non-clinical samples respond to objective self-report inventories. That research often supports clinical observations. Ronningstam points out, for instance, that the distinction between arrogant and shy forms of NPD is paralleled in factor analytic studies by a differentiation between measures of overt and covert narcissism [1].

Frequently mentioned by Ronningstam is a dimensionality in narcissistic functioning that has been substantiated in personality research as well. The relevant studies initially rested upon use of the 54-item version of the

[1] *Psychology/Department #2803, 350 Holt Hall—615 McCallie Avenue, University of Tennessee at Chattanooga, TN 37403, USA*

Narcissistic Personality Inventory and the leadership/authority, superiority/ arrogance, self-absorption/self-admiration, and exploitativeness/entitlement factors that are found within it [2]. Correlations with other variables, including self-esteem, typically identified exploitativeness/entitlement as a fairly clear index of maladjusted overt narcissism, whereas the other three dimensions tended to reflect an at least somewhat adjusted form of overt narcissism [3–6].

Such mental health implications often became more obvious in partial correlations in which maladjusted overt narcissism was reexamined after controlling for adjusted overt narcissism and vice versa. These results appeared, for example, in the relationship between narcissism and empathy [7], which Ronningstam has described as "one of the least empirically explored characteristics for NPD", but which has in fact been analysed at least to some degree in a number of studies [3,5,7,8]. Later investigations also revealed that partial correlations controlling for self-esteem largely eliminated linkages that appeared between adjusted overt narcissism and greater mental health [9–11]. In addition, they demonstrated that similar patterns of zero-order and partial correlational data could be obtained with clinical samples, that such results were not specific to the Narcissistic Personality Inventory, and that they could be observed with clinical assessment and not only with self-report data [12].

One effort to organize the complexity of these findings has been based on the suggestion that a self functions along a psychological continuum that is related to the strength and stability of self-esteem [9–12]. A fully healthy self-esteem theoretically anchors the more adjusted pole of a continuum that is defined next by adjusted overt narcissism, then by maladjusted overt narcissism, and perhaps finally by covert narcissism. Self-report measures of narcissism are presumed to represent different amalgamations of self-functioning along this hypothetical continuum. Partial correlations consequently produce their effects by removing the relatively more adjusted or relatively more maladjusted features of narcissistic functioning from those representations. Relative to this hypothesis, the self of each individual would operate along a "bandwidth" of self-esteem regulation defined by an average level of functioning, by a leading edge of emerging self-potentials that would develop out of sustaining interpersonal relationships, and by a trailing edge of immaturity to which an individual would regress during distressing social interactions [8].

Emphasis has been placed on how this conceptualization of narcissism is deeply compatible with Kohut's [13] psychoanalytic psychology of the self [8,12], but the hypothesis is consistent with other clinical approaches to narcissism as well [11]. Direct comparisons between the continuum hypothesis and other empirically derived interpretations of narcissism have also demonstrated its superior predictability with regard to at least some issues

[9]. The continuum hypothesis, therefore, appears to depict the complexity of narcissism in a manner that has some potential for integrating and clarifying both clinical and non-clinical perspectives on narcissistic pathology. At the same time, the hypothesis is presented solely as a heuristic device. In its early stages of development, the hypothesis undoubtedly is characterized by imprecision and incompleteness. Much more research is clearly needed.

REFERENCES

1. Wink P. (1991) Two faces of narcissism. *J. Person. Soc. Psychol.*, **61**: 590–597.
2. Emmons R.A. (1984) Factor analysis and construct validity of the Narcissistic Personality Inventory. *J. Person. Assess.*, **48**: 291–300.
3. Watson P.J., Grisham E.O., Trotter M.V., Biderman M.D. (1984) Narcissism and empathy: validity evidence for the Narcissistic Personality Inventory. *J. Person. Assess.*, **48**: 301–305.
4. Watson P.J., Taylor D., Morris R.J. (1987) Narcissism, sex roles, and self-functioning. *Sex Roles*, **16**: 335.
5. Watson P.J., McKinney J., Hawkins C., Morris R.J. (1988) Assertiveness and narcissism. *Psychotherapy*, **25**: 125–131.
6. Watson P.J., Biderman M.D. (1993) Narcissistic Personality Inventory factors, splitting, and self-consciousness. *J. Person. Assess.*, **61**: 41–57.
7. Watson P.J., Little T., Sawrie S.M., Biderman M.D. (1992) Measures of the narcissistic personality: complexity of relationships with self-esteem and empathy. *J. Person. Disord.*, **6**: 434–449.
8. Watson P.J., Biderman M.D., Sawrie S.M. (1994) Empathy, sex role orientation, and narcissism. *Sex Roles*, **30**: 701–723.
9. Watson P.J., Hickman S.E., Morris R.J. (1996) Self-reported narcissism and shame: testing the defensive self-esteem and continuum hypotheses. *Person. Indiv. Diff.*, **21**: 253–259.
10. Watson P.J., Morris R.J., Miller L. (1997–98) Narcissism and the self as continuum: correlations with assertiveness and hypercompetitiveness. *Imagination, Cognition, and Personality*, **17**: 249–259.
11. Watson P.J., Varnell S.P., Morris R.J. (1999–2000) Self-reported narcissism and perfectionism: an ego-psychological perspective and the continuum hypothesis. *Imagination, Cognition, and Personality*, **19**: 59–69.
12. Watson P.J., Sawrie S.M., Greene R.L., Arredondo R. (2002) Narcissism and depression: MMPI-2 evidence for the continuum hypothesis in clinical samples. *J. Person. Assess.*, **79**: 85–109.
13. Kohut, H. (1977). *The Restoration of the Self*. International Universities, New York.

4.5
Narcissism: Psychodynamic Theme and Personality Disorder

Robert Michels[1]

Narcissistic personality disorder is a relatively recent diagnostic category. Unlike most other personality disorders, it is not based on an extrapolation from the hypothetical psychodynamics of a symptomatic neurosis, or on a description of the non-psychotic features of a psychotic disorder, or even on a cluster of maladaptive behaviour traits. It began with psychoanalysts and psychoanalytic psychotherapists struggling to understand a group of particularly troublesome patients, neither psychotic nor classically neurotic, in general not responsive to traditional psychotherapeutic interventions, and characterized not so much by observable psychopathologic phenomenology as by inferred psychodynamic patterns. The other personality disorder with a similar history is borderline, but while borderline patients were early recognized to exhibit a characteristic cluster of affective instability, chaotic relationships and life course, and at times deficits in autonomous ego functions, narcissistic patients were often viewed by the world as high functioning and without apparent psychopathology. Their problems were internal and related to the way in which they experienced themselves and others. They suffered, although they often denied it; the rest of the world often failed to recognize it, and only their therapists realized its depth. It was clear from the beginning that narcissism was more of a theme in mental life than a distinct nosological category, that it was essentially universal, although more prominent in some than in others, and that it could be associated with a wide range of pathology, from relatively healthy to seriously disturbed.

Elsa Ronningstam attempts to treat narcissism much as one might discuss any other personality disorder, emphasizing signs and symptoms, diagnostic criteria, comorbidities, etc. This approach organizes a great deal of information, but it threatens to emphasize attributes rather than essence. For example, the range of prevalence rates she reports (less than 1% to 17% in general samples, as high as 47% in selected samples, and with poor correlation between DSM diagnosis and clinician usage) suggests that the official criteria are only loosely associated with the meaning of the concept as used in clinical practice. Narcissism and narcissistic personality disorder are concepts developed by psychoanalytic clinicians and found useful by them. A diagnostic system that avoids psychodynamic inferences and emphasizes the observable surface rather than the inferred depth is unlikely to capture the concept or to be useful to those who most often employ it.

_____
[1] *Cornell University, 418 East 71st Street, Suite 41, New York, NY 10021, USA*

This is particularly true since the underlying psychological conflict can lead to surface manifestations that may be disparate or even contradictory. A single category that includes as subtypes "arrogant" and "shy", without specifying the latent theme that unites them, is likely to confuse more than it explains.

Another limitation of a phenomenological emphasis is that it limits the range of associated issues to be explored. For example, in her discussion of comorbidities, Elsa Ronningstam discusses antisocial, borderline, bipolar spectrum, and even eating disorders and substance abuse, but there is no mention of masochism, a closely linked entity which also is defined more by a core dynamic than by surface phenomenology, which is also found in normals as well as in a wide range of psychopathology, and which is also of particular interest to psychoanalytic clinicians. Another example is the absence of any mention of the developmental dynamics or childhood precursors of narcissism. We are told that the pathologic constellation is found in children, and that childhood history is one of the features that differentiates it from borderline personality, but there is no mention of the developmental origins of what will become narcissistic dynamics, traits, or personalities. There are, of course, few systematic studies, but there are many clinical reports, and considerable conjecture by the two clinical theorists whom she cites at length, Kernberg and Kohut. Perhaps most important, there is considerable experience with the effect of reconstructive developmental interpretations in psychodynamic psychotherapy. This information is critical in understanding our evolving concepts of narcissism and narcissistic personality, although it may be only distantly related to the DSM category of narcissistic personality disorder.

In summary, Elsa Ronningstam approaches narcissistic personality disorder as one of the DSM categories, attempting to consider it apart from the theoretical context in which the concept developed, and focusing on its reliably observable characteristics and their correlation with other reliably observable phenomena. She does an excellent job of assembling and analysing the available information relevant to these questions. However, the discussion of this particular disorder is severely limited by these constraints. The core concept of narcissism is not an observable cluster of phenomena but rather an inferred psychodynamic theme. Its surface manifestations are, accordingly, variable and inconsistent. Its most important comorbidities are not only with other phenomenologic clusters, but also with other dynamic themes. Its understanding requires a developmental model as well as a cross sectional description. Her review outlines what we know from the perspective of one important tradition, the empirical psychological and psychiatric study of the phenomenology of personality disorders, but at the same time unwittingly reveals the limitations of this approach, particularly when addressing an entity that derives from the experience of psychoanalytic clinicians. The psychoanalyst reader will find much that is of interest, but also much that is missing, and perhaps most bewildering, no discussion of why it is not included.

4.6
Of Narcissism, Narcissistic Personality Disorder and Normal Personality

Mark A. Blais[1]

Pathological narcissism and narcissistic personality disorder (NPD) are important clinical conditions that are beginning to receive increased attention from clinicians and researchers. As a complex personality construct, narcissism exists on a continuum from the healthy to the pathological. As such, research into this condition holds promise for improving our understanding of personality development and for integrating models of normal and abnormal personality. Ronningstam's comprehensive review provides an informative and clear presentation of the developmental psychodynamic theories of pathological narcissism.

Developing an accurate stable self-image and methods for effective ongoing regulation of self-esteem are two crucial components of personality functioning in general [1]. As Ronningstam points out, NPD can be understood primarily as a disorder of self-image development and self-esteem regulation. Using the DSM-IV NPD criteria, my colleagues and I [2] identified three primary features of NPD: grandiose self-image, lack of empathy and the excessive reliance on external factors to regulate self-esteem. Patients with NPD develop unrealistic exaggerated views of their abilities, importance and worth (i.e. grandiose self-image), and learn to value other people almost exclusively in terms of how they help support or maintain their grandiose image (i.e. lack of empathy). Additional research has revealed that it is their grandiose sense of self or exaggerated self-image that is unique to NPD patients relative to patients with other Cluster B personality disorders (borderline and antisocial personality disorders) [3]. Other aspects of the disorder reviewed by Ronningstam, such as affect dysregulation and interpersonal exploitiveness, have been shown to be less specific to NPD. For example, affective dysregulation is a quality shared by virtually all of the Cluster B personality disorders and interpersonal exploitiveness is common to both NPD and antisocial personality disorder [3]. Therefore, focusing future research on exploring the unique NPD features of grandiosity

[1] Blake 11, Massachusetts General Hospital, 55 Fruit Street, Boston, MA 02114, USA

and pathological self-esteem regulation would be the most effective means for increasing our understanding of the DSM version of NPD.

The study of NPD is also important because it offers the opportunity for advancing our understanding of personality disorders by linking them to the increasingly accepted five-factor model (FFM) of normal personality. Consistent with other researchers and theorists, we [4] have shown that the DSM-IV NPD has a strong positive association to the FFM trait of extraversion. Extraversion is one of the most prominent normal personality traits, with representation in almost every multi-scale self-report personality inventory. The association of NPD to extraversion has the potential to both bridge the domains of normal and abnormal personality and to connect NPD to an underlying neurobiological structure, as extraversion has been shown to have a strong association to the behavioural activating system and the dopamine system [5]. Continued research into the relationship of NPD to extraversion might further the integration of normal and abnormal personality research, while also bringing the methodologies of cognitive neuroscience and neuroimaging more fully into the study of personality disorders.

I found Ronningstam's portrayal of the "shy narcissist" most interesting and a promising area of continued study in this field. The shy narcissist appears most similar to earlier references such as the "closet narcissists" or "deflated narcissists". These patients tend to enter therapy with chronic dysphoria and excessive sensitivity to shame. Initially they look more avoidant or inhibited interpersonally than narcissistic, but over time they reveal their underlying grandiose fantasies and latent sense of superiority. In fact, once comfortable in the therapy relationship, their narcissistically coloured inner life themes are evident even when their external behaviour remains highly constricted. These patients appear to have the first essential feature of narcissism, a grandiose self-image, but do not actively seek admiration or evidence a true lack of empathy towards others. As such, their narcissism remains behaviourally silent. It seems too early to say whether or not this condition is a true variant of pathological narcissism, but it is clearly a frequently encountered clinical condition and certainly worthy of further study.

REFERENCES

1. Livesley J.W. (2001) Conceptual and taxonomic issues. In *Handbook of Personality Disorders* (Ed. J.W. Livesley), pp. 3–39. Guilford, New York.
2. Blais M.A., Hilsenroth M.J., Castlebury F.D. (1997) Content validity of the DSM-IV borderline and narcissistic personality disorder criteria sets. *Compr. Psychiatry*, **38**, 31–37.

3. Holdwick D.J., Hilsenroth M.J., Castlebury F.D., Blais M.A. (1998) Identifying the unique and common characteristics of the DSM-IV antisocial, borderline and narcissistic personality disorders. *Compr. Psychiatry*, **39**, 277–286.
4. Blais M.A. (1997) Clinician ratings of the five-factor model of personality and the DSM-IV personality disorders. *J. Nerv. Ment. Dis.*, **185**, 388–393.
5. DePue R.A., Lenzenweger M.F. (2001) A neurobehavioral dimensional model. In *Handbook of Personality Disorders* (Ed. J.W. Livesley), pp. 136–176. Guilford, New York.

4.7
Narcissistic Personality Disorder: The Cassel Hospital Experience
Kevin Healy[1]

In this commentary I report my experience of working at the Cassel Hospital in London. I describe some of the research undertaken there on individuals diagnosed as having severe disorders of personality functioning. I question the relevance of a diagnosis of narcissistic personality disorder with no co-morbidity to my psychiatric practice in a national health service.

The Cassel Hospital in London is a national health service hospital, whose services are primarily aimed at helping individuals of all ages, couples and families to live with the consequences of disordered personality functioning. Three clinical services provide a number of differing assessment and treatment programmes, and help families, young people and adults with diagnoses of personality disorder find a better fit between their own needs and their ability to find ways to have their needs met appropriately. Supporting consultancy, training, research and development services prepare professional networks to better meet the needs of the patients for whom they are clinically responsible.

The Cassel Personality Disorder Study [1] has been very influential in making improvements to the work of our clinical services. This outcome study used measures of symptom change, social adjustment and global functioning to monitor outcome of interventions at 6 months, 12 months, 24 months, 36 months and at 5 year follow up [2]. A study of health service utilization patterns by individuals with diagnoses of personality disorder was completed [3]. Economic evaluation demonstrated the high economic cost of untreated individuals with personality disorders, individuals treated as usual in mainstream psychiatric settings, and individuals treated in services specializing in the management of individuals with disorders of

¹ *Cassel Hospital, 1 Ham Common, Richmond, Surrey, UK*

personality. The Adult Attachment Interview was used as the main measure to detect structural change and attachment status pre- and post-treatment [4].

This research has shown the importance of transitions into and out of hospital, and into and out of other treatment programmes, in the lives of patients with disorders of personality functioning. The importance of such transitions to the well being of the professionals trying to provide services to appropriately meet the needs of this patient group, has also become very clear. This patient group has significant and continuing needs that are best met by continuing, co-ordinated, comprehensive and integrated care provision.

However, our patients were repeatedly telling us this over many years. They knew what aspects of our treatment programmes were not benefiting them, and what aspects they valued. We did not choose to listen to them directly. We did however build listening to their views and to their accounts of their experiences into our research programme with important results [5,6]. Taking considered and specific actions in response to these views had a direct impact on the drop out rate from our treatment programmes [7]. Listening to the views of patients, or "experts by experience" as now known in Department of Health documentation, is now a central pillar in the planning and provision of services for people suffering from disorders of personality functioning in the United Kingdom [8].

Who and where are the patients described by Elsa Ronningstam in her review of narcissistic personality disorder? My experience in national health service practice of assessing and treating individuals with severe disorders of personality functioning suggests that it is very rare to find individuals who only meet diagnostic criteria for a single personality disorder. Such an individual is unlikely to pose significant problems for society and for mental health services in particular. The mean number of diagnoses of personality disorder was 3.5 per patient in the Cassel Personality Disorder study. Narcissistic personality disorder never existed just on its own [9], but was usually associated with borderline personality disorder, paranoid personality disorder, and/or personality disorders of avoidant, self defeating, dependent, obsessive–compulsive and passive–aggressive types.

The value of diagnosis from a clinical perspective is that it enables planning of interventions to relieve pain and suffering for the patient, for their family and carers, and importantly for their professional networks. A diagnosis based on observable symptoms is probably too narrow a perspective from which to plan effective treatment of complex personality disordered functioning. A trans-theoretical model of change considers a pre-contempla-tion stage, a contemplation stage, a preparation stage, an action stage, and a maintenance stage. As a participant progresses through the stages, positive change becomes more stable, internalized and sustainable [10]. Assessment and strengthening of a patient's motivation for change, a patient's engagement in a treatment setting and programme, and consideration of a patient's likely impact on the professionals working with them are central elements of a good psychodynamic formulation [11]. The elements described in Ronningstam's review seem to me to be largely static, unchanging, unchangeable, non-dynamic, and consequently less clinically helpful.

Within the world of office psychotherapy and private practice, Elsa Ronningstam's review raises some important questions. How do we determine the best fit between an individual with narcissistic personality spectrum disorder and a particular therapist, so that the patient can be helped to address and change some of his difficulties? Some patient/ therapist fits may survive for a long time without evident change in either patient or therapist. Do individuals with narcissistic spectrum pathology make good psychodynamic psychotherapists? Does a healthy degree of narcissism help a therapist to work primarily in the transference and counter-transference paradigm, where self-referential actions and thinking are central? What level of narcissism ideally facilitates a therapist to focus on the work of understanding and attempting to change a patient's difficulties?

REFERENCES

1. Chiesa M., Fonagy P. (2000) Cassel personality disorder study: methodology and treatment effects, *Br. J. Psychiatry*, **176**: 485–491.
2. Chiesa M., Fonagy, P. (2003) Cassel personality disorder study: a 36-month follow-up. *Br. J. Psychiatry*, **183**: 356–362.
3. Chiesa M., Fonagy P., Holmes J., Drahorad C., Harrison-Hall A. (2002) Health service use costs by personality disorder following specialist and non-specialist treatment: a comparative study. *J. Person. Disord.*, **16**: 160–173.
4. Chiesa M. (2004) Assessment of structural change and attachment status in personality disorder, following specialist psychosocial treatment: work in progress. Paper in preparation.
5. Drahorad C. (1999) Reflections on being a patient in a therapeutic community. *Therapeutic Communities*, **20**: 227–236.
6. Chiesa M., Pringle P., Drahorad C. (2003) Users' views of therapeutic community treatment: a satisfaction survey at the Cassel Hospital. *Therapeutic Communities*, **24**: 129–143.
7. Chiesa M., Drahorad C., Longo S. (2000) Early termination of treatment in personality disorder treated in a psychotherapy hospital: quantitative and qualitative study. *Br. J. Psychiatry*, **177**: 107–111.
8. National Institute for Mental Health in England (2003) *Personality Disorder; No Longer a Diagnosis of Exclusion*. National Institute of Mental Health, London.
9. Chiesa M., Bateman A., Wilberg T., Friis S. (2002) Patients' characteristics, outcome and cost-benefit of hospital-based treatment for patients with personality disorder: a comparison of three different programmes. *Psychology and Psychotherapy: Theory, Research and Practice*, **75**: 381–392.
10. Prochaska J., DiClemente C. (1986) Towards a comprehensive model of change. In *Treating Addictive Behaviours* (Eds W.R. Miller, N. Heather), pp. 2–37. Plenum, New York.

11. Healy K. (2004) Is a psychodynamic formulation of use in predicting inter-
    action between members of the multi-disciplinary team. Presented at the
    Annual Meeting of the Royal College of Psychiatrists, Harrogate, July 6–9.

4.8
Narcissistic Personalities: Pathobiographies and Research Findings from Latin America

Ramon U. Florenzano[1]

Ronningstam underscores some interesting clinical differences between
arrogant and shy narcissists. We have recently published two patho-
biographies of South American forefathers [1,2]. Both presented strong
narcissistic traits. One, Lord Thomas Cochrane, belonged to the arrogant
and boastful type; the other, Don Diego Portales, to the shy one. The first
was dismissed from Her Majesty's Navy after an attempt to gain money in
the London stockmarket in a very doubtful manner: a friend, dressed as a
French officer, entered the City stating Napoleon was dead. The market
rose swiftly until the lie was uncovered. Lord Cochrane made a hefty gain,
until he was publicly exposed and the Regent expelled him from the Order
of the Bath. This narcissistic blow was too much for him: he accepted the
offer of the Chilean Government to become the first Admiral of the new
country Navy. In Chile, he defeated the Spaniard fleet using tricks he had
already perfected against the French, allowing Chileans and Peruvians to
become free. After feeling unrecognized by his new country, he went first to
Brazil and then to Greece and to England and today is buried in the Abbey of
Westminster. The second, a First Minister in the 1830s during the organization
of Chile as an independent nation, resigned at the minor criticism or
disapproval of his policies, to be recalled to duty when his services were
needed again. Only after his death he was recognized as the organizer of the
future Republic. He presented clear-cut obsessional character traits,
reviewing in depth the military cadres in the Chilean army, preparing
them for a future victorious campaign against Peru. When told he was to be
ambushed by a rebellious faction of the Army, he did not believe they
would dare to imprison him, but they did. He was killed and became a
symbol of civilian bravery against the military. Both heroes had many of the
traits that Ronningstam describes. Lord Cochrane's diagnosis is in-between
antisocial and narcissistic personality disorder. The shy Diego Portales has
an obsessional disorder with shy narcissistic traits. They put the issue of the

[1] Chair of Psychiatry, Hospital del Salvador, Santiago de Chile, Chile

social need, in times of upheaval, for people that think highly of themselves and are able to take a stance against the societal beliefs. Contextual factors influence the characteristics and the consequences of narcissistic prone personalities and their behaviours. In post-modern times, appearance is for many much more important than being. This applies to Latin America in sociological and individual terms. Globalization of culture puts people in touch with Western values and hierarchies. The structure that was fixed for a long time has changed dramatically in the last fifty years. Rosaria Stabili [3] has underscored how an aristocratic and hierarchical society has been replaced by a much more mobile one. The prior pre-dominantly Catholic *weltanschauung*, which valued austerity, humility and sobriety in food and dress, has turned into a boastful milieu where cars, clothing and exhibition of the body are central.

Our research group has validated in Chile the Ego Development Scale, which orders individuals from early, pre-conformist stages where impulsive behaviours prevail, through a conformist period where the person respects societal norms, to a post-conformist stage where the individual defines his behaviour in a self-reflective and personal manner. Following Hauser's research on adolescent and their families [4], we have documented how in Chile youth risk behaviours appear when parents (and especially fathers) are absent or not fulfilling a socializing role. We believe that Latin-American *machismo* was a local name for narcissism in a society that did not recognize women as full human beings. The structure of many antisocial personalities was much more socially acceptable in rural Hispano-American environments. Urbanization and globalization of cultures require mentalization and a psychological sophistication that corresponds to a conformist, and hopefully to a post-conformist ego development. Our data using the Chilean version of the Ego Development Scale show that many adolescents remain at the pre-conformist stages, most achieve the conformist one, but very few attain a post-conformist developmental period [5]. This can be related to an upbringing that treats children as appendixes of their parents until a certain age, and then puts a strong distance among them, as Paulina Kernberg has described [6].

We agree with Ronningstam about the need to compare narcissistic personalities in different social and geographical contexts. This is a research area which remains to be explored.

REFERENCES

1. Florenzano R. (2001) DJPP: una personalidad anancástica que influyó en la historia de Chile. *Folia Psiquiátrica*, 7: 12–18.

2. Florenzano R. (2003) TAC: ¿Trastorno impulsivo o compulsión a la repetición? *Folia Psiquiátrica*, **8**, 7–14.
3. Stabili M.R. (2002) *El Sentimiento Aristocrático en Chile*. Andres Bello, Santiago de Chile.
4. Valdés M., Florenzano R., Serrano T., Roizblatt A., Rodriguez J. (1999) Factores protectores, resiliencia, conductas de riesgo adolescente: relación con el desarrollo yoico (1999) *Boletín de Investigaciones en Educatión, Facultad de Educación, Pontificia Universidad Católica de Chile*, **12**: 131–150.
5. Florenzano R., Valdés M., Serrano T., Rodríguez J., Roizblatt A. (2001) Desarrollo yoico, familia y adolescencia. Presented at the XI Jornadas de Psiquiatría Universidad de Valparaíso, April 20–21.
6. Kernberg P. (1989) Los padres de niños y adolescentes narcisistas. *Rev. Chil. Psicoanalisis*, 9–19.

5

The Anxious Cluster of Personality Disorders: A Review

Peter Tyrer

Department of Psychological Medicine,
Imperial College (Charing Cross Campus), Claybrook Centre,
St. Dunstan's Road, London W6 8RP, UK

INTRODUCTION

Personality disorders have had a chequered history but they are an excellent exemplar of the phrase "there is nothing new under the sun". Cluster C personality disorders are a group of these conditions that also appear to be new, but their descriptions were well established over 100 years ago, and we have only rediscovered and repackaged them. In this review it will be argued that people who are often described in lay terms as "neurotic" and who in the past were subsumed under the chapter headings of "neurosis and personality disorder" in standard textbooks, are really equivalent to Cluster C personality disorders. The development and justification of the Cluster C concept, the characteristics of the conditions making up its categories, the comorbidity of Cluster C with other (Axis I) disorders, the implications of this comorbidity on short- and long-term outcome, and the treatment of Cluster C personality disorders will be described.

HISTORY

The notion of personality disorders being aggregated into clusters is a relatively recent one. In the early classification of personality disorder there was a general notion of degeneracy attached to all personality abnormality [1], but no general classification of types, although the germ of such a

Personality Disorders. Edited by Mario Maj, Hagop S. Akiskal, Juan E. Mezzich and Ahmed Okasha.
©2005 John Wiley & Sons Ltd: ISBN 0-470-09036-7

classification had been present since Theophrastus in early Greece [2]. Freud and the early psychoanalysts made further progress in identifying "character" as a predisposition to many other disorders, and what is now described as anankastic or obsessive-compulsive disorder was first described accurately by Freud as the "anal character" [3]. Then Kurt Schneider appeared on the scene, and his ability to encapsulate types of clinical psychopathology bedazzled his contemporaries so much that his description of the now standard personality types such as paranoid, schizoid and dependent groups (all described under the general rubric of "psycho-pathic") became the acknowledged psychiatric classification almost overnight. I have argued previously that this has been a highly counter-productive initiative [4], because although it popularized personality disorder it also devalued it scientifically and ever since then we have struggled to get a reliable and valid system of classification for these disorders.

The cluster notion arose because of the perceived need to rationalize the description of personality disorders, as there was such extensive comorb-idity between them. When a condition such as borderline personality disorder occurred nine times more often as a comorbid condition than as a single one [5], something had to be done to improve matters, and although borderline personality disorder is perhaps the worst comorbidity offender because of its heterogeneity [6], other personality disorders are not much better. The problem was that there was little alternative for the dissatisfied. The dimensional classification was clearly superior to the categorical one [7], but it was difficult to unite with normal diagnostic conventions, and the diagnostic criteria for the individual personality disorders showed little internal consistency and so could not be regarded as prototypical [8]. The possibility of reducing the numbers of personality disorders to around four—dependent, antisocial, schizoid and obsessional—was suggested by factor analytical studies [9,10] and the same was considered appropriate for normal personality, except that an additional factor, openness, was included as well to make the Big Five [11]. The studies of normal and pathological personality variation have come together in the development of personality clusters.

VALIDITY OF THE CLUSTER MODEL, WITH SPECIAL REFERENCE TO CLUSTER C

The cluster notion followed soon after the introduction of DSM-III. The reformulation of the 11 DSM-III personality disorders into Cluster A (odd and eccentric personalities), Cluster B (flamboyant and erratic personalities) and Cluster C (anxious and fearful personalities) was supported by initial factor analytic studies (e.g. [12,13]), but not always to the same extent by later studies [14]. In particular, the notion that clusters might represent a better categorization of personality disorders than the 11 group model was not really supported, as diagnostic comorbidity of personality disorders occurs across the range of the 11 disorders, not just within clusters.

However, the cluster notion has persisted, not least because it represents a grouping of personality disorders that has face validity. Cluster C is the least clear of the three clusters and this is illustrated by the description of personality disorders in this book. The obsessive-compulsive category, although at first appearing to be part of this group, is separately identified in factor analytic studies and across the range of personality measurement [10,11,15–17] and will not be discussed elsewhere in this chapter except in connection with the general neurotic syndrome (where it is one of the postulated components).

The other major difficulty associated with this group of personality disorders is the obvious overlap with the equivalent mental states of anxiety and depression that are part of mental state disorders (called Axis I disorders in the rest of this chapter). The central features of timidity, persistent tension, proneness to anxiety, dependence, lack of confidence, and the constant expectation of distress and disaster in these personality disorders are very similar to the nervous apprehension, muscular and nervous tension of anxiety disorders, and to the avoidant behaviour of social anxiety disorder (a subject discussed at greater length later) and illustrate that what used to be called neuroticism but is now described as "negative affectivity" [18] encompasses both the states of depression and anxiety and the predisposition to develop them. It is therefore not surprising that this group of personality disorders shows less reliability in assessment than others [19]. This probably also accounts for the almost universal finding, first demonstrated nearly 40 years ago [20], that when individuals are in states of depression and/or anxiety they show different personality features than when they are well.

Although it has been common for researchers to claim that the personality assessment is artifactually altered in some way in such instances—it is suggested that the assessment of personality is "contaminated", "distorted" or "flawed" by the mental state—Clark et al. [21] have suggested that the distortion may be a real finding and that the personality is temporarily, but genuinely, influenced by the state. Indeed, these authors go further and, after finding in a treatment study that the main component predicting late depression severity is a general one—with variance shared across personality and psychosocial variables—conclude that this general component (probably a trait component linked to personality) is the prime determinant of mood outcome rather than any specific factor linked to treatment [22]. If the personality was distorted by the mental state this finding would not have been demonstrated, as the mood state would have had predictive primacy.

DESCRIPTION OF CONDITIONS COMPRISING THE ANXIOUS CLUSTER

Avoidant personality disorder has been the most studied condition in this group and in most people's minds the term "anxious personality disorder" identifies the same condition. Indeed, in ICD-10 the adjective "anxious" is followed by "avoidant" in the description of anxious personality disorder, implying that they are the same disorder. However, the description of avoidant personality disorder overlaps a little more with the Cluster A personalities than anxious personality disorder, and at least one classification system separates them on this basis following a cluster analysis procedure [15,23]. Avoidant personality disorder was originally classified with the Cluster A personalities and there is some clear sharing of its characteristics with schizotypal personality disorder [24].

The avoidant category is one of the few personality disorders derived recently and not discussed by Schneider or other pioneers. It was proposed by Millon [25] and has clear face validity, but has been put under some stress by the concern over its overlap with social phobia, now called social anxiety disorder. It describes a persistent behavioural pattern of avoidance created by anxiety, which leads to a highly restricted life style and limited social interaction. This clearly overlaps with the dependent group, which also tends to be characterized by limited social interaction, except that in the latter group there is perceived incompetence with the vicissitudes of life, so that help from others is always perceived to be necessary. The ICD-10 and DSM-IV criteria for this group are shown in Table 5.1. It could be argued that other conditions vying for inclusion in the personality disorder grouping could also be included in the anxious cluster. These include hypochondriacal personality disorder [26], depressive personality disorder [27] and dysthymic personality disorder [15]. However, these conditions remain controversial categories and need further work.

MEASUREMENT OF ANXIOUS PERSONALITY DISORDERS

It is common to measure all personality disorders with a standard instrument, such as the Structured Interview to Diagnose Personality Disorders (SIDP) [28] or the International Personality Disorder Examination

TABLE 5.1   Characteristics of personality disorders of the anxious cluster in the current ICD and DSM classifications

ICD-10 personality disorders	DSM-IV personality disorders
F 60.6 *Anxious*—Persistent uncertainty and fear in relationships because of (i) excessive self-consciousness, (ii) hypersensitivity to rejection (therefore avoids new relationships), (iii) exaggeration of risks in social situations leading to restricted life-style, (iv) reluctance to enter into relationships unless there is certainty of acceptance	*Avoidant*—Pervasive social 301.82 inhibition and discomfort leading to (i) avoidance of occupational activities involving significant interpersonal contact, (ii) unwillingness to be involved with people unless there is certainty of being liked, (iii) restraint due to fear of being ridiculed or shamed in intimate relationships, (iv) preoccupation with being criticized or rejected in social situations, (v) inhibition in new social situations because of perceived inadequacy, (vi) belief that one is socially inept, personally unappealing or inferior to others and (vii) reluctance to take personal risks or engage in new activities because of embarrassment
F 60.7 *Dependent*—Failure to take responsibility for actions, with subordination of personal needs to those of others, excessive dependence with need for constant reassurance and feelings of helplessness when a close relationship ends	*Dependent*—A persistent need 301.60 for support and care characterized by (i) inability to make everyday decisions without advice, (ii) need for others to take responsibility for major areas of life, (iii) fear of disagreeing with others because of fear of disapproval or loss of support, (iv) unable to carry out tasks because of lack of self-confidence, (v) going to excessive lengths to obtain support from others, (vi) feeling helpless when alone because of exaggerated feelings of incompetence, (vii) urgent need for new relationships as source of support when old relationship ends, (viii) unrealistic preoccupation with fears of having to care for oneself alone

(IPDE) [29]. The problem of personality interacting with mental state and influencing the assessment is stronger with the anxious cluster than any of the other personality disorders, and even the most stringent of the assessment instruments, the IPDE, is not completely free of its effect [30]. The alteration with mental state is most marked with self-rating assessments (as no significant allowance can be made for present state by the rater) and so it is gratifying that one recent self-rated assessment, the Dependent Personality Questionnaire (DPQ) [31], shows temporal stability over a six-month period in health anxious patients, with preliminary data showing a mean change of less than 5% (mean of 10 at baseline, 9.54 at 6 months) [32].

In discussing measurement, it is important to recognise the importance of comorbidity of personality disorders and the relative rarity of single disorders only being present. This can sometimes be defined in personality assessment, in which personality disorders from different clusters are given greater prominence in terms of overall severity [33].

EPIDEMIOLOGY OF THE ANXIOUS CLUSTER

There have been very few large scale studies of the epidemiology of the anxious cluster of personality disorders, mainly because of the length of time it takes to complete an assessment and the training necessary for interviewers. The studies described in Table 5.2 are all dwarfed by the very large study of Torgersen *et al.* [40], in which 2053 people aged between 18 and 65 years were studied in Oslo between 1994 and 1997. This study was exceptional in that a full interview (the Structured Interview for DSM-III-R Personality Disorders) was used in the assessment and in most cases subjects were interviewed at home. The overall prevalence of personality disorder was 13.4% and avoidant personality disorder was the most prevalent at 5%.

This could be a local effect. Norway is well known for its independent spirit and averseness to closeness and it is no coincidence that Oslo covers a larger surface area than almost any other capital city in the world. However, when considering all the studies described in Table 5.2, the overall prevalence of avoidant personality disorder is a very high 4.3%. By contrast, dependent personality disorder is at a lower level of 2.4%, but this is still higher than many other disorders.

THE ANXIOUS CLUSTER AND AGE

The long-standing definition of personality disorder states that it begins in adolescence and early adult life and is persistent, although sometimes showing attenuation towards middle and old age [41,42]. This view is becoming increasingly untenable, as evidence accumulates that personality

TABLE 5.2   Prevalence of avoidant (anxious) and dependent personality disorders in normal populations

Authors	Population (n)	Prevalence (%) Avoidant	Prevalence (%) Dependent
Drake and Vaillant [34]	Normal controls for population comparison with juvenile delinquency (456)	4.6	7.9
Casey et al. [35]; Casey [36]	Random sample of patients registered with a general practitioner (200)	1	2
Black et al. [37]	Matched controls for population with obsessive–compulsive personality disorder (127)	3.2	2.4
Blanchard et al. [38]	Matched controls for post-traumatic stress disorder (93)	1.1	2.2
Maier et al. [39]	Random population (109)	1.3	1.6
Torgersen et al. [40]	Random sample of urban population (Oslo) aged 18–65 (2053)	5.0	1.5
	Mean	4.3	2.4

status fluctuates both in the short term (see below) and in the longer term. The data are not fully clear, but it appears likely that the anxious cluster of personalities becomes more pronounced with increasing age. This is hinted at by the epidemiological studies showing a greater proportion of anxious personalities in older people, which is partly influenced by the lower number of Cluster B personalities in this age group [43], and also by specific studies. Thus, for example, Loranger [44] found that, of 3640 consecutive hospital admissions 342 had a diagnosis of dependent personality disorder, but more than half of these were over 40 years of age compared with 26% of those with other personality disorders.

Change in personality status can only be determined directly by recording personality at different times in the same subjects. In our work we have found that, in those with common anxiety and depressive disorders, personality status changes over time in a fairly consistent fashion. Those with Cluster B personalities tend to improve with age, but others, and this includes avoidant but not dependent personality disorder, become more disordered 12 years after original assessment [45]. It is important to note that these findings were demonstrated in a population with mood symptomatology at baseline; replication is desirable in those with no psychiatric pathology.

The implications of a change in personality with increasing age are considerable for a population whose mean age is gradually increasing, and the favourable notion that, as we all get older, our less attractive personality features improve or, in this context, "mellow", is not likely to be an accurate one, except for antisocial and impulsive features.

THE ANXIOUS CLUSTER AND NEUROTICISM

The word "neurotic" was air-brushed out of all diagnostic descriptions in the United States after the love affair with psychodynamic psychiatry broke up in acrimony in the 1970s [46]. The new atheoretical system of DSM-III disorders had no place for the diffuse concept of neuroticism and its implications of unconscious motivation, so it had to go. However, the notion was too well established to be extinguished entirely. The ideas of neuroticism and extraversion originally described by Jung were developed by Eysenck as personality types and led to the identification of three dimensions of personality: N (neuroticism–stability), E (extraversion–introversion) and P (psychoticism–normality). The first inventory designed to measure neuroticism, the Maudsley Medical Questionnaire (MMQ), distinguished normal and neurotic soldiers, and was the stimulus for the Maudsley Personality Inventory (MPI), designed to measure both neuroticism and extraversion [47]. Later, the Eysenck Personality Inventory (EPI) was introduced [48], and subsequently refined to the Eysenck Personality Questionnaire [49].

Although Eysenck's scales have fallen into disuse, their fundamental concepts of personality have been supported by other workers approaching personality from completely different standpoints (e.g. [16,50]). The equivalent concept in the United States, negative affectivity [18], is an equally attractive and necessary concept for those studying normal personality variation. Its neglect by those involved in the study of personality disorder has been recently criticized [51].

The confusion, or overlap, between the personality and mental state features of anxiety and depression is perhaps the best known form of all relationships between mental state and personality and stems back to the early days of psychoanalysis [52]. Anxious, dependent and "oral" personality features are commonly associated with anxiety disorders and could be part of the overlapping comorbidity model described by Lyons *et al.* [53], in which the Axis I and Axis II conditions could be perceived as all part of the same syndrome. The co-occurrence of a personality disorder in the anxious/ fearful cluster and any anxiety or non-psychotic depressive diagnosis is common but by no means universal, and it has been suggested that this condition could be a single coaxial diagnosis formulated as the general neurotic syndrome [54–56].

Examining the merits of the arguments for and against the general neurotic syndrome depend on whether you are a "splitter" or a "lumper" when it comes to psychiatric classification. This difference is often felt to be one that depends on a fundamental philosophical dichotomy between the two approaches, but it is really one of timing. Splitters see tremendous potential in separating disorders early in their investigation, whereas lumpers are reluctant to effect separation until there is good evidence for their validity as distinct entities.

The main characteristics of the syndrome are the simultaneous presence of anxiety and depressive disorders, at least one change in the primacy of anxiety and depression at different times, the presence of dependent and/ or anankastic (obsessive–compulsive) personality features, and a family history of a similar disorder [54] . This has been incorporated into a scale for the diagnosis of the general neurotic syndrome [57]. There is some evidence that this syndrome persists and leads to a poorer outcome than in those who do not have the condition [58,59].

The general neurotic syndrome is not a conventional diagnosis and it appears atavistic in this age when we have a single diagnosis for every ill. However, it is a useful concept that unites the anxious cluster of personality disorders and the symptoms of anxiety and depression, and is recognizable to every clinician closely involved with the treatment of these disorders. It is a concept that has received support in the assessment of those with common mental disorders in the elderly [60,61], in primary care [62], and in epidemiological studies [55], but it is a "lumping" diagnosis that is against the spirit of the age. Despite some support for a unified syndrome from genetic studies [63], the prevailing climate sees merit in splitting anxiety, depression and personality into smaller and smaller groups; an activity that would be meritorious if it was founded on the basis of greater understanding. Unfortunately, it may be stimulated more by commercial pressure than by scientific ones [64].

COMORBIDITY OF THE ANXIOUS CLUSTER WITH AXIS I DISORDERS

Generalized Social Phobia and the Avoidant Personality Disorder

One of the strongest Axis I/Axis II relationships in psychiatry is between social phobia, particularly the generalized form of the condition, and avoidant personality disorder. There are strong arguments against the two conditions being usefully separated [65,66] and this is relevant to the current great interest in social anxiety disorder, the new term for social phobia. This condition is now recognized to be increasingly common, with rates around 8% in the community, often occurring as a precursor of other common mental disorders [67]. To clarify whether avoidant personality disorder reflects a personality variant of generalized social phobia, research is needed to show that the avoidant disorder precedes generalized social phobia and that they have a shared form of familial, presumably genetic, transmission. There is no such evidence and it is reasonable to regard the two conditions as part of a single spectrum of disorder in which the personality component leads to greater maladjustment and handicap [68].

An interesting cultural variant of avoidant personality disorder is the Japanese *taijin kyofu*, a condition in which there is crippling social anxiety leading to almost total isolation [69].

Eating Disorders and the Anxious Cluster

It has long been claimed that anorexia nervosa was associated with personality abnormality, with histrionic features lying behind the excessive self-absorption that is so characteristic of the condition, and obsessional features associated with determination to continue dieting to excessive thinness [70]. Since formal assessments have been made in patients having both anorexia and bulimia nervosa, this association has been confirmed, but the Cluster C association is much stronger with anorexia nervosa than with bulimia nervosa. Anorexia has a clear association with obsessional as well as avoidant features [71], whereas bulimia nervosa tends to be associated more strongly with the impulsive features of Cluster B personality disorder [72–74].

Anxiety and Depressive Disorders and the Anxious Cluster

Many studies have been carried out into the relationship between anxiety and depressive disorders and a range of Axis II conditions, and the results are not universally consistent. Patients with generalized anxiety disorder have been found to have a higher association with antisocial personality disorder in one study [75], whereas in another the association was strongest with avoidant personality disorder [76]. Panic disorder is more commonly associated with Cluster C personalities [66], particularly with dependent personality disorder [76]. Agoraphobic patients also have links with dependent personality disorder, and those without panic are more likely to have avoidant personality disorder [77].

Not surprisingly, the results of personality assessment with depressed patients show that what used to be called neurotic depression, now euphemistically called non-melancholic or (even less satisfactory) mild depression, has a greater association with personality disorder than psychotic or melancholic depression, particularly with avoidant personality disorder [78]. The adjective "neurotic" in the old classifications was almost a code for an association with the anxious cluster.

Many of the somatoform disorders, particularly somatization disorder, are associated with major personality disturbance. In almost all published studies in secondary care, most of those with somatization disorders have some personality disorder also [79–81]. The specific association with the anxious cluster is not especially strong—there is a significant component from Cluster B personality disorders—but in one group, hypochondriasis (or health anxiety), there is a closer association with the Cluster C group [82].

Somatization disorder may be a persistent condition and often begins in early adult life. It has been argued that this disorder may be a form of personality disorder [81]. This may be true, but the chronicity and temporal stability of somatization disorder may of course be quite independent of personality.

There is now good evidence that dependent (Cluster C) and antisocial and impulsive (Cluster B) personality disorders predispose to an increased rate of life events in patients with neurotic disorder and adjustment disorders [83–86] and therefore such personality disorders might be expected to be associated with more serious stress disorders such as post-traumatic stress disorder (PTSD). Over the last few years, there has been increasing evidence that those who, through their personality abnormality, put themselves at greater risk are more likely to develop PTSD. It is fair to add that most of these have one or more of the Cluster B disorders rather than Cluster C ones [87].

IMPLICATIONS OF COMORBIDITY OF THE ANXIOUS CLUSTER WITH AXIS I DISORDERS

Baseline Differences in Symptom Severity

It is generally, but not universally, demonstrated that, when comparisons of Axis I disorders are made between those with and without personality disorder, those in the former group have greater severity of symptoms [23,88–91]. One consequence of this is that improvement in those without personality disorder could be exactly to the same degree as those who have personality disorder, but the outcome may still appear to be more favourable in those with no disorder. If the analysis of outcome (whether or not it is linked to specific treatment) makes allowance for the initial difference in pathology (most commonly by analysis of covariance with adjustment of baseline scores), then any initial differences are taken into account. However, if there is an absolute level of improvement regarded as necessary for success (e.g. a score of less than 10 on the Beck Anxiety Inventory), then the results would unfairly favour those who had no personality at onset, because more of these would go below this threshold at the time that outcome is measured. It is therefore wise to check whether the outcomes recorded are ones that can be affected by these baseline differences. Particularly in systematic reviews, it is popular to have outcomes that are dichotomous (e.g. recovered/not recovered) and these tend to favour error in interpretation.

Confusion Between Symptoms and Cluster C Personality Traits

As discussed earlier, the problem of confounding or distorting of personality status by anxious or depressive symptoms has been a constant irritant to those who maintain that personality is a persistent characteristic pattern of behaviour and should therefore show temporal reliability. Common sense tells us that this is indeed the case; personality may not be as unique and as reproducible as a fingerprint, but it is a recognizable marker in an ever-shifting sea of change and its fundamental components do not change radically. So, why do all instruments recording personality status show so many changes over a short time scale, so that the kappa value measuring temporal reliability over a period such as 6 months is no higher than 0.5 [92]? As Clark et al. [21] have suggested, the distortion is probably a real phenomenon: using a combination of factor-analytic and regression techniques, they showed that only trait, not state, variance in depression predicted later depression symptomatology. This is not a simple relationship, however, and further work has elicited some of its subtleties.

In Clark et al.'s later study [22], we have an indication that during treatment (in this case cognitive behaviour therapy for depression) some aspects of personality can change independently of the general trait factor over time. Thus, the trait of dependence is found to behave differently from others such as self-harm and detachment, in that it shows a difference between its general common factor, the factor shared with the psychosocial and personality variables (the within-type factor) and the factor unique to the individual measure (the scale-specific factor). These authors found that whereas the general component of dependency correlated positively with depression severity, the within-type and scale-specific components both correlated inversely with depression severity at early assessment, but had correlations close to zero later. The authors speculate that "increased dependency early in therapy is a sign of involvement in the therapeutic alliance, a willingness on the part of a patient to form a close relationship with the therapist, which in and of itself reduces depression. Later in therapy, the therapeutic alliance may change to a more collaborative relationship so dependency and depression severity become uncoupled" [22].

The significance of this work is that different components of personality seem to constitute a dynamic mixture in which some can change independently of others and also be situation-specific or individual-specific. It moves us towards the notion that while some personality attributes—we would like to think of them as core ones—are stable, others are sensitive to changes in relationships and setting and so show fluctuation. Such fluctuation should not be regarded as measurement error and, if we were able to separate it reliably, it may help to understand how genuine personality change can be created as a consequence of psychological or pharmacological interventions.

Improvement of Personality as a Consequence of Intervention for an Axis I Disorder

There is a literature, gradually growing, which shows that some interventions are effective in personality disorder, even if most of these are used in a heterogeneous group, borderline personality disorder, which is regarded by some as an unsatisfactory diagnosis [6,93] and which shows much greater fluctuation than other personality disorders. In examining the impact of personality disorder on outcome of Axis I mental disorders, it is therefore quite possible that the treatment of the Axis I disorder—primarily acting on symptoms—may also influence personality.

In my personal experience, I have found this to be most commonly found with the monoamine oxidase inhibitor (MAOI) phenelzine. Although generally MAOIs are not particularly effective in those with depression who also have personality disorder [94], they can produce quite marked changes in symptoms when all other drug treatments seem to have failed. However, some people, while seeming to benefit greatly in terms of their perceived well-being, also undergo apparent personality change at the same time, and this is not such a positive experience. The typical Cluster C personality of cautious over-concern may be replaced by cavalier risk-taking behaviour that troubles the relatives and friends of the patient to a degree that far outweighs the benefit of the drug. This change in behaviour, nicely summarized by Parker *et al.* [95] as one of "acting-in" to "acting-out", can sometimes be interpreted as a consequence of relief of symptoms, but it needs not necessarily take place. Standard forms of clinical and research assessment do not take adequate notice of such changes and so to a large extent they remain unrecorded.

In examining the outcome of comorbid mental state and personality disorder, we therefore have to be conscious of personality as well as symptom impact. One consequence is that a treatment for the mood disorder might also improve the personality disorder, so that the outcome could be better in those with personality disorder than in those without; a rare event but one that has been postulated in one study [96].

Results of Studies Examining Cluster C Comorbidity and Outcome

The general interpretation of the literature on personality disorder and treatment is that the co-existence of a personality disorder and a mental illness handicaps response to treatment. This began as an impressionistic notion, exemplified by my former teacher, William Sargant, who stated, somewhat dogmatically, that antidepressants and other drugs were only effective in those of "good previous personality" [97], but has been gradually reinforced by a series of studies in which personality status was recorded at the onset of a treatment programme and then examined as a predictor of response. These studies have, in general, shown that the presence of a personality disorder impairs response to treatment for a wide range of interventions [72,98–102], although in some this was explained by greater baseline levels of pathology [103].

However, this has been thrown into debate by a robust review of the subject by Mulder [104], who, concentrating on personality and the outcome of depression, argued that many of these studies were flawed methodologically and concluded that comorbid personality disorder should "not be seen as an impediment to good treatment response" and that "the best-designed studies report the least effect of personality pathology on treatment outcome". Much of the literature supporting Mulder's contention comes from studies with Cloninger's Tridimensional Personality Questionnaire [105].

However, Mulder did not carry out a full systematic review and, in particular, did not allow for sample size in giving weight to the different studies, so that small studies with negative results were given equal prominence to larger ones showing a positive relationship. In a recent review we attempted to determine response dichotomously in a set of 2 by 2 tables (i.e. response/no response and personality disorder/no disorder) and then to combine them in a meta-analysis.

This study [106] showed that the results of many investigations are insufficient to be analysed in this way. An on-line search displayed 890 potentially useful papers, but 769 were rejected as unsuitable. Of the remainder, 22 were found to have suitable data for this separation of outcome and the analysis of these showed a clear and consistent negative association between comorbid personality disorder (not just confined to Cluster C) and the outcome of depression. This conclusion clearly can only apply to the subject of depression, but similar studies should be possible for other mental state disorders.

SPECIFIC TREATMENT OF THE ANXIOUS CLUSTER OF PERSONALITY DISORDERS

There have been remarkably few studies of the treatment of the anxious cluster of personality disorders and most have methodological flaws or cannot really be described as research enquiries in the formal sense. However, they are still worth describing individually as I suspect they will be the forerunners of many more (Table 5.3).

Pharmacological Treatments

Antidepressant drugs have been used, or at least evaluated, for the treatment of personality disorders and, in most of these instances, Cluster C personalities are the focus of interest. In an early work, Deltito and Stam [107] suggested that selective serotonin reuptake inhibitors (SSRIs) and MAOI might be effective in avoidant personality disorder. Now the conventional view might be that they are efficacious only in social anxiety disorder, in which the value of these drugs has been shown in controlled trials. However, when separate examination of avoidant personality traits is made, it seems that these are influenced also [108].

Selective serotonin reuptake inhibitors have also been suggested to be effective in a study carried out by Ekselius and von Knorring [109,110]. Sertraline and citalopram were used for 24 weeks and the improvement in symptoms was accompanied by improvement not just in avoidant and dependent personality features but also in paranoid and borderline ones. Unfortunately there was no control group.

TABLE 5.3   Potential specific treatments of the anxious cluster of personality disorders

Authors	Type of study	Treatment	Outcome
Deltito and Stam [107]	Open	Fluoxetine, phenelzine	Suggested improvement of avoidant personality disorder independent of mood pathology
Fahlen [108]	Randomized controlled trial	Brofaromine (reversible selective monoamine oxidase inhibitor)	Fall in prevalence of avoidant personality disorder from 60% to 20% after 12 weeks treatment
Ekselius and von Knorring [109,110]	Randomized controlled trial (of two active drugs)	Selective serotonin reuptake inhibitors (sertraline and citalopram)	After 24 weeks, significant reductions in the frequency of paranoid, borderline, avoidant and dependent personality disorder diagnoses in both treatment groups
Tyrer et al. [111]	Randomized controlled trial	Tricyclic antidepressants, cognitive behaviour therapy and self-help	Improvement in personality disordered patients significantly better in those treated with antidepressants
Karterud et al. [112]	Cohort study	Day hospital therapeutic community	Better improvement for Cluster C personality disorders than others after 6 months
Gude et al. [113]	Cohort study	Schema focused therapy	Some indications of responsiveness to treatment in those with Cluster C personality disorders
Tyrer [114,115]	Open case studies	Nidotherapy	Presumptive evidence of improvement

Psychological Treatments

Psychological and pharmacological treatments were compared in a two-year study of anxious and depressive disorders [111]. Among personality disordered patients, the improvement was significantly higher in those treated with the tricyclic antidepressant dothiepin than in those receiving psychological treatments (cognitive-behaviour therapy and self-help).

Day hospital care linked to different forms of psychotherapy has also been evaluated, but lack of comparison with a control group limits interpretation. However, there is good evidence that those with the anxious cluster engage in treatment and there may be specific benefits of this approach [112,113]. Cognitive behaviour therapy has been extended to include personality disorders [116], but has yet to be formally tested in Cluster C personality disorders. Another psychological treatment, nido-therapy, has been introduced for those who find it difficult to change and who might be better helped by creating a better adaptive fit with their environment. Nidotherapy, named after the Latin *nidus* (nest), attempts to systematically alter the environment, both physical and social, so that a better fit is created, but at present its benefit is confined to case reports [114,115].

Adherence to Treatment

One of the positive aspects of the anxious cluster of personality disorders, exemplified in the Norwegian studies, is that those with these disorders are more likely to stay in contact with services and to engage than many others. Certainly the tempestuous relationships that therapists have with border-line patients are much less common in this group. In a classification of personality disorders, Type S (treatment seeking) cases have been separated from treatment resisting ones (Type R) [117]. Those with avoidant and dependent personality disorder have a much higher proportion of Type S cases than other personality disorders, and this may be important when engaging in a programme of intensive treatment.

A MOOD DIATHESIS

One way of explaining the strong comorbidity of anxiety and mood disorders with the anxious cluster is to regard the anxious or dependent personality disorders as a mood diathesis, an Achilles heel that makes the individual more likely to suffer from a specific mental disorder when exposed to certain stressful events [53]. In order to study this adequately, we need many more long-term follow-up studies in which good rates of contact can be established and in which life events can be noted prospectively.

In our own work, we have found that the anxious cluster is associated with more diagnostic change over time and with a rate of life events twice that of those with no personality disorder [118]. This supports the mood diathesis and also suggests that the life events in this group are either created by the personality style of the individual (as one of my patients puts it: "why does trouble always have to follow me around?") or are overtly manifest as significant events by the exaggerated response to them. The diathesis is represented by Clark's general trait factor and explains the poor outcome in the long term, particularly when outcome is measured longitudinally rather than at a single point in time.

In the short term, the effect of personality is relatively small and in the Nottingham Study of Neurotic Disorder this was not significant over the course of the initial 10 weeks of a randomized controlled trial [88]. However, with each successive relapse or recrudescence of symptoms, the amount of improvement is diminished. Thus, when longitudinal outcome is measured over a five or 12 year period, the presence of personality disorder (and in this study most were in the anxious cluster) is one of the strongest predictors of a poor outcome as measured by global outcome scales and social functioning [58,119]. Those with anxiety and depression and diffuse or complex personality disorder (a personality disorder from more than one cluster) have somewhat worse symptoms after 12 years than at baseline. This indicates that, if a successful treatment was available for the personality disturbance in such patients, it would be likely to have a important influence on long-term morbidity.

FUTURE PERSPECTIVES

Among the personality disorders, the anxious cluster is relatively neglected. It does not have the same prominence that is attached to its flamboyant equivalent, particularly borderline personality disorder, and it does not carry the hint of excitement and implied greater understanding that schizotypal and paranoid personality disorder impart. Nevertheless, it is the largest group of personality disorders and is associated with more morbidity than others.

It is deficient in several respects and so is not widely used in clinical discourse. Its boundaries are not as clear as they should be, and in particular the evidence that assessments can be influenced by current mood state should lead to caution in interpreting any assessment carried out when anxiety and depression symptoms are prominent. Its overlap with other related personality disorders, of which obsessive-compulsive (anankastic) and histrionic are the most prominent, is considerable and cannot be described as true comorbidity. The links with both anxiety and depression and their mixed combination, cothymia [120], are also very marked and, as the behavioural and symptomatic presentations of both personality traits and symptoms are so similar, it is often difficult to separate Axis I and Axis II.

Indeed, the inconsistent value of the separate personality diagnosis is a strong argument for promoting the "alternative version" of personality description, in which Axis II would be represented by personality traits or dispositions rather than disorders [121], allowing several dispositions to coexist without invoking multiple comorbid categories. The roughly similar hereditable and environmental components to these traits [122] is also in keeping with this approach.

The alternative view is to retain the category of the anxious cluster or its individual components (the latter is more difficult to argue) and use the co-axial approach when describing the common anxiety and depressive disorders. Describing an anxiety or depressive condition without describing the personality component also gives very limited information and covers a wide range of potential intervention and outcomes. By at least pointing out the possibility of a personality aspect (and initially it would be wise to call this "possible" rather than "probable" because of our uncertainty when there is strong mental pathology), the clinician is at least "wised up" to the idea that something else may need to be addressed apart from the simple relief of symptoms. When anxiety and depressive symptoms coexist with suspected personality abnormality, we are in the territory of the general neurotic syndrome, and whilst this may have to be bowdlerized into a term such as "general negative affectivity disposition" to satisfy the sensitivity of our American colleagues, the condition is out there in clinical practice and cannot be ignored.

A good diagnosis, as Kendell [123] has constantly reminded us, is a useful one and, once there is an effective treatment for the anxious cluster or one of its constituents, the point of the distinction between personality and mental state will become clear immediately [124]. Of course, if the distinction is a phoney one, it will never be found but, even in that situation, every clinician will need to be aware of the range that covers those common mental disorders extending from brief stress reactions at one extreme through to a paralysing state of anxiety and anhedonia in which any relief is short-lived and the extent of lifetime suffering incalculable.

SUMMARY

Consistent Evidence

There is now reasonable agreement between clinicians and researchers that the anxious cluster of personality disorders describes a significant clinical grouping. Even though there may be arguments about its boundaries and exact description, there can be no doubt that the combination of general anxiousness and fearfulness with a proneness to help-seeking is indepen-dent from the general symptomatology of anxiety and needs some form of general description. There is also now a reasonable body of evidence, but not completely uniform, that the presence of this condition makes individuals more prone to relapse and have recurrent morbidity of anxious and associated disorders. In the short term these differences are much less pronounced than in the longer term.

There is also consistency in the view that, although we have some clues as to treatment of this condition, we have no evidence-based interventions. This is a major handicap preventing full acceptance of the condition.

Incomplete Evidence

The boundaries of the anxious cluster remain extremely fuzzy and, even accepting that this group of conditions constitutes a continuum, there is a need for much greater clarity. On the positive side, the presence of a group variously described as anxious/dependent, neurotic, negative affective by different authors is robust and persistent in studies of both normal and abnormal personality and cannot be ignored. The separation of this trait grouping from those with just anxious symptomatology is still extremely difficult and this explains why, for example, social anxiety disorder is so difficult to separate from anxious or avoidant personality disorder. Both conditions are manifest early in life, tend to be persistent, are associated with secondary morbidity, and lead to marked persistent behavioural disturbance. A toss of a coin seems to be an accurate way as any of allocating a patient to a diagnosis, and what is chosen seems more likely to be determined by the choice of treatment. As this is an area where pharmaceutical companies are increasingly influential in diagnostic practice [64], both clinicians and researchers need to be vigilant and not be led too much by epidemiologists finding large areas of unmet need in surveys.

Areas Still Open to Research

The anxious cluster of personality disorders is still not a fully established diagnostic entity and may never achieve such status. However, if one examines the psychiatric diagnoses in the current classification using an independent measure of diagnostic validity [125], very few come up to an acceptable standard. In order to improve the utility of this diagnostic category, at least four goals have to be achieved:

(a) A better way of separating the personality (Axis II) elements of anxiousness and propensity to negative mood states from the states themselves. Although a start has been made to this [22], we have much further to go. Because the states and traits are so similar, they do create a spectrum of morbidity in which the personality component becomes more prominent with greater severity, but it is still perfectly possible to argue on the basis of what we know currently that severity of symptoms alone may be just as good a separator as the identification of a specific personality abnormality.

(b) Some independent way of diagnosing these disorders as the separation of personality from symptom remains at best a probability exercise which is of limited value in an individual case. The biological underpinnings of the diagnosis do not yet exist, and studies to date do not support any clear distinction [126].

(c) At least some evidence in favour of treatment effects for the anxious cluster. The list of treatments in Table 5.3 is a potential list only. We need to have definitive evidence of efficacy from one or more of these.

(d) A better classification of personality disorders in general. Clearly, if the present system of classification is inadequate, as indeed we are all aware, clustering of wrong single diagnoses will led to wrong clusters, whatever else is gained. Whether or not the obsessive-compulsive group needs to be kept separate from the others is also an open question that can only be answered once we have a new classification.

REFERENCES

1. Koch J.L.A. (1891) *Die Psychopathischen Minderwertigkeiten.* Ravensburg, Dorn.
2. Adlington R. (1925) *A Book of Characters.* Rutledge, London.
3. Freud S. (1908) Character and anal-eroticism. In *Complete Psychological Works*, pp. 167–175. Hogarth Press, London.
4. Tyrer P. (2001) Personality disorder. *Br. J. Psychiatry*, **179**: 81–84.
5. Fyer M.R., Frances A.J., Sullivan T., Hurt S.W., Clarkin J. (1988) Co-morbidity of borderline personality disorder. *Arch. Gen. Psychiatry*, **45**: 348–352.
6. Akiskal H.S., Chen S.E., Davis G.C., Puzantian V.R., Kashgarian M., Bolinger J.M. (1985) Borderline: an adjective in search of a noun. *J. Clin Psychiatry*, **46**: 41–48.
7. Widiger T.A. (1991) Personality disorder dimensional models proposed for DSM-IV. *J. Person. Disord.*, **5**: 386–398.
8. Livesley W.J. (1991) Classifying personality disorders: ideal types, prototypes, or dimensions? *J. Person. Disord.*, **5**: 52–59.
9. Walton H.J., Presly A.S. (1973) Use of a category system in the diagnosis of abnormal personality. *Br. J. Psychiatry*, **122**: 259–268.
10. Tyrer P., Alexander J. (1979) Classification of personality disorder. *Br. J. Psychiatry*, **135**: 163–167.
11. Costa P.T., McCrae R.R. (1985) *The NEO Personality Inventory Manual.* Psychological Assessment Resources, Odessa.
12. Kass F., Skodol A.E., Charles E., Spitzer R.L., Williams J.B.W. (1985) Scaled ratings of DSM-III personality disorders. *Am. J. Psychiatry*, **143**: 627–630.
13. Hyler S., Lyons M. (1988) Factor analysis of the DSM-III personality disorder clusters: a replication. *Compr. Psychiatry*, **29**: 304–308.

14. Oldham J.M., Skodol A.E., Kellman H.D., Hyler S.E., Rosnick L., Davies M. (1992) Diagnosis of DSM-III-R personality disorders by two semistructured interviews: patterns of comorbidity. *Am. J. Psychiatry*, **149**: 213–220.
15. Tyrer P., Alexander J., Ferguson B. (1988) Personality Assessment Schedule. In *Personality Disorders: Diagnosis, Management and Course* (Ed. P. Tyrer), pp. 140–167. Butterworth/Wright, London.
16. Cloninger C.R. (1987) A systematic method for clinical description and classification of personality variants. *Arch. Gen. Psychiatry*, **44**: 573–588.
17. Cloninger C.R., Svrakic D.M., Pryzbeck T.R. (1993) A psychobiological model of temperament and character. *Arch. Gen. Psychiatry*, **50**: 975–990.
18. Watson D., Clark L.A. (1984) Negative affectivity: the disposition to experience aversive emotional states. *Psychol. Bull.*, **96**: 465–490.
19. Hassiotis A., Tyrer P., Cicchetti D. (1997) Detection of personality disorders by a community mental health team: a study of diagnostic accuracy. *Irish J. Psychol. Med.*, **14**: 88–91.
20. Coppen A.L., Metcalfe H. (1965) The effect of a depressive illness on MMPI scores. *Br. J. Psychiatry*, **111**: 236–239.
21. Clark L.A., Vittengl J., Kraft D., Jarrett R.B. (2003) Separate personality traits from states to predict depression. *J. Person. Disord.*, **17**: 152–172.
22. Clark L.A., Vittengl J.R., Kraft D., Jarrett R.B. (in press) Shared, not unique, components of personality and psychosocial functioning predict depression severity after acute-phase cognitive therapy. *J. Person. Disord.*
23. Tyrer P., Alexander J., Ferguson B. (2000) Personality Assessment Schedule. In: *Personality Disorders: Diagnosis, Management and Course* (Ed. P. Tyrer), pp. 132–159. Arnold, London.
24. Fogelson D.L., Nuechterlein K.H., Asarnow R.F., Payne D.L., Subotnik K.L., Giannini C.A. (1999) The factor structure of schizophrenia spectrum personality disorders: signs and symptoms in relatives of psychotic patients from the UCLA family members study. *Psychiatry Res.*, **87**: 137–146.
25. Millon T. (1969) *Modern Psychopathology: A Biosocial Approach to Maladaptive Learning and Functioning.* Saunders, Philadelphia.
26. Tyrer P., Fowler Dixon R., Ferguson B., Kelemen A. (1990) A plea for the diagnosis of hypochondriacal personality disorder. *J. Psychosom. Res.*, **34**: 637–642.
27. Gunderson J.G., Phillips K.A., Triebwasser J., Hirschfeld R.M. (1994) The Diagnostic Interview for Depressive Personality. *Am. J. Psychiatry*, **151**: 1300–1304.
28. Pfohl B., Blum N., Zimmerman M. (1997) *Structured Interview for DSM-IV Personality Disorders (SIDP-IV).* American Psychiatric Press, Washington.
29. Loranger A.W., Susman V.L., Oldham J.M., Russakoff L.M. (1987) *International Personality Disorder Examination (PDE). A Structured Interview for DSM-III-R and ICD-10 Personality Disorders. WHO/ADAMHA Version.* The New York Hospital, Cornell Medical Center, New York.
30. Loranger A.W., Lenzenweger M.F., Gartner A.F., Susman V.L., Herzig J., Zammit G.K., Gartner J.D., Abrams R.C., Young R.C. (1991) Trait-state artifacts and the diagnosis of personality disorders. *Arch. Gen. Psychiatry*, **48**: 720–728.
31. Tyrer P., Morgan J., Cicchetti D. (in press) The Dependent Personality Questionnaire (DPQ): a screening instrument for dependent personality. *Int. J. Soc. Psychiatry.*
32. Seivewright N. Personal communication.
33. Tyrer P., Johnson T. (1996) Establishing the severity of personality disorder. *Am. J. Psychiatry*, **153**: 1593–1597.

34. Drake R.E., Vaillant G.E. (1985) A validity study of Axis II of DSM-III. *Am. J. Psychiatry*, **142**: 553–558.

35. Casey P.R., Tyrer P.J. (1986) Personality, functioning and symptomatology. *J. Psychiatr. Res.*, **20**: 363–374.

36. Casey P. (1988) The epidemiology of personality disorder. In *Personality Disorders: Diagnosis, Management and Course* (Ed. P. Tyrer), pp. 74–81. Wright, London.

37. Black D.W., Noyes R., Pfohl B., Goldstein R.B., Blum N. (1993) Personality-disorder in obsessive–compulsive volunteers, well comparison subjects, and their 1st-degree relatives. *Am. J. Psychiatry*, **150**: 1226–1232.

38. Blanchard E.B., Hickling E.J., Taylor A.E., Loos W. (1995) Psychiatric morbidity associated with motor vehicle accidents. *J. Nerv. Ment. Dis.*, **183**: 495–504.

39. Maier W., Lichtermann D., Klinger T., Heun R. (1995) Prevalences of personality disorders (DSM-III-R) in the community. *J. Person. Disord.*, **6**: 187–196.

40. Torgersen S., Kringlen E., Cramer V. (2001) The prevalence of personality disorders in a community sample. *Arch. Gen. Psychiatry*, **58**: 590–596.

41. World Health Organization (1968) *ICD-9: Classification of Mental and Behavioural Disorders*. World Health Organization, Geneva.

42. World Health Organization (1992) *ICD-10: Classification of Mental and Behavioural Disorders*. World Health Organization, Geneva.

43. Cohen B.J., Nestadt G., Samuels J.F., Romanoski A.J., McHugh P.R., Rabins P.V. (1994) Personality disorder in later life: a community study. *Br. J. Psychiatry*, **165**: 493–499.

44. Loranger A.W. (1996) Dependent personality disorder. Age, sex, and axis I comorbidity. *J. Nerv. Ment. Dis.*, **184**: 17–21.

45. Seivewright H., Tyrer P., Johnson T. (2002) Change in personality status in neurotic disorders. *Lancet*, **359**: 2253–2254.

46. Bayer R., Spitzer R.L. (1985) Neurosis, psychodynamics and DSM-III: a history of the controversy. *Arch. Gen. Psychiatry*, **42**, 187–196.

47. Eysenck H.J. (1959) *The Maudsley Personality Inventory*. University of London Press, London.

48. Eysenck H.J., Eysenck S.B.G. (1964) *Manual of the Eysenck Personality Inventory*. University of London Press, London.

49. Eysenck H.J., Eysenck S.B.G. (1975) *The Eysenck Personality Questionnaire*. University of London Press, London.

50. Tellegen A. (1985) Structures of mood and personality and their relevance to assessing anxiety, with an emphasis on self report. In *Anxiety and the Anxiety Disorders* (Eds A.H. Tuema, J.D. Maser), pp. 681–706. Erlbaum, Hillsdale.

51. Duggan C., Milton J., Egan V., McCarthy I., Palmer B., Lee A. (2003) Theories of general personality and mental disorder. *Br. J. Psychiatry*, **182** (Suppl. 44): s19–s23.

52. Freud S. (1916) Some character types met with in psychoanalytic work. In *The Standard Edition of the Complete Psychological Works of Sigmund Freud, Vol. 14*, pp. 309–333. Hogarth Press, London.

53. Lyons M.J., Tyrer P., Gunderson J., Tohen M. (1997) Heuristic models of comorbidity of axis I and axis II disorders. *J. Person. Disord.*, **11**: 260–269.

54. Tyrer P. (1985) Neurosis divisible? *Lancet*, **i**, 685–688.

55. Andrews G., Stewart G., Morris-Yates A., Holt P., Henderson S. (1990) Evidence for a general neurotic syndrome. *Br. J. Psychiatry*, **157**: 6–12.

56. Tyrer P., Seivewright N., Ferguson B., Tyrer J. (1992) The general neurotic syndrome: a coaxial diagnosis of anxiety, depression and personality disorder. *Acta Psychiatr. Scand.*, **85**: 201–206.

57. Tyrer P. (1989) *Classification of Neurosis.* Wiley, Chichester.

58. Seivewright H., Tyrer P., Johnson T. (1998) Prediction of outcome in neurotic disorder: a five year prospective study. *Psychol. Med.,* **28**: 1149–1157.

59. Tyrer P., Seivewright H., Johnson T. (2003) The core elements of neurosis: mixed anxiety-depression (cothymia) and personality disorder. *J. Person. Disord.,* **17**: 109–118.

60. Lindesay J. (1991) Phobic disorders in the elderly. *Br. J. Psychiatry,* **159**: 531–541.

61. Larkin B.A., Copeland J.R.M., Dewey M.E., Davidson I.A., Saunders P.A., Sharma V.K., McWilliam C., Sullivan C. (1992) The natural history of neurotic disorder in an elderly urban population: findings from the Liverpool study of continuing health in the community. *Br. J. Psychiatry,* **160**: 681–686.

62. Boulenger J.P., Lavallee Y.J. (1993) Mixed anxiety and depression: diagnostic issues. *J. Clin. Psychiatry,* **54** (Suppl. 8), 3–8.

63. Roy M.A., Neale M.C., Pedersen N.L., Mathe A.A., Kendler K.S. (1995) A twin study of generalized anxiety disorder and major depression. *Psychol. Med.,* **25**: 1037–1049.

64. Shorter E., Tyrer P. (2003) The separation of anxiety and depressive disorders: blind alley in psychopharmacology and the classification of disease. *Br. Med. J.,* **327**: 158–160.

65. Herbert J.D., Hope D.A., Bellack A.S. (1992) Validity of the distinction between generalized social phobia and avoidant personality disorder. *J. Abnorm. Psychol.,* **101**: 332–339.

66. Sanderson W.C., Wetzler S., Beck A.T., Betz F. (1994) Prevalence of personality disorders among patients with anxiety disorders. *Psychiatry Res.,* **51**: 167–174.

67. Stein M.B., Fuetsch M., Muller N., Hofler M., Lieb R., Wittchen H.U. (2001) Social anxiety disorder and the risk of depression—A prospective community study of adolescents and young adults. *Arch. Gen. Psychiatry,* **58**: 251–256.

68. Kessler R.C. (2003) The impairments caused by social phobia in the general population: implications for intervention. *Acta Psychiatr. Scand.,* **108**: 19–27.

69. Ono Y., Yoshimura K., Sueoka R., Yamauchi K., Mizushima H., Momose T., Nakamura K., Okonogi K., Asai M. (1996) Avoidant personality disorder and taijin kyofu: sociocultural implications of the WHO/ADAMHA international study of personality disorders in Japan. *Acta Psychiatr. Scand.,* **93**: 172–176.

70. Dally P., Gomez J. (1979) *Anorexia Nervosa.* Heinemann, London.

71. Diaz-Marsa M., Carrasco J.L., Saiz J. (2000) A study of temperament and personality in anorexia and bulimia nervosa. *J. Person. Disord.,* **14**: 352–359.

72. Herzog D.B., Keller M.B., Lavori P.W., Kenny G.M., Sacks N.R. (1992) The prevalence of personality disorders in 210 women with eating disorders. *J. Clin. Psychiatry,* **53**: 147–152.

73. Fahy T.A., Eisler I., Russell G.F.M. (1993) Personality disorder and treatment response in bulimia nervosa. *Br. J. Psychiatry,* **162**: 765–770.

74. Skodol A.E., Oldham J.M., Hyler S.E., Kellman H.D., Doidge N., Davies M. (1993) Comorbidity of DSM-III-R eating disorders and personality disorders. *Int. J. Eat. Disord.,* **14**: 403–416.

75. Blashfield R., Noyes R., Reich J., Woodman C., Cook B.L., Garvey M.J. (1994) Personality disorder traits in generalized anxiety and panic disorder patients. *Compr. Psychiatry,* **35**: 329–334.

76. Noyes R. Jr., Woodman C.L., Holt C.S., Reich J.H., Zimmerman M.B. (1995) Avoidant personality traits distinguish social phobic and panic disorder subjects. *J. Nerv. Ment. Dis.,* **183**: 145–153.

77. Hoffart A., Thornes K., Hedley L.M. (1995) DSM-III-R Axis I and II disorders in agoraphobic inpatients with and without panic disorder before and after psychosocial treatment. *Psychiatry Res.*, **56**: 1–9.

78. Parker G., Roussos J., Austin M.P., Hadzi-Pavlovic D., Wilhelm K., Mitchell P. (1998) Disordered personality style: higher rates in non-melancholic compared to melancholic depression. *J. Affect. Disord.*, **47**: 131–140.

79. Fink P. (1995) Psychiatric illness in patients with persistent somatisation. *Br. J. Psychiatry*, **166**: 93–99.

80. Rost K.M., Akins R.N., Brown F.W., Smith G.R. (1992) The comorbidity of DSM-III-R personality disorders in somatization disorder. *Gen. Hosp. Psychiatry*, **14**: 322–326.

81. Stern J., Murphy M., Bass C. (1993) Personality disorders in patients with somatisation disorder: a controlled study. *Br. J. Psychiatry*, **163**: 785–789.

82. Barsky A.J., Wyshak G., Klerman G.L. (1992) Psychiatric comorbidity in DSM-III-R hypochondriasis. *Arch. Gen. Psychiatry*, **49**: 101–108.

83. Andrews G., Tennant C. (1978) Life event stress and psychiatric illness. *Psychol. Med.*, **8**: 545–549.

84. Seivewright N. (1987) Relationship between life events and personality in psychiatric disorder. *Stress Med.*, **3**: 163–168.

85. Seivewright N. (1988) Personality disorder, life events and onset of mental illness. In *Personality Disorders: Diagnosis, Management and Course* (Ed. P. Tyrer), pp. 82–92. Butterworth, London.

86. Poulton R.G., Andrews G. (1992) Personality as a cause of adverse life events. *Acta Psychiatr. Scand.*, **85**: 35–38.

87. Gray N.S., Carman N.G., Rogers P., MacCulloch M.J., Hayward P., Snowden R.J. (2003) Post-traumatic stress disorder caused in mentally disordered offenders by the committing of a serious violent or sexual offence. *J. Forensic Psychiatry Psychol.*, **14**: 27–43.

88. Tyrer P., Seivewright N., Ferguson B., Murphy S., Darling C., Brothwell J., Kingdon D., Johnson A.L. (1990) The Nottingham Study of Neurotic Disorder: relationship between personality status and symptoms. *Psychol. Med.*, **20**: 423–431.

89. Tyrer P., Gunderson J., Lyons M., Tohen M. (1997) Extent of comorbidity between mental state and personality disorders. *J. Person. Disord.*, **11**: 242–259.

90. Boone M.L., McNeil D.W., Masia C.L., Turk C.L., Carter L.E., Ries B.J., Lewin M.R. (1999) Multimodal comparisons of social phobia subtypes and avoidant personality disorder. *J. Anxiety Disord.*, **13**: 271–292.

91. Kendler K.S., McGuire M., Gruenberg A.M., O'Hare A., Spellman M., Walsh D. (1993) The Roscommon Family Study. III. Schizophrenia-related personality disorders in relatives. *Arch. Gen. Psychiatry*, **50**: 781–788.

92. Clark L.A., Harrison J.A. (2001) Assessment instruments. In *Handbook of Personality Disorders: Theory, Research and Treatment* (Ed. W.J. Livesley), pp. 277–306. Guilford, New York.

93. Tyrer P. (1999) Borderline personality disorder: a motley diagnosis in need of reform. *Lancet*, **354**: 2095–2096.

94. Shawcross C.R., Tyrer P. (1985) Influence of personality on response to monoamine oxidase inhibitors and tricyclic antidepressants. *J. Psychiatr. Res.*, **19**: 557–562.

95. Parker G., Roy K., Wilhelm K., Mitchell P. (2000) 'Acting out' and 'acting in' behavioural stress responses: the relevance of anxiety and personality style. *J. Affect. Disord.*, **57**: 173–177.

96. Ansseau M., Troisfontaines B., Papart P., Von Frenckell R. (1991) Compulsive personality as predictor of response to serotonergic antidepressants. *Br. Med. J.*, **303**: 760–761.
97. Sargant W. (1966) Psychiatric treatment in general teaching hospitals: a plea for a mechanistic approach. *Br. Med. J.*, **2**: 257–262.
98. Shea M.T., Widiger T.A., Klein M.H. (1992) Comorbidity of personality disorders and depression: implications for treatment. *J. Consult. Clin. Psychol.*, **60**: 857–868.
99. Diguer L., Barber J.P., Luborsky L. (1993) Three concomitants: personality disorders, psychiatric severity, and outcome of dynamic psychotherapy of major depression. *Am. J. Psychiatry*, **150**: 1246–1248.
100. Piper W.E., Joyce A.S., Azim H.F., Rosie J.S. (1994) Patient characteristics and success in day treatment. *J. Nerv. Ment. Dis.*, **182**, 381–386.
101. Tyrer P., Merson S., Onyett S., Johnson T. (1994) The effect of personality disorder on clinical outcome, social networks and adjustment: a controlled clinical trial of psychiatric emergencies. *Psychol. Med.*, **24**: 731–740.
102. Viinamaki H., Hintikka J., Honkalampi K., Koivumaa-Honkanen H., Kuisma S., Antikainen R., Tanskanen A., Lehtonen J. (2002) Cluster C personality disorder impedes alleviation of symptoms in major depression. *J. Affect. Disord.*, **71**: 35–41.
103. Hardy G.E., Barkham M., Shapiro D.A., Stiles W.B., Rees A., Reynolds S. (1995) Impact of Cluster C personality disorders on outcomes of contrasting brief psychotherapies for depression. *J. Consult. Clin. Psychol.*, **63**: 997–1004.
104. Mulder R.T. (2002) Personality pathology and treatment outcome in major depression: a review. *Am. J. Psychiatry*, **159**: 359–371.
105. Cloninger C.R. (1987) *Tridimensional Personality Questionnaire (TPQ)*. Department of Psychiatry and Genetics, Washington University School of Medicine, St. Louis.
106. Newton-Howes G., Tyrer P., Johnson T. Association between personality disorder and the outcome of depression: a meta-analysis of studies. Submitted for publication.
107. Delito J.A., Stam M. (1989) Psychopharmacological treatment of avoidant personality disorder. *Compr. Psychiatry*, **30**: 498–504.
108. Fahlen T. (1995) Personality traits in social phobia, II: Changes during drug treatment. *J. Clin. Psychiatry*, **56**: 569–573.
109. Ekselius L., von Knorring L. (1998) Personality disorder comorbidity with major depression and response to treatment with sertraline or citalopram. *Int. Clin. Psychopharmacol.*, **13**: 205–211.
110. Ekselius L., von Knorring L. (1999) Changes in personality status during treatment with sertraline or citalopram. *Br. J. Psychiatry*, **174**: 444–448.
111. Tyrer P., Seivewright N., Ferguson B., Murphy S., Johnson A.L. (1993) The Nottingham Study of Neurotic Disorder: effect of personality status on response to drug treatment, cognitive therapy and self help over three years. *Br. J. Psychiatry*, **162**: 219–226.
112. Karterud S., Vaglum S., Friis S., Irion T., Johns S., Vaglum P. (1992) Day hospital therapeutic-community treatment for patients with personality-disorders: an empirical-evaluation of the containment function. *J. Nerv. Ment. Dis.*, **180**: 238–243.
113. Gude T., Monsen J.T., Hoffart A. (2001) Schemas, affect consciousness, and Cluster C personality pathology: a prospective one-year follow-up study of patients in a schema-focused short-term treatment program. *Psychother. Res.*, **11**: 85–98.

114. Tyrer P. (2002) Nidotherapy: a new approach to the treatment of personality disorder. *Acta Psychiatr. Scand.*, **105**: 469–471.
115. Tyrer P. (2003) Nidotherapy as a treatment strategy in stress. *Stress and Health*, **19**: 127–128.
116. Beck A.T., Freeman A. (1990) *Cognitive Therapy of Personality Disorders*. Guilford, New York.
117. Tyrer P., Mitchard S., Methuen C., Ranger M. (2003) Treatment-rejecting and treatment-seeking personality disorders: Type R and Type S. *J. Person. Disord.*, **17**: 265–270.
118. Seivewright N., Tyrer P., Ferguson B., Murphy S., North B., Johnson T. (2000) Longitudinal study of the influence of life events and personality status on diagnostic change in three neurotic disorders. *Depress. Anxiety*, **11**: 105–113.
119. Seivewright H., Tyrer P., Johnson T. (in press) Persistent social dysfunction in anxious and depressed patients with personality disorder. *Acta Psychiatr. Scand.*
120. Tyrer P. (2001) The case for cothymia: mixed anxiety and depression as a single diagnosis. *Br. J. Psychiatry*, **179**: 191–193.
121. Livesley W.J. (1998) Suggestions for a framework for an empirically based classification of personality disorder. *Can. J. Psychiatry*, **43**: 137–147.
122. Livesley W.J., Jang K.L., Jackson D.N., Vernon P.A. (1993) Genetic and environmental contributions to dimensions of personality disorder. *Am. J. Psychiatry*, **150**: 1826–1831.
123. Kendell R.E. (1989) Clinical validity. *Psychol. Med.*, **19**: 45–55.
124. Kendell R.E. (2002) The distinction between personality disorder and mental illness. *Br. J. Psychiatry*, **180**: 110–115.
125. Tyrer P., Silk K. (2003) The diagnostic validity of personality disorders. In *Abstracts Book of the 8th International Society for the Study of Personality Disorders Congress*, pp. 6–7. Scaramuzzi, Florence.
126. Laasonen-Balk T., Viinamaki H., Kuikka J., Husso-Saastamoinen M., Lehtonen J., Halonen P., Tiihonen J. (2001) Cluster C personality disorder has no independent effect on striatal dopamine transporter densities in major depression. *Psychopharmacology*, **155**: 113–114.

Commentaries

5.1
Theory, Contexts, Prototypes and Subtypes
Theodore Millon[1]

The prevalence and chronicity of the anxiety cluster, be they clinical syndromes or personality disorders, attests to their significance as major and pervasive human conditions. Peter Tyrer's comprehensive survey well illustrates the diversity and empirical grounding of these impairments.

I should like to comment on three aspects of our thinking—the value of theory, the role of sociocultural contexts, and the need to employ the concepts of prototypes and subtypes—that are only tangentially discussed in Tyrer's authoritative review.

No one should argue against the view that theories that float, so to speak, on their own, unconcerned with the empirical domain, should be seen as the fatuous achievements they are. However, even a reasonable speculative framework can be a compelling instrument for helping coordinate and give consonance to complex and diverse observations. By probing beneath surface impressions to inner or hidden processes, previously isolated facts and difficult to fathom data may yield new relationships and expose clearer meanings. Progress does not advance by "brute empiricism" alone, that is, by merely piling up more descriptive and more experimental data. What is elaborated and refined in theory is understanding—an ability to see relations more plainly, to conceptualize categories more accurately, and to create greater overall coherence in a subject, that is, to integrate its elements in a more logical, consistent, and intelligible fashion.

The value systems and nosological schemas generated in Western societies, such as seen in the ICD and the DSM, reflect particular models of thought that may be at variance with numerous cultures and subcultures around the world. The perspectives of Western and Eurocentric schemas are oriented to the patient's personal experiences and, secondly, are grounded in an infectious disease model, one driven by contemporary biomedical technologies and, more particularly, that of pharmacologic therapies. These perspectives contrast with many cultural orientations that are

---

[1] *Institute for Advanced Studies in Personology and Psychopathology, 5400 Fairchild Way, Coral Gables, FL 33156, USA*

centred more on social and relational contexts, as well as interpersonal methods of intervention that reflect humane and preventive public health systems [1].

Prototypes are a relatively recent diagnostic innovation; they are neither categorical nor dimensional, but a synthesis of both. Prototypal conceptions should become the preferred schema for representing not only personality disorders, but also clinical syndromes. Most advocates of the dimensional approach to clinical practice choose to overlook the fact that the concept of "categories" is used very loosely in the DSM and ICD. The prototype construct explicitly recognizes the heterogeneity of patients; most patients meet criteria for several clinical syndromes and may have significant features of a number of personalities, as well. Indeed, the problems imputed to categorical models largely evaporate when categories are conceived as prototypes, given that they do not employ discrete boundaries [2]. Horowitz *et al.* [3] describe the construct succinctly: "A prototype consists of the most common features or properties of members of a category and thus describes a theoretical ideal or standard against which real people can be evaluated. All of the prototype's properties are assumed to characterize at least some members of the category, but no one property is necessary or sufficient for membership in the category.... Different people approximate it to different degrees. The more closely a person approximates the ideal, the more closely the person typifies the concept".

Each theoretically-generated prototype can serve usefully as a conceptually relevant anchoring point, a logically rational and cohesive framework of descriptors around which clinically realistic variants take form. Numerous variants are encountered in clinical work which give evidence of the core features of each prototype. These variants or subtypes differ to some degree and in certain of their particulars, e.g. not all tables are rectangular or have four legs, though the construct "table" is well understood as distinct from a chair or a lamp. In a like manner, the prototype "avoidant personality" comprises consensually agreed upon descriptive clinical features, whatever the theoretical schema is from which it was derived. The widely publicized categorical versus dimensional debate may, in part, be resolved by identifying the numerous subtype variants that exist among each prototypal personality disorder.

Which set of theoretical constructs should be employed to formulate the prototypes of the anxious cluster remains an issue for future research and scholarly thought. Only further work will tell whether a five-factor model, based on a lexical approach to descriptors [4,5], Cloninger's dimensional schema, derived from ostensive neurobiologic substrates [6], Freud's intrapsychic model, grounded in conflicts among the mind's fundamental structures [7], or Millon's evolutionary model, framed in terms of survival and adaptational polarities [8], will prove most fruitful and enduring.

REFERENCES

1. Alarcón R.D., Foulks E.F., Vakkur M. (1998) *Personality Disorders and Culture. Clinical and Conceptual Interactions.* Wiley, New York.
2. Cantor N., Genero N. (1986) Psychiatric diagnosis and natural categorization: a close analogy. In *Contemporary Directions in Psychopathology. Towards the DSM-IV* (Eds T. Millon, G.L. Klerman), pp. 233–256. Guilford, New York.
3. Horowitz L.M., Post D.L., French R. de S., Wallis K.D., Siegelman E.Y. (1981) The prototype as a construct in abnormal psychology: 2. Clarifying disagreement in psychiatric judgments. *J. Abnorm. Psychol.*, **90**: 575–585.
4. Davis R., Millon T. (1993) The five-factor model for personality disorders: apt or misguided? *Psychol. Inquiry*, **4**: 104–110.
5. Widiger T.A., Trull T.J., Clarkin J.F., Sanderson C., Costa P.T. (1994) A description of the DSM-IV personality disorders within the five-factor model of personality. In *Personality Disorders and the Five-Factor Model of Personality* (Eds P.T. Costa Jr., T.A. Widiger), pp. 89–99. American Psychological Association, Washington.
6. Cloninger C.R., Svrakic D.M., Przybeck T.R. (1993) A psychobiological model of temperament and character. *Arch. Gen. Psychiatry*, **50**: 975–990.
7. Freud S. (1931/1950) Libidinal types. In *Collected Papers, Vol. 5*. Hogarth, London.
8. Millon T. (1990) *Toward a New Personology: An Evolutionary Model*. Wiley, New York.

5.2
Anxious Cluster Personality Disorders: Perspectives from the Collaborative Longitudinal Personality Disorders Study

Andrew E. Skodol[1]

Tyrer's chapter on anxious cluster personality disorders (PDs) raises interesting and important questions about cluster membership, reliability of diagnosis, consistency of criteria sets, comorbidity, stability of disorders over time, relationship to normal personality traits, and clinical significance, among others. The National Institute of Mental Health (NIMH)-supported Collaborative Longitudinal Personality Disorders Study (CLPS) [1] sheds light on all of these issues for two putative Cluster C disorders: avoidant personality disorder (AVPD) and obsessive-compulsive personality disorder (OCPD).

Cluster membership. Confirmatory factor analysis of DSM-IV diagnostic criteria obtained from semi-structured intake interviews of 668 patients with schizotypal personality disorder (STPD), borderline personality disorder

[1] *Department of Personality Studies, New York State Psychiatric Institute, 1051 Riverside Drive, New York, NY 10032, USA*

(BPD), AVPD, or OCPD, or with major depressive disorder (MDD) and no PD, showed that OCPD was separable from AVPD. A four-factor "disorder model" was more strongly supported than a three-factor "cluster model", both at intake and at blinded follow-up interviews two years later [2].

Reliability of diagnosis. Interrater (IR) and test-retest (TRT) reliabilities (kappas) respectively were as follows: AVPD, IR = 0.68, TRT = 0.73; OCPD, IR = 0.71, TRT = 0.74 [3]. Both disorders were diagnosed at or above the median for all PDs according to each type of reliability.

Internal consistency of criteria. Internal consistency (Cronbach's alpha) of criteria for AVPD was 0.83 and for OCPD was 0.69 [4]. Coefficient alpha for AVPD was higher than the median for all PDs, but for OCPD was lower than the median.

Comorbidity. Lifetime social phobia was found to co-occur significantly with AVPD (compared to other PDs); no lifetime Axis I disorder was found to co-occur significantly with OCPD. Antisocial PD was diagnosed at a significantly *lower* rate in patients with OCPD; no Axis II disorder was diagnosed more or less frequently in patients with AVPD [5].

Stability over time. Although most patients with PDs did not remain at full criteria for their disorders every month of a one-year follow-up period, more patients with AVPD (56%) remained at full criteria than did patients in any of the three other CLPS PD groups. OCPD (42%) had the second highest stability rate [6]. On blinded re-interview at two-year follow-up, kappas for agreement with baseline diagnosis, adjusted for rater reliability, were 0.53 for AVPD and 0.51 for OCPD. These stability rates were similar to those for the other two study PDs. "Remission" rates, defined as falling to 2 or fewer criteria for 12 consecutive months over the two-year period, were 31% for AVPD and 38% for OCPD. These rates were not significantly different from the other PD groups [7].

Relationship to normal personality traits. Patients with AVPD and OCPD were characterized by higher levels of neuroticism than were community controls, but OCPD had lower levels than other PDs, including AVPD. AVPD was characterized by more introversion than community controls and other PDs. Patients with AVPD had lower levels of conscientiousness than community controls, but not lower than patients with other PDs. Patients with OCPD had lower levels of agreeableness than community subjects, but not lower than patients with other PDs, and higher levels of conscientiousness than other PDs, but marginally lower levels than persons in the community [8].

Clinical significance. Patients with OCPD experienced less functional impairment in work, social relationships, leisure, and global functioning than did patients with severe PDs, such as STPD or BPD. Patients with AVPD experienced levels of impairment in between those of patients with severe PDs and those with OCPD [9]. Patients with OCPD were more likely to have received individual psychotherapy than were patients with MDD and no PD during their lives, but not other psychosocial or psycho-pharmacological treatments. They received fewer months of individual psychotherapy than patients with BPD, however. Patients with AVPD were no more (or less) likely than depressed patients to receive any particular type of treatment, but they received more months of group psychotherapy [10].

Conclusions. From the perspective of the CLPS, AVPD and OCPD appear to be distinct PDs, which represent reasonably coherent constructs that can be reliably diagnosed. Neither disorder is as stable over time as the DSM construct of a PD would imply, but both have more trait-based criteria and are more stable than other PDs. Both disorders have a complex relationship to normal personality traits, and AVPD may have a special relationship to social phobia, suggesting a common underlying endophenotype. OCPD is the least impairing Cluster C disorder, yet it leads to considerable amounts of individual treatment; AVPD is associated with more impairment, but not to the extent of severe Cluster A or B PDs. Cluster C PDs are probably the least studied and much more research is needed before they can be optimally defined and their impact fully understood.

REFERENCES

1. Gunderson J.G., Shea M.T., Skodol A.E., McGlashan T.H., Morey L.C., Stout R.L., Zanarini M.C., Grilo C.M., Oldham J.M., Keller M.B. (2000) The Collaborative Longitudinal Personality Disorders Study: development, aims, design, and sample characteristics. *J. Person. Disord.*, **14**: 300–315.
2. Sanislow C.A., Morey L.C., Grilo C.M., Gunderson J.G., Shea M.T., Skodol A.E., Stout R.L., Zanarini M.C., McGlashan T.H. (2002) Confirmatory factor analysis of DSM-IV borderline, schizotypal, avoidant and obsessive-compulsive person-ality disorders: findings from the Collaborative Longitudinal Personality Disorders Study. *Acta Psychiatr. Scand.*, **105**: 28–36.
3. Zanarini M.C., Skodol A.E., Bender D., Dolan R., Sanislow C., Schaefer E., Morey L.C., Grilo C.M., Shea M.T., McGlashan T.H. *et al.* (2000) The Collaborative Longitudinal Personality Disorders Study: reliability of Axis I and II diagnoses. *J. Person. Disord.*, **14**: 291–299.
4. Grilo C.M., McGlashan T.H., Morey L.C., Gunderson J.G., Skodol A.E., Shea M.T., Sanislow C.A., Zanarini M.C., Bender D., Oldham J.M. *et al.* (2001) Internal consistency, intercriterion overlap and diagnostic efficiency of criteria sets for DSM-IV schizotypal, borderline, avoidant and obsessive-compulsive personality disorders. *Acta Psychiatr. Scand.*, **104**: 264–272.
5. McGlashan T.H., Grilo C.M., Skodol A.E., Gunderson J.G., Shea M.T., Morey L.C., Zanarini M.C., Stout R.L. (2000) The Collaborative Longitudinal Person-ality Disorders Study: baseline Axis I/II and II/II diagnostic co-occurrence. *Acta Psychiatr. Scand.*, **102**: 256–264.
6. Shea M.T., Stout R.L., Gunderson J.G., Morey L.C., Grilo C.M., McGlashan T.H., Skodol A.E., Dolan-Sewell R.T., Dyck I.R., Zanarini M.C. *et al.* (2002) Short-term diagnostic stability of schizotypal, borderline, avoidant, and obsessive-compul-sive personality disorders. *Am. J. Psychiatry*, **159**: 2036–2041.

7. Grilo C.M., Shea M.T., Sanislow C.A., Skodol A.E., Gunderson J.G., Stout R.L., Pagano M.E., Yen S., Morey L.C., Zanarini M.C. *et al.* (in press) Two-year stability and change in schizotypal, borderline, avoidant and obsessive-compulsive personality disorders. *J. Consult. Clin. Psychol.*
8. Morey L.C., Gunderson J.G., Quigley B.D., Shea M.T., Skodol A.E., McGlashan T.H., Stout R.L., Zanarini M.C. (2002) The representation of borderline, avoidant, obsessive-compulsive, and schizotypal personality disorders by the five-factor model. *J. Person. Disord.*, **16**: 215–234.
9. Skodol A.E., Gunderson J.G., McGlashan T.H., Dyck I.R., Stout R.L., Bender D.S., Grilo C.M., Shea M.T., Zanarini M.C., Morey L.C. *et al.* (2002) Functional impairment in patients with schizotypal, borderline, avoidant, or obsessive-compulsive personality disorder. *Am. J. Psychiatry*, **159**: 276–283.
10. Bender D.S., Dolan R.T., Skodol A.E., Sanislow C.A., Dyck I.R., McGlashan T.H, Shea M.T., Zanarini M.C., Oldham J.M., Gunderson J.G. (2001) Treatment utilization by patients with personality disorders. *Am. J. Psychiatry*, **158**: 295–302.

5.3
Personality in Anxiety Disorders
Matig R. Mavissakalian[1]

Clinical reality supports Tyrer's notion of a general neurotic syndrome and the need to "lump" sooner or later. Lumping at the level of a functional phenomenology appears to be preferable, due to the parsimony that a syndromal conceptualization provides, compared to lumping artificially created myriad morbidities as comorbidities or spectra of disorders. Indeed, the so-called comorbidity is the rule rather than the exception between DSM anxiety disorders, depression and some personality disorders (PDs), especially but not exclusively from the anxious cluster. Further, the generalized effectiveness of exposure based cognitive behavioural treatments, serotonergic antidepressants and, with rare exceptions, benzo-diazepines—which transcends DSM Axis I and II anxiety categories—is consistent with the syndromal approach as a clinically valid conceptual framework for practice and for inquiry of psychopathological dimensions and pathophysiological processes.

In a series of articles, my colleagues and I explored the relationship and the specificity of the link between personality and panic disorder with agoraphobia (PAD/AG), obsessive-compulsive disorder (OCD) and general-ized anxiety disorder (GAD), using the Personality Diagnostic Questionnaire (PDQ) [1], a self rating questionnaire of 163 true or false items designed to

[1] *Case Western Reserve University, Anxiety Disorders Program, University Hospitals of Cleveland, 11100 Euclid Avenue, Cleveland, OH 44106, USA*

assess the eleven PDs from Axis II of the DSM-III. Three variables were derived from the PDQ: a diagnosis for each of the disorders, the presence or absence of each personality trait irrespective of diagnostic category and a personality profile obtained by calculating the percentage of items endorsed within each PD category.

We found that the personality profiles of PAD/AG, OCD and GAD samples had a similar composition and that the major features identified—namely avoidant, dependent and histrionic dimensions—were more pronounced in patients with OCD [2]. The greater personality dysfunction in OCD was generalized and not limited to a specific PD, such as compulsive PD. Moreover, whereas avoidant characteristics did not significantly differ between the diagnostic groups, dependent characteristics were highest in OCD, lowest in GAD and intermediate in PAD/AG. Because GAD lacks the prominent phobic, panic and obsessive-compulsive symptoms, the overwhelming similarities pointed to a common personality profile in these anxiety disorders. The generalized greater personality dysfunction in OCD and the more pronounced dependent features in PAD/AG were thought to reflect level of interference with daily activities, which is usually highest in OCD and higher in PAD/AG than GAD.

Stepwise regression analyses were conducted separately in each of these diagnostic groups [3–5] and supported the hypothesis of a nonspecific link between PD traits or characteristics and anxiety disorders. In all instances, the most important correlates of personality traits in general and of specific clusters or PD dimensions consisted of dysphoria/depression and the interpersonal sensitivity scale of the Hopkins Symptoms Checklist and Neuroticism (PAD/AG and GAD samples only) rather than duration or severity of anxiety, panic, phobic or obsessive-compulsive symptoms. Further analysis in GAD [5] revealed that four personality traits, each from a separate Axis II disorder, were consistently associated with dysphoria and interpersonal sensitivity: social withdrawal from avoidant, lacks self-confidence from dependent, feeling empty and bored from borderline and undue social anxiety from schizotypal. It was suggested that in anxiety disorders, personality disorder in the sense of serious interpersonal dysfunction and unhappiness is most likely to occur when a cluster of traits from those depicted above accompany an avoidant personality style.

Interestingly, a study of PAD/AG patients in stable and marked remission led to the same conclusion [6]. Although such an approach might not have eliminated the impact of having been ill, it was thought to represent the best possible characterization of enduring personality features in clinical samples. There was an impressive stability of the personality profiles during remission. Secondly, the personality profile was predominated by avoidant PD traits. Finally, although overall personality functioning, as measured by general PDQ measures, resembled normative samples, the remitted patients' endorsements of eight individual PDQ items were consistently more like the response of symptomatic panic disorder patients than normal controls: (a) I often act very emotional when little things go wrong (histrionic); (b) Criticism often makes me feel ashamed, inferior, or humiliated (narcissistic); (c) I often get so angry that I lose control (borderline); (d) I often feel rejected (avoidant); (e) I am overly critical of myself (avoidant); (f) I am often unsure of myself (dependent); (g) It takes me too long to make decisions (compulsive); (h) I often feel that people push me around (passive aggressive).

Thus, even during stable and virtually symptom-free remitted states, PD/AG patients see themselves as unassertive, indecisive, self critical and as emotional individuals who are easily frustrated and feel rejected when criticized. Now, one can talk of avoidant PD, cluster C and comorbidity between these and cluster B disorders, but these enduring characteristics fit closely the description of the neurotic personality that can be found, as Tyrer says, in old textbooks and which may well be the most basic clinical manifestation of a temperamental and perhaps constitutionally based proneness to anxiety and depression.

REFERENCES

1. Hyler S.E., Rieder R.O., Spitzer R.L., Williams J.B. (1983) *Personality Diagnostic Questionnaire (PDQ)*. New York State Psychiatric Institute, New York.
2. Mavissakalian M.R., Hamann M.S., Haider S.A., deGroot C.M. (1993) DSM-III personality disorders in generalized anxiety, panic/agoraphobia, and obsessive compulsive disorders. *Compr. Psychiatry*, **34**: 243–248.
3. Mavissakalian M., Hamann M.S. (1988) Correlates of DSM-III personality disorder in panic disorder with agoraphobia. *Compr. Psychiatry*, **29**: 535–544.
4. Mavissakalian M., Hamann M.S., Jones B. (1990) Correlates of DSM-III personality disorder in obsessive-compulsive disorder. *Compr. Psychiatry*, **31**: 481–489.
5. Mavissakalian M.R., Hamann M.S., Haidar S.A., deGroot C.M. (1995) Correlates of DSM-III personality disorder in generalized anxiety disorder. *J. Anxiety Disord.*, **9**: 103–115.
6. Mavissakalian M.R., Hamann M.S. (1992) DSM-III personality characteristics of panic disorder with agoraphobia patients in stable remission. *Compr. Psychiatry*, **33**: 305–309.

5.4
"Minima Moralia" on Cluster C Personality Disorders

Carlo Faravelli[1]

Peter Tyrer's review of cluster C is comprehensive and full of constructive critical remarks. His starting point "there's nothing new under the sun" is justified by his view that there is a continuity between the old paradigm of neurosis and the present anxious cluster of personality disorders. In his conclusions, Tyrer contends that "the anxious cluster is deficient under several respects" and that there is a strong argument for promoting the abolition of Axis II disorders, with their substitution with traits or dispositions (here again nothing new under the sun). I would like to propose a few comments on Tyrer's paper, going a little further on the way of criticism.

Operational diagnostic systems obviously focus on diagnostic criteria, i.e. those features which delimit the disorders and make them different from the others. Diagnostic criteria are aimed at distinguishing, not at describing. The characteristics that are common to groups of disorders are less emphasized (if not ignored) by definition. This notwithstanding, the usual inappropriate habit of considering diagnostic criteria as an exhaustive description of a disorder is supported even by most present textbooks.

In pre-DSM-III psychiatry, the descriptions of mental disorders contained: (a) a general definition, (b) the description of premorbid personality, (c) the typical symptoms and their course, (d) the short- and long-term outcome, (e) the differential diagnoses, as well as (f) other relevant information. For neuroses, the general definition was "a *quantitative* alteration of otherwise normal aspects of psychic life, such as anxiety, fears, etc." (psychoses were defined as *qualitative* abnormalities). The concept of continuity between normality and neurosis was clearly implicit in the definition. Furthermore, in the classical description of neuroses, the central, most prominent feature, to which the greatest emphasis was given, was the enduring attitude of anxiety, indecision, fear, insecurity, hypochondriasis, etc. (referred to as personality, traits, attitudes or other). Single, specific symptoms were not emphasized. In no other area as in that of neuroses the distinction between personality and symptoms was so weak and in no other disorder or group of disorders personality characteristics were given such a high priority.

In the debate "splitters vs. lumpers" mentioned by Tyrer, the former clearly won the battle for anxiety, whereas the latter had the best in the field of depression. The result is that on the one hand we have a DSM-IV diagnosis of major depressive episode which is highly criticised for being

---

[1] Chair of Psychiatry, University Medical School, Florence, Italy

excessively heterogeneous, while, on the other, there is a group of several anxiety disorders characterized by an impressive degree of overlap and comorbidity with each other, and yet lacking an unitary concept. Axis II has obviously followed the same route, so that we have now three anxiety personality disorders that clearly mimic their senior brothers.

In the continuum from normal to pathological that characterizes this group of personality disorders, the epidemiological rates rely heavily on the threshold chosen for defining the pathological level. Minor changes in the recognition threshold may induce large variations in the prevalence figures. In this respect, the distinction between "normal" and "pathological" is probably mainly based on the criterion C of the general diagnostic criteria for personality disorders ("significant distress or impairment in social, occupational, or other important areas of functioning"). It should not be neglected, however, that social/occupational distress/impairment is heavily dependent on the social and cultural context where the subject lives. In a highly competitive society, being insecure, passive, reluctant to fight, is a disadvantage for getting a socially prominent position, but in other cultures these attitudes may even be appropriate and adaptive.

Cluster C personality disorders often fail to meet criteria B ("the enduring pattern is inflexible and pervasive"), D ("stable and of long duration") and perhaps E ("not better accounted for as a manifestation or consequence of another disorder") of the general diagnostic criteria for personality disorders. In fact, as Tyrer points out, they are changeable and subject to improvement following treatment.

Cluster C personality disorders are: (a) clinically not distinguishable from their corresponding Axis I disorders if not for their supposed (but not certain) milder severity and their usually (but not always) longer duration; (b) responsive to treatment. Moreover, it is a common experience, even if scarcely documented in the literature, that people with enduring "personality" anxious features at one point in their lives develop a full anxiety disorder for which they are treated. Quite often they not only recover from their Axis I disorder, but their premorbid functioning level is also improved. All this seems clearly to support the hypothesis that the so-called personality pattern is made up of mild chronic symptoms.

Among the possible interpretations of the relationship between Axis I and Axis II anxiety, Tyrer seems to favour Clark's concept of diathesis. Diathesis is an old medical concept, very fashionable one century ago, that combines predisposition and constitution. There are other grossly equivalent models, not to count those emphasizing the role of early (childhood) relationships. Now the question is: is such a distinction between predisposing factors and overt symptoms necessary? Or is it simply the inheritance of (or, the compromise with) those positions (originally psychodynamic) that conceive psychiatric disorders as descending from something already written in the personality? The equivalent phenomenon of an alteration that stays in between normality and illness, and is likely both to worsen (thus becoming an illness) and to lead to other diseases is common in medicine (e.g. hypertension, hypercholesterolemia). No particularly sophisticated theory is required to explain it.

The outcome of these reflections is a strong doubt on the usefulness of the paradigm of personality disorders for clinical psychiatry. The hypothesis of combining Axis I and Axis II into a single Axis could be taken into consideration in order to obtain stronger prototypes. One could also question whether the concept itself of personality is useful in psychiatry or represents an unnecessary complication.

5.5
Anxious Cluster Personality Disorders and Axis I Anxiety Disorders: Comments on the Comorbidity Issue

M. Tracie Shea[1]

Peter Tyrer's review of the anxious cluster of personality disorders touches upon many of the vexing issues confronting personality disorder classification and research more broadly. Central to many of these issues is the problem of diagnostic overlap, including with other personality disorders and with Axis I disorders, particularly anxiety and depressive disorders. Tyrer notes that the boundaries of the anxious cluster of personality disorders "... are not as clear as they should be..." and that "it is often difficult to separate Axis I and Axis II". This commentary will expand upon some of the overlap issues.

One issue concerns the influence of mental state on personality assessment. It has been argued that the presence of a depressed or anxious state may result in inaccurate assessments, in the direction of elevated psychopathology or false positive diagnoses. Tyrer considers whether what has been assumed to be a distortion may rather be a real phenomenon—personality may in fact be influenced by the mental state. The term "state" effect has been used in different ways and it may be helpful to consider the multiple ways that current mental state may (or may not) influence findings and their interpretations. One finding that is reasonably consistent is that when depressed, many individuals report their "usual self" differently than when they are not depressed. Reporting higher levels of neuroticism when

[1] Department of Psychiatry and Human Behavior, Brown University Medical School, Veterans Affairs Medical Center, Providence, RI, USA

depressed is a strong predictor of course, and in that sense it is a "real" and clinically meaningful phenomenon, whether or not the reported levels are consistent with the actual premorbid levels. However, if the goal is to determine "true" cases of high neuroticism (or personality disorders), then the influence of current mental state may result in false positives. This can lead to erroneous conclusions about the influence of treatments, for example, on personality traits or disorders. It may be that the level of personality psychopathology at the end of treatment is actually the same as it was prior to the depressed (or anxious) state, rather than an "improvement" from what was (erroneously) reported at the start of treatment.

With regard to the overlap with Axis I disorders, one of the features believed to distinguish between Axis I and II disorders is stability over time: personality disorders should be stable over time, in contrast to Axis I disorders, which may be variable in duration and have generally been considered more "episodic". As noted in this book's commentary by Skodol, findings from the Collaborative Longitudinal Personality Study (CLPS) [1,2] have shown that the four personality disorders being followed are less diagnostically stable than the definition of personality disorder implies. Recently, we [3] compared the stability findings for the CLPS personality disorders, including the two Cluster C disorders of avoidant and obsessive-compulsive, with published findings from studies of depressive and anxiety disorders that used similar methodology. Based on the same definition of "remission" (minimum of two consecutive months with minimal or no symptoms/criteria), four of the five anxiety disorders actually had *lower* rates of "remission" than the four personality disorders. The exception was panic disorder without agoraphobia, which had a rate of remission (0.40) only slightly higher than the rates for avoidant and obsessive–compulsive personality disorders (0.30 and 0.38, respectively) at the one-year follow-up. While mood disorders had the highest remission rates, the probability of recurrence was also high. Consistent with so many other findings, the absence of temporal distinctions points to the need for improvements in our conceptualizations and definitions of Axis I and Axis II disorders.

Why do the personality disorders show such low stability? One factor is the nature of the criteria. Some criteria are broader traits, while others are more specific behaviours [4]. Some of these behavioural criteria, while perhaps good markers for personality disorder, are not good indicators of change. For example, the avoidant personality disorder criteria "Avoids occupational activities that involve significant interpersonal contact..." is just one way that fear of rejection may be manifested, and may be irrelevant to some individual circumstances.

Of greater relevance to the need for improvement in classification are the dimensional models that have been proposed. Tyrer discusses the dimensional models of neuroticism and introversion/extraversion (more recently described by Clark and Watson as negative and positive affectivity) [5]. A different model that has been proposed focuses on "cross-cutting" psychobiological dimensions that may underlie Axis I and II disorders [6], including a dimension of anxiety/inhibition proposed to underlie the Cluster C personality disorders and the Axis I anxiety disorders. There is clearly overlap among these models: the anxiety/inhibition dimension is conceptually related to facets of the temperamental dimension of "neuroticism" or negative affectivity. The idea that the Cluster C personality disorders and the anxiety disorders may share an underlying temperamental trait dimension helps to explain the overlap among the disorders, as well as the apparent lack of distinction in terms of stability. Using longitudinal data from the CLPS, we investigated time-varying associations among the personality disorders and Axis I disorders, i.e. whether change in one predicted change in the other within a one-month time frame [7]. We found significant associations for avoidant personality disorder with both social phobia and obsessive-compulsive disorder, consistent with the idea of a shared dimension of psychopathology. On the other hand, less than half of the avoidant personality disorder subjects had an initial diagnosis of either social phobia or obsessive-compulsive disorder. And while change in course was correlated, more than half of the avoidant personality disorder subjects whose social phobia remitted continued to have avoidant personality disorder. Thus, these disorders are far from concordant. These findings highlight the multi-dimensional nature of the personality disorders—some dimensions may be shared with Axis I disorders, while others may not. Interestingly, we did not find any significant time-varying associations for obsessive–compulsive personality disorder with any of the anxiety (or other Axis I) disorders. This finding is consistent with Tyrer's observations that obsessive–compulsive personality disorder may not be well characterized as a disorder of the "anxious-inhibited" cluster.

In conclusion, it seems clear that the Cluster C personality disorders are capturing clinically significant features. It also seems clear that their current classification is not optimal. Dimensional approaches offer promise of improved understanding of this realm of psychopathology, including the nature of the overlap with anxiety disorders.

REFERENCES

1. Shea M.T., Stout R., Gunderson J.G., Morey L.C., Grilo C.M., McGlashan T., Skodol A.E., Dolan-Sewell R., Dyck I., Zanarini M.C. et al. (2002) Short-term diagnostic stability of schizotypal, borderline, avoidant, and obsessive-compulsive personality disorders. Am. J. Psychiatry, 159: 2036–2041.

2. Grilo C.M., Shea M.T., Sanislow C.A., Skodol A.E., Gunderson J.G., Stout R.L., Pagano M.E., Yen S., Morey L.C., Zanarini M.C. *et al.* (in press) Two-year stability and change in schizotypal, borderline, avoidant and obsessive-compulsive personality disorders. *J. Consult. Clin. Psychol.*
3. Shea M.T., Yen S. (2003) Stability as a distinction between Axis I and Axis II disorders. *J. Person. Disord.*, **17**: 373–386.
4. Shea M.T. (1992) Some characteristics of the Axis II criteria sets and their implications for assessment of personality disorders. *J. Person. Disord.*, **6**: 377–381.
5. Clark L.A., Watson D., Mineka S. (1994) Temperament, personality, and the mood and anxiety disorders. *J. Abnorm. Psychol.*, **103**: 103–116.
6. Siever L.J., Davis K.L. (1991) A psychobiological perspective on the personality disorders. *Am. J. Psychiatry*, **148**: 1647–1658.
7. Shea M.T., Stout R.L., Gunderson J.G., Skodol A.E., Yen S., Morey L.C. (2002) Personality disorders and Axis I disorders: longitudinal associations of course. Presented at the American Psychiatric Association 155th Annual Meeting, Philadelphia, May 18–23.

5.6
Cluster C Personality Disorders: Utility and Stability
Timothy J. Trull and Stephanie D. Stepp[1]

Peter Tyrer presents a wide-ranging review of issues related to Cluster C personality disorders. He notes the history of the disorders now represented in this cluster, the features and prevalence rates of these disorders, their comorbidity and overlap with other disorders (especially Axis I disorders), and a variety of issues related to treatment and outcome. We will elaborate on two issues that Tyrer raises.

Tyrer notes that Cluster C personality disorders and "neurotic disorders" overlap to a great extent, perhaps calling into question the need for Cluster C disorders (given the existence of Axis I diagnoses for anxiety and depressive disorders). Clearly there is a strong relationship between the neuroticism and Cluster C disorders. However, an interesting and largely under-explored question is whether Cluster C disorders can account for important outcomes or clinical correlates that cannot be accounted for by neurotic disorders (e.g. Axis I anxiety disorders and depressive disorders). Such a test of incremental validity directly assesses the utility of Cluster C diagnoses. In a recent investigation [1], we found that an Axis II factor largely defined by Cluster C disorders accounted for a significant amount of the variance in educational outcome two years later, even after controlling

[1] *Department of Psychological Sciences, University of Missouri–Columbia, 106C McAlester Hall, Columbia, MO 65211, USA*

for a number of variables, including Axis I internalizing pathology (which included anxiety and depressive disorders). Thus, at least for certain outcomes, it appears that Cluster C disorders may uniquely account for important outcomes, suggesting that they should not be abandoned or subsumed by Axis I diagnoses. We encourage others to conduct similar studies that are designed to investigate these kinds of incremental validity issues.

Tyrer also describes the maturational trends of the anxious cluster personality disorders. He reports his general impression (based on several clinical studies and his clinical experience) that anxious cluster personality disorders "become more pronounced" with age. However, there are problems with basing this claim only on research or contact with psychiatric populations. For example, older patients presenting for treatment are likely to be more distressed ("neurotic") than those that do not present for treatment. Therefore, in addition to examining research on clinical populations, it is important to consider research regarding personality and aging in normative samples to determine if the traits associated with the anxious cluster personality disorders do become significantly more pronounced with age.

Costa and McCrae [2] reported that personality throughout adulthood (i.e. age 35–80) is relatively stable. They provide evidence summarizing the developmental trends of the five factors of personality, i.e. neuroticism (N), extraversion (E), openness to experience (O), agreeableness (A), and conscientiousness (C). Several studies using non-clinical samples in the United States have found that N, E, and O show declines over the adult lifespan [3,4]. However, these effect sizes are small, suggesting only slight changes in these personality traits. The most recent and parsimonious conclusion regarding the A and C factors are that they do not change significantly in adulthood [2,4].

Cross-cultural studies of the maturational development of personality traits generally replicate this pattern. Researchers investigated the maturational trends in the five factor personality traits from adolescence to mid-life (i.e. 14–50+) across German, British, Spanish, Czech, and Turkish non-psychiatric samples [5]. They found significant cross-sectional decreases in neuroticism and extraversion and increases in conscientiousness with increasing age. Results were mixed for the agreeableness and openness to experience dimensions across the five cultures. In German, Czech, and Turkish samples, agreeableness significantly increased with age. Openness to experience was found to significantly decrease with age in the Spanish, Czech, and Turkish samples. However, even though these changes in personality traits across the lifespan are significant, the magnitude of these effects is quite small. Similar patterns were also found in Italian, Portuguese, Croatian, and South Korean non-psychiatric samples [6]. Overall, these studies point to a relatively stable personality style in adulthood, suggesting that one would not expect anxious cluster personality disorder traits to be exacerbated in the later years. Therefore, we urge caution in assuming that cluster C traits become more pronounced with age.

REFERENCES

1. Bagge C., Nickell A., Stepp S., Durrett C., Jackson K., Trull T. (in press). Borderline personality disorder features predict negative outcomes two years later. *J. Abnorm. Psychol.*
2. Costa P.T. Jr, McCrae R.R. (2002) Looking backward: changes in the mean levels of personality traits from 80 to 12. In *Advances in Personality Science* (Eds D. Cervone, W. Mischel), pp. 219–237. Guilford, New York.
3. Costa P.T. Jr, McCrae R.R., Zonderman A.B., Barbano H.E., Lebowitz B., Larson D.M. (1986) Cross-sectional studies of personality in a national sample: 2. Stability in neuroticism, extraversion, and openness. *Psychol. Aging*, 1: 144–149.
4. Costa P.T. Jr, Herbst J.H., McCrae R.R., Siegler I.C. (2000) Personality at midlife: stability, intrinsic maturation, and response to life events. *Assessment*, 7: 365–378.
5. McCrae R.R., Costa P.T. Jr, Ostendorf F., Angleitner A., Hřebíčková M., Avia M.D., Sanz J., Sánchez-Bernandos M.L., Kusdil M.E., Woodfield R. *et al.* (2000) Nature over nurture: temperament, personality, and life span development. *J. Person. Soc. Psychol.*, 78: 173–186.
6. McCrae R.R., Costa P.T. Jr, Lima M.P., Simões A., Ostendorfr F., Angleitner A., Marušić I., Bratko D., Caprara G.V., Barbaranelli C. *et al.* (1999) Age differences in personality across the adult life span: parallels in five cultures. *Develop. Psychol.*, 35: 466–477.

5.7

Anxiety, Avoidance and Personality—A Dynamic Borderland

Dusica Lecic-Tosevski and Mirjana Divac-Jovanovic[1]

The state/trait dilemma seems to be particularly prominent in the anxious personality cluster. The confusion still prevailing in the field might be overcome by the concept of "levels of personality functioning" (normal, neurotic, borderline, psychotic), instead of the prevailing concept of personality disorders types [1]. The core issue is that personality disorder exists whenever there is splitting as a central defence mechanism, whatever traits are predominant. This holds true for the anxiety cluster as well as for the other two clusters. Anxious personalities can be positioned on both neurotic and borderline level of functioning. However, true anxious personality disorders are most of the time on the borderline level of functioning.

---

[1] *Institute of Mental Health, School of Medicine, University of Belgrade, Serbia and Montenegro*

Symptoms of an Axis I disorder may exaggerate the clinical picture of a personality disorder, but very soon in therapy it becomes easy to differentiate the two. When the symptoms are removed, we either finish therapy or are faced with the underlying level of personality functioning, which then might need a long-term treatment. It should be stressed that the level of personality functioning can be transient and provoked by an affective state (depression or anxiety). Inability to metabolize affect leads to a transient regression to the borderline level of functioning, which is improved after remission of symptoms, either spontaneous or produced by treatment with antidepressants [2]. This is in accordance with Tyrer's notion that some personality attributes are stable (core ones), while others are sensitive to changes in relationships and setting and show fluctuation.

Theoretically, clinically and therapeutically, it is less important *what* type of personality disorder we are dealing with, as long as we have to deal with the consequences of splitting, which are: disturbed relationships (because of partial and inconstant inner objects), affective instability and cognitive contaminations. These are common throughout the personality disorders spectrum and for all three clusters. If there are no manifestations of splitting, we suggest the use of an Axis I diagnosis (e.g. general neurotic syndrome with mixed symptomatology of anxiety and depression [3], social anxiety disorder, etc.).

In avoidant and dependent personality disorders, avoidance and dependence are coping strategies an individual uses to overcome splitting, or to adjust to a painful and unbearable reality. They are partly biologically based [1,4] and often combined. Avoidance might be a healthy coping of biologically anxious people. It should be noted, however, that all personality disorders might have avoidant, passive and dependent features.

Personality traits, previous stressful experience and recent life events may have an independent and direct influence on developing anxiety and avoidant behaviour. However, the effect of these factors cannot just be added up, since the factors interact in their impact on psychopathology [5].

Anxious personality disorders are more treatment seeking (Tyrer's type S personalities). However, this does not mean that their treatment is easier. On the surface they do seek treatment, since they want to get rid of their anxiety. But, they usually have passive-aggressive defences, tend to be treatment resistant and to engage in long-term therapies because of their frequent and prominent dependence.

The heterogeneity of anxious features and the wide differences in severity found in patients with a diagnosis of avoidant personality disorder make the categorical diagnosis of limited value. Dimensional diagnostics is much closer to nature in personality disorders. This holds especially true for the anxious personality cluster, since it has many faces and might be understood as a level of functioning, rather than a fixed type of personality disorder [1,6]. It finds its place on a continuum which goes from slight anxious traits, to true anxious, i.e. avoidant personality disorder, with paralysing symptoms, on the borderline level of functioning [1]. The last resembles the "discouraged borderline", recently described by Millon and Davis [7].

REFERENCES

1. Divac-Jovanovic M., Svrakic D., Lecic-Tosevski D. (1993) Personality disorders: model for conceptual approach and classification. Part I: General model. *Am. J. Psychother.*, **47**: 558–571.
2. Lecic-Tosevski D., Divac-Jovanovic M. (1996) The effect of dysthymia on personality assessment. *Eur. Psychiatry*, **11**: 244–248.
3. Tyrer P., Seivewright N., Ferguson B., Tyrer J. (1992) The general neurotic syndrome: a coaxial diagnosis of anxiety, depression and personality disorder. *Acta Psychiatr. Scand.*, **85**: 201–206.
4. Cloninger C.R., Svrakic D.M., Pryzbeck T.R. (1993) A psychobiological model of treatment and character. *Arch. Gen. Psychiatry*, **50**: 975–990.
5. Lecic-Tosevski D., Gavrilovic J., Knezevic G., Priebe S. (2003) Personality factors and posttraumatic stress: associations in civilians one year after air attacks. *J. Person. Disord.*, **17**: 537–549.
6. Lecic-Tosevski D. (2000) Description of specific personality disorders. In *New Oxford Textbook of Psychiatry* (Eds M. Gelder, J.J. Lopez-Ibor, N. Andreasen), pp. 927–953. Oxford University Press, Oxford.
7. Millon T., Davis R. (2000) *Personality Disorders in Modern Life*. Wiley, New York.

5.8
A Theoretical Model of Cluster C Personality Disorders
Joel Paris[1]

The overall concept of classifying personality disorder into clusters is in concordance with data showing that personality disorders are dysfunctional amplifications of normal personality traits [1]. The basic dimensions of personality have been most often described as four or five factors [2,3], a number closer to the three clusters in the DSM Axis II system than to ten categories. Moreover, the clusters are conceptually coherent. It is generally accepted in research in child psychiatry that symptoms tend to fall into externalizing or internalizing clusters [4]. It has been shown that almost all adult disorders on Axis I can be factor analysed in much the same way [5].

[1] *Department of Psychiatry, McGill University, Research and Training Building, 1033 Pine Avenue West, Montreal, Québec H3A 1A1, Canada*

Thus, Cluster B corresponds to an externalizing dimension of psychopathology, while Cluster C corresponds to an internalizing dimension [6]; Cluster A picks up the dimension of cognitive dysfunction. While there are problems with overlap between clusters and categories across clusters, these could be attributable to the specific way that disorders are classified. There is no reason why the criteria cannot be changed to make the clusters more distinct.

The problem is that personality disorders, both in DSM-IV and ICD-10, have been classified from clinical tradition rather than from systematic empirical investigation. The muddle that our present system finds itself in may be resolved when we understand more about the aetiology and pathogenesis of personality pathology as a whole.

The comorbidity of personality disorders in no way reduces their validity. Patients rarely present with "pure" egodystonic personality pathology, but come to clinical attention because of symptoms. The principle behind making a personality disorder diagnosis is that there is a developmental process that underlies the development of overt psychopathology. For example, the overlap between cluster C disorders and Axis I anxiety disorders only represents a distinction between current symptoms and underlying personality patterns. Similarly, the fact that patients with anorexia nervosa have strong compulsive traits [7] shows that traits associated with perfectionism in young women can express themselves as an eating disorder.

A theoretical model of cluster C personality disorders should be based on developmental psychopathology. These disorders are probably rooted in anxious traits that develop early in life. While we need prospective studies to confirm this relationship, there is some longitudinal data on highly anxious children [8]. It will be illuminating to see whether this cohort eventually develops Cluster C personality disorders in adult life.

We can apply a stress-diathesis (or biopsychosocial) model to Cluster C disorders [9]. These conditions probably develop through gene-environment interactions. The biological risk factors would consist of genetic-temperamental predispositions that shape vulnerability to anxiety. Although compulsive traits have sometimes been considered to be ways of coping with anxiety, some research suggests they may constitute a separate personality dimension [2]. The presence of genetic predispositions to Cluster C disorders is confirmed by the fact that anxious traits are heritable [10], as well as by the finding from a Norwegian twin study [11].

The psychological factors in Cluster C disorders have not been well researched, but would likely consist of life experiences that either amplify these traits or fail to modulate them. The social factors in Cluster C disorders might consist of social and cultural demands that make it difficult for anxious individuals to develop adequate coping skills [9].

In contrast with Cluster B disorders, which generally improve with age [6], Cluster C disorders tend to persist over time [12]. One possible explanation is that impulsive traits tend to modulate with time and experience, while anxious traits cause vicious cycles that maintain psychopathological patterns.

Diagnosing a Cluster C disorder is important for planning treatment. Whereas pharmacological agents have been useful for the management of anxiety disorders, there is little evidence that they reduce trait anxiety. However, some studies suggest that social skills training [13], which addresses the personality pathology behind overt symptoms, is effective for patients with Cluster C disorders.

REFERENCES

1. Rutter M. (1987) Temperament, personality, and personality development. *Br. J. Psychiatry*, **150**: 443–448.
2. Livesley W.J., Jang K.L., Vernon P.A. (1998) Phenotypic and genetic structure of traits delineating personality disorder. *Arch. Gen. Psychiatry*, **55**: 941–948.
3. Costa P.T., Widiger T.A. (eds) (2001) *Personality Disorders and the Five Factor Model of Personality*, 2nd edn. American Psychological Association, Washington.
4. Achenbach T.M., McConaughy S.H. (1997) *Empirically Based Assessment of Child and Adolescent Psychopathology: Practical Applications*, 2nd edn. Sage, Thousand Oaks.
5. Krueger R.F. (1999) The structure of common mental disorders. *Arch. Gen. Psychiatry*, **56**: 921–926.
6. Paris J. (2003) *Personality Disorders Over Time: Precursors, Course, and Outcome.* American Psychiatric Press, Washington.
7. Vitouske K., Manke F. (1994) Personality variables and disorders in anorexia nervosa and bulimia nervosa. *J. Abnorm. Psychol.*, **103**: 137–147.
8. Kagan J. (1994) *Galen's Prophecy.* New York, Basic Books
9. Paris J. (1998) Anxious traits, anxious attachment, and anxious cluster personality disorders. *Harv. Rev. Psychiatry*, **6**: 142–148.
10. Jang K.L., Livesley W.J., Vernon P.A., Jackson D.N. (1996) Heritability of personality traits: a twin study. *Acta Psychiatr. Scand.*, **94**: 438–444.
11. Torgersen S., Lygren S., Oien P.A., Skre I., Onstad S., Edvardsen J., Tambs K., Kringlen E. (2000) A twin study of personality disorders. *Compr. Psychiatry*, **41**: 416–425.
12. Seivewright H., Tyrer P., Johnson T. (in press) Persistent social dysfunction in anxious and depressed patients with personality disorder. *Acta Psychiatr. Scand.*
13. Stravynyski A., Belisle M., Macouiller M., Lavallée Y.-V., Elie R. (1994) The treatment of avoidant personality disorder by social skills training in the clinic or in real-life settings. *Can. J. Psychiatry*, **39**: 377–383.

5.9
Anxious Cluster Personality Disorders:
The Need for Further Empirical Data
Julien Daniel Guelfi[1]

The relationships that exist between mental and personality disorders still need to be clarified. No suitable classification has been found for personality disorders yet. The superiority of the dimensional model on the categorial one is an attractive hypothesis. In spite of many favourable arguments (stable distribution of personality traits, data loss in individuals under the diagnostic threshold, etc....), one has to admit that this hypothesis is still lacking sufficient experimental justification.

The relationships that exist between episodic phenomena and the characteristics of "long-term" functioning or, in other words, the relationships between DSM Axes I and II are necessarily complex. Some patients suffer from chronic disorders; in others, long-term behaviour can be qualified as pathological under certain circumstances and these patients will, along their lives, develop a variety of anxious and/or depressive pathological episodes with psychological repercussions. As an example, recurrent depressive episodes modify long-term psychological functioning and it is not surprising that no straightforward classification system is available to reflect that complexity.

Depression is one of the examples described in detail in Peter Tyrer's review. The relationship between depressive mood and behavioural inhibition or between anxiety and situation avoidance is inevitably made up by a multiplicity of interactions. Depression increases emotional dependence and promotes defensive regression. A variety of therapeutic processes may modify long-term psychological functioning, reduce behavioural inhibition, either transient or durable, reduce emotional instability and mental tensions, alter vegetative functioning or even modify thinking patterns. It may not be necessary, however, to classify them as "treatments of personality and personality disorders".

Recent dissatisfactions in classification users concerning avoidant and dependent personality disorders may have been produced by some changes made without any real experimental justification from the DSM-III and DSM-III-R.

For instance, to the question "can avoidant personality disorder be differentiated from other disorders with which it shares certain features?", Millon [1] replied that social phobia can covariate with avoidant personality

_____
[1] Clinique des Maladies Mentales et de l'Encéphale, Hôpital Sainte-Anne, 100 rue de la Santé, 75674 Paris, France

disorder, but that a distinction is still possible, because avoidant personality disorder is essentially a problem of interpersonal relationships, whereas social phobia is a problem of "performing on situation". By dropping some DSM-III criteria for avoidant personality disorder and introducing common phobia criteria, the DSM-III-R committee inadvertently made avoidant personality disorder and social phobia highly comparable.

Other authors have indeed argued differently, but again without any real experimental justification. This was the case with Cloninger and Svrakic [2], who strongly advocated the attractive psychobiological dimension model, stating that: "avoidant personality disorder is very difficult to distinguish from social phobia. Many authors believe these are alternative labels for the same or similar conditions".

Concerning dependent personality disorder, several clinical investigations by Hirschfeld since 1976 [3] have assessed composite traits in normal and clinical samples and have examined them psychometrically. The clinical findings were consistent, distinguishing two components of dependent personality disorder, i.e., attachment on the one side and general dependency with lack of self confidence on the other. The emotional dependence concept as well as the dimensional subdivision would appear to be of heuristic interest. In any case, it justifies further clinical and psychometric research along that line.

REFERENCES

1. Millon T. (1996) Avoidant personality disorder. In *DSM-IV Sourcebook, Vol. 2*, pp. 757–765. American Psychiatric Association, Washington.
2. Cloninger C., Svrakic D.M. (2000) Personality disorders. In *Comprehensive Textbook of Psychiatry*, 7th edn. (Eds B.J. Sadock, V.A. Sadock), pp. 1723–1764. Lippincott Williams and Wilkins, Philadelphia.
3. Hirschfeld R.M.A., Shea T., Talbot K.M. (1996) Dependent personality disorder. In *DSM-IV Sourcebook, Vol. 2*, pp. 767–775, American Psychiatric Association, Washington.

5.10
Quest for a Clinically Useful Diagnosis
Marco Antonio Alves Brasil[1] and Luiz Alberto B. Hetem[2]

Why do we change psychiatric nomenclature, especially the one concerning personality disorders, from time to time? For two main reasons: the search for diagnostic entities which are more representative of the groups of patients we see in clinical practice and the need to integrate new data originated in research settings (including epidemiological and pharmacological findings). Dimensional classification, even being superior to the categorical one, does not fit in with modern diagnostic systems. This is the reason why we have seen several tentative developments of personality clusters in the last decades.

As Peter Tyrer very clearly shows in his review, the anxious cluster probably is the most prevalent and the most problematic one. It includes anxious/avoidant, dependent and anankastic/obsessive–compulsive personality disorders. Not to discuss the latter in this chapter was a wise decision. It does not seem to be related to anxiety and depressive disorders as the other two, in terms of premorbid traits and predictive value. Moreover, this position supports the ICD-10's proposition that its mental disorder counterpart, obsessive–compulsive disorder, must be considered separately from anxiety disorders.

A second point in the review, perhaps the most important one, is the emphasis on the idea of the so-called "general neurotic syndrome", which has an undeniable importance, because it represents many patients seen in the primary care and psychiatric outpatient settings. Formerly understood as a syndrome characterized by a mixture of depressive and anxious symptoms and anxious personality features, it can be now viewed as the final common result of several possible combinations of Axis I and II diagnostic categories (comorbidity of anxiety disorders and depression, comorbidity of anxious personality with anxiety and/or depressive disorders, residual symptoms of clinical entities not completely resolved), requiring different therapeutic approaches depending on its components. The acceptance of this syndrome would represent a clinically useful exception to the general prevalent tendency of splitting mental disorders in smaller and more "specific" groups and, at the same time, a consequence of the movement towards categorization.

In Brazil, a considerable proportion of the people who come to our outpatient general hospital services complain of a condition whose clinical

[1] Federal University of Rio de Janeiro, Brazil
[2] Faculdade de Medicina de Ribeirão Preto, Universidade de São Paulo, Brazil

symptoms are hard to fit into a traditional nosography: the "nervous disease". The name "nervous disease" is given to a syndrome characterized by vague and migratory symptoms, such as dizziness, palpitations, chest pain, weakness, amnesia, back pain, etc. Differently from the "ataques de nervios" described in other Latin American countries, it is not acute, but usually chronic. Patients with "nervous disease" have hardly been studied from the point of view of a more exact clinical diagnosis. In a study conducted in a general hospital outpatient clinic [1,2], it was observed that a substantial part of these patients, besides multiple, non-specific and varied complaints, were reporting domestic conflicts, violence and housing problems. As for diagnosis, anxiety disorders, followed by mood and somatoform disorders, predominated. The most common diagnosis was generalized anxiety disorder. After a close analysis of the results, it became clear that an exact clinical diagnosis was practically useful only for some of the patients. This shows the limitations of the current diagnostic classifications. The "general neurotic syndrome" is an attempt to reunify syndromes which are separated in our present classifications. In this comprehensive approach, anxiety and depression are associated with specific personality features and regarded as reflecting overreactivity to various stressful situations.

Our late Professor Leme Lopes used to say that it is almost impossible to make a unidirectional diagnosis. In 1954 he proposed a multidimensional diagnostic system [3,4]: the dimensions or axes presented were the syndrome, the premorbid personality, and the aetiological constellation. Differently from the multiaxial system introduced by DSM-III, the three levels of diagnostic evaluation brought to one single psychiatric diagnosis. Leme Lopes' work became an important reference amongst Brazilian psychiatrists and over many years was used for resident training in psychiatry. The introduction of the multiaxial classification scheme of DSM-III in our clinical practice did not imply a more comprehensive approach to psychiatric diagnosis. Actually, what we have seen is a tendency to use only the Axis I categories and an abandonment of the other axes. We believe this could be one of the reasons of the paucity of research on personality disorders in our country.

REFERENCES

1. Brasil M.A., Furlanetto L.A. (1997) A atual nosologia psqiuátrica e sua adequação aos hospitais gerais. *Cadernos do IPUB*, **6**.
2. Brasil M.A. (1995) Pacientes com queixas difusas. Um estudo nosológico de pacientes com queixas múltiplas e vagas. Doctorate thesis, Instituto de Psiquiatria, Federal University of Rio de Janeiro.

3. Leme Lopes J. (1954) *As Dimensões do Diagnóstico Psiquiátrico.* Agir, Rio de Janeiro.
4. Leme Lopes J. (1988) Brazilian contributions to diagnostic systems in psychiatry. In *International Classification in Psychiatry: Unity and Diversity* (Eds J.E. Mezzich, M. von Cranach), pp. 30–36. Cambridge University Press, Cambridge.

5.11
The "Anxious Cluster": A Descriptive Disguise for Diversity in Personality Classification

Fuad Antun[1]

The concept of "anxious" personality depicts a behavioural pattern which emanates from an intricate variety of characteristics of a personality in its dynamic interaction with the environment. It is therefore quite appropriate to refer to this concept as a cluster of individual personality types, conventionally identified as "Cluster C". The dilemma is what to include under this heading and how such subcategories influence the causality, course and outcome of mental illness. Peter Tyrer's review, in its introductory and historical sections, clearly pays tribute to early thinkers and shows the obvious problems with accuracy and conclusiveness of later and ongoing research.

If we move away from the cluster concept to individual personality disorders, we find that all the attempts to synchronize personality test results to classification of personality disorders (ICD and DSM) have not yielded a meaningful and helpful aid to the clinician, who is unable to match the test results to a single personality type.

The attempt to reduce the number of personality types [1] did not solve the problem of diversity. Maybe it is wise to describe the personality clinically through its behavioural pattern, without referring to an Axis I diagnosis. Having said that, one faces two major problems: (a) how to delineate the boundaries of an Axis II diagnosis (i.e. avoidant, dependent, obsessive) without much overlap, and (b) where to draw the line with respect to Axis I disorders (i.e. social anxiety disorder, panic anxiety and obsessive-compulsive disorder in its mild form). Such controversy, that needs further elucidation, justifies a more flexible approach to the classification of personality types, as indicated in Tyrer's review.

The anxious personality is in several ways related to the physiological threshold of the hypothalamic neuroendocrine axis [2–4]. Such threshold is genetically influenced in its reaction to environmental and developmental

[1] *Antun Building, Zouk Mikhael, P.O. Box 135098, Beirut, Lebanon*

factors, which determines its response to outside events or stressors. A frequent feature of the "anxious" cluster is the hyperexcitability of the hypothalamic neuroendocrine axis in handling life events. In a clinical setting, we see a lot of similarity of response in various family members in stressful situations. Perhaps comorbidity, as illustrated in the review, between the "anxious" cluster and Axis I disorders is part of this dualism of genetically determined neuronal physiology, upbringing and environmental factors.

Personality type is important in all psychiatric illness, especially in affecting the course and outcome of the condition and the patient's quality of life. In many instances the treatment of the Axis II conditions with pharmacotherapy and/or psychotherapy can lessen or prevent transition to an Axis I disorder. In the "anxious" cluster this is particularly relevant, because of the unclear boundary between Axis I and II.

The "anxious" cluster covers a broad area of overlap between Axis I and II, but the boundaries between them are not well demarcated. Problems in the classification of personality disorders are particularly evident in this area. "Anxiety" is a term denoting a psychological state, yet is used here to group a variety of personality types sharing some common and ill-defined features under the same umbrella.

REFERENCES

1. Walton H.J., Presly A.S. (1973) Use of a category system in the diagnosis of abnormal personality. *Br. J. Psychiatry*, **122**: 259–268.
2. Mason J.W. (1975) Emotion as reflected in patterns of endocrine integration. In *Emotions. Their Parameters and Measurement* (Ed. L. Levi), pp 163–181. Raven Press, New York.
3. Persky H. (1975) Adrenocortical function and anxiety. *Psychoneuroendocrinology*, **1**: 37–44.
4. Emrich H.M., Millan M.J. (1982) Stress reactions and endorphinergic systems. *J. Psychosom. Res.*, **26**: 101–104.

5.12
Beyond the Anxious Traits
Miguel Márquez[1]

The concept of an anxious cluster poses several issues such as the need to rationalize the description of Cluster C personality disorders, to explain the large co-morbidity among them and to give sense to the frequent overlap between personality disorders and their equivalent anxiety and mood Axis I disorders. The chapter by Peter Tyrer is a synthesis of all these issues.

Most of Tyrer's statements are confirmed by everyday clinical experience. For example, the anxious personality cluster is often seen together not just with Axis I anxiety disorders, but also with mood disorders (non-psychotic and non-melancholic). It is also observed that the personality features are contaminated or distorted by Axis I symptoms, particularly so in cluster C than in any other type of personality disorders. On the other hand, in several clinical settings, the clinical weakness of the diagnosis of a single personality disorder stimulates clinicians to consider Axis II features as a personality trait or disposition, rather than a disorder.

According to Tyrer, the concept of general neurotic syndrome goes against the tide, but is supported by modern neuropsychological conceptions. Our investigations [1] allow us to suggest that under obsessive–compulsive, dependent and probably avoidant traits, we may find deficits of executive functions that limit the adaptive capacities of the subject for interpersonal relationships and performance in the very complex world in which we live, generating behavioural patterns eventually observed as personality traits or Axis I disorder symptoms. When dealing with patients with Axis I and Axis II anxiety disorders, we often find cognitive rigidity, lower processing speed, attentional and motivational bias and visuoconstructive deficits. Executive function failure is critical: attention, working memory and set-shifting deficits, perseverative behaviour in the Wisconsin Card Sorting Test, failure in planning and strategy and qualitatively altered decision making profiles, are clear indicators of these executive dysfunctions. The dysfunctions may not be specific, but each disorder seems to have a neuropsychological profile that is characteristic.

In patients with Axis I generalized anxiety disorder and Axis II dependent personality disorder, we found deficits in context exploration, especially when the patient is dealing with complex tasks. Deficits in organizational strategies, planning, generalized anticipation and, especially, in organizing behaviour, disrupt decision making and problem solving. These subjects perform as controls on verbal memory tasks for words, but

[1] *Department of Psychiatry, Hospital Francés, Juramento 1805, Buenos Aires, Argentina*

when dealing with phrases their performance decreases, perhaps as a result of task complexity. In episodic verbal memory the results are poor if the information to encode is aversive. Testing their performance on episodic memory tasks (Baddeley/Signoret), we found clear differences with respect to controls, that can be attributed to attentional and emotional bias, which impairs the information encoding and especially disrupts encoding of aversive information.

Poor anticipation and planning resources, strategic deficit and excessive but inefficient monitoring lead to poor performance in non-verbal fluency tasks and impact on information processing speed.

Probably the neuropsychological abnormalities, and the resulting dysexecutive profile, precede the anxious and depressive symptomatic expressiveness. They could be considered as the basis of some dispositions and vulnerabilities, characteristic of Cluster C personality disorders, especially in the case of dependent, avoidant and obsessive–compulsive subjects, and the triggering factor or facilitator of pathological traits of personality and Axis I disorders. It is possible that these neuropsychological dysfunctions and Axis I and II symptoms and traits are not entities of different universes and that there is a close relationship—sometimes a causal relationship—between these dysexecutive profiles and clinical symptomatology. The rehabilitation of neuropsychological dysfunctions may represent a new target for treatment, in addition to the Axis I symptoms and the personality abnormal traits [2].

REFERENCES

1. Márquez M. (2002) Bases to nosography of obsessive-compulsive disorder. *Anxia, Journal of Argentine Association of Anxiety Disorders*, **6**: 28–35.
2. Figiacone S., Márquez M. (2002) The obsessive-compulsive disorder: bases for a rational therapeutic; toward a third therapeutic approach. Presented at the 1st Virtual Congress of the Argentine College of Neuropsychopharmacology, November 1–30.

6

Obsessive–Compulsive Personality Disorder: A Review

Paul Costa, Jack Samuels, Michael Bagby, Lee Daffin and Hillary Norton

National Institute on Aging, Intramural Research Program, 5600 Nathan Shock Drive, Baltimore, MD 21224, USA

INTRODUCTION

In this chapter, we review the research on obsessive–compulsive personality disorder (OCPD) as a discrete disorder on Axis II of the DSM-IV. The many difficulties surrounding the Axis II disorders are especially evident in the case of OCPD. The terms "obsessive" and "compulsive" are so much a part of the ordinary vernacular that their clinical and conceptual meanings are easily obscured. The DSM-IV-TR [1] enumerates five to nine criteria for each of the ten personality disorders (PDs), but operationalization is not validation [2]. OCPD is not necessarily a valid, clinically coherent personality type because, in part, it encompasses many different constructs, features, and individuals.

We will attempt to demonstrate that not all the criteria used to define OCPD are associated with maladaptive consequences, as some are adaptive and valued by society. Particularly challenging is the attempt to understand the circumstances that make for impairment or disorder. Whether the collection of criteria used to diagnose OCPD represents a valid disorder, one that reflects true psychopathology, or is better conceptualized as a problem in living, is one among a number of issues that must await future research and clinical consensus.

This paper consists of three major sections. In the first, we present a historical review of the OCPD construct, from the perspectives of the early psycho-analysts, various editions of the DSM, and ICD. In the second, we review

Personality Disorders. Edited by Mario Maj, Hagop S. Akiskal, Juan E. Mezzich and Ahmed Okasha.
©2005 John Wiley & Sons Ltd: ISBN 0-470-09036-7

problems of validity of the DSM construct, including convergent validity, discriminant validity, temporal stability and functional impairment. In the third, we present dimensional approaches to understanding this personality construct. Our focus will be on the Five Factor Model (FFM), which is a well-studied hierarchical model of the structure of personality traits. The five higher order dimensions of the FFM are neuroticism, extraversion, openness to experience, agreeableness, and conscientiousness. These factors represent the most basic dimensions underlying personality traits. Finally, in the summary, we discuss areas of consistent evidence, areas of incomplete evidence, and areas still open to investigating OCPD as a personality disorder.

HISTORICAL REVIEW

Pre-DSM: Freud's Anal Type and Psychoanalytical Perspectives

Modern conceptualizations of OCPD are heavily influenced by the theories and clinical observations of early 20th century psychoanalysts, especially Sigmund Freud [3]. In 1908, Freud described a triad of "anal erotic" characteristics—orderliness, parsimony, and obstinacy—that tended to co-occur in some of his patients. "Orderliness" included concerns about bodily cleanliness, conscientiousness in carrying out duties, and trustworthiness; "parsimony", or miserliness, in the most extreme form could manifest itself as "avarice"; "obstinacy" could extend to "defiance, rage, and revengefulness"[4]. Freud hypothesized that these characteristics were either sublimations of, or reaction formations against, anal-erotic instincts of childhood.

Ernest Jones [5] elaborated on this description of "anal-erotic character traits" by expanding the number of associated traits and by emphasizing the theme of control underlying them. Jones noted that such individuals are prone to procrastination in work but, once a project is begun, they are extremely persistent, sensitive to interference, and reluctant to delegate tasks to others. They particularly focus on tedious chores, have a "special sense of duty", and are "pathologically intolerant" of other views on issues of morality. Furthermore, they are imbued with a sense of perfection, and are "extremely sensitive to any disturbing or disharmonious element in a situation". They insist on orderliness, organization, and cleanliness, are parsimonious, and dislike throwing anything away.

On the one hand, Jones noted the negative social aspects of this character type, which included low amounts of positive affect, high amounts of negative affect, and antagonism. On the other hand, Jones recognized that some traits, especially those related to conscientiousness and persistence, are likely to be adaptive.

Karl Abraham [6] put even greater emphasis on the demand for control as a fundamental theme underlying the "anal character". Abraham also noted that such individuals do not work well with others unless they are in control of the situation. Furthermore, as such individuals focus on smaller details, they may often lose sight of a project's main focus. Unlike Freud or Jones, Abraham noted that these individuals often have a peculiar, eccentric quality.

Although the psychoanalytic theory for the genesis of this character type is without empirical support, these authors provided rich clinical descriptions of what would later become known as compulsive or obsessive–compulsive personality disorder, and several of the traits, as well as speculation about their origin, were incorporated into later diagnostic criteria. For instance, DSM-IV criterion 1 (preoccupation with details and lists to the extent that the point of the activity is lost) is rooted in the anal characteristic of exceptional orderliness, criterion 5 (hoarding) in fascination with retention, criterion 7 (miserliness) in stinginess, and criterion 8 (rigidity) in obstinacy. Less clear is how these and other clinicians conceived of the relationship among these characteristics and psychiatric symptoms (i.e. obsessions and compulsions) and psychiatric disorders (i.e. compulsive neurosis and, later, obsessive–compulsive disorder, OCD).

Emil Kraepelin [7] suggested that personality features preceded the appearance of psychiatric symptoms. He noted many of the same characteristics described by the psychoanalysts. In "Obsessions and Psychasthenia", Pierre Janet considered what we would call personality traits fundamental to the early stage ("the psychasthenic state") of "psychasthenic illness" (i.e. OCD). These traits included perfectionism, indecisiveness, orderliness, authoritarianism, and restricted emotional expression [8,9].

Revisions to DSM Nomenclature and Criteria for OCPD

In 1952, DSM-I [10] described several personality disorders as being maladaptive manifestations of normal personality structure which, in most instances, do not negatively affect the individual emotionally. Personality disorders were divided into three main groups with an additional group. The text went on to state that the groupings were "largely descriptive, made partially on the basis of the dynamics of personality development". The second grouping, "personality trait disturbance", referred to those individuals whose personality dispositions led them to be easily upset by minor or major stressors. It was suggested that this classification should only be applied to those whose personality is maladaptive and who have a minimum of anxiety.

It is in the "personality trait disturbance" grouping that compulsive personality is found, along with emotionally unstable personality, passive-aggressive personality, and personality trait disturbance, other (perhaps akin to DSM-IV's personality disorder not otherwise specified, PDNOS). From DSM-I to DSM-II [11], there was little change in the core clinical description of OCPD. One definite change was in the name. DSM-I termed it compulsive personality, while DSM-II named it obsessive–compulsive personality. The key features of the disorder for both versions included: excessive or chronic concern for adherence to standards of conscience, overinhibited, overconscientious, an inordinate capacity for work, rigidity, and being unable to relax easily. DSM-I noted that compulsive personality may "appear as a persistence of an adolescent pattern of behavior, or as a regression from more mature functioning as a result of stress".

Of note, there are several consistencies between the phenomenological picture of the obsessive–compulsive person in DSM-I and DSM-II. First, the obsessive–compulsive person is characterized by excessive superego control, concern with conformity and morality or standards of conscience. Second, the DSM-II suggested that obsessive–compulsive neurosis (corresponding to current OCD) may be co-morbid with other disorders and indicated that it may be difficult distinguishing the neurosis from the personality. Third, the term "anankastic personality" appeared in the second edition of the DSM as an alternative label to avoid the confusion with OCD, but was deleted from subsequent editions.

From a clinical perspective, the DSM-III [12] represented a sea change. The emphasis of the description of OCPD changed from excessive efforts or concerns at self-control, conformity and morality, to affective constriction and the inability to express warm and tender emotions. Clinically, cold and uncaring traits replaced overinhibited, overconscientious features. From the FFM perspective, the OCPD patients were closed to feelings, low in warmth, and possibly agreeableness. DSM-III lists five criteria, any four of which were necessary for an OCPD diagnosis. These criteria included: (1) emotional constriction; inability to express warm and tender emotions; (2) perfectionism that interferes with completing larger goals; (3) insistence that others submit to his or her way of doing things and lack of awareness of the feelings elicited by this behaviour in others; (4) excessive devotion to work and productivity to the exclusion of pleasure and the value of interpersonal relationships; and (5) indecisiveness: decision-making is either avoided, postponed or protracted due to fear of making a mistake.

The transition from DSM-III to DSM-III-R [13] saw a radical change in the core description to "a pervasive pattern of perfectionism and inflexibility, beginning by early adulthood and present in a variety of contexts". Affective constriction was reduced to an associated feature in DSM-III-R. Several new criteria were added, including a preoccupation with details, rules, lists,

TABLE 6.1   DSM-IV-TR [1] Criteria for obsessive–compulsive personality disorder (OCPD) (listed in descending order of prototypicality)

1. Is preoccupied with details, rules, lists, order, organization, or schedules to the extent that the major point of the activity is lost.
2. Shows perfectionism that interferes with task completion.
3. Is excessively devoted to work and productivity to the exclusion of leisure activities and friendships.
4. Is overconscientious, scrupulous, and inflexible about matters of morality, ethics, or values.
5. Is unable to discard worn-out or worthless objects even when they have no sentimental value.
6. Is reluctant to delegate tasks or to work with others unless they submit to exactly his or her way of doing things.
7. Adopts a miserly spending style toward both self and others. Money is viewed as something to be hoarded for future catastrophes.
8. Shows rigidity and stubbornness.

order, organization, or schedules to the extent that the major point of the activity is lost; overconscientousness, scrupulousness, and inflexibility about matters of morality, ethics, or values; lack of generosity in giving time, money, or gifts when no personal gain is likely to result; and an inability to discard worn-out or worthless objects even when they have no sentimental value. To receive this diagnosis, five of the nine criteria needed to be met.

The core description changed again from DSM-III-R to DSM-IV [14] and DSM-IV-TR [1]. The emphasis returned to original definitions which focused on preoccupations with order, perfection, and control at the expense of flexibility, openness, and efficiency [1]. The DSM-IV added criteria such as rigidity, stubbornness, and hoarding, whereas DSM-III conceptualized the latter as being a lack of generosity. Also, the DSM-IV-TR dropped DSM-III-R's criterion 7 (restricted expression of affection) and criterion 5 (indecisiveness), moving the latter down to an associated feature. Finally, the DSM-IV lists the criteria in descending order of prototypicality (Table 6.1).

International Classification of Diseases (ICD)

The equivalent of OCPD in the International Classification of Diseases, 10th edition (ICD-10) [15] is anankastic personality disorder, characterized by "feelings of doubt, perfectionism, excessive conscientiousness, checking and preoccupation with details, stubbornness, caution and rigidity". The person must first meet the general criteria for a personality disorder and then, like in the DSM-IV, must display four of eight listed criteria: (1) feelings of excessive doubt and caution; (2) preoccupation with details, rules, lists, order, organization or schedule; (3) perfectionism that interferes with task completion; (4) excessive conscientiousness and scrupulousness; (5) undue preoccupation with productivity to the exclusion of pleasure and interpersonal relationships; (6) excessive pedantry and adherence to social conventions; (7) rigidity and stubbornness; and (8) unreasonable insistence by the individual that others submit to exactly his or her way of doing things, or unreasonable reluctance to allow others to do things.

Agreement between the DSM-IV and ICD-10 definitions of OCPD is high ($\kappa = 0.91$) [16]. Ottosson et al. [17] reported similar results ($\kappa = 0.75$) and a high correlation between the number of fulfilled criteria in each system ($r = 0.89$). Starcevic et al. [18] note that ICD-10 tends to overdiagnose anankastic personality disorder, due to the "excessive doubt and caution" criterion, which is frequently endorsed by patients but yields low specificity. They also report a kappa of 0.79 for diagnostic agreement between the ICD and DSM.

VALIDITY OF OCPD CRITERIA

We agree with Livesley's [19] assertion that, when assessing the validity of PDs, construct validity and not face validity is key. Construct validity refers to the degree to which OCPD and the other PDs predict important external variables including aetiology and prognosis. Unfortunately, there is a paucity of studies addressing this issue and fewer studies utilizing the DSM-IV criteria for OCPD. One study, the Collaborative Longitudinal Personality Disorders Study (CLPS) [20], will be examined in detail as it represents the largest, most carefully done study on these issues.

Interrater Agreement

We have reviewed studies that provided statistical measures of agreement such as the kappa coefficient across various structured interviews. Clark and Harrison [21] summarized interrater reliabilities for five well-known diagnostic interviews and concluded that each of the measures met the standard cut-off of 0.70 for good interrater reliability. The interrater reliability "for any personality disorder" is a remarkably consistent 0.70 to 0.71. Test-retest reliability even over short-term intervals is lower: 0.50 for the Structured Clinical Interview for DSM-IV Axis II Personality Disorders (SCID-II), 0.58 for the Diagnostic Interview for DSM-IV Personality Disorders (DIPD) and 0.66 for the Structured Interview for the DSM-III Personality Disorders (SIDP). Mean kappas for individual diagnoses were also lower: 0.49 (SCID-II) 0.68 (DIPD) and 0.66 (SIDP).

Is the OCPD diagnosis more reliable than the mean kappas reported by Clark and Harrison [21]? Table 6.2 presents kappa coefficients for studies that compare structured interviews to self-report measures (hetero-method approach) or two structured interviews (mono-method approach).

The five studies comparing interviews to self-reports yielded low kappas for OCPD, regardless of the instrument or version of the DSM. Kappa values ranged from −0.10 [27] to 0.38 [22,25], with a mean value of 0.10.

In a comparison of the Personality Diagnostic Questionnaire (PDQ) with an unstructured clinical interview ($n = 552$), Hyler *et al.* [23] obtained a kappa of 0.08 for OCPD. Zimmerman and Coryell [24] examined the agreement between the SIDP and the PDQ ($n = 697$) and found that the kappa for OCPD was 0.13.

Hyler *et al.*'s [25] comparison of the Personality Diagnostic Questionnaire—Revised (PDQ-R) with two different structured interview instruments yielded slightly better results. When PDQ-defined OCPD was compared to SCID-defined OCPD, agreement was moderate ($\kappa = 0.30$); agreement of the Personality Disorder Examination (PDE) and the PDQ-R was slightly higher ($\kappa = 0.38$). Nevertheless, the herero method kappas were well below the benchmark kappa of 0.70.

Finally, in a sample of 97 patients, Soldz *et al.* [27] found that the PDE and the Millon Clinical Multiaxial Inventory (MCMI-II) had poor to moderate agreement in assigning personality disorder diagnoses. Diagnostic agreement of $k > 0.30$ was achieved concerning antisocial, borderline, avoidant, and dependent personality disorders for "definite plus probable PDE diagnoses", but only borderline and avoidant personality disorders had kappas above 0.30 for "definite PDE". The agreement for OCPD was near zero (definite: $\kappa = -0.07$; definite or probable: $\kappa = -0.10$). Further analysis of specificity, sensitivity, and positive and negative predictive power showed that the scales agreed on the absence of a diagnosis but failed to agree on its presence.

In studies comparing structured inverviews, the interrater agreement for the diagnosis of OCPD is better, but still below acceptable levels. Skodol *et al.*'s [28] study produced three comparisons and varying results depending on which instruments were compared. Comparing the SCID-II and PDE yielded the greatest agreement ($\kappa = 0.50$). The agreement of the SCID-II and the Longitudinal Expert Evaluation Using All Available Data (LEAD) was much lower ($\kappa = 0.30$). Finally, agreement dropped further still when

TABLE 6.2   Kappa coefficients for obsessive–compulsive personality disorder (OCPD)

Study	Diagnostic system	Instruments compared	Kappa(s)
Hetero-Method Approach			
Hyler *et al.* [22,23]	DSM-III	PDQ vs. clinical interview	0.08
Zimmerman and Coryell [22,24]	DSM-III	SIDP vs. PDQ	0.13
Hyler *et al.* [22,25]	DSM-III-R	PDQ-R vs. SCID	0.30
Hyler *et al.* [22,25]	DSM-III-R	PDQ-R vs. PDE	0.38
Jackson *et al.* [22,26]	DSM-III	SIDP vs. MCMI	0.00
Soldz *et al.* [27]	DSM-III-R	MCMI-II vs. PDE	PDE definite −0.07 PDE definite and probable −0.10
		Mean	*0.10*
Mono-Method Approach			
Skodol *et al.* [22,28]	DSM-III-R	SCID-II vs. PDE	0.50
Skodol *et al.* [22,28]	DSM-III-R	LEAD vs. SCID-II	0.30
Skodol *et al.* [22,28]	DSM-III-R	LEAD vs. PDE	0.06
Hyler *et al.* [29]	DSM-III-R	PDE vs. SCID-II	0.36
Bronisch and Mombour [30]	DSM-III-R	IPDE vs. IDCL-P	0.30
Pilkonis *et al.* [31]	DSM-III-R	PDE and SIDP-R	PDE 0.51 SIDP-R 0.40
Zanarini *et al.* [32]	DSM-IV	SCID-I vs. DIPD-IV	Test 0.71 Retest 0.74
		Mean	*0.43*

DIPD-IV, Diagnostic Interview for DSM-IV Personality Disorders; IDCL-P, International Diagnostic Checklist for the Assessment of DSM-III-R and ICD-10 Personality Disorders; IPDE, International Personality Disorder Examination; LEAD, Longitudinal Expert Using All Available Data; MCMI, Millon Clinical Multiaxial Inventory; MCMI-II, Millon Clinical Multiaxial Inventory—II; PDE, Personality Disorder Examination; PDQ, Personality Diagnostic Questionnaire; PDQ-R, Personality Diagnostic Questionnaire—Revised; SCID-I, Structured Clinical Interview for DSM-IV Axis I Disorders; SCID-II, Structured Clinical Interview for DSM-IV Axis II Personality Disorders; SIDP, Structured Interview for the DSM-III Personality Disorders; SIDP-R, Structured Interview for the DSM-III Personality Disorders—Revised.

comparing the LEAD to the PDE ($\kappa = 0.06$). These results suggest problems with the LEAD.

Bronisch and Mombour [30] undertook a study in which the International Diagnostic Checklist for the Assessment of DSM-III-R and ICD-10 Personality

Disorders (IDCL-P) and the International Personality Disorder Examination (IPDE) were administered to forty inpatients over two consecutive days. There was acceptable agreement with regard to the presence of a PD, but low agreement for the specific types of PDs. The OCPD kappa was moderate ($\kappa = 0.30$).

Pilkonis *et al.* [31] examined the reliability and validity of Axis II disorders in 108 patients with non-psychotic Axis I disorders, comparing the Structured Interview for the DSM-III Personality Disorders—Revised (SIDP-R) and the PDE. Kappas were computed by comparing the interview diagnosis from the primary rater's protocol against the best estimate consensus. The kappa for any PD was 0.18 for the PDE and 0.37 for the SIDP-R. Kappas for OCPD were $\kappa = 0.51$ on the PDE and $\kappa = 0.40$ on the SIDP-R.

To summarize, Table 6.2 reports the diagnostic agreement expressed as kappa coefficient for the studies that examined OCPD via hetero-methods (interview vs. self-report) and mono-methods (interview vs. interview). The mean kappa for interview vs. self-report across six studies primarily dealing with DSM-III and DSM-III-R is a dismal 0.10. In contrast, the mean kappa for structured interviews vs. structured interviews across five studies is considerably higher ($\kappa = 0.43$), although still far from the 0.70 value of kappa considered to be acceptable. From these data one could justifiably conclude that the diagnosis of OCPD is an illusive and perhaps illusory construct. If these were the only results available, the weight of the empirical evidence would suggest that OCPD is not a valid diagnosis insofar as trained clinicians cannot reach acceptable levels of agreement when identifying individuals with the disorder.

However, Zanarini *et al.* [32], as part of the CLPS [20], reported the first kappas above the 0.70 threshold. Utilizing the SCID-I and the DIPD, they found that OCPD displayed a median interrater kappa of 0.71 at test and a kappa of 0.74 at retest. They further note that the dimensional levels of Axis II reliability are much higher than the categorical ones, suggesting that there is interrater agreement on whether a subject displays character pathology on a specific dimension but disagreement on the number of diagnostic criteria met.

Diagnostic Efficiency of Criterial Items

Another study by the CLPS group [33] examined the internal consistency and diagnostic efficiency of the specific criterial items of OCPD. Within-category inter-relatedness was evaluated in two ways: Cronbach's alpha and the median intercriterion correlations (MIC). Cronbach's alpha for OCPD was 0.69 and the MIC was 0.20. To examine criterion-overlap among

PD categories, they calculated an inter-category median intercriterion correlation (ICMIC) [33]. For OCPD, ICMIC values ranged from 0.00 (antisocial) to 0.07 (narcissistic), suggesting that OCPD criteria are more related to each other than to criteria for other PDs. Thus, in the CLPS data set, the OCPD diagnosis seems to possess an adequate degree of discriminant validity. Grilo *et al.* [33] concluded that the absence of three criteria for OCPD (#8, rigid and stubborn, #2, perfectionism, and #6, reluctant to delegate) is generally predictive of the absence of the diagnosis.

Table 6.3 lists how frequently each of the criterial items for OCPD is endorsed (base rate). Only one item, miserly, had an extremely low base rate (0.14). The positive predictive power (PPP) reveals that the eight criteria are of moderate usefulness in terms of their ability to predict a diagnosis, despite the fact that two criteria (1 and 7) show high values. Overall, we can identify a few of the items as bad (miserly and workaholic) and suggest they be replaced or deleted from the OCPD criteria. Criteria 1, 2, 6, and 8 are more useful than the others.

Confirmatory factor analysis of the CLPS data [34] suggested reorienting the criteria according to their prototypicality. Under this scheme, the DSM-IV's sixth and eighth criteria would be advanced to first and fourth place, respectively, suggesting that "reluctant to delegate tasks" and "rigid and stubborn" are more prototypic features of OCPD than "workaholic" and "pack rat".

COMORBIDITY OF OCPD WITH CERTAIN AXIS I AND AXIS II DISORDERS

OCD

The relationship between OCD and OCPD has long been of great interest to clinicians. Later psychoanalysts suggested a common aetiology, viz. fixation or regression to the anal stage of development [35]. As noted above, Kraepelin [7] and especially Janet [8,9] considered that specific personality traits precede the development of what we would call OCD and are part of the condition. In contrast, Aubrey Lewis [36] rejected the notion of obsessional personality features specific to patients with obsessive neurosis, noting that, while many obsessional patients have features of excessive cleanliness, orderliness, pedantry, conscientiousness, and uncertainty (which, in some cases, may be obsessional symptoms rather than character traits), these characteristics are also commonly found among patients without obsessions. Instead, Lewis suggested that there were two types of personality in individuals with chronic, severe obsessional neurosis, one

TABLE 6.3 Diagnostic efficiency of criterial items of obsessive–compulsive personality disorder (OCPD). Reproduced by permission of Blackwell Publishing Ltd. from Grilo *et al.* [33]

DSM-IV criteria	BR	SEN	SPE	PPP	NPP	Item total	Factor score weights [34]	Proto-typicality ranking of criteria [34]
Criterion 1: Details rules lists and order	0.29	0.60	0.92	0.83	0.78	0.43	0.65	3
Criterion 2: Perfectionism	0.43	0.78	0.80	0.72	0.85	0.45	0.77	2
Criterion 3: Workaholic	0.27	0.51	0.88	0.73	0.73	0.31	0.42	6
Criterion 4: Inflexible about morality	0.31	0.58	0.86	0.73	0.76	0.37	0.53	5
Criterion 5: Pack rat	0.40	0.64	0.75	0.62	0.76	0.29	0.35	7
Criterion 6: Reluctant to delegate tasks	0.46	0.82	0.78	0.71	0.87	0.52	0.67	1
Criterion 7: Miserly	0.14	0.29	0.96	0.82	0.68	0.27	0.27	8
Criterion 8: Rigid and stubborn	0.45	0.79	0.77	0.69	0.85	0.43	0.57	4
Mean	0.34	0.62	0.84	0.73	0.79	0.38	—	—

BR, Base rate; SEN, Sensitivity; SPE, Specificity; PPP, Positive Predictive Power; NPP, Negative Predictive Power.

being characterized by negative affect, stubbornness, and irritability, and the other more characterized by uncertainty in themselves or decision-making, and submissiveness.

It is instructive to trace the changes across editions of the DSM in the conceptualization of the relationship between OCD and OCPD. There was a trend from the DSM-I [10] to the DSM-III [12] to emphasize the potential relationship between OCD and OCPD. However, the DSM-IV [14] de-emphasized the likelihood of such a relationship and suggested that the two conditions were distinct, as OCD was marked by the presence of real obsessions and compulsions. In contrast, ICD-9 [37] is fuzzier in its distinction between anankastic personality disorder (i.e. OCPD) and obsessional neurosis (i.e. OCD), noting that the difference is one of degree, i.e. the unwelcome cognitions in the former are not as severe. Such differences in conceptualization and diagnostic criteria may explain why there are differences between studies in the reported comorbidity of OCPD in OCD.

Black and Noyes [38] reviewed studies on the co-occurrence of OCPD and OCD. Results from studies conducted before 1974 indicated that 64–84% of patients with OCD had premorbid obsessional traits; however, standardized diagnostic instruments were rarely used. In addition, family studies [36,39–41] found that relatives of OCD patients frequently had obsessional personality traits. However, it is difficult to conclude that this occurrence was unexpectedly high, since the occurrence of personality traits in relatives of non-OCD control groups, using comparable diagnostic methods, was not reported.

Other recent studies, which used standardized personality disorder assessment instruments (SIDP, PDQ, SCID, or MCMI), found a relatively high co-occurrence of DSM-III compulsive or DSM-III-R obsessive–compulsive personality disorder in persons with OCD. The co-occurrence ranged from 16% to 44% [42–47], but, again, the co-occurrence of these personality disorders in comparable control groups, using comparable diagnostic instruments, was not reported [38].

More recently, the Hopkins OCD Family Study, in which OCD cases were matched on age, sex, race, and telephone exchange to non-OCD community controls, reported a rate of 32% of DSM-IV OCPD in case probands, compared to 6% for control probands, and in 12% of case relatives, compared to 6% of control relatives [48].

In contrast, other studies also using standardized diagnostic instruments found a low co-occurrence (2–6%) of compulsive or obsessive–compulsive personality disorder in individuals with OCD [49–53]. If OCPD was not found to be the most common comorbid disorder with OCD, then what PDs, if any, do they find? Most frequently reported in OCD subjects are avoidant, dependent, and passive-aggressive PDs, which are classified along with OCPD in the DSM-III "anxious" cluster. A Brazilian study of 40 DSM-III-R diagnosed OCD patients and 40 non-psychiatric controls found similar results. Two Cluster C disorders (avoidant and dependent) were much more common in OCD than OCPD (52.5% for avoidant and 40% for dependent versus 17.5% for OCPD) [54].

Although most studies suggest that OCPD occurs more frequently in OCD than in non-OCD cases, OCPD is not found in the majority of OCD cases, which might be expected if they were intrinsically comorbid. This leads one to conclude that OCPD is not an intrinsic feature of OCD and that the nature of the relationship between OCPD and OCD remains unresolved. Normal personality dimensions may provide greater insight into the personality features of individuals with OCD. Few studies have assessed the prevalence of obsessive–compulsive traits, as opposed to OCPD, in OCD cases and their relatives.

An exception is a study by Samuels *et al.* [48] in 72 OCD cases and 72 control probands and 198 case and 207 control first degree relatives. They found that all facets of neuroticism were higher in case probands. Case probands were also significantly higher in openness to fantasy and feelings. OCD case probands scored lower in two facets of conscientiousness (competence and self-discipline). These trait differences between OCD case probands and controls are substantially different from the expected trait profile of individuals with OCPD. The finding of low conscientiousness scores in those with OCD was replicated by Rector *et al.* [55], who studied 98 patients with a primary diagnosis of OCD and 98 major depressives using the NEO Personality Inventory—Revised (NEO-PI-R) domains and facets. OCD patients were more extraverted, including significant facet differences in the desire to express warm and tender emotions, but these significant differences were lost when depression severity was controlled. Again, these results highlight the importance of investigating concomitant anxiety and depression symptoms for future studies for OCPD.

Eating Disorders

In several studies, OCPD has been shown to be the most common Axis II disorder comorbid with eating disorders (binge eating disorder, BED or anorexia nervosa, AN). Co-occurrence rates range from 15.2% [56] to 26% [57,58] for BED and 20% [59] to 61% [60] for AN. Zaider *et al.* [61] reported that, after controlling for other PDs, only OCPD independently predicted the presence of eating disorder symptoms.

One problem unresolved by these studies is that they cannot address the direction of causation, i.e. whether personality traits predispose a person to develop eating disorders, or whether eating disorders result in the exaggeration of certain personality traits or disorders; or whether eating disorders and personality traits are caused by a common third variable [62]. Lilenfeld *et al.* [63], in a study of 26 anorexic probands and their first-degree relatives, found evidence for shared familial transmission of AN and OCPD.

Anderluh *et al.* [60] used a sample of 44 women with AN to investigate the frequency of childhood traits reflecting obsessive–compulsive personality and their effect on the development of eating disorders. These traits included perfectionism, inflexibility, rule-boundness, doubt and cautiousness, and the drive for order and symmetry. Two-thirds of women reported perfectionism and at least one of the two traits reflecting rigidity in childhood. A logistic regression analysis showed that for every additional childhood trait that is present, the estimated odds ratio for the development of an eating disorder increased by 6.9%. Hence, retrospective childhood OCPD traits increase the likelihood of the co-occurrence of OCPD in adulthood.

Grilo [56] conducted a principal components factor analysis with varimax rotation on the eight DSM-IV criteria for OCPD. Results showed that three of the OCPD criteria accounted for 65% of the variance in BED. They were: rigid and stubborn, which made up 39.3% of the variance; perfectionism, which accounted for 13.8%; and miserly, which accounted for 11.8%. The author notes that these three criteria may reflect distinct interpersonal control (rigidity), intrapersonal control (perfectionism), and behavioural features (miserliness) of OCPD. This study confirms Anderluh *et al.*'s [60] emphasis on childhood rigidity and perfectionism and its influence on the development of eating disorders.

Other DSM-III-R Axis I Disorders

Among patients with either DSM-III-R depressive or bipolar disorders, Rossi *et al.* [64] found that OCPD (30%) and borderline diagnoses were very common (about 30%). In one of the few studies of DSM-III-R defined panic disorder with agoraphobia, Brooks *et al.* [65] reported that OCPD (27%), along with avoidant (26%) and paranoid (20%), was the most common PD.

Other DSM-IV Axis I Disorders

McGlashan *et al.* [66], in the Collaborative Longitudinal Personality Disorders (CLPD) Study, examined the diagnostic co-occurrence of OCPD with Axis I disorders. A significant number of OCPD patients (75.8%) were diagnosed with major depression. Also of significance, 29.4% were diagnosed to have comorbid generalized anxiety disorder (GAD), 29.4% alcohol abuse/dependence, and 25.7% drug abuse/dependence. In another study [67], OCPD was the most common personality disorder (17.1%) in elderly patients with dysthymic disorder.

The frequent co-occurrence of a mood disorder, especially major depressive disorder, with OCPD is likely to have significant influences on individuals' personality traits. Specifically, mood disorder is likely to elevate a patient's neuroticism and lower his extraversion and conscientiousness. One implication of this finding is that predictions based solely on the FFM [68] are likely to be seriously in error as they do not take into account mood disorder.

DSM-III Axis II Co-occurrence

There have been several studies of the occurrence of other PDs in individuals with OCPD. In the study by Zimmerman and Coryell [69] discussed above, of 16 non-patient subjects with DSM-III compulsive personality disorder, half had another PD; the most frequent co-occurring PDs were histrionic ($n = 3$), paranoid ($n = 2$), and avoidant, borderline, and passive-aggressive (each with $n = 2$). Zimmerman and Coryell also reported the correlations among personality disorder dimensions, which were the numbers of personality criteria present for each disorder. The compulsive score correlated most strongly with scores on histrionic, narcissistic, avoidant, borderline, and passive-aggressive (all $rs \sim 0.33$).

By contrast, in the clinical reappraisal [70] sample of eastern Baltimore residents, Nestadt *et al.* found that only one subject with DSM-III PD had another PD (schizotypal). The compulsive score, derived by summing the scores of each of the compulsive traits, was most strongly correlated with the histrionic score ($r = 0.28$). The CLPD Study [67] showed that among 153 patients with OCPD, 8% had DSM-IV paranoid, 9% borderline, 7% narcissistic, 28% avoidant, and 23% research diagnosis depressive PD. Also, the presence of OCPD was related to absence of antisocial PD. The authors note that this is logical, since the trademarks of OCPD are steadiness, careful planning, and a proclivity toward work, the antithesis of antisocial PD. Finally, no significant co-occurrence between OCD and OCPD was found.

DSM-III-R Axis II Co-occurrence

Pfohl and Blum [3] noted that the primary problem with DSM-III-R defined OCPD is its overlap with other PDs. But, as Morey [71] pointed out, this problem extends beyond OCPD. The primary difficulty with DSM-III-R PD criteria is that revisions significantly increased the amount of diagnostic overlap between PDs. Morey [71] noted that, while the DSM-III had four PDs with a considerable co-occurrence, the DSM-III-R had six disorders with co-occurrence rates of 20% or greater. OCPD displayed the greatest overlap with avoidant (56.5%) and narcissistic (30.4%) PDs. Widiger and Trull [72], across a variety of different semi-structured interviews, observed DSM-III-R defined OCPD cases to co-occur with six other PDs at the 20% or greater level: avoidant (37.2%), dependent (27.2%), histrionic (21.1%), paranoid (30.5%), passive-aggressive (23%) and borderline (24.6%).

In contrast to the limitations of the previous two studies (small sample sizes, infrequently occurring personality disorders limiting detection of patterns of co-occurrence), Stuart *et al.* [73] studied over 1000 inpatients and outpatients in four US and one Italian clinic, all using the SIDP-R. In this large series of patients, the most common PDs were avoidant, histrionic and dependent, the least common were schizoid, schizotypal and sadistic. The co-occurrence percentages between OCPD and other Axis II disorders were, in descending magnitude, schizoid (43.8%), paranoid (39.4%), schizotypal (36.4%), avoidant (35%), passive-aggressive (32.3%), dependent (30.8%) and borderline (25.7%). Interestingly, OCPD had higher percentages of co-occurrence with some of the least common PDs, namely the Cluster A diagnoses of schizoid and schizotypal, than with avoidant or dependent PDs. But, of course, these rates do not take into account the degree of overlap or co-occurrence that would occur by chance.

For that, Stuart *et al.* turned to the odds ratio statistic. Odds ratios are an informative index of co-occurrence. Odds ratios greater than 4.0 were considered to be clinically significant, i.e. beyond that expected simply by chance. Of the 11 PDs, significant odds ratios were observed only for three PDs: avoidant (4.72), paranoid (4.46) and schizoid (4.21). The significant co-occurrence with avoidant is not surprising, but the lack of co-occurrence with dependent is.

Even more surprising or unexpected is the beyond chance co-occurrence of OCPD with the two Cluster A PDs of paranoid and schizoid. The authors remark that "Though very few of the subjects diagnosed with either avoidant or obsessive–compulsive PD were diagnosed with schizoid PD, nearly two-thirds of the subjects diagnosed with schizoid PD met criteria for avoidant PD and over 43% met criteria for obsessive–compulsive PD". Interestingly, when the Iowa and Italy samples were analysed separately and odds ratios compared within samples, the largest odds ratio was within the Iowa sample and was 8.41 between OCPD and paranoid PD.

DSM-IV Axis II Co-occurrence

McGlashan *et al.* [67] from the CLPS study group, using the DIPD, reported co-occurrence rates between OCPD and the other Axis II disorders. Of the 86 schizotypal patients, 27 or 31.4% also received an OCPD diagnosis. Of the 175 borderlines, 45 or 25.7% met OCPD criteria. Of the 157 avoidant patients, 36 or 22.9% also obtained an OCPD diagnosis. These results are quite similar to those obtained by Stuart *et al.* [73], also showing higher co-occurrence rates of OCPD with a Cluster A diagnosis (schizotypal, 31%)

than a Cluster C disorder (avoidant 22.9%). In the CLPS data set, when the other Axis II diagnoses received by the 153 OCPD patients were considered, for five of the PDs the co-occurrences were near zero or zero (schizoid 0%, schizotypal 0%, antisocial 2%, histrionic 2% and, surprisingly, dependent 2.6%). The remaining three disorders showed co-occurrences of 27.5% (avoidant), 9.2% (borderline) and 7.9% (paranoid). Whether these dramatically lower co-occurrence rates reflect changes in DSM-IV criteria, or the diagnostic interview employed, or the particular sample, or the sample cell-assignment design, will need to be determined by subsequent research.

TEMPORAL STABILITY OF OCPD

There are little data to support the DSM-IV assumption of a persistent pattern of maladaptive traits throughout adulthood for PDs. Many of the studies that did examine diagnostic stability did not report rates for individual PDs because of study group size [74]. The only study that specifically investigated the stability of OCPD was again from the CLPS group. In a sample of 146 OCPD patients, Shea *et al.* [74] report that 60% of patients stayed at threshold or above at six months. However, a majority of patients failed to maintain their diagnosis over a 12-month period. In fact, only 42% of patients showed diagnostic stability from the first to the twelfth month.

Shea and Yen [75] have reported that individuals with OCPD have higher recovery rates than the other PDs (57%, versus 47% for avoidant, 42% for borderline and 34% for schizotypal) at 2 years. Surprisingly, rates of remission/recovery from OCPD were higher than rates for Axis I anxiety disorders. Far from being enduring and reflecting personality and character, OCPD, as well as other PDs, appears to be similar to other episodic psychiatric syndromes.

Another index of temporal instability is the number of criteria that individuals diagnosed with OCPD display at different time points. In the CLPS data set, the mean number of criteria met at baseline was 5.2 and fell to 4.0 at six months and 3.4 at twelve months. Even though the individuals at twelve months do not meet the threshold to receive the OCPD diagnosis, they still carry many of the traits. This highlights the problematic nature of the diagnostic threshold, and efforts to make the number of criteria more appropriate should be undertaken. It may also be necessary to lower the number of criteria necessary to receive the diagnosis and, as Grilo and McGlashan [58] note, the impact of Axis I psychiatric disorders on PD course needs to be explored to see if any effect, whether positive or negative, can be discerned.

FUNCTIONAL IMPAIRMENT AND OCPD

According to the DSM-IV, personality traits are indicative of PDs only if they lead to functional impairment or distress. Although one can conceive of situations—particularly work activities—in which extreme orderliness, perfectionism, and conscientiousness are useful, one might expect that obsessive–compulsive traits are not adaptive in many interpersonal situations. However, because many individuals with OCPD traits may not present for treatment in the absence of co-occurring psychopathology, the impact of these traits on social functioning has not been investigated. Furthermore, to our knowledge, there has been little study of the relationship between OCPD traits and social impairment in community samples.

We investigated this issue in analyses of the Hopkins Epidemiology of Personality Study (HEPS). Subjects ($n = 730$) were sampled from the Baltimore Epidemiologic Catchment Area Follow-up survey that has been described previously. The sample was overselected for subjects with specific mood disorders, anxiety disorders, and alcohol and drug use disorders, but most individuals in the sample did not have these disorders [76]. A total of 742 subjects were examined by clinical psychologists, using the IPDE [77].

Prior to the IPDE interview, clinical psychologists asked questions about relationships with parents, siblings, children, and spouses or partners; performance at work, school, and home; and use of free time, all over the past six months. Scales for six areas of functioning were derived by summing scores for each of the questions comprising the area of functioning. Subjects were also asked to give overall ratings of their functioning in the three areas of social, family, and work lives over the past six months. Ratings of functioning were correlated with the psychologists rating of the subjects' OCPD score, derived by summing the score for each of the DSM-IV OCPD traits, based on responses by the subject as well as knowledgeable informants.

As shown in Table 6.4, OCPD scores showed small negative correlation coefficients to relationships with spouse/partner and siblings, self-rated performance at work/school/home, and use of free time. Considering the three overall areas of functioning, OCPD scores were again significantly though modestly related to social and family life but not work life. Finally, OCPD scores were not related to the psychiatrist-rated current Global Assessment of Functioning (GAF) (Axis IV of DSM-IV).

OCPD traits in the HEPS data set do not impair or otherwise correlate to relations with children or parents, but do significantly impair relations with spouse or partner. The impact of OCPD on social functioning might thus be less negative for individuals who are unmarried or have no partner.

There may be other areas of interpersonal interaction and performance, not measured in the HEPS study, in which OCPD traits are maladaptive or

TABLE 6.4   Obsessive–compulsive personality disorder (OCPD) score correlations with functioning domains

Scale	Pearson correlation coefficient	p value
Relationship with spouse/partner	−0.20	<0.001
Relationship with children	−0.03	0.41
Relationship with parents	−0.08	0.19
Relationship with siblings	−0.13	0.001
Performance at work, school, home	−0.12	0.001
Use of free time	−0.12	0.002
Overall functioning in social life	−0.15	<0.001
Overall functioning in family life	−0.09	0.02
Overall functioning in work life	−0.04	0.29
Global Assessment of Functioning	0.06	0.14

even adaptive. This issue and that of interactions between these traits and the environment (e.g. degree of job stress; proximity to family members) need to be explored.

The CLPS group [78] also evaluated functional impairment in patients with schizotypal, borderline, avoidant PDs or OCPD via interviewer-administered and self-report measures. 5-point ratings (1 = high level of functioning or very good functioning; 2 = no impairment, satisfactory or good functioning; 3 = mild impairment or fair functioning; 4 = moderate impairment or poor functioning, and 5 = severe impairment or very poor functioning) were used in four specific areas of functioning: employment, household duties, student work, and recreation. A fifth area of functioning, interpersonal relationships, was subdivided into six sub-areas of parents, siblings, spouse/mate, children, relatives and friends. Importantly, the highest rating of impairment in all of these areas of functioning was 2.7, indicating less than mild impairment in the arena of interactions with friends and recreation. None of the areas of functioning, including global satisfaction ratings, had moderate or severe impairment ratings. Even the global social adjustment ratings were in the mild impairment or fair functioning range (3.2). These results shed interesting light on the limited degree of social impairment of OCPD.

Lastly, in terms of GAF scores, Skodol et al. [78] found that OCPD was associated with the least degree of functional impairment (score of 64.7 as compared to 54.1 for schizotypal, 54.3 for borderline, 60.4 for avoidant, and 60.7 for major depressive disorder).

These findings suggest that while OCPD patients are not without any degree of impairment, they appear to be generally well functioning in terms of social, occupational, school and interpersonal functioning.

Another study by Costa *et al.* [79] investigated the degree to which OCPD traits cause or are related to significant impairment in a large sample of depressed outpatients undergoing treatment at the Center for Addiction and Mental Health in Toronto, Canada. In their sample of 203 patients, none of the OCPD criterial items correlated significantly with GAF ratings. These results are consistent with the CLPS results [78] and raise the possibility that OCPD may not be a diagnosis that causes moderate or severe impairment.

TREATMENT OF OCPD

Like other PDs, the treatment of OCPD presents considerable challenges to the clinician. These patients often are rigid and inflexible, seek absolute clarity, have a strong need for control, are resistant to change, and suppress expression of emotions and feelings. Moreover, it is difficult for them to recognize that their personality features are maladaptive, and they come into treatment only at the insistence of an exasperated spouse or supervisor, or because of symptoms of depression, anxiety, or somatic complaints [80].

The traditional approach to treatment is intensive psychoanalysis. During the long course of interaction with the therapist and interpretation by the therapist of transference feelings and behaviours, it is hoped that the patient will become aware of the defences he marshals to control anxiety (intellectualization, isolation, displacement, and reaction formation) and how these interfere with a satisfying interpersonal life [81]. Given the length and cost of this approach, more focused, time-limited treatment approaches have been proposed, including brief [82] and group psychotherapy [83].

More recently, cognitive-behavioural therapies have been the treatment of choice for OCPD. Cognitive therapy aims to identify and change patients' maladaptive interpretations and meanings that they associate with experience [84]. For example, some maladaptive cognitive "schemas" of OCPD patients are: "There are right and wrong behaviors, decisions and emotions; I must avoid mistakes to be worthwhile; to make mistakes is to have failed; loss of control is intolerable; I must be perfectly in control of my environment as well as of myself" [85]. Behavioural therapy aims to increase adaptive and decrease maladaptive behaviour patterns, by using behavioural techniques such as graded exposure to increase the patient's rewards and tolerance for novelty, increase emotional awareness and expression, and decrease avoidance tendencies. In practice, these modalities are often used together [86].

Stone [87] suggested that OCPD patients respond best to treatment when they are characterized mainly by an inability to experience positive affect, and have few antagonistic features. However, it must be emphasized that, apart from clinical observation, there is little empirical evidence and no rigorous efficacy trials of any approach for the treatment of OCPD [88,89]. Indeed, the weight of the clinical literature suggests that, as for other PDs, treatment of OCPD is difficult, requiring patience and flexibility on the part of patient and therapist. Even in resistant cases, however, the clinician can encourage patients to capitalize on adaptive aspects of their personalities [90].

DIMENSIONAL APPROACHES TO OCPD

DSM-IV OCPD and the FFM

The FFM [91] provides one possible dimensional approach to PD diagnosis. The continuing and growing consensus on the model, as well as the fact that the alternative dimensional models can be understood within the FFM framework, make it a logical choice. The comprehensiveness, temporal stability, heritability, and universality of the FFM dimensions are additional positive features. Specifically, the hypothesis that PDs are maladaptive problems associated with general personality traits of the FFM has been supported by several studies that showed significant correlations between the five broad dimensions and PD scales.

The volume Personality Disorders and the Five-Factor Model of Personality [92] focused explicitly on the relationship of the FFM to PD symptomatology. A key chapter by Widiger et al. [93] translated the DSM-III-R PDs (using both criterial items and associated features) into the more specific facet scales of the NEO-PI-R. The criteria for each PD were first translated into one or more of the 30 facets of the NEO-PI-R and the facets were hypothesized to be either positively related (marked as an expected high score) or negatively related (marked as an expected low score) on the respective NEO-PI-R facet scale. Between the first [92] and second [91] editions of this volume, a substantial amount of empirical research, indeed over 50 studies, showed empirical support for these hypothesized links [91].

Focusing only on the DSM-IV criteria items, Widiger et al. [68] mapped 10 DSM-IV PDs in terms of the FFM. OCPD is primarily seen as "a disorder of excessive conscientiousness, including such facets as order (preoccupation with details, rules, lists, order), achievement striving (excessive devotion to work and productivity), dutifulness (overconscientious, scrupulousness about matters of ethics and morality), and competence (perfectionism)". Adaptively conscientious people tend to be organized, self-disciplined, hardworking, reliable, and punctual. On the other hand, maladaptively conscientious people (i.e. OCPD individuals) are excessively devoted to work; perfectionist to such a degree that tasks are often not completed; and preoccupied with details, lists, and rules [68]. They are also closed to values, manifested in the DSM-IV criteria as rigid and stubborn and inflexible about matters of morality, ethics, or values. Finally, the authors note that the OCPD person's reluctance to delegate tasks or work with others unless they submit to his or her way of doing things may be a manifestation of low compliance and high assertiveness.

Empirical Tests of DSM-III-R and DSM-IV Hypothesized OCPD-FFM Facet Predictions

Early studies that assessed the relationship of the FFM to PD symptomatology largely focused on the broad domains (N, E, O, A, and C). Table 6.5 provides results in terms of coefficients of correlation between four different measures of DSM-III-R defined OCPD and the five factors or domains of the NEO PI-R [93].

For neuroticism, significant Pearson rs ranged from 0.16 [95] to 0.52 [94]. Only one DSM-III-R study [95] yielded a significant negative correlation ($r = -0.39$, $p < 0.001$), which was obtained on the MCMI-I, and the correlations for the two other studies utilizing either the MCMI-II or MCMI-III [95,96], though non-significant, were also negative. Only the three forms of the MCMI yielded negative correlations with neuroticism, possibly suggesting a problem with the instrument.

Considering extraversion, all reported correlations were negative, though less than half were significant. Significant correlations ranged from -0.29 [94] to -0.62 [95].

Conceptually, the domain most related to OCPD from DSM-III-R facet level predictions is conscientiousness. Haigler and Widiger [97] rationalized its role: "It is not unreasonable to hypothesize that persons who are excessively conscientious will be overconscientious; will engage in excessive deliberation; will be excessively devoted to their work to the detriment of social and leisure activities; will be perfectionistic to the point that tasks are not completed; or will be preoccupied with order, organization, rules, and details". However, the domain and facet level studies have not consistently demonstrated this. For DSM-III-R studies, only one self-report instrument, the MCMI, shows large positive correlations with conscientiousness. Dyce and O'Connor [96], in a large undergraduate student sample, also found a significant correlation (0.62) for MCMI-III OCPD scale and NEO-PI-R conscientiousness, and the more specific facets of conscientiousness were all moderate in magnitude, as well ranging from 0.38 for competence to 0.51 for self-discipline.

Trull *et al.* [98], utilizing the Structured Interview for the Five-Factor Model (SIFFM) to evaluate DSM-IV OCPD-FFM predictions, observed significant correlations on all six neuroticism facets. DSM-IV OCPD symptom severity scores studied by Trull *et al.* [98] were also correlated with high introversion whether measured by the SIFFM or the standard self-report NEO-PI-R measure. DeClercq and Fruyt [99], in an adolescent student sample, found that low extraversion scores were negatively correlated with OCPD scores, with five of the six facets ranging from −0.22 to −0.17.

Considering the domains and facets of openness, agreeableness and conscientiousness, Trull *et al.* found OCPD symptom counts to be positively related to fantasy and ideas, but negatively related to actions. OCPD symptom counts tended to be negatively related to the facets of agreeableness, particularly trust (−0.26). Regarding the facets of conscientiousness, all were negatively correlated, but only the coefficients for competence and self-discipline were −0.20 or higher.

TABLE 6.5 Correlations between DSM-III-R obsessive–compulsive personality disorder (OCPD) and FFM domains

Study	Assessment tool used	FFM tool used	N	E	O	A	C
Trull [94]	MMPI	NEO-PI	0.52*	−0.29*	0.03	−0.27	−0.01
Costa and McCrae [95]	MMPI Self-Report	NEO-PI	0.16*	−0.62*	0.06*	−0.12*	0.14*
Trull [94]	SIDP-R	NEO-PI	0.29*	−0.28*	0.01	−0.53*	0.02
Trull [94]	PDQ-R	NEO-PI	0.38*	−0.05	0.26	−0.34*	−0.12
Costa and McCrae [95]	MCMI-I	NEO-PI	−0.39*	−0.09	−0.19*	0.09	0.38*
Costa and McCrae [95]	MCMI-II	NEO-PI	−0.05	−0.03	−0.11	0.15	0.52*
Dyce and O'Connor [96]	MCMI-III	NEO-PI-R	−0.14	−0.03	−0.15	0.22*	0.62*

*Significant correlation.
MMPI, Minnesota Multiphasic Personality Inventory; SIDP-R, Structured Interview for the DSM-III Personality Disorders—Revised; PDQ-R, Personality Diagnostic Questionnaire—Revised; MCMI, Millon Clinical Multiaxial Inventory; NEO-PI, NEO Personality Inventory; NEO-PI-R, NEO Personality Inventory—Revised; FFM, Five Factor Model; N, Neuroticism; E, Extraversion; O, Openness; A, Agreeableness; C, Conscientiousness.

Blais [100] found a moderate (0.21) correlation between OCPD and the FFM marker scales. He further notes that a principal component factor analysis showed OCPD to have loadings on a factor including openness and conscientiousness. Yang *et al.* [101], in a study of over 1900 Chinese psychiatric patients, found that 5 of the 6 facets of conscientiousness were non-significant and only one, achievement-striving, showed a small r of 0.1. This latter finding, along with the negative correlations found by Trull *et al.* (98) between OCPD symptom counts and competence and self-discipline, suggests the need to reexamine the hypothesis that DSM-defined OCPD can be measured or understood as extreme conscientiousness. Similar arguments were put forth by Morey and colleagues [102], who suggested that interactions between domains such as neuroticism and conscientiousness might better represent OCPD than single domain or facet level scores.

It might be argued, as several critics have, that the FFM is inadequate to capture the symptomology of the PDs. The more general claim is not supported, as there is substantial evidence that the FFM and especially its 30 facets more than adequately account for important disorders such as borderline and avoidant PDs [103,104]. But it may be the case that conscientiousness and its facets are not tapping the key elements of OCPD. Evidence against this particular argument is provided by convergence between Clark's [105] and Livesley's [106] models of personality pathology.

Clark's Schedule for Nonadaptive and Adaptive Personality (SNAP) resulted from comprehensive efforts to find empirical symptom clusters from all the DSM PD criteria as well as criteria from influential non-DSM conceptualizations of PD and from selected Axis I disorders noted to resemble PDs. In a study of 194 students enrolled in an introductory psychology course, the SNAP workaholism scale correlated strongest with conscientiousness ($r = 0.54$). This is the SNAP scale most similar to the DSM description of OCPD. SNAP impulsivity ($r = -0.51$), manipulativeness ($r = -0.44$), and dependency ($r = -0.41$) all correlated negatively with conscientiousness, while propriety ($r = 0.26$) correlated positively. A principal factor analysis was also utilized to investigate the combined structure of normal and abnormal personality traits. Clark *et al.* [105] reported that the results show "that the SNAP scales contain content relevant to all five factors and, furthermore, that the dimensions of the FFM account for much of the variance in traits of personality disorder". SNAP workaholism loaded heavily on conscientiousness (0.69), while SNAP impulsivity also had a significant negative loading (-0.66). OCPD's high conscientiousness manifestation in the NEO-PI-R seems to be represented here as well through workaholism.

Another dimensional approach is that of the Dimensional Assessment of Personality Pathology—Basic Questionnaire (DAPP-BQ) of Livesley [106]. Rather than begin with the DSM criteria symptoms of PDs, Livesley began the development of the DAPP-BQ by conducting a content analysis of the PD literature and compiling a comprehensive list of trait descriptors and behavioural acts. OCPD is captured in the DAPP-BQ dimension of compulsivity (orderliness, precision, and conscientiousness). In an obliquely rotated factor pattern for combined analysis of the NEO-PI factors and DAPP-BQ dimensions, compulsivity and passive-oppositionality (defined as difficulties in planning, organizing, and completing tasks) loaded most heavily on the NEO domain of conscientiousness (0.72 and −0.55 respectively). Schroeder et al. [106] also reported a large canonical correlation of 0.86 between compulsivity and conscientiousness. Finally, a multiple regression analysis, like the factor analysis, showed that conscientiousness related most strongly to compulsivity (0.69) and passive-oppositionality (−0.60).

Clark and Livesley [107] used the FFM as a common metric to compare the two trait structures of PD. The empirical correspondence of the matched scales was quite good. DAPP-BQ compulsivity correlated 0.63 with NEO conscientiousness and DAPP-BQ passive oppositionality correlated −0.71. Similar results were obtained for the corresponding SNAP scales: passive aggressiveness correlated −0.60 using the NEO Five Factor Inventory (FFI) and conventionality-rigidity correlated 0.32. The lower value for SNAP conventionality-rigidity compared to DAPP-BQ compulsivity may be due to the shorter version of the NEO being employed, or it may be that the relations between conscientiousness and conventionality-rigidity are lower in patient samples.

But in either case, these results demonstrate that NEO conscientiousness scores do relate meaningfully to maladaptive measures of compulsivity in community and patient samples. As Clark and Livesley [107] concluded, "In summary, the factor scales of the DAPP-BQ and the SNAP-based personality disorder symptom clusters are themselves highly convergent and yield an elaborated picture of the FFM that is quite consistent with previous descriptions of these domains".

Thus, alternative measures of personality pathology show that the FFM and NEO-PI-R scales can capture OCPD-relevant symptoms and dimensions. Perhaps the problems reside in the DSM definitions of the construct of OCPD. One possible way to approach this issue is to compare expert clinicians' prototypical OCPD ratings using the facets of the NEO-PI-R [93] for OCPD patients. Recent studies by Lynam and Widiger [108] and by Sprock [109] in fact did just that. Lynam and Widiger [108] generated an expert consensus prototype for each of the ten DSM-IV PDs by having a panel of 120 experts rate prototypic cases of the various PDs with respect to the 30 facet scales of the NEO-PI-R [93]. Experts were asked to rate the prototypic case of a specified personality disorder on a 1–5 scale. Taking any facet with a mean score of 2 and lower or 4 and higher as a relevant characteristic, it is possible to describe each PD with the facets of the NEO-PI-R. The experts' ratings are summarized in the first column of Table 6.6.

The second column in Table 6.6 summarizes the result of Sprock's study [109]. 181 doctoral-level licensed psychologists rated three case vignettes, one from each of the three clusters of PDs, including a mix of prototypic and nonprototypic cases. One group was asked to rate the case using only the five factors of the FFM and a second group was asked to rate using the 30 facets of the FFM.

The correlation of Sprock's OCPD prototype based on the 30 facets with Widiger and colleagues [68] DSM-III-R predictions for OCPD was a rather large 0.66. The convergences with the Lynam and Widiger [108] expert prototype were even greater. Sprock's [109] first group of clinicians who used only the broad factors correlated 0.79 with Lynam and Widiger and the correlation rose to 0.86 when the 30 facets were used. These are impressive levels of agreement between expert prototypes. As Sprock observed, "the prototypic obsessive–compulsive case was distinguished by high conscientiousness at the domain and facet level, low warmth, high assertiveness, and relatively low altruism, as suggested by Widiger and colleagues. However, it did not demonstrate the proposed associated features (i.e. low compliance, high hostility, depressiveness and self-consciousness), which may vary depending on severity or other features unique to the case".

SUMMARY

Consistent Evidence

Most of the consistent evidence alludes to problems with OCPD. Kappas have repeatedly been shown to be poor (0.10 for hetero-method and 0.43 for mono-method approaches), falling short of the 0.70 threshold. There is also a lack of empirical support for the number of diagnostic criteria needed to receive an OCPD diagnosis, that is highlighted by problems with temporal stability. In addition, the fact that OCPD shares its criteria with several other PDs (i.e. avoidant) is problematic, since the disorders are no longer orthogonal. On a positive note, antisocial PD, conceptually the direct opposite of OCPD, is consistently the lowest in terms of diagnostic overlap. Finally, OCPD is found to be highly comorbid with Axis I major depressive disorder, AN, and GAD, and Axis II avoidant PD. The lack of comorbidity with OCD is also consistently supported in the literature, with a few exceptions.

TABLE 6.6 Comparison of two sets of experts on the Five Factor Model (FFM) domains and facets for obsessive–compulsive personality disorder (OCPD)

	Lynam and Widiger's [108] experts	Sprock's [109] experts	Agreement between the two groups of experts
Neuroticism		H	
Extraversion			
Openness	L	L	Yes
Agreeableness		L	
Conscientiousness	H	H	Yes
N1: Anxiety	H		
N2: Angry-hostility			
N3: Depression			
N4: Self-consciousness			
N5: Impulsiveness	L	L	Yes
N6: Vulnerability			
E1: Warmth		L	
E2: Gregariousness			
E3: Assertiveness		H	
E4: Activity		H	
E5: Excitement-seeking	L		
E6: Positive emotions			
O1: Fantasy		L	
O2: Aesthetics		L	
O3: Feelings	L	L	Yes
O4: Actions	L	L	Yes
O5: Ideas	L	L	Yes
O6: Values	L	L	Yes
A1: Trust		L	
A2: Straightforwardness			
A3: Altruism			
A4: Compliance			
A5: Modesty			
A6: Tender mindedness		L	
C1: Competence	H	H	Yes
C2: Order	H	H	Yes
C3: Dutifulness	H	H	Yes
C4: Achievement striving	H	H	Yes
C5: Self-discipline	H	H	Yes
C6: Deliberation	H	H	Yes

Incomplete Evidence

The areas where evidence is incomplete include the following:

- The impact of Axis I disorders on the course and treatment of OCPD needs to be examined for its effect on temporal stability, since an Axis I disorder could worsen, improve, or have no effect on the course of an Axis II PD.

- In one study, the prototypicality of DSM-IV OCPD criteria was shown to be questionable and this finding [34] needs to be replicated. The implications for the DSM-V may be significant.

- The relationship of OCPD and eating disorders needs to be further explored to see if OCPD is an expression of AN or vice versa.

- Inconsistencies across studies exist in the extent to which ICPD is related to functional impairment. Future research is needed to resolve this issue.

Areas Still Open to Research

The areas still open to research included the following:

- Treatment approaches for OCPD need to be tested empirically.

- Comorbidity needs to be examined, to see if it is artifactual, or due to a cross-cutting underlying dimension, or caused by something else.

- Little attention has been paid to the frequency of obsessive–compulsive traits (as distinct from OCPD) in individuals with OCD. This relationship should be explored further.

- The diagnostic threshold for receiving an OCPD diagnosis was consistently shown to be problematic. Efforts need to be undertaken to firmly establish an empirically based threshold that takes into account the course, treatment, and impairment.

- The results of the correlational analyses undertaken to measure expert agreement between the Lynam and Widiger [108] and Sprock [109] studies suggest an intriguing new direction for future research. OCPD cases might be defined by a person's personality profile that matches the Sprock or Lynam and Widiger prototypic NEO-PI-R profile, not by meeting DSM criteria. Psychiatrists would then blindly interview patients whose personality profiles match OCPD consensus profile. It would be of interest to see which if any criteria they would all meet and what possible impairments they might possess.

REFERENCES

1. American Psychiatric Association (2000) *Diagnostic and Statistical Manual of Mental Disorders* (4th edn, text revision). American Psychiatric Association, Washington.
2. McHugh S. (1998) *The Perspectives of Psychiatry*, 2nd edn. Johns Hopkins University Press, Baltimore.
3. Pfohl B, Blum N. (1991) Obsessive–compulsive personality disorder: a review of available data and recommendations for DSM-IV. *J. Person. Disord.*, **5**: 363–375.
4. Freud S. (1908) Character and anal eroticism. In *The Standard Edition of the Complete Psychological Works of Sigmund Freud, Vol. 9* (Ed. J. Strachey), pp. 169–175. Hogarth, London.
5. Jones E. (1918) Anal-erotic character traits. In *Papers on Psycho-analysis*, 2nd edn, pp. 664–668. Baillière Tindall, London.
6. Abraham K. (1966) Contribution to the theory of the anal character. In *On Character and Libido Development* (Ed. B.D. Lewin), pp. 165–187. Basic Books, New York.
7. Kraepelin E. (1990) *Psychiatry, Vol. 2* (Ed. J.M. Quen). Science History, Canton.
8. Pitman R.K. (1984) Janet's obsessions and psychasthenia: a synopsis. *Psychiatr. Quarterly*, **56**: 291–314.
9. Pitman R.K. (1987) Pierre Janet on obsessive–compulsive disorder (1903). *Arch. Gen. Psychiatry*, **44**: 226–232.
10. American Psychiatric Association (1952) *Diagnostic and Statistical Manual of Mental Disorders*, 1st edn. American Psychiatric Association, Washington.
11. American Psychiatric Association (1968) *Diagnostic and Statistical Manual of Mental Disorders*, 2nd edn. American Psychiatric Association, Washington.
12. American Psychiatric Association (1980) *Diagnostic and Statistical Manual of Mental Disorders*, 3rd edn. American Psychiatric Association, Washington.
13. American Psychiatric Association (1987) *Diagnostic and Statistical Manual of Mental Disorders*, 3rd edn, revised. American Psychiatric Association, Washington.
14. American Psychiatric Association (1994) *Diagnostic and Statistical Manual of Mental Disorders*, 4th edn. American Psychiatric Association, Washington.
15. World Health Organization (1992) *The ICD-10 Classification of Mental and Behavioural Disorders. Clinical Descriptions and Diagnostic Guidelines*. World Health Organization, Geneva.
16. Ekselius L., Tillfors M., Furmark T., Fredrikson M. (2001) Personality disorders in the general population: DSM-IV and ICD-10 defined prevalence as related to sociodemographic profile. *Person. Indiv. Diff.*, **30**: 311–320.
17. Ottosson H., Ekselius L., Grann M., Kullgren G. (2002) Cross-system concordance of personality disorder diagnoses of DSM-IV and diagnostic criteria for research of ICD-10. *J. Person. Disord.*, **16**: 283–292.
18. Starcevic V., Bogojevic G., Kelin K. (1997) Diagnostic agreement between the DSM-IV and ICD-10-DCR personality disorders. *Psychopathology*, **30**: 328–334.
19. Livesley W.J. (2001) Conceptual and taxonomic issues. In *Handbook of Personality Disorders: Theory, Research, and Treatment* (Ed. W.J. Livesley), p. 17. Guilford, New York.
20. Gunderson J.G., Shea M.T., Skodol A.E., McGlashan T.H., Morey L.C., Stout R.L., Zanarini M.C., Grilo C.M., Oldham J.M., Keller M.B. (2000) The Collaborative Longitudinal Personality Disorders Study: development, aims, design, and sample characteristics. *J. Person. Disord.*, **14**: 300–315.

21. Clark L.A., Harrison J.A. (2001) Assessment instruments. In *Handbook of Personality Disorders: Theory, Research, and Treatment* (Ed. W.J. Livesley), pp. 277–306. Guilford, New York.

22. Perry J.C. (1992) Problems and considerations in the valid assessment of personality disorders. *Am. J. Psychiatry*, **149**: 1645–1653.

23. Hyler S.E., Rieder R.O., Williams J.B., Spitzer R.L., Lyons M., Hendler J. (1989) A comparison of clinical and self-report diagnoses of DSM-III personality disorders in 552 patients. *Compr. Psychiatry*, **30**: 170–178.

24. Zimmerman M., Coryell W.H. (1990) Diagnosing personality disorders in the community: a comparison of self-report and interview measures. *Arch. Gen. Psychiatry*, **47**: 527–531.

25. Hyler S.E., Skodol A.E., Kellman H.D., Oldham J.M., Rosnick L. (1990) Validity of the Personality Disorder Questionnaire Revised: comparison with two structured interviews. *Am. J. Psychiatry*, **147**: 1043–1048.

26. Jackson H.J., Gazis J., Rudd R.P., Edwards J. (1991) Concordance between two personality disorder instruments with psychiatric inpatients. *Compr. Psychiatry*, **32**: 252–260.

27. Soldz S., Budman S., Demby A., Merry J. (1993) Diagnostic agreement between the Personality Disorder Examination and the MCMI-II. *J. Person. Assess.*, **60**: 486–499.

28. Skodol A., Oldham J., Rosnick L., Kellman H.D., Hyler S. (1991) Diagnosis of DSM-III-R personality disorders: a comparison of two structured interviews. *Int. J. Methods Psychiatr. Res.*, **1**: 13–26.

29. Hyler S., Skodol A., Oldham J., Kellman H., Doidge N. (1992) Validity of the Personality Diagnostic Questionnaire—Revised: a replication in an outpatient sample. *Compr. Psychiatry*, **33**: 73–77.

30. Bronisch T., Mombour W. (1994) Comparison of a diagnostic checklist with a structured interview for the assessment of DSM-III-R and ICD-10 personality disorders. *Psychopathology*, **27**: 312–320.

31. Pilkonis P., Heape C., Proietti J., Clark S., McDavid J., Pitts T. (1995) The reliability and validity of two structured diagnostic interviews for personality disorders. *Arch. Gen. Psychiatry*, **52**: 1025–1033.

32. Zanarini M.C., Skodol A.E., Bender D., Dolan R., Sanislow C., Schaefer E., Morey L.C., Grilo C.M., Shea M.T., McGlashan T.H. *et al.* (2000) The Collaborative Longitudinal Personality Disorders Study: reliability of Axis I and II diagnoses. *J. Pers. Disord.*, **14**: 291–299.

33. Grilo C.M., McGlashan T.H., Morey L.C., Gunderson J.G., Skodol A.E., Shea M.T., Sainslow C.A., Zanarini M.C., Bender D., Oldham J.M. *et al.* (2001) Internal consistency, intercriterion overlap and diagnostic efficiency of criteria sets for DSM-IV schizotypal, borderline, avoidant, and obsessive–compulsive personality disorders. *Acta Psychiatr. Scand.*, **104**: 264–272.

34. Sanislow C.A., Morey L.C., Grilo C.M., Gunderson J.G., Shea M.T., Skodol A.E., Stout R.L., Zanarini M.C., McGlashan T.H. (2002) Confirmatory factor analysis of DSM-IV borderline, schizotypal, avoidant, and obsessive–compulsive personality disorders: findings from the collaborative longitudinal personality disorders study. *Acta Psychiatr. Scand.*, **105**: 28–36.

35. Kline P. (1968) Obsessional traits, obsessional symptoms, and anal eroticism. *Br. J. Med. Psychol.*, **41**: 299–305.

36. Lewis A. (1935) Problems of obsessional illness. *Proc. Roy. Soc. Med.*, **29**: 325–336.

37. World Health Organization (1980) *The International Classification of Diseases*, 9th edn. World Health Organization, Geneva.
38. Black D.W., Noyes R., Pfohl B., Goldstein R.B., Blum N. (1993) Personality disorder in obsessive–compulsive volunteers, well comparison subjects, and their first-degree relatives. *Am. J. Psychiatry*, **150**: 1226–1232.
39. Kringlen E. (1965) Obsessional neurotics: a long-term follow-up. *Br. J. Psychiatry*, **111**: 709–722.
40. Rasmussen S.A., Tsuang M.T. (1986) Clinical characteristics and family history in DSM-III obsessive–compulsive disorder. *Am. J. Psychiatry*, **143**: 317–322.
41. Lenane M.C., Swedo S.E., Leonard H., Pauls D.L., Sceery W., Rapoport J.L. (1990) Psychiatric disorders in first-degree relatives of children and adolescents with obsessive–compulsive disorder. *J. Am. Acad. Child Adolesc. Psychiatry*, **29**: 407–412.
42. Alnaes R., Torgerson S. (1988) The relationship between DSM-III symptom disorders (axis I) and personality disorders (axis II) in an outpatient population. *Acta Psychiatr. Scand.*, **78**: 485–492.
43. Pfohl B. (1996) Obsessiveness. In *Personality Characteristics of the Personality Disordered* (Ed. C.G. Costello), pp. 91–119. Wiley, New York.
44. Stanley M.A., Turner S.M., Bordern J.W. (1990) Schizotypal features in obsessive–compulsive disorder. *Compr. Psychiatry*, **31**: 511–518.
45. Baer L., Jenike M.A., Black D.W., Treece C., Rosenfeld R., Greist J. (1992) Effect of axis II diagnoses on treatment outcome with clomipramine in 55 patients with obsessive–compulsive disorder. *Arch. Gen. Psychiatry*, **49**: 862–866.
46. Ravizza L., Barzega G., Bellino S., Bogetto F., Maina G. (1995) Predictors of drug treatment response in obsessive–compulsive disorder. *J. Clin. Psychiatry*, **56**: 368–373.
47. Diaferia G., Bianchi I., Bianchi M.L., Cavedini P., Erzegovesi S., Bellodi L. (1997) Relationship between obsessive–compulsive personality disorder and obsessive–compulsive disorder. *Compr. Psychiatry*, **38**: 38–42.
48. Samuels J., Nestadt G., Bienvenu O., Costa P.T., Riddle M., Liang K., Hoehn-Saric R., Grados M., Cullen B. (2000) Personality disorders and normal personality dimensions in obsessive–compulsive disorder. *Br. J. Psychiatry*, **177**: 457–462.
49. Joffe R.T., Swinson R.P., Regan J.J. (1988) Personality features of obsessive–compulsive disorder. *Am. J. Psychiatry*, **145**: 1127–1129.
50. Baer L., Jenike M.A., Ricciardi J.N., Holland A.D., Seymour R.J., Minichiello W.E., Buttolph M.L. (1990) Standardized assessment of personality disorders and obsessive–compulsive disorders. *Arch. Gen. Psychiatry*, **47**: 826–830.
51. Mavissakalian M., Hamann M.S., Jones B. (1990) A comparison of DSM-III personality disorders in panic/agoraphobia and obsessive–compulsive disorder. *Compr. Psychiatry*, **31**: 238–244.
52. Mavissakalian M., Hamann M.S., Jones B. (1990) DSM-III personality disorders in obsessive–compulsive disorder: changes with treatment. *Compr. Psychiatry*, **31**: 432–437.
53. Mavissakalian M., Hamann M.S., Jones B. (1990) Correlates of DSM-III personality disorder in obsessive–compulsive disorder. *Compr. Psychiatry*, **31**: 481–489.
54. Torres A.R., Del Porto J.A. (1995) Comorbidity of obsessive–compulsive disorder and personality disorders: a Brazilian controlled study. *Psychopathology*, **28**: 322–329.

55. Rector N.A., Hood K., Richter M.A., Bagby R.M. (2002) Obsessive–compulsive disorder and the five-factor model of personality: distinction and overlap with major depressive disorder. *Behav. Res. Ther.*, **40**: 1205–1219.

56. Grilo C.M. (2004) Factor structure of DSM-IV criteria for obsessive–compulsive personality disorder in patients with binge eating disorder. *Acta Psychiatr. Scand.*, **109**: 64–69.

57. Karwautz A., Troop N., Rabe-Hesketh S., Collier D., Treasure J. (2003) Personality disorders and personality dimensions in anorexia nervosa. *J. Person. Disord.*, **17**: 73–85.

58. Grilo C.M., McGlashan T.H. (2000) Convergent and discriminant validity of DSM-IV axis II personality disorder criteria in adult outpatients with binge eating disorder. *Compr. Psychiatry*, **41**: 163–166.

59. Nilsson E.W., Gillberg C., Gillberg C., Rastam M. (1999) Ten-year follow-up of adolescent-onset anorexia nervosa: personality disorders. *J. Am. Acad. Child Adolesc. Psychiatry*, **38**: 1389–1395.

60. Anderluh M., Tchanturia K., Rabe-Hesketh S., Treasure J. (2003) Childhood obsessive–compulsive personality traits in adult women with eating disorders: defining a broader eating disorder phenotype. *Am. J. Psychiatry*, **160**: 242–247.

61. Zaider T., Johnson J., Cockell S. (2000) Psychiatric comorbidity associated with eating disorder symptomatology among adolescents in the community. *Int. J. Eat. Disord.*, **28**: 58–67.

62. Wonderlich S., Mitchell J. (2001) The role of personality in the onset of eating disorders and treatment implications. *Psychiatr. Clin. North Am.*, **24**: 249–258.

63. Lilenfeld L., Kaye W., Greeno C., Merikangas K., Plotnicov K., Pollice C., Rao R., Strober M., Bulik C., Nagy L. (1998) A controlled family study of anorexia nervosa and bulimia nervosa. *Arch. Gen. Psychiatry*, **55**: 603–610.

64. Rossi A., Marinangeli M.G., Butti G., Scinto A., DiCicco L., Kalyvoka A., Petruzzi C. (2001) Personality disorders in bipolar and depressive disorders. *J. Affect. Disord.*, **65**: 3–8.

65. Brooks R., Baltazar P., McDowell D., Munjack D., Bruns J. (1991) Personality disorders co-occurring with panic disorder with agoraphobia. *J. Person. Disord.*, **5**: 328–336.

66. McGlashan T.H., Grilo C.M., Skodol A.E., Gunderson J.G., Shea M.T., Morey L.C., Zanarini M.C., Stout R.L. (2000) The collaborative longitudinal personality disorders study: baseline axis I/II and II/II diagnostic co-occurrence. *Acta Psychiatr. Scand.*, **102**: 256–264.

67. Devanand D.P., Turrett N., Moody B., Fitzsimons L., Peyser S., Mickle K., Nobler M., Roose S. (2000) Personality disorders in elderly patients with dysthymic disorder. *Am. J. Geriatr. Psychiatry*, **8**: 188–195.

68. Widiger T.A., Trull T.J., Clarkin J.F., Sanderson C., Costa P.T. (2002) A description of the DSM-IV personality disorders with the five-factor model of personality. In *Personality Disorders and the Five Factor Model of Personality* (Eds P.T. Costa, T.A. Widiger), pp. 89–99. American Psychological Association, Washington.

69. Zimmerman M., Coryell W. (1989) DSM-III personality disorder diagnoses in a nonpatient sample. *Arch. Gen. Psychiatry*, **46**: 682–689.

70. Nestadt G., Romanoski A.J., Brown C.H., Chahal R., Merchant A., Flostein M.F., Gruenberg E.M., McHugh P.R. (1991) DSM-III compulsive personality disorder: an epidemiological survey. *Psychol. Med.*, **21**: 461–471.

71. Morey L.C. (1988) Personality disorders in DSM-III and DSM-III-R: convergence, coverage, and internal consistency. *Am. J. Psychiatry*, **145**: 573–577.

72. Widiger T., Trull T. (1998) Performance characteristics of the DSM-III-R personality disorder criteria sets. In *DSM-IV Sourcebook* (Eds T. Widiger, A. Frances, H. Pincus, R. Ross, M. First, W. Davis, M. Kline), pp. 357–373, American Psychiatric Association, Washington.

73. Stuart S., Pfohl B., Battaglia M., Bellodi L., Grove W., Cadoret R. (1998) The co-occurrence of DSM-III-R personality disorders. *J. Pers. Disord.*, **12**: 302–315.

74. Shea M.T., Stout R., Gunderson J., Morey L.C., Grilo C.M., McGlashan T., Skodol A.E., Dolan-Sewell R., Dyck I., Zanarini M.C. et al. (2002) Short-term diagnostic stability of schizotypal, borderline, avoidant, and obsessive–compulsive personality disorders. *Am. J. Psychiatry*, **159**: 2036–2041.

75. Shea M.T., Yen S. (2003) Stability as a distinction between axis I and axis II disorders. *J. Person. Disord.*, **17**: 373–386.

76. Samuels J., Eaton W.W., Bienvenu O.J. III, Brown C.H., Costa P.T., Nestadt G. (2002) Prevalence and correlates of personality disorders in a community sample. *Br. J. Psychiatry*, **189**: 536–542.

77. Loranger A.W. (1999) *International Personality Disorder Examination: DSM-IV and ICD-10 Interviews*. Psychological Assessment Resources, Odessa.

78. Skodol A., Gunderson J., McGlashan T., Dyck I., Stout R., Bender D., Grilo C., Shea M., Zanarini M., Morey L. et al. (2002) Functional impairment in patients with schizotypal, borderline, avoidant, or obsessive–compulsive personality disorder. *Am. J. Psychiatry*, **159**: 276–283.

79. Costa P.T., Bagby M., Ryder A., Bacchiochi J., Marshall M. (2003) Evaluation of the SCID-II personality disorders diagnostic criteria sets. Presented at the Conference of the International Society of Personality Disorders, Florence, October 9–12.

80. Harper R.G. (2003) Compulsive personality. In *Personality-guided Therapy in Behavioural Medicine* (Ed. R.G. Harper), pp. 251–276. American Psychological Association, Washington.

81. McCullough P.K., Maltsberger J.T. (2001) Obsessive–compulsive personality disorder. In *Treatments of Psychiatric Disorders* (Ed. G.O. Gabbard), pp. 2341–2352. American Psychiatric Press, Washington.

82. Suess J.F. (1972) Short-term psychotherapy with the compulsive personality and the obsessive–compulsive neurotic. *Am. J. Psychiatry*, **129**: 270–275.

83. Schwartz E.K. (1972) The treatment of the obsessive patient in the group therapy setting. *Am. J. Psychother.*, **26**: 352–361.

84. Beck A.T., Weeshar M. (1989) Cognitive therapy. In *Comprehensive Handbook of Cognitive Therapy* (Eds A. Freeman, K.M. Simon, L.E. Beulter, H. Arkowitz), pp. 21–36. Plenum, New York.

85. Beck A.T., Freeman A. (1990) *Cognitive Therapy of Personality Disorders*. Guilford, New York.

86. Kyrios M. (1998) A cognitive-behavioural approach to the understanding and management of obsessive–compulsive personality disorder. In *Cognitive Psychotherapy of Psychotic and Personality Disorders* (Eds C. Perris, P.D. McGorry), pp. 351–378. Wiley, Chichester.

87. Stone M.H. (1993) *Abnormalities of Personality*. Norton, New York.

88. Turkat I.D. (1990) *The Personality Disorders: A Psychological Approach to Clinical Management*. Pergamon, Elmsford.

89. Fleming B., Pretzer J.L. (1990) Cognitive–behavioral approaches to personality disorders. In *Progress in Behavioral Modification*, Vol. 25 (Eds M. Hersen, R.M. Eisler) pp. 119–151. Sage, Thousand Oaks.

90. Dowson J.H., Grounds A.T. (1995) *Personality Disorders: Recognition and Clinical Management.* Cambridge University Press, Cambridge.
91. Costa P.T., Widiger T.A. (Eds) (1994) *Personality Disorders and the Five Factor Model of Personality.* American Psychological Association, Washington.
92. Costa P.T., Widiger T.A. (Eds) (2002) *Personality Disorders and the Five Factor Model of Personality*, 2nd edn. American Psychological Association, Washington.
93. Costa P.T., McCrae R. (1992) *Professional Manual: Revised NEO Personality Inventory (NEO-PI-R) and NEO Five-factor Inventory (FFI).* Psychological Assessment Resources, Odessa.
94. Trull T. (1992) DSM-III-R personality disorders and the five-factor model of personality: an empirical comparison. *J. Abnorm. Psychol.*, 103: 553–560.
95. Costa P.T., McCrae R. (1990) Personality disorders and the five-factor model of personality. *J. Person. Disord.*, 4: 362–371.
96. Dyce J., O'Connor B. (1998) Personality disorders and the five-factor model: a test of facet-level predictions. *J. Person. Disord.*, 12: 31–45.
97. Haigler E.D., Widiger T.A. (2001) Experimental manipulation of NEO-PI-R items. *J. Person. Assess.*, 77: 339–358.
98. Trull T., Widiger T., Burr R. (2001) A structured interview for the assessment of the five-factor model of personality: facet-level relations to the Axis II personality disorders. *J. Person.*, 69: 175–198.
99. DeClercq B., DeFruyt F. (2003) Personality disorder symptoms in adolescence: a five-factor model perspective. *J. Person. Disord.*, 17: 269–292.
100. Blais M. (1997) Clinician ratings of the five-factor model of personality and the DSM-IV personality disorders. *J. Nerv. Ment. Dis.*, 185: 388–394.
101. Yang J., Dai X., Yao S., Cai T., Gao B., McCrae R., Costa P.T. (2002) Personality disorders and the five-factor model of personality in Chinese psychiatric patients. In *Personality Disorders and the Five Factor Model of Personality* (Eds P.T. Costa Jr, T.A. Widiger), pp. 215–221. American Psychological Association, Washington.
102. Morey L.C., Gunderson J.G., Quigley B.D., Shea M.T., Skodol A.E., McGlashan T.H., Stout R.L., Zanarini M.C. (2002) The representation of borderline, avoidant, obsessive–compulsive, and schizotypal personality disorders by the five-factor model. *J. Person. Disord.*, 16: 215–234.
103. Wilberg T., Urnes O., Friis S., Pedersen G., Karterud S. (1999) Borderline and avoidant personality disorders and the five-factor model of personality: a comparison between DSM-IV diagnoses and NEO-PI-R. *J. Person. Disord.*, 13: 226–240.
104. Trull T.J., Widiger T.A., Lynam D.R., Costa P.T. (2003) Borderline personality disorder from the perspective of general personality functioning. *J. Abnorm. Psychol.*, 112: 193–202.
105. Clark L.A., Vorhies L., McEwen J.L. (2002) Personality disorder symptomatology from the five-factor model perspective. In *Personality Disorders and the Five Factor Model of Personality* (Eds P.T. Costa Jr., T.A. Widiger), pp. 125–147. American Psychological Association, Washington.
106. Livesley W.J., Jackson D.N., Schroeder M.L. (1992) Factorial structure of traits delineating personality disorders in clinical and general population samples. *J. Abnorm. Psychol.*, 101: 432–440.
107. Clark L.A., Livesley W.J. (2002) Two approaches to identifying the dimensions of personality disorder: convergence on the five-factor model. In *Personality*

Disorders and the Five Factor Model of Personality (Eds P.T. Costa Jr, T.A. Widiger), pp. 161–176, American Psychological Association, Washington.
108. Lynam D., Widiger T. (2001) Using the five-factor model to represent the DSM-IV personality disorders: an expert consensus approach. *J. Abnorm. Psychol.*, **110**: 401–412.
109. Sprock J. (2002) A comparative study of the dimensions and facets of the five-factor model in the diagnosis of cases of personality disorder. *J. Person. Disord.*, **16**: 402–423.

Commentaries

6.1
Obsessive–Compulsive Personality Disorder:
Elusive for Whom?

Glen O. Gabbard[1]

The elegant review by Costa *et al.* provides a superb summary of what is known about obsessive–compulsive personality disorder (OCPD). As they note, the criteria for the disorder are problematic in some regards, because one must make a judgment regarding which of these features are adaptive and maladaptive with any one particular individual. Moreover, some of the features may be maladaptive for the individual but extremely useful for society. We see many persons with OCPD who are high-functioning professionals like physicians [1]. For groups such as physicians, society benefits by having a person who will be excessively conscientious, check and recheck diagnoses, and have an exaggerated responsibility for patients under his or her care. Nevertheless, a physician may have great difficulty in interpersonal relationships and family harmony as a result of this personality style at work. One could even argue that certain traits listed among the OCPD criteria in DSM-IV-TR are necessary for success in many professional fields.

The authors also are concerned that OCPD may not actually constitute an identifiable personality disorder, based on their survey of the research that looks at diagnostic agreement. They note for example that, based on five studies using structured interviews, one could "justifiably conclude that the diagnosis of OCPD is an elusive and perhaps illusory construct".

The other possibility, of course, is that the diagnostic instruments are less than optimal in their capacity to diagnose personality disorders. It is noteworthy, in this regard, that OCPD is a time-honoured construct that clinicians have identified and treated for many decades. Westen [2] examined the extent to which instruments used to assess Axis II conditions diverged from clinical diagnostic procedures. In a national sample of 1901 experienced psychiatrists and psychologists, he found that the majority of clinicians eschew direct questions derived from DSM-IV diagnostic categories when trying to assess personality disorders. These clinicians preferred to make

[1] *Department of Psychiatry and Behavioral Sciences, Baylor College of Medicine, 6655 Travis, Houston, TX 77030, USA*

the diagnoses by listening to patients describe how they relate to others and by observing their behaviour with the interviewer. Experienced clinicians have generally found it reasonably straightforward to identify the patient with OCPD. Hence the empirical evidence questioning the validity of the diagnosis may say more about instruments than about the construct itself.

Costa *et al.* also raise some questions about the way the criteria are regarded within the current DSM-IV-TR diagnosis. Confirmatory factor analysis of the Collaborative Longitudinal Personality Disorders Study (CLPS) data suggests reorienting the criteria according to how prototypical they are. The authors suggest that the current criteria of "reluctant to delegate tasks" and "rigid and stubborn" are more prototypical of OCPD than "workaholic" and "packrat" features. This finding is no surprise, as the "workaholic" item is one riddled with suggestive value judgments. There is also considerable irony in that many researchers who are making the assessment probably work excessive hours and are in academic cultures where such work conditions are highly valued. The "packrat" item has also been highly problematic in terms of where it belongs in our current diagnostic understanding. The work of Frost *et al.* [3] has demonstrated that hoarding is probably not a good fit with either obsessive–compulsive disorder (OCD) or OCPD and probably constitutes an entity into itself. Moreover, hoarding does not appear to respond well to treatments that are effective for OCD or OCPD.

The authors rightly point out that the relationship between OCPD and OCD continues to vex most researchers and clinicians. I agree with their conclusion that, based on a host of studies seeking to answer the question of comorbidity, one can only say that the relationship between OCD and OCPD "remains unresolved". While traditionally we regard OCPD as involving ego-syntonic character traits while we think of OCD as characterized by ego-dystonic obsessions and rituals, even that distinction may not hold up in actual clinical work. Some OCD patients become so accustomed to the rituals that they cease to cause distress. Similarly, some OCPD patients who have had longstanding features of the disorder may start to suffer as a consequence of the disorder and experience their "drivenness" as ego-dystonic [4]. The difficulty distinguishing the two disorders does not prevent the recognition that different treatment approaches are now being tailored to persons who present with a predominant picture of OCD compared to those who present with a primary clinical picture of OCPD. Behaviour therapy and selective serotonin reuptake inhibitors are used for OCD, while either dynamic therapy or cognitive therapy is used for OCPD [4].

A recent study not cited by the authors [5] seeks to look at which types of personality disorders were prevalent among a severely disordered OCD population of 65 subjects. They used three different methods of assessing personality disorders: structured interview, questionnaire, and clinical diagnosis. With clinical diagnosis, only 10.8% of the OCD patients had OCPD; using the Structured Clinical Interview for DSM-IV Personality Disorders (SCID-II), 24.6% had OCPD; and using the Assessment of the DSM-IV Personality Disorders (ADP-IV), only 29.2% could be categorized as OCPD. Hence this study, like most others cited by the authors, suggests that less than 1/3 of OCD patients are likely to have OCPD as a comorbid diagnosis. I suspect that the continued use of the term "obsessive–compulsive" for both disorders is a remnant of psychoanalytic jargon in the early years of the development of psychoanalysis, when problems with personality were thought to be nothing more than characterological manifestations of neuroses. Hence, in the early literature, the obsessive–compulsive neurosis was regarded as obsessive–compulsive character neurosis if certain signs appeared as personality patterns rather than a symptomatic neurosis.

The authors give remarkably short shrift to considerations of treatment. The results of recent clinical trials are encouraging. Winston et al. [6] conducted a controlled trial of 25 patients with Cluster C personality disorders, many of whom had OCPD, who were treated in dynamic therapy with a mean length of 40.3 sessions. The sample improved significantly on all measures compared with control patients on a wait list. At follow-up 1.5 years later, the patients demonstrated continued benefit.

Svartberg et al. [7] randomly assigned 50 patients who met criteria for Cluster C personality disorders to 40 sessions of either dynamic psychotherapy or cognitive therapy. The therapists were all experienced in manual guided supervision. The outcomes were assessed in terms of symptom distress, interpersonal problems, and core personality pathology. The full sample of patients showed statistically significant improvements on all measures during treatment and during the two-year follow-up period. Patients who received cognitive therapy did not report significant change in symptom distress after treatment, whereas patients who underwent dynamic therapy treatment did. Two years after the treatment, 54% of the dynamic therapy patients and 42% of the cognitive therapy patients had recovered symptomatically. Investigators concluded that there was reason to think that improvement persists after treatment with dynamic psychotherapy. These investigations are confirming what clinicians have known for many years—namely, that patients with OCPD are highly amenable to psychotherapy and there is every reason for optimism in terms of the prognosis. However, as Costa et al. point out, some of these patients are not characterologically disposed to enter treatment. In many cases, they are pressured into treatment by family members who are "fed up" or colleagues in the workplace who are concerned about work habits.

REFERENCES

1. Gabbard G.O. (1985) The role of compulsiveness in the normal physician. *JAMA*, **254**: 2926–2929.
2. Westen D. (1997) Divergences between clinical and research methods for assessing personality disorders: implications for research and the evolution of Axis II. *Am. J. Psychiatry*, **154**: 895–903.
3. Frost R.O., Steketee E.G., Williams L.F., Warren R. (2000) Mood, personality disorder symptoms, and disability in obsessive–compulsive hoarders: a comparison with clinical and non-clinical controls. *Behav. Res. Ther.*, **38**: 1071–1081.
4. Gabbard G.O., Newman C. (in press) Psychotherapy of obsessive–compulsive personality disorder. In *Concise Oxford Textbook of Psychotherapy* (Eds G. Gabbard, J. Beck, J. Holmes). Oxford University Press, New York.
5. Tenney N.H., Schotte C.K.W., Denys D.A.J.P., van Megen H.J.G.M., Westenberg H.G.M. (2003) Assessment of DSM-IV personality disorders and obsessive–compulsive disorder: comparison of clinical diagnosis, self-report, questionnaire, and semi-structured interview. *J. Person. Disord.*, **17**: 550–561.
6. Winston A., Laikin M., Pollack J., Samstag L.W., McCullough L., Muran J.C. (1994) Short-term psychotherapy of personality disorders. *Am. J. Psychiatry*, **151**: 190–194.
7. Svartberg M., Stiles T.C., Seltzer M.H. (in press) Effectiveness of short-term dynamic psychotherapy and cognitive therapy for cluster C personality disorders: a randomized controlled trial. *Am. J. Psychiatry*.

6.2
Clinical Challenges of Obsessive–Compulsive Personality Disorder
Albert Rothenberg[1]

A longstanding problem with the diagnosis and management of obsessive–compulsive personality (OCPD) is the misleading attempt to squeeze, in a metaphorical sense, a square peg into a round hole. This is shown quite vividly by the lack of any firm conclusions from the Costa *et al.*'s encyclopedic and multifaceted review of diagnostic studies and approaches. As a square peg essentially unlike all other personality disorders, the attributes of OCPD consist entirely of excessive expressions of highly valued and socially adaptive characteristics, especially of Western cultures. Although Costa *et al.* note this adaptability of features, the diagnosis and clinical management implications are not fully pursued. Despite historical variations in specific criteria included in the diagnosis, the core feature is maladaptiveness due to excessiveness of otherwise adaptive factors. Thus, conscientiousness and devotion to work, reliability and care for details, adherence to rules, morality,

[1] *Department of Psychiatry, Harvard Medical School, Boston, MA, USA*

self reliance, firmness, drive for achievement and perfection, striving and maintaining mastery, orderliness, cleanliness, looking at both sides of an issue, thriftiness, preference for balance, are in OCPD turned respectively into overconscientiousness and workaholism, preoccupation with details, over-compliance with rules, scrupulousness, inability to delegate to others and self righteousness, rigidity and stubbornness, perfectionism that interferes with task completion or diffuse and unrelenting perfectionism, preoccupation with control, order, spotlessness and purity, and rumination, miserliness, concern with symmetry. Because the diagnosis depends on such assessment of excess, a matter of degree rather than kind, accuracy and consistency is difficult for evaluating clinicians using either structured or unstructured interviews as well as research studies employing standard diagnostic instruments, especially those involving self-report. As indicated in Costa *et al.*'s review, the best judgment reliability comes from the domain investigations of Sprock [1] and Linam and Widiger [2], which focus directly on excess, that is, degree and severity.

From the clinical perspective, all of the designated OCPD extreme factors produce suffering and are therefore psychopathological. The picture is, however, often complex, because, despite suffering and disability, some adaptive factors may be retained with compensatory better functioning. This produces confusion both for clinicians and patients, leading not only to diagnostic oversights but sometimes reinforcing these patients' not uncommon fear of, or resistance to, treatment. The clinical challenge here is to elicit information carefully about degree of excessiveness of each feature and overall level of maladaptive functioning. Also important is exploration of connections with other intercurrent or comorbid conditions. Persons with OCPD may not manifest overall impairment until they develop other disorders, the main ones being obsessive–compulsive disorder (OCD), eating disorder, mood disorders, and alcoholism.

The frequent connection of the personality disorder with other morbid conditions emphasizes the psychopathological nature of the OCPD constellation. Rather than suggesting a third underlying factor or disorder, co-occurrence and co-morbidity presents clinically as an interactive relationship. Despite varying correlations between OCPD and OCD in research studies, for instance, connections are often observed clinically and, to our knowledge, there have been no longitudinal studies of the relationship or assessments of developmental interactions. Features of OCPD often appear changed or reduced when OCD develops, e.g. scrupulousness becomes ritualistic behaviour, and retrospective diagnosis of the personality disorder is difficult.

We have shown, in our studies of eating disorders, interconnections with OCPD. On the basis of long-term assessment, we described particular OCPD factors having distinct intercurrent psychopathological effects. Eating disorder patients, in comparison with controls, significantly manifested both premorbid and morbid habitual controlling, rumination, excessive perfectionism, extreme cleanliness, orderliness, rigidity, rumination, and scrupulous self-righteousness [3,4]. Each of these characteristics contributed to the manifestations of their eating disorders: perfectionism was involved in the striving for unqualified thinness, cleanliness with inner sanitation and purging, orderliness in careful amassing of caloric lists and (often bogus) food characteristics, stubbornness in rock bound dieting and weight loss, excessive morality as preoccupations with good and bad foods and practices. Similar OCPD features were documented in our diagnostic eating disorder literature review [5].

Although mood disorder patients manifest a variety of personality disorders, or none at all, OCPD is especially frequent. Again, maladaptiveness and suffering induced by the OCPD component is distinct, and assessment of extensiveness of each feature is important both for psychotherapy and pharmacological treatment. When patients with dysthymia or major depression manifest debilitating OCPD features, dual acting antidepressants—i.e. fluoxetine, paroxetine, sertraline—are beneficial for both immediate and prolonged effects [6]. On the other hand, with absent or minimal OCPD features, other types of antidepressants may be satisfactorily used. With respect to psychotherapy, OCPD features seem clearly to play an aetiological role in mood disorder together with, or regardless of, genetic or chemical factors. Persons who are excessively or diffusely perfectionistic are bound to be subject to deep disappointments with their strivings that produce both mild and severe depressive diatheses. Similarly, in the face of losses and stresses, stubbornness, rigidity, and concern with control readily give way to extreme self-reproach. Excessive morality leads often to pervasive preoccupations with guilt.

Sociocultural biases tend to obscure connections between OCPD and alcohol abuse [6]. The latter condition is most commonly associated, by both laity and professionals, with images of persons who are down and out, disorderly, and often unclean, a far cry from any of the over-adaptive characteristics listed earlier. But a closer look at the high incidence of closet alcoholism among hard driving business executives, entertainment celebrities, and the incessant alcohol imbibing revels of other rich and famous people indicates that the same personality features that lead to success can, with OCPD excess, lead to alcoholic abuse and eventual rack and ruin. Again, in addition to possible biological and genetic factors, anxiety generated by need for control, perfectionism, rigidity, and the setting of virtually impossible goals leads to pathological self-medicating attempts at control through a substance. Alcohol abuse in these cases produces a psychopathological spiral where total abandonment of perfectionistic values leads to self-loathing and further abuse.

The extreme and socially alienating nature of otherwise adaptive facets of OCPD contributes to another complication in diagnosis and clinical management: patient shame and secrecy. Seldom will OCPD patients volunteer descriptions of their excessive characteristics but they will instead be evasive or righteously defend seemingly irrational behaviour. If asked about excessive perfectionism, for example, they will often insist they simply try to do things well. This shame and secrecy, which may be intrinsic also to formative factors in OCPD psychopathology, accounts in part for difficulties in obtaining treatment collaboration with such patients. It also plays a significant role in the marked variability in research results, as well as miscalculations about the true incidence of the condition (along with OCD which shares the secrecy problem) in the population at large. Developing patient confidence, multiple assessments, long-term contact, gathering broad information about degree of impairment, are critically important for both recognition and effective care of OCPD.

REFERENCES

1. Sprock J. (2002) A comparative study of the dimensions and facets of the five-factor model in the diagnosis of cases of personality disorder. *J. Person. Disord.*, **16**: 402–423.
2. Linam D., Widiger T. (2001) Using the five-factor model to represent the DSM-IV personality disorders. An expert consensus approach. *J. Abnorm. Psychol.*, **110**: 401–412.
3. Rothenberg A. (1986) Eating disorder as a modern obsessive–compulsive syndrome. *Psychiatry*, **49**: 45–53.
4. Rothenberg A. (1990) Adolescence and eating disorder: the obsessive–compulsive syndrome. *Psychiatr. Clin. North Am.*, **13**: 469–488.
5. Rothenberg A. (1988) Differential diagnosis of anorexia nervosa and depressive illness: a review of eleven studies. *Compr. Psychiatry*, **29**: 427–432.
6. Rothenberg A. (1998) Diagnosis of obsessive–compulsive illness. *Psychiatr. Clin. North Am.*, **21**: 791–801.

6.3
Obsessive–Compulsive Character
David Shapiro[1]

The conditions that will be considered here as obsessive–compulsive character include those that are often, and variously, diagnosed as obsessive–compulsive neurosis, obsessive–compulsive disorder (OCD) and obsessive–compulsive personality. Thus the term obsessive–compulsive character, as I will use it, encompasses a somewhat wider range than that considered by Costa *et al.* All these diagnostic categories share certain general principles of their psychological organization and qualities of subjective life. They can therefore be understood as variations within a kind of personality. The variety of diagnostic names for this general form of neurotic character reflects the fact that, although its traits or symptoms share essential subjective and objective qualities, they may vary widely in their particulars. It is not only that, for example, the content of specific rituals or specific obsessive ideas varies widely. The condition may be severe or mild and characteristic traits or personality features may be conspicuous and odd-seeming in one case and hardly noticeable in another, subjectively distressing or troublesome or, again, hardly noticeable. Thus, although sharing essential qualities, character features may be recognized as symptoms in one case, but no more than ordinary personality differences in another. It frequently seems, also, that particular symptoms will be easily recognized, while the distinctive qualities of mind from which these particular symptoms emerge will not, leading the observer to the misconception that the particular symptoms are quite isolated from the personality as a whole.

It should be added, also, that no psychopathology, apart from unambiguously organic ones, appears as a pure and discrete type, as physical diseases usually do. Obsessive–compulsive conditions are no exception and, even where obsessive–compulsive characteristics predominate in a personality, symptoms or characteristics of other diagnostic categories will be found.

The fundamental characteristic of this condition, present in all its forms and, as Costa *et al.* point out, noted by clinical observers and researchers of virtually all theoretical persuasions, is a certain kind of conscientiousness. This conscientiousness is reflected not only in obvious obsessive–compulsive traits such as perfectionism, compulsive work habits, obsessive cleanliness, and such. It is also reflected less obviously in various symptoms such as indecisiveness in matters of personal choice, where it demands a critical and inevitably prejudiced review of whichever leaning is presently in mind, leading then to a higher valuation of the alternative, until it, too, is subjected

[1] *Graduate Faculty of Political and Social Science, Clinical Psychology Program, 65 Fifth Avenue, New York, NY 10003, USA*

to critical review. The same conscientiousness is present in obsessive worry, where it requires continual and exaggerated attention to any possibility of misfortune. This kind of conscientiousness is almost always referred to in psychiatry and psychology as excessive, too strict, or too severe. That characterization is not quite correct, although it is easily understandable. Actually, what distinguishes the conscientiousness of obsessive–compulsive character is its rigidity. It is based on rules, not conviction. It does not have the subjective form of an unambivalent or wholehearted devotion to principle or good works that marks a healthy conscience. Instead, it typically has the subjective form of a nagging feeling of "I should..." according to some rule that is only grudgingly respected. That this conscientiousness is one of rules rather than conviction is frequently evident in its legalistic nature, in which the letter of the rule must be obeyed even when it makes no realistic sense. One sees this especially in formalistic compulsive rituals, where any semblance of conviction of adaptive value is lost. On the other hand, compulsive traits often have adaptive value. In this, obsessive–compulsive conditions are no different from any other non-psychotic psychopathology. Any neurotic style has adaptive aspects. The hysteric's spontaneity is socially engaging; even the psychopath's spur-of-the-moment way of living permits him to be unusually and sometimes adaptively decisive in certain circumstances, where he is a "man of action". Thus the question "Is this condition adaptive or maladaptive?" can be answered "It can be both, even in the same individual, at least until the condition becomes so severe, as may happen with a fanatical and formalistic perfectionism, that it makes life very difficult and work impossible".

As Costa *et al.* point out, the early psychoanalysts followed Freud's lead in understanding obsessive and compulsive conditions in terms of early drive-related fantasies and conflicts. That was the conceptual equipment available to them at the time. It should be added, however, that in later psychoanalytic development, specifically with the development in the 1920s of the concept of the "ego", a concept which included wider aspects of the personality, a much broader conception of these conditions emerged. I am referring particularly to the work of Wilhelm Reich [1]. Reich described the obsessive–compulsive condition as a kind of character; he described it in terms of general attitudes, as a "way of being", notable for example for its orderliness and "evenness of living". This point of view, now stripped of its supposed connection with early drive-related fantasies, has more recently been developed by Shapiro [2–4].

Obsessive–compulsive conditions have traditionally been regarded by psychoanalysts and analytically-influenced psychotherapists as particularly difficult to treat. Unfortunately the responsibility for this difficulty has often been laid at the doorstep of the patient or the nature of the patient's problems rather than the limitations of the therapy. Or, if the difficulty is recognized as a limitation of the therapy, it may be regarded as a limitation of psychotherapy in general rather than a particular method of psychotherapy. In fact, however, psychodynamic therapy that is attentive to present attitudes and ways of thinking finds obsessive and compulsive symptoms not easy to treat, but no more difficult than other neurotic symptoms [5].

REFERENCES

1. Reich W. (1933) *Character Analysis*. Orgone Institute Press, New York.
2. Shapiro D. (1965) *Neurotic Styles*. Basic Books, New York.
3. Shapiro D. (1981) *Autonomy and Rigid Character*. Basic Books, New York.
4. Shapiro D. (2000) *Dynamics of Character*. Basic Books, New York.
5. Shapiro D. (1989) *Psychotherapy of Neurotic Character*. Basic Books, New York.

6.4

Understanding and Measuring Obsessive–Compulsive Personality Disorder: The Jury is Still Out

Lucy Serpell[1] and Varsha Hirani[2]

We would like to raise four issues concerning Costa *et al.*'s excellent and thorough review of obsessive–compulsive personality disorder (OCPD).

Firstly, the review considers adaptive and maladaptive personality traits and whether features of OCPD are merely maladaptive "problems in living" or are "psychopathological". Many of the criteria used to define OCPD, such as DSM-IV criteria, consist of both adaptive and maladaptive traits, or alternatively, they can be considered adaptive if present to a certain degree, but maladaptive when they are extreme. However, our understanding of a personality *disorder* is as a maladaptive manifestation of normal personality, hence in order to be diagnosed with a personality disorder the person would need to present with traits which are maladaptive rather than adaptive [1]. Deciding which traits are maladaptive is complex and controversial, but lies at the heart of the definition of personality disorder. We would add that difficulty in distinguishing between "normal" and "abnormal" levels of pathology also occurs in Axis I disorders, for example in defining an abnormal level of weight preoccupation in the diagnosis of an eating disorder.

[1] *Institute of Psychiatry, London, UK*
[2] *St. George's Hospital Medical School, London, UK*

A second issue we would like to highlight is the presence of many inconsistencies in definitions of OCPD and its characteristic features. Many of the studies in the area either fail to define their terms or use different definitions. For example, perfectionism described as a feature of OCPD in DSM-IV is referred to as competence in the five-factor model (FFM) of personality disorders, and excessive devotion to work productivity is categorized as achievement striving in the FFM. These vital differences directly affect the validity of comparing findings across studies. Further to this, some of the terms used seem to connote more maladaptive/negative traits (for example, the use of words such as "excessive") whereas others appear more adaptive and positive (for example, competence). Clinicians should move towards agreement in the criteria they use to diagnose OCPD and researchers need to have more consensus in the definitions they use and subsequently the tools used to measure the disorder. This will ensure greater validity in comparisons made across clinical studies conducted in this area.

A third issue is the paucity of literature concerning OCPD compared to the other personality disorders. We would perhaps disagree with Costa *et al.*'s comment that OCPD may not be a valid category. This is not because we think it has been shown to be valid, but because we would suggest that the research bearing on this issue has not yet been done. A search of the Medline database (1996–2004) revealed only 55 articles concerned with OCPD, compared with 760 concerning borderline personality disorder.

What are possible reasons for the lack of interest in OCPD as a category? Firstly, it seems unlikely, given the nature of the condition, that individuals with OCPD will seek treatment. Secondly, it is possible that OCPD is seen as a less interesting and dramatic personality disorder, and hence researchers are less willing to study it, choosing instead to focus on the more exciting presentations such as those in Cluster B. Alternatively, it may be that OCPD is considered less of a problem than other personality disorders, because it has less of an effect on others. However, our experience, supported by the findings of the 1997 study by Loranger *et al.* [2] is that OCPD can be extremely disabling to the individual with the condition, as well as to those in his or her immediate environment (family members, work colleagues, etc.). Furthermore, we would suggest that none of the possibilities suggested above are good reasons to neglect the disorder when considering future research. We would agree with Costa *et al.* that important focus for such research would be establishing which of the features of OCPD (as listed in DSM-IV-TR) are core to the condition and which are more peripheral.

Finally, we would wish to extend comments on the comorbidity of OCPD with eating disorders. As mentioned in the review, it appears that eating disorders sufferers, especially those with anorexia nervosa, may show several features of OCPD [3,4]. Two aspects of the diagnosis which are currently the focus of research are perfectionism [5,6] and inflexibility or rigidity [7–9]. As Costa *et al.* point out, the direction of causation has not yet clearly been established. However, it is possible that personality features like inflexibility may explain why some people progress from normal dieting into anorexia nervosa and others do not.

It may be that understanding comorbidity requires more than simply measuring the coincidence of two disorders. Instead, work in eating disorders aims to understand how features of an Axis II condition such as OCPD might be inextricably linked to the development of an Axis I condition.

REFERENCES

1. Arntz, A. (1999) Do personality disorders exist? On the validity of the concept and its cognitive–behavioural formulation and treatment. *Behav. Res. Ther.*, **37**: S97–S134.
2. Loranger A., Janca A., Sartorius N. (1997) *Assessment and Diagnosis of Personality Disorders: the ICD-10 International Personality Disorder Examination (IPDE)*. Cambridge University Press, Cambridge.
3. Serpell L., Livingstone A., Neiderman M., Lask B. (2002) Anorexia nervosa: obsessive compulsive disorder, obsessive compulsive personality or neither. *Clin. Psychol. Rev.*, **22**: 647–669.
4. Serpell L., Hirani V., Willoughby K., Neiderman M., Lask B. Personality or pathology?: Obsessive–compulsive symptoms in children and adolescents with anorexia nervosa. Submitted for publication.
5. Shafran R., Cooper Z., Fairburn C. (2002) Clinical perfectionism: a cognitive behavioural analysis. *Behav. Res. Ther.*, **40**: 773–791.
6. Shafran R., Cooper Z., Fairburn C.G. (2003) "Clinical perfectionism" is not "multidimensional perfectionism": a reply to Hewitt, Flett, Besser, Sherry & McGee. *Behav. Res. Ther.*, **41**: 1217–1220.
7. Tchanturia K., Brecelj Anderluh M., Morris R., Rabe-Hesketh S., Collier D., Sanchez P. (in press) Cognitive flexibility in anorexia nervosa and bulimia nervosa. *J. Int. Neuropsychol. Soc.*
8. Tchanturia K., Morris R., Surguladze S., Treasure J. (2002) An examination of perceptual and cognitive set shifting tasks in acute anorexia nervosa and following recovery. *Eat. Weight Disord.*, **7**: 312–315.
9. Tchanturia K., Serpell L., Troop N., Treasure J. (2002) Perceptual illusions in eating disorders: rigid and fluctuating styles. *Behav. Ther. Exper. Psychiatry*, **32**, 107–115.

6.5
Obsessive–Compulsive Personality Disorder:
Not Just a Mere Problem in Living
Eric Hollander and Lisa Sharma[1]

Costa *et al.* provide a thorough review of the research on obsessive–compulsive personality disorder (OCPD) and call to question OCPD's place as a valid and maladaptive disorder. The main question at hand is whether OCPD can be validated as a debilitating psychopathology or if it would be better conceptualized as a maladaptive problem in living.

While a number of the disorder's characteristics (perfectionism, attention to detail, devotion to work and productivity) are valued within society and the workplace, one must ask: what happens when these characteristics go too far? Take, for example, the case of a surgeon who must suture and re-suture a muscle until it is perfect, even at the expense of several extra hours in the operating room.

Although the relationship of OCPD traits to social functioning and impairment has not been extensively studied, through our clinical experience as psychiatrists we can vouch for the extreme anguish faced by those of our patients suffering from OCPD. This debilitating disorder is one in which perfectionism and devotion to work takes over one's life to the extent of sacrificing personal relationships. Intimate relationships, friendships and parent–child relationships are strained due to discomfort in expression of emotions, insistence on perfection and excessive devotion to work. The disorder affects the sufferer's children as well; as the parent expects extreme compliance to rules and absolute perfection of tasks (i.e. sports are to be played to win, not just for the fun of the game).

Work relations also suffer, as this population does not work well with others and as a result is very difficult in group or team situations. They plan ahead with meticulous detail and are unwilling to consider changes suggested by other members of the group. Deadlines are missed because of their need for perfection. When especially stressed at work, all focus is honed on perfection of the task at hand, so much so that other aspects of life fall to shambles.

For those that do present for treatment, most are resistant to change, challenging to treat and tend not to comply with doctors' recommendations. OCPD traits often overlap with typical "type A" personality traits, which may put these individuals at higher risk for stress related health problems (myocardial infarction, high blood pressure). As discussed in Costa *et al.*'s review, preliminary results suggest that obsessive–compulsive

---

[1] *Mount Sinai School of Medicine, New York, NY, USA*

personality traits negatively impact self-reported social functioning in several areas. Specifically, they found increased OCPD traits to be negatively correlated to relationships with spouse/partner and siblings, performance at work, school and home, use of free time, and overall functioning in social and family life [1]. It is also important to note that, although Skodol *et al.* [2] found OCPD to have the least amount of functional impairment of all personality disorders assessed, the amount of impairment was still well below "normal" Global Assessment of Functioning (GAF) scores (OCPD mean GAF score = 64.7, SD = 10.6).

With regards to the diagnostic overlap of DSM-defined OCPD and other Axis II disorders, although all personality disorders have some features in common, there are concrete distinctions to aid in diagnosis. For example: those with narcissistic personality disorder also display perfectionism and hold the idea that others cannot perform tasks as well, but are not self-critical like those with OCPD. Both those with narcissistic and antisocial personality disorder lack generosity, but, unlike those with OCPD, they will indulge themselves. Lastly, while those with schizoid personality disorder also possess apparent formality and social detachment, this is due to a lack of capacity for intimacy, rather than discomfort with emotions and excessive devotion to work that is commonly exhibited in OCPD. Regarding OCPD's similarity to avoidant personality disorder, according to the Collaborative Longitudinal Personality Disorders Study [3], only 27% of patients had co-morbid OCPD. Although this was the highest co-occurrence of DSM-IV personality disorders, the co-occurrence was still low enough to consider both as distinct disorders.

Considering OCPD's high comorbidity and similarities to other personality disorders, the current DSM-IV-TR diagnostic criteria may be too vague to ensure proper diagnosis, especially for those who are mildly symptomatic. As evidenced in the above study, OCPD may also involve a substantial anxiousness, a controlled restraint (low impulsiveness) and an excessive cautiousness (low excitement seeking) that are not recognized by the DSM-IV criteria. Therefore, as suggested by Lynam and Widiger [4] and Sprock [5], the comprehensive (30 facet) five-factor model (FFM) or NEO Personality Inventory—Revised (NEO-PI-R) may be more viable options for accurate diagnosis of OCPD. This, of course, would need to be studied empirically to compare validity with the DSM-IV diagnosis construct.

REFERENCES

1. Samuels J., Eaton W.W., Bienvenu O.J. III, Brown C.H., Costa P.T., Nestadt G. (2002) Prevalence and correlates of personality disorders in a community sample. *Br. J. Psychiatry*, **189**: 536–542.

2. Skodol A., Gunderson J., McGlashan T., Dyck I., Stout R., Bender D., Grilo C., Shea M., Zanarini M., Morey L. *et al.* (2002) Functional impairment in patients with schizotypal, borderline, avoidant, or obsessive–compulsive personality disorder. *Am. J. Psychiatry*, **159**: 276–283.
3. McGlashan T.H., Grilo C.M., Skodol A.E., Gunderson J.G., Shea M.T., Morey L.C., Zanarini M.C., Stout R.L. (2000) The collaborative longitudinal personality disorders study: baseline axis I/II and II/II diagnostic co-occurrence. *Acta Psychiatr. Scand.*, **102**: 256–264.
4. Lynam D., Widiger T. (2001) Using the five-factor model to represent the DSM-IV personality disorders: an expert consensus approach. *J. Abnorm. Psychol.*, **110**: 401–412.
5. Sprock J. (2002) A comparative study of the dimensions and facets of the five-factor model in the diagnosis of cases of personality disorder. *J. Person. Disord.*, **16**: 402–423.

6.6
Psychiatry Trapped in Obsessive–Compulsive Overdiagnosing?

Iver Hand and Susanne Fricke[1]

In a recent issue of World Psychiatry, the official journal of the WPA, the forum addressed "the challenge of psychiatric comorbidity", reflecting on a possible inflation of diagnosing comorbidities, "dimensional" versus "categorical" models, differences between disorders and diseases, and diagnostic hierarchies [1]. Over the past decades, we have developed a huge diagnostic armamentarium. We have refined the description and counting of disorder symptomatology in the DSM and ICD systems, possibly at the costs of aetiological understanding. What for? Sure, the collection of descriptive data in categorical systems has greatly improved comparability of national and international studies. But what has happened with regard to treatment? Enhancing patients' treatment should be a major objective of diagnosing. With the development of diagnosing over the past two decades, haven't we finally set ourselves a trap? Particularly the assessment of personality disorders is still under extensive debate (see [2]). "A dominant example of excessive comorbidity in the DSM-IV resulting in widespread dissatisfaction among clinicians is in the area of personality disorders" [1]. Let us investigate this issue a little further focusing on obsessive–compulsive behaviours.

We have created quite a variety of "diagnoses" to differentiate obsessive–compulsive behaviours: obsessive–compulsive ("anancastic") personality

---
[1] *Behaviour Therapy Unit, Clinic for Psychiatry and Psychotherapy, University Hospital Eppendorf/ Hamburg, Martinistrasse 52, D-20246 Hamburg, Germany*

traits [3,4]; obsessive–compulsive personality accentuation [2], obsessive–compulsive personality disorder (OCPD) and obsessive–compulsive disorder (OCD). Already some 25 years ago, the literature on the role of OCPD for the development and treatment of OCD was quite contradictory (see [4] for a review). Here are some examples of controversial positions: OCPD has different quality in normals as compared to OCPD in patients with OCD [5]; in "normals" OCPD is integrated into the personality, whereas in OCD patients OCPD changes over time as OCD develops [6]; there is no clearly defined OCPD as a precondition for the development of OCD [10]; OCPD is a predictor of negative treatment outcome in OCD [7]; "anancastic personality" is a predictor of positive treatment outcome in OCD [8].

Doesn't it require already definite anancastic personality traits (or more than that?) for us to understand what we are doing? And, why do we have to do this? If all diagnostic obsessive–compulsive entities do represent different developmental stages of obsessive–compulsive behaviours, would that not question the diagnostic dichotomy present–not present (or, in the medical system: ill–not ill; treatment necessary–treatment not necessary; reimbursement of treatment costs recommended–not recommended)?

OCD and OCPD are now accepted as disorders in the medical sense. However, as Costa et al. point out, not all criteria of OCPD are maladaptive, some criteria are functional and valued by society. And the question remains open as to what extent and under what circumstances obsessive–compulsive personality traits are to be considered maladaptive. Recent research provides evidence that some aspects of personality disorders and traits could have a positive impact on treatment outcome in OCD [9], and the study of Moritz et al. [10] showed that only a subset of criteria were antecedents for treatment failure in OCD. If we believe that already specific personality traits, accentuations and disorders can become a decisive factor for treatment outcome of an Axis I disorder would this not, by itself, indicate the necessity of a "personality-specific" treatment to improve the outcome of the Axis I disorder? And, would this not require to label even a personality variant as a disorder, in order to help the patient to get reimbursement for treatment? If so, then we would give up completely our current dichotomy of sick–not sick. The decade-long criticism of psychiatry by sociologists and psychologists (and even some psychiatrists) that with our diagnoses we invade the normal population to make them feel in need of treatments would be reactivated.

With an endless variety of rating questionnaires, are we now in danger of overdiagnosing and undertreating our patients? The more complex our assessments, the higher the pressure has become to simplify and shorten treatments, particularly psychotherapy, with manual guided, "evidence-based", highly standardized and preferably (very) short-term interventions for Axis I and II disorders.

As diagnosing becomes more and more complex, treatment does not seem to follow the same trend. Recent developments, e.g. those concerning selective serotonin reuptake inhibitors (SSRIs), seem to move in the opposite direction: these drugs are able to reduce depression, anxiety and panic, compulsions and obsessions, several impulse control disorders etc., and sometimes they even induce anxiety, panic attacks, restlessness and the like for shorter or longer periods of time. And, in the same individual, one of these drugs may have aversive and another one highly beneficial effects. On the level of the individual patient, we cannot reliably predict the effects of the drug on the patient's emotion and behaviour. SSRIs are regarded to be pharmacologically "cleaner" and much more selective (in receptor affinity) than tricyclics. Yet, their potential effects are rather unspecific regarding Axis I diagnoses and individually difficult to predict.

The differentiation between OCD, OCPD and obsessive–compulsive traits is still under discussion, as pointed out by Costa *et al*. The more pieces of diagnostic entities we create, the higher the probability to hit significant correlations. These are then given clinical value, and we may create a new myth until enough external replications have proven that our results were statistical artefacts of an unrepresentative sample of patients.

Haven't we put ourselves in a kind of Sisyphus position, rolling "new stones again and again up the hill" (watching the old one rolling down) with the never ending hope that one may stay on top as "the stone of wisdom"? More than a hill or a mountain, life is like a river, continuously flowing through ever changing environments, thus changing quality, direction and speed depending on its interaction with the changing environment. Are personality traits, accentuations or disorders the "causes" for the development of Axis I disorders or a response to them? So what does it mean, if these variables seem to influence treatment outcome?

REFERENCES

1. Pincus H.A., Tew J.D., First M.B. (2004) Psychiatric comorbidity: is more less? *World Psychiatry*, 3: 18–23.
2. Fricke S., Moritz S., Andresen B., Hand I., Jacobsen D., Kloss M., Rufer M. (2003) Impact of personality disorders on treatment outcome in obsessive–compulsive disorders—Part I: problems. *Verhaltenstherapie*, 13: 166–171.
3. Donath J. (1987) Zur Kenntnis des Anancasmus (psychische Zwangszustände). *Archiv für Psychiatrie und Nervenkrankheiten*, 29: 211–224.
4. Zaworka W., Hand I. (1981) Die "anankastische Persönlichkeit"—Fakt oder Fiktion? *Zeitschrift für Differentielle und Diagnostische Psychologie*, 2: 31–54.
5. Lewis A.-J., Mapother E. (1941) Obsessional disorder. In *Textbook of the Practice of Medicine* (Ed. J. Price), pp. 1140–2001. Oxford University Press, London.
6. Sandler J., Hazari A. (1960) The obsessional: on the psychological classification of obsessional character traits and symptoms. *Br. J. Med. Psychol.*, 33: 113–122.

7. Lewis A.-J. (1965) A note on personality and obsessional illness. *Psychiatry and Neurology*, **150**: 299–305.
8. Kringlen E. (1965) Obsessional neurotics. *Br. J. Psychiatry*, **111**: 709–722.
9. Lo W.H. (1967) A follow-up study of obsessional neurotic in Hongkong Chinese. *Br. J. Psychiatry*, **113**, 823–832.
10. Fricke S., Moritz S., Andresen B., Hand I., Jacobsen D., Kloss M., Rufer M. (2003) Impact of personality disorders on treatment outcome in obsessive–compulsive disorders—Part II: results of an empirical study. *Verhaltenstherapie*, **13**: 172–182.
11. Moritz S., Fricke S., Jacobsen D., Kloss M., Wein C., Rufer M., Katenkamp B., Farhumand R., Hand I. (2004) Positive schizotypal symptoms predict treatment outcome in obsessive–compulsive disorder. *Behav. Res. Ther.*, **42**: 217–227.

6.7
Obsessive–Compulsive Personality Disorder: Personality or Disorder?

Gerald Nestadt and Mark Riddle[1]

The diagnosis of obsessive–compulsive personality disorder (OCPD) and its treatment has a long tradition in clinical psychiatry. In fact, the construct has remained relatively consistent both over time and across psychological orientation. However, as Costa *et al.* report, the diagnostic reliability and psychometric properties of the OCPD diagnostic category leave much to be desired. They propose that this disorder, and in particular its diagnosis, should be supplanted by a more reliable dimensional approach and suggest that the five-factor model (FFM) of normal personality is the most practical choice. They also suggest that the factor (i.e. dimension) conscientiousness (C) most closely approximates the OCPD construct.

The construct, proposed by Costa *et al.*, that OCPD is a dimension of normal personality that can adequately be represented by the FFM, is supported by a body of work that they review comprehensively. However, there are at least three alternate hypotheses that have yet to be excluded. OCPD could, as the DSM-IV describes, be a discrete category of personality pathology in which the defined criteria cluster together with greater specificity than any of the other personality disorder criteria; patients with this diagnosis would have a unique set of risk factors and outcome. Another possibility is that there are adverse personality characteristics that are dimensionally distributed in the population. Finally, OCPD may be an interpersonal feature of an axis I disorder, OCD, much in the way that schizotypal personality disorder and schizophrenia relate to one another.

[1] *Johns Hopkins Medical Institutions, Baltimore, MD, USA*

Costa *et al.*'s proposal provides the basis for a series of testable hypotheses, several of which are proposed in the review. A critical issue is, however, which external (independent/predictive) validating criteria are most suitable for this purpose. The ultimate test is the definition of a distinct and specific biology that underlies the construct and differentiates it from other like-constructs. In the absence of a gold standard of this sort, as with other disorders (Axis I or II), we must rely upon the accumulation of evidence from disparate sources such as specific risk factors, response to treatment, course, and outcome. This approach is complicated in the case of OCPD. If it is construed as a personality "disorder" (as in the DSM-IV), these criteria would or should apply. However, if, as Costa *et al.* propose (and we concur), OCPD is construed as a dimension distributed in a graded fashion throughout the population, then it is likely that its expression in the clinic, as well as its course and outcome, will be substantially influenced by additional (unrelated) factors such as personal circumstances and other psychopathology. Although this does not prevent study of the validity of the construct, it does require additional care be taken in research of this kind.

The functional outcome of OCPD may be an important example of this complexity. Costa *et al.* report evidence to the effect that OCPD is unrelated to Global Assessment of Functioning (GAF) score, a global measure of adaptive functioning. This is consistent with our own finding, in a general population sample, that a dimensional construal of OCPD did not predict a reduction of the GAF score 13–17 years later, in contradistinction to other personality disorder dimensions [1]. It is just such evidence that leads other researchers in the field (e.g. [2]) to conclude that compulsivity ought not be included in the personality disorder rubric, as it is an adaptive personality dimension, in contrast to the other primary personality disorder dimensions that they identify in factor analytic studies. However, Costa *et al.* are circumspect in this conclusion; they acknowledge that there may be specific areas of dysfunction that are more relevant to individuals with OCPD such as interpersonal relationships. It is also relevant that certain assets that accrue to the compulsive individuals, consequent on their personality style, may mitigate against certain outcomes. For example, the hard working compulsive individual may persist at work despite adversity, yet manifest emotional sequelae such as anxiety and depression. This is illustrated in a study we conducted [3] which found that compulsivity is related in a dose-response fashion to generalized anxiety disorder, whereas it is protective for alcohol use disorders (the latter was not significant, but suggestive).

Costa *et al.* state that "the lack of comorbidity with OCD is also consistently supported in the literature with a few exceptions". This is in such opposition to our own work that we must mention it. In a general population sample we found that the prevalence of obsessions and compulsions increased in a dose-response fashion with increasing compulsivity [4]. In the Hopkins OCD

Family Study we found that there was a considerably higher frequency of OCPD in the cases than controls [5]. More importantly, we found that the prevalence of OCPD was greater in the first degree relatives of cases than those of controls, suggesting that there is a familial relatedness of OCPD and OCD. Finally, we found that, among the relatives of OCD probands, the frequency of OCPD increased with increasing neuroticism scores, but this was not the case for relatives of control probands. This suggested to us that OCPD may, in some forms of OCD, be a clinical phenotype indicative of a vulnerability to OCD, possibly a subclinical form of the disorder.

In conclusion, the clinical observation, borne out over time, is that individuals presenting to clinicians often have this (OCPD) constellation of traits and behaviours; that these traits and behaviours often lead to specific difficulties in and of themselves (though not necessarily so); and that these traits and behaviours are frequently associated with other psychopathology. It remains to be established whether OCPD is best construed as an aspect of normal personality, a personality disorder, or a subclinical or associated feature of Axis I psychopathology.

REFERENCES

1. Hong J.P., Samuels J., Bienvenu O.J., Hsu F.C., Eaton W.W., Costa P.T., Nestadt G. (in press) The longitudinal relationship between personality disorder dimensions and subsequent global functioning in a community residing population. *Psychol. Med.*
2. Livesley W.J., Jang K.L., Vernon P.A. (1998) Phenotypic and genotypic structure of traits delineating personality disorder. *Arch. Gen. Psychiatry*, **55**: 941–948.
3. Nestadt G., Romanoski A.J., Samuels J.F., Folstein M.F., McHugh P.R. (1992) The relationship between personality and axis I disorders in the population: results from an epidemiological survey. *Am. J. Psychiatry*, **149**: 1228–1238.
4. Nestadt G., Samuels J.F., Romanoski A.J., Folstein M.F., McHugh P.R. (1994) Prevalence and correlates of obsessions and compulsions: results from a community survey. *Acta Psychiatr. Scand.*, **89**: 219–224.
5. Samuels J., Nestadt G., Bienvenu O.J., Costa P.T. Jr, Riddle M., Liang K.-Y., Hoehn-Saric R., Grados M.A., Cullen B. (2000) Personality disorders and normal personality dimensions in obsessive–compulsive disorder. Results from the Johns Hopkins OCD Family Study. *Br. J. Psychiatry*, **177**: 457–462.

6.8
Cognitive Therapy for the Perfectionism Dimension?
Jean Cottraux[1]

The review by Costa *et al.* describes in depth the move from psychoanalytic interpretations of obsessive–compulsive personality disorder (OCPD) to more reliable forms of conceptualization based upon experimental studies. They finely underline that OCPD is in continuity with "normal" personality, meaning that this type of personality is the more adapted to contemporary civilization. In the same vein, Oldham and Morris [1] contended humorously that OCPD was the "backbone of America", made of faithful husbands, reliable workers, scrupulous parents and overachievers.

One may also reflect on several early studies, published in Europe. Two studies, one from the UK [2] and one from France [3], have been carried out in so-called neurotic patients. The French study represents a replication of the British one. These two studies, using factorial analysis, demonstrated that anal character and obsessive–compulsive symptoms represented two orthogonal dimensions.

More recently, a review by Summerfeldt *et al.* [4] did not find any correlation between anal character and obsessive–compulsive symptoms in the vast majority of recent experimental studies. In contrast an anankastic cluster, including a constellation of traits such as incompleteness feelings, indecision, doubt and perfectionism, may be shared by obsessive–compulsive disorder (OCD) and OCPD. Several studies quoted by these authors demonstrated that doubt and indecision are not linked to anal character. These findings strongly support the concept of psychasthenia put forward a century ago by Janet [5], which was centred around the incompleteness feeling, doubt and abulia. They support also the concept of anankastic personality as described by the ICD-10. Hence, the DSM-IV could be criticized if one considers OCPD as the equivalent of the anal character, while the bulk of the British, French and American studies pointed to perfectionism (or psychasthenia) as being the dimension underlying OCD.

Costa *et al.* point out that cognitive therapy [6,7] seems more suitable for the treatment of OCPD than more traditional approaches as psychoanalysis. However, there is a dearth of hard data on its effectiveness. From a practical standpoint, cognitive therapy requires considerable resources. Trained therapists are required who can follow patients for one or two years. Such resources are not available everywhere. The main counterindication is the absence of motivation by the patient. One may also add the predominance

[1] *Anxiety Disorder Unit, Hôpital Neurologique, 59 bd. Pinel, 69394 Lyon, France*

of Axis I problems requiring immediate and proper treatment: for instance depression. Priorities have to be set with the patient. The clinical experience suggests that OCPD patients are requesting therapy because they are depressed after a negative life event. OCPD patients may suffer from depression whenever the basic schema of perfectionism is confronted to the "slings and arrows" that plague any overachieving person's life. On the other side, any cognitive therapist knows that in case of depression the basic unconditional schemas of the depressed patient are often about failure, perfectionism, and high and unreachable standards.

Validated instruments measuring self-schemas are available. Young's Schema Questionnaire (SQII), revised version [8] has been used to study the schematic structure in healthy individuals and personality disorders. A factor analysis yielded a three-factor solution [9]. The three factors were labelled loss of interpersonal relations (abandonment, abuse, emotional deprivation, mistrust, personal defectiveness, emotional inhibition, fear of losing control); social dependence (functional dependence, enmeshment, vulnerability, incompetence/inferiority); perfectionism (unrelenting standards, self-sacrifice). Insufficient self-control had high loadings on each of these three factors. Another study [10] replicated these findings.

From this point of view, one may expect that future cognitive therapy studies will show a correlation between OCPD improvement and the modification of the perfectionism factor measured by the SQII. An epidemiological study on OCPD as antecedent of depression could be also of great interest.

REFERENCES

1. Oldham J.M., Morris L.B (1990) *Personality Self-Portrait*. Bantam, New York.
2. Sandler J., Hazari A. (1960) The "obsessional": on the psychological classification of obsessional character traits and symptoms. *Br. J. Med. Psychol.*, **33**: 113–122.
3. Delay J., Pichot P., Perse J. (1962) Personnalité obsessionnelle et caractère dit obsessionnel. Etude clinique et psychométrique. *Revue de Psychologie Appliquée*, **12**: 233–262.
4. Summerfeldt L.J., Huta V., Swinson R.P. (1998) Personality and obsessive–compulsive disorder. In *Obsessive Compulsive Disorder: Theory, Research and Treatment* (Eds R. Swinson, M. Anthony, S. Rachman, M. Richter), pp. 79–119. Guilford, New York.
5. Janet P. (1903) *Les Obsessions et la Psychasthénie*. Alcan, Paris.
6. Beck A.T., Freeman A. (1990) *Cognitive Therapy of Personality Disorders*. Guilford, New York.
7. Cottraux J., Blackburn I.M. (1999) Cognitive therapy of personality disorder. In *Handbook of Personality Disorder* (Ed. J. Livesley), pp. 377–399. Guilford, New York.

8. Young J. (1994) *Cognitive Therapy for Personality Disorders: A Schema Focused Approach*. Professional Resource Exchange, Sarasota.
9. Schmidt N.B., Joiner T.E., Young J.E., Telch M.J. (1995) The schema questionnaire: investigation of psychometric properties and the hierarchical structure and measure of maladaptive schemas. *Cogn. Ther. Res.*, **19**: 295–321.
10. Lee C.W., Taylor G., Dunn J. (1999) Factor structure of the schema questionnaire in a large clinical sample. *Cogn. Ther. Res.*, **23**: 441–451.

6.9
Anankastic and Obsessive–Compulsive Personality Disorder in ICD-10 and DSM-IV-TR

Charles Pull and Marie-Claire Pull[1]

The basic positions on personality disorders (PDs) are almost identical in ICD-10 and DSM-IV-TR. Both systems adopt a categorical approach to PDs, the diagnostic process uses explicit descriptive criteria and algorithms for defining each PD, and both systems recommend the use of structured interview procedures for making diagnoses. The descriptions of the individual PDs are, however, not identical in ICD-10 and DSM-IV-TR. In their masterly review, Costa *et al.* focus on obsessive–compulsive PD as defined in DSM-IV-TR. In our comments, we will concentrate on the similarities as well as the differences between the descriptions provided for the individual PDs in ICD-10 and DSM-IV, and in particular on anankastic PD (ICD-10) and obsessive–compulsive PD (DSM-IV-TR).

In a recent article, we have published the results of a systematic comparison between the PDs in the two systems [1]. Major differences include: (a) the naming of several PDs, (b) the total number of criteria listed for each disorder as well as the minimum number of criteria required to make a diagnosis, and (c) the content of the individual criteria defining each disorder.

Differences in the naming of PDs include "dissocial" (ICD-10) versus "antisocial" (DSM-IV-TR), anxious (ICD-10) versus avoidant (DSM-IV-TR) and anankastic (ICD-10) versus obsessive–compulsive (DSM-IV-TR) PD. For the latter category, the labelling chosen in DSM-IV-TR suggests that there may be a systematic link between obsessive–compulsive disorder and obsessive–compulsive PD. There is no such suggestion in the term "anankastic" as proposed in ICD-10.

There are differences in the number of required criteria, and total number of criteria proposed, for a diagnosis of schizoid PD (4/9 in ICD-10 versus 4/7 in DSM-IV-TR); schizotypal disorder (4/7 in ICD-10) versus schizotypal PD (5/9 in DSM-IV-TR); dissocial/antisocial PD (3/6 in ICD-10 versus 4/7

[1] Department of Neurosciences, Centre Hospitalier de Luxembourg, 1210 Luxembourg, Luxembourg

in DSM-IV-TR); emotionally labile PD, borderline type (5/10 in ICD-10) versus borderline personality disorder (5/9 in DSM-IV-TR); histrionic PD (4/6 in ICD-10 versus 5/8 in DSM-IV-TR); anxious/avoidant PD (4/6 in ICD-10 versus 4/7 in DSM-IV-TR); and dependent PD (4/6 versus 5/7 in DSM-IV-TR). There are only two disorders for which the total number of criteria proposed for the diagnosis as well as the minimum number of criteria required to make a diagnosis are identical in ICD-10 and DSM-IV-TR: one is anankastic (ICD-10) or obsessive–compulsive PD (DSM-IV-TR) PD (4/8), the other paranoid PD (4/7).

There are many differences in the content of the individual criteria defining each PD in ICD-10 and DSM-IV-TR. There are major differences between the criteria for paranoid disorder (four of the criteria listed in ICD-10 are not listed in DSM-IV-TR, and four criteria listed in DSM-IV-TR are not listed in ICD-10); schizoid PD (although only one of the ICD-10 criteria is not listed in DSM-IV-TR, three of the DSM-IV-TR criteria are not listed in ICD-10); schizotypal disorder/schizotypal PD (three ICD-10 criteria are not listed in DSM-IV-TR and three DSM-IV-TR criteria are not listed in ICD-10); dissocial/antisocial PD (three ICD-10 criteria are not listed in DSM-IV-TR and three DSM-IV-TR criteria are not listed in ICD-10); anxious/avoidant PD (two ICD-10 criteria are not listed in DSM-IV-TR and three DSM-IV-TR criteria are not listed in ICD-10); dependent PD (two ICD-10 criteria are not listed in DSM-IV and four DSM-IV-TR criteria are not listed in ICD-10). There are also at least some differences between the two systems for the remaining disorders, i.e. emotionally labile PD, borderline type/borderline PD (two ICD-10 criteria are not listed in DSM-IV-TR and one of the DSM-IV-TR criteria is not listed in ICD-10) and histrionic PD (two of the DSM-IV-TR criteria are not listed in ICD-10). Concerning anankastic/obsessive–compulsive PD, two of the ICD-10 criteria for anankastic PD are not listed in DSM-IV-TR and two of the DSM-IV-TR criteria for obsessive–compulsive disorder are not listed in ICD-10. The two ICD-10 criteria not listed in DSM-IV-TR are "feelings of excessive doubt and caution" and "excessive pedantry and adherence to social conventions", and the two DSM-IV-TR criteria not listed in ICD-10 are "is unable to discard worn-out or worthless objects even when they have no sentimental value" and "adopts a miserly spending style toward both self and others, money is viewed as something to be hoarded for future catastrophes".

On the whole, and although the content of the criteria is not identical in ICD-10 and DSM-IV-TR, anankastic/obsessive–compulsive PD is among those PDs for which consensus is highest between the two systems.

While we do share the opinion expressed by Costa et al. that "most of the consistent evidence alludes to problems with obsessive–compulsive PD", we are less pessimistic with regard to the reliability and temporal stability of the various PDs in general, and with regard to the interrater reliability and temporal stability of anankastic/obsessive PD in particular. In 1992–1994, we participated in the International Pilot Study of Personality Disorders, a joint project sponsored by the World Health Organization and the Alcohol, Drug Abuse, and Mental Health Administration [2]. In this study, 716 patients were assessed in clinical facilities at 14 participating centres in 11 countries, using the International Personality Disorder Examination (IPDE). The IPDE demonstrated an interrater reliability and temporal stability for PDs (ICD-10 and DSM-III-R criteria) roughly similar to instruments used to diagnose the psychoses, mood, anxiety, and substance use disorders. In particular, the kappas used to measure the interrater agreement and temporal stability were 0.73 and 0.74 for anankastic PD (ICD-10), and 0.82 and 0.75 for obsessive–compulsive PD (DSM-III-R).

REFERENCES

1. Pull C.B., Pull M.C. (2002) Critères diagnostiques des troubles de la personnalité. In *Les Troubles de la Personnalité* (Eds A. Féline, J.D. Guelfi, P. Hardy), pp. 81–97. Flammarion, Paris.
2. Loranger A.W., Sartorius N., Andreoli A., Berger P., Buchheim P., Channaba-savanna S.M., Coid B., Dahl A., Diekstra R.F.W, Ferguson B. *et al.* (1994) The International Personality Disorder Examination. The World Health Organization/Alcohol, Drug Abuse, and Mental Health Administration International Pilot Study of Personality disorders. *Arch. Gen. Psychiatry*, **51**: 215–224.

6.10
Obsessive–Compulsive Personality Disorder: A Discrete Disorder?

Tom G. Bolwig[1]

Is obsessive–compulsive personality disorder (OCPD) a valid disorder, reflecting true psychopathology, or should it be considered a maladaptive problem in living? When comparing the DSM-IV and the ICD-10 definitions the agreement between the two systems is high and there is also a high correlation between the number of fulfilled criteria in each system. The main difference seems to be the emphasis of ICD-10 on "excessive doubt and caution". Regarding diagnostic agreement, a kappa coefficient of 0.79 between the two systems has been reported [1]. However, in studies on convergent and discriminant validity of the OCPD construct, the standard

[1] *Department of Psychiatry, Rigshospitalet, Copenhagen, Denmark*

cut-off of 0.70 for good interrater reliability and test-retest reliability is far from reached. Also hetero-method approaches versus mono-method approaches, as described in the Costa *et al.* review, yield meagre results of 0.10 and 0.43, respectively. Only the Collaborative Longitudinal Personality Disorder Study (CLPS) found that the first kappa was above the 0.70 threshold [2].

Another major problem is the co-occurrence of OCPD with Axis I disorders. This is particularly significant with major depression, but also with generalized anxiety disorder (GAD) and substance dependence/ abuse. Of particular interest is the relationship between obsessive– compulsive disorder (OCD) and OCPD, a relationship which was regarded as fundamental by early clinicians such as Janet, Freud and Kraepelin, who considered specific personality traits essential for the development of what today is called OCD. With the appearance of DSM-IV the likelihood of such a relationship was de-emphasised. Studies from before 1970 found up to 80% of patients with OCD having premorbid obsessional traits, but with standardized diagnostic instruments this co-occurrence dropped to below 45%. Several studies have shown that OCPD also occurs in many cases of OCD, yet it is in a minority. Further, it is of interest that among patients with anorexia nervosa (AN) an important co-occurrence with OCPD has been reported, and that among all personality disorders only OCPD seemed to predict the presence of eating disorder symptoms [3].

Another major problem related to the OCPD construct is its lack of temporal stability, a feature normally considered essential for the diagnosis of personality disorder. In the case of OCPD, one study showed that the stability of the diagnosis dropped from 60% at six months to a mere 42% at 12 months [4].

Since no epidemiological studies have pointed to a high prevalence of OCPD in community samples, the question of social impairment in OCPD becomes pertinent. As pointed out the Costa *et al.* review, people with OCPD rarely present for treatment unless there is a co-occurrent psychopathology (i.e. depression, panic disorder, AN) and Axis I disorders may either dominate or enhance certain features of OCPD, for instance perfectionism, raising problems for evaluation of this personality disorder. If OCPD does not produce functional impairment, it will be considered normal and maybe even valuable by the individual, who therefore does not suffer and may resist treatment, which in that case also seems questionable.

Costa *et al.* [5] emphasise the five factor model (FFM) as one possible dimensional approach to diagnosis of personality disorder. They base this emphasis on studies that look at the comparison of two sets of experts on the FFM domains and facets for OCPD. These two sets of experts observed interesting agreement on a number of items and this approach may perhaps make way for clinicians to blindly interview patients whose personality profiles match the OCPD consensus profile.

In spite of the many efforts so carefully described by Costa *et al.*, it still seems to be an unanswered question whether OCPD is a valid disorder or should be considered a maladaptive problem in living.

REFERENCES

1. Starcevic V., Bogojevic G., Kelin L. (1997) Diagnostic agreement between the DSM-IV and ICD-10-DCR personality disorders. *Psychopathology*, **30**: 328–334.
2. McGlashan T.H., Grilo C.M., Skodol A.E., Gunderson J.G., Shea M.T., Morey L.C., Zanarini M.C., Stout R.L. (2000) The collaborative longitudinal personality disorders study: baseline axis I/II and II/II diagnostic co-occurrence. *Acta Psychiatr. Scand.*, **102**: 256–264.
3. Zaider T., Johnson J., Cockell S. (2000) Psychiatric comorbidity associated with eating disorder symptomatology among adolescents in the community. *Int. J. Eat Disord.*, **28**: 58–67.
4. Shea M.T., Stout R., Gunderson J., Morey L.C., Grilo C.M., McGlashan T., Skodol A.E., Dolan-Sewell R., Dyck I., Zanarini M.C. *et al.* (2002) Short-term diagnostic stability of schizotypal, borderline, avoidant, and obsessive–compulsive personality disorders. *Am. J. Psychiatry*, **159**: 2036–2041.
5. Costa P.T., Widiger T.A. (Eds) (1994) *Personality Disorders and the Five Factor Model of Personality*. American Psychological Association, Washington.

6.11
Obsessive–Compulsive Personality Disorder or Negative Perfectionism?

Stefano Pallanti[1]

The term "obsessive–compulsive" (OC) has been overused in the last ten years, partly because the criterion of ego-dystonia is no longer used for the diagnosis of the obsessive–compulsive disorder (OCD) and partly because of the broad definition of the OCD spectrum [1], which includes a large number of disorders on the basis of both clinical and neurobiological similarities.

The OCD spectrum has been both a clinical point of reference, encouraging the use of selective serotonin reuptake inhibitors (SSRIs) for these supposedly related disorders, and a scientific concept which has stimulated research aimed at validation.

At the clinical level, comorbidity studies have been one of the means of verification of this "working hypothesis" and, as pointed out by Costa *et al.*,

[1] *Department of Neuroscience, University of Florence, Italy*

recent reports have shown a higher rate of obsessive–compulsive personality disorder (OCPD) in bipolar disorder than in OCD [2].

A core feature of OCPD is perfectionism [3]. Research data regarding the relationship between perfectionism and anxiety have provided little support to the notion of a unique relationship between OCPD and OCD: studies about perfectionism in anxiety disorders [4,5] have found few differences between OCD, panic disorder and social phobia. On the other hand, the impact of perfectionism has also been documented in depression [6] and bipolar disorder [7,8]. Specifically, it seems that the maladaptive evaluation aspects of perfectionism are associated with negative affectivity rather than anxiety per se [3].

Morality concern, preoccupation with order, scrupulosity and perfectionism are essential features of both Tellenbach's typus melancholicus [9] and OCPD, as well as of the prototype of the highly rewarded subjects belonging clinically to the area of the so-called "soft bipolar spectrum".

Specific dimensions of perfectionism have been candidates for empirical validation: perfectionism directed towards oneself, others, generalized beliefs and the entire world. The latter is a global concept that introduces specific irrational beliefs bridging the OC and the schizotypic area.

The interest of psychiatrists has focused only on "negative" perfectionism. In order to better understand the phenomenon, future research should include non-clinical samples and should not neglect "positive" perfectionism, in other words perfectionism that is not associated with social or interpersonal impairments.

In an unpublished study, we found that a diagnosis of OCPD was attributed to 40% of newly graduated physicians following assessment by the Structured Clinical Interview for DSM-IV (SCID), but without a true social or relational impairment [10]. Anecdotally, OC or perfectionistic personality features have been reported in leading scholars (e.g. A. Einstein, L. Wittgenstein, W.B. Yeats, L. Carroll, F.W. Taylor). This has been shown so conclusively that it calls into question the adoption of the OC terminology, implying the existence of a psychopathology, to describe them.

Two main conclusions may be drawn. The inclusion of OCPD amongst the OCD-related disorders, as a "semantic" consequence of its denomination, is questionable for at least two main reasons: first, because its pertinence has not been documented so far; and second, because in this way the term is restricted to the OC area, while the presence of this condition has to be assessed and targeted in several other disorders, particularly in the area of anxiety and mood disorder. For the time being, the adoption of a multidimensional construct—negative, maladaptive perfectionism—is advisable. This is specifically domain-oriented and could represent a target for empirical research and for behavioural and pharmacological intervention in mood, anxiety, eating and somatoform disorders.

468 PERSONALITY DISORDERS

REFERENCES

1. Hollander E. (1993) *Obsessive–compulsive and related disorders*. American Psychiatric Association, Washington.
2. Rossi A., Marinangeli M.G., Butti G., Scinto A., DiCicco L., Kalyvoka A., Petruzzi C. (2001) Personality disorders in bipolar and depressive disorders. *J. Affect. Dis.*, **65**: 3–8.
3. Flett G., Hewitt P.L. (2002) *Perfectionism: Theory, Research and Treatment*. American Psychologist Association, Washington.
4. Frost R.O., Steketee G. Perfectionism in obsessive–compulsive disorder patients. *Behav. Res. Ther.*, **35**: 291–296.
5. Antony M.M., Purdon C.L., Huta V., Swinson R.P. (1998) Dimensions of perfectionism across the anxiety disorders. *Behav. Res. Ther.*, **36**: 1143–1154.
6. Hewitt P.L., Flett G.L. (1991) Perfectionism in the self and social contexts: conceptualization, assessment, and association with psychopathology. *J. Person. Soc. Psychol.*, **60**: 456–470.
7. Scott J., Stanton B., Garland A., Ferrier I.N. (2000) Cognitive vulnerability in patients with bipolar disorder. *Psychol. Med.*, **30**: 467–472.
8. Scott J., Pope M. (2003) Cognitive styles in individuals with bipolar disorders. *Psychol. Med.*, **33**: 1081–1088.
9. Tellenbach H. (1967) Endogenicity as the cause of melancholia and of typus melancholicus. *Folia Psychiatr. Neurol. Jpn*, **21**: 241–249.
10. Pallanti S., Quercioli L., Giordani B., Sassi C. (1998) Personalità, temperamento e disturbo ossessivo-compulsivo. Presented at the 8th Congress of the Italian Society of Biological Psychiatry, Naples, September 29–October 3.

6.12
Obsessive–Compulsive Personality Disorder: Response to Pharmacological Treatment

Marc Ansseau[1]

The pharmacological treatment of obsessive–compulsive disorder (OCD) is currently well established and is based on antidepressants acting on the serotonergic system, such as the tricyclic clomipramine or selective serotonin reuptake inhibitors (SSRIs). In contrast, pharmacological agents are generally considered of negligible interest in the treatment of obsessive–compulsive personality disorder (OCPD). There are, however, several links between the two conditions. First, in the traditional psychoanalytic explanation of obsessional disorders, OCPD has been seen as a feature predisposing to OCD: according to this view, the two conditions exist side by side in a continuum, and persons with OCPD differ from those with OCD only in

[1] *Department of Psychiatry and Medical Psychology, University of Liège, CHU du Sart Tilman (B35), B-4000 Liège, Belgium*

that they are symptomatic. Second, most studies using standardized personality disorder assessment instruments found a relatively high co-occurrence of OCPD in patients with OCD [1]. Based on this possible relationship between OCPD and OCD, we hypothesized that OCPD could also be associated to some forms of serotonergic dysfunction and improved by serotonergic antidepressants.

In a pilot open study, we included 4 male outpatients with OCPD [2] without any significant depressive symptomatology. The subjects received fluvoxamine at the dose of 50 mg/day during the first week and 100 mg/day throughout the remainder of a 3-month study period. Initial and final assessments were performed by rating each of the nine features of DSM-III-R OCPD on a 5 point scale (0 = absent, 1 = mild, 2 = moderate, 3 = severe, 4 = very severe). All four patients completed the trial. The mean total score for OCPD features improved significantly during the study, from an initial score of 16.2 ± 2.9 to a final score of 11.7 ± 3.6 ($t = 7.0$, $p = 0.006$). The results of this preliminary open study supported a beneficial activity of SSRIs in OCPD. Therefore, we decided to validate this finding in a more controlled study.

In the second trial, 24 outpatients with OCPD without significant depressive symptomatology were randomly assigned to either fluvoxamine (50 mg/day during the first week, then 100 mg/day) ($n = 12$) or placebo ($n = 12$) in double-blind conditions. The duration of the study was 3 months. Initial and final assessments were performed by rating each of the eight features of DSM-IV OCPD on a 5 point scale as detailed above. Three patients did not complete the study, 2 in the fluvoxamine group and 1 in the placebo group. Changes over time in OCPD scores showed a significant superiority of fluvoxamine over placebo: from 18.6 to 13.7 in the fluvoxamine group vs from 18.5 to 17.7 in the placebo group ($t = 4.39$, $p = 0.0003$).

A case series of 8 children confirmed recently the benefical effect of SSRIs in OCPD. These children, characterized by an "obsessive difficult tempera-ment", improved significantly as a result of serotonergic medication [3].

These results therefore support a beneficial activity of SSRIs in OCPD. They favour the possibility that at least some elements of personality disturbances have a biological component. In the case of OCPD, serotonergic dysfunction could play a role. These findings should however be confirmed in further studies.

Based on the hypothesis that major depressive patients with an underlying OCPD preferentially exhibit a serotonergic depression and therefore respond better to a serotonergic antidepressant, we compared the outcome following 8 weeks of fluvoxamine (100–200 mg/day) of 22 major depressive outpatients exhibiting OCPD with 24 major depressive outpatients which did not exhibit more than one OCPD feature [4]. Results showed significantly better improvement of depressive symptomatology in the OCPD subgroup at the end of the treatment period, suggesting that a comorbid OCPD could be used as a predictive parameter in the treatment response of major depressive patients to serotonergic antidepressants. These results were confirmed in a study with 119 depressed outpatients, where a comorbid OCPD was associated with a greater chance of recovery [5].

Three studies have evaluated the influence of an underlying OCPD on the outcome of OCD patients following pharmacotherapy by serotonergic antidepressants. The first study used clomipramine [6]. Among a total sample of 54 patients, 10 (17%), exhibited a DSM-III compulsive personality disorder. This subgroup did not exhibit any significant correlation with outcome, measured by the Yale–Brown Obsessive–Compulsive Scale ($r = 0.11$) or the National Institute of Mental Health Global Improvement Scale ($r = 0.21$). In contrast, schizotypal personality disorder was found to be negatively related to outcome on both dependent variables; avoidant, borderline, and paranoid personality disorders were also negatively related to outcome on several variables. The second study used fluoxetine [7]. Among 67 patients, only 3 (4 %) exhibited a DSM-III compulsive personality disorder. Again, this subgroup was not significantly related to any of the outcome measures ($r = -0.18$ for the Yale–Brown Obsessive–Compulsive Scale and $r = 0.01$ for the Maudsley Obsessional Compulsive Inventory). Surprisingly, in this study, the presence of avoidant personality disorder was related to greater improvement on Yale–Brown Obsessive–Compulsive Scale. The third study was performed with clomipramine and fluvoxamine in 30 OCD patients [8]. At the end of a 10-week study, the presence of OCPD, along with the total number of personality disorders, predicted poorer outcome of pharmacological treatment.

In sum, the presence of an underlying obsessive–compulsive personality seems to represent a predictor of response to serotonergic antidepressants and possibly to antidepressants in general in major depressive patients. In contrast, a comorbid OCPD does not appear to be associated with a better response to serotonergic antidepressants in OCD and could even represent a negative predictor.

REFERENCES

1. Samuels J., Nestadt G., Bienvenu O., Costa P.T., Riddle M., Liang K., Hoehn-Saric R., Grados M., Cullen B. (2000) Personality disorders and normal personality dimensions in obsessive–compulsive disorder. *Br. J. Psychiatry*, **177**: 457–462.
2. Ansseau M., Troisfontaines B., Papart P., von Frenckell R. (1993) Compulsive personality and serotonergic drugs. *Eur. Neuropsychopharmacol.*, **3**: 288–289.
3. Garland E.J., Weiss M. (1996) Obsessive difficult temperament and first response to serotonergic medication. *J. Am. Acad. Child Adolesc. Psychiatry*, **35**: 916–920.

4. Ansseau M., Troisfontaines B., Papart P., von Frenckell R. (1991) Compulsive personality as predictor of response to serotoninergic antidepressants. *Br. Med. J.*, **303**: 760–761.
5. Hoencamp E., Haffmans P.M.J., Duivenvoorden H., Knegtering H., Dijken W.A. (1994) Predictors of (non-) response in depressed outpatients treated with a three-phase sequential medication strategy. *J. Affect. Disord.*, **31**: 235–246.
6. Baer L., Jenike M.A., Black D.W., Treece C., Rosenfeld R., Greist J. (1992) Effects of axis II diagnoses on treatment outcome with clomipramine in 55 patients with obsessive–compulsive disorder. *Arch. Gen. Psychiatry*, **49**: 862–866.
7. Baer L., Jenike M.A. (1990) Personality disorders in obsessive–compulsive disorder. In *Obsessive–Compulsive Disorders: Theory and Management*, 2nd edn (Eds M.A. Jenike, L. Baer, W.E. Minichiello) pp. 76–88. Year Book Medical Publishers, Littleton.
8. Cavedini P., Erzegovesi S., Ronchi P., Bellodi L. (1997) Predictive value of obsessive–compulsive personality disorder in antiobsessional pharmacological treatment. *Eur. Neuropsychopharmacol.*, **7**: 45–49.

6.13
Obsessive–Compulsive Personality Disorder: Relationship to Childhood Onset OCD and Diagnostic Stability

Per Hove Thomsen[1]

The concept of obsessive–compulsive personality disorder (OCPD) is still under intense debate. Its relationship to other personality disorders and Axis I disorders—in particular depression, dysthymia, obsessive–compulsive disorder (OCD) and eating disorders—and its diagnostic criteria have been the focus of attention for years.

Studies on OCD patients with onset of obsessions and compulsions in early childhood may contribute significantly to the understanding of the developmental aspects of OCD and OCPD. OCPD is not a necessary basis for the development of OCD, as shown by Mavissakalian *et al.* [1]. However, based on our clinical experience, we know that children who later develop OCD often show personality traits like conscientiousness, need for sameness, a tendency to feel guilty (even pathological), ambitiousness, self-criticism, and focus on details.

Do OCD patients with early onset—compared to OCD patients with later onset (i.e. late adolescence or adulthood)—have a higher prevalence of OCPD? Few studies actually concentrate on this issue [2]. In general, only very few studies on long-term course of OCD with childhood onset have been performed [3].

[1] *Psychiatric Hospital for Children and Adolescents, Harald Selmersvej 66, DK-8240 Risskov, Denmark*

One other problem with OCPD, as well as with other personality disorders, is that treating the often coexisting Axis I disorder (for instance OCD) will in some cases make the personality disorder disappear as well. So, what do we, in fact, measure when looking for personality traits (supposed to be stable) in patients with severe Axis I disorders? One explanation could be that personality traits may be accentuated by the Axis I disorder, thereby fulfilling diagnostic criteria for a personality disorder at evaluation. They could then decrease in intensity when the Axis I disorder is successfully treated. On the other hand, it should be taken into account that the diagnostic criteria for some personality disorders, such as OCPD, overlap with those of some axis I disorders (in the case of OCPD, in particular dysthymia, OCD, and eating disorders). Shea *et al.* [4] have questioned the stability over time of OCPD. They found a decrease over 6 and 12 months of the number of criteria met compared to baseline. However, they found a considerably high number of similar personality characteristics at follow-up.

In conclusion, more data are warranted on the long-term stability of the criteria defining OCPD (either from a categorical or a dimensional point of view). To what extent are personality traits sensitive to the influence of treatment or of changes in the life situation?

More studies on children are also needed. What characteristics or personality style predict later OCPD? These studies should be conducted longitudinally, to avoid recall bias, and they should be carried out in large samples. According to current diagnostic systems, the diagnosis of personality disorder should not be made in children. However, trained child psychiatrists are able to detect early manifestations of personality traits or style that can be predictors of later personality disorder. A more systematic, evidence based knowledge of this relationship is, however, needed. The inclusion of clinical populations may enable us to illustrate how different Axis I disorders influence the development of personality both in paediatric and adolescent patients.

REFERENCES

1. Mavissakalian M.R., Hamann M.S., Jones B. (1990) DSM-III personality disorders in obsessive–compulsive disorder: changes with treatment. *Compr. Psychiatry*, **31**: 432–437.
2. Pauls D.L., Alsobrook II J.P. (1999) The inheritance of obsessive–compulsive disorder. *Child Adolesc. Psychiatr. Clin. North Am.*, **8**: 481–496.
3. Skoog G., Skoog I. (1999) A 40-year follow-up of patients with obsessive–compulsive disorder. *Arch. Gen. Psychiatry*, **56**: 121–127.
4. Shea M.T., Stout R., Gunderson J., Morey L.C., Grilo C.M., McGlashan T., Skodol A.E., Dolan-Sewell R., Dyck I., Zanarini M.C. *et al.* (2002) Functional impairment in patients with schizotypal, borderline, avoidant, or obsessive–compulsive personality disorder. *Am. J. Psychiatry*, **159**: 276–283.

6.14
Figure and Background: Challenges in Trying to Understand Axis I and Axis II Interactions

Albina Rodrigues Torres[1]

Personality traits are dimensional constructs and it is quite difficult to draw lines between normal (adaptive) and abnormal traits, as well as between types of personality disorders (PDs) or PDs and "axis I" disorders. For practical reasons, arbitrary boundaries have been established in our categorical nosologies and, therefore, "comorbidity" is now the rule rather than the exception when we deal with personality psychopathology.

The differential diagnosis between psychiatric symptoms and personality traits is an important and complex issue, especially in chronic disorders with early age of onset, when the personality development occurs in the context of an already existing mental disorder. The phenomenological overlap is sometimes so remarkable that it is impossible (and even pointless) to differentiate symptoms from traits, as in social phobia and avoidant PD, probably just two different names for the same condition. In obsessive–compulsive disorder (OCD), whose onset also frequently occurs early in life, many longstanding personal characteristics initially considered personality traits simply vanish when appropriate and successful treatment is applied to the Axis I disorder [1].

Some current diagnostic criteria for obsessive–compulsive personality disorder (OCPD) overlap a great deal with OCD symptoms, as is the case, for example, of "difficulty in throwing away objects" and hoarding compulsions, "preoccupation with order and cleanliness" and contamination obsessions, washing and ordering rituals. Not to mention the problem of ICD-10 criteria, that include "intrusive thoughts" as a diagnostic criterion for anankastic personality. A central aspect here is the classic distinction based on the supposed egodistonicity of OCD symptoms versus the egosintonicity of OC personality traits. However, the patients' insight about their obsessive–compulsive (OC) symptoms is not a black and white phenomenon, but also a dimensional one, a continuum of degrees of insight varying considerably from patient to patient, and in the same patient, in different occasions [2]. Therefore, a distinction between OC symptoms and traits based solely on this criterion can be misleading. A possibly helpful difference comes from the cognitive perspective, that emphasizes the meaning behind the patients' actions: OCD sufferers overestimate risks and their own sense of responsibility, with all actions being taken in order to feel

---

[1] Departamento de Neurologia e Psiquiatria, Botucatu, Brazil

safer or to avoid being responsible for catastrophic events, even in a way considered unreasonable by themselves [3].

As clearly pointed by Costa *et al.*, despite the similarity in names, OCPD is not specifically related to OCD, occurring in many other clinical conditions, such as depressive and eating disorders. In fact, recent studies, using more reliable instruments of assessment, have shown that only a minority of OCD patients has comorbid OCPD, as currently conceptualized, with avoidant and dependent characteristics prevailing [4]. Indeed, in clinical practice we rarely see OCD patients that are inflexible, stubborn, assertive, hostile, stingy and cold. Most of them are inhibited, insecure, submissive, generous and caring, resembling the second type of personality style described in OCD by Lewis [5]. The latter characteristics are better captured by the current avoidant/dependent PD prototypes. As also emphasized by Costa *et al.*, the ever-changing diagnostic criteria and the different instruments of assessment are partially responsible for the low agreement between studies in this area. An additional problem is that persons with OCPD do not usually look for treatment, unless they have an associated Axis I disorder of any kind, due to the fact that, to some extent, anankastic traits are socially desirable. Of note is that antisocial PD is the only one whose essence is considered clearly opposite to OCPD, but it is included in the highly heterogeneous "obsessive–compulsive spectrum" group, while OCPD is not [6].

As expected, most psychiatric patients, including those with OCD, present a combination of abnormal traits belonging to more than one type of PD. The current prototypical model also adds to the diversity of presentations that are possible within each type and to the overlap of different PD categories, with several criteria being less specific to the construct.

Besides these difficulties in differential diagnoses, OCPD is frequently accompanied by some Axis I disorder and the determination of which condition (if any) is primary is still largely unsolved. Causal relationships are not easy to establish, but it seems reasonable to consider that a mutual and permanent interplay is likely to occur between symptoms and traits, each influencing the other. Only well-conducted longitudinal studies, taking into account stressful life events and response to treatment, can shed some light over this important question.

Understandably, Costa *et al.*'s comprehensive review only discusses psychological treatments for OCPD, not mentioning possible pharmacological interventions, which is another quite unexplored area of study not only for OCPD, but also for all PDs. I believe we should consider that personality traits could be changed not only by psychotherapy, but also by biological approaches.

Personality functioning is a relatively new area of study for psychiatrists. Therefore, we still have many challenges to face and a long way to go to improve the validity of the constructs, the instruments of assessment and the classifying systems in this area. A further step would be to better understand the influence of personality features on the development, presentation, treatment response and prognosis of our patients. Nevertheless, oversimplifications should be avoided in the approach to this important, fascinating and inevitably complex area of study.

REFERENCES

1. Ricciardi J.N., Baer L., Jenike M.A., Fischer S.C., Scholtz D., Buttolph L. (1992) Changes in DSM-III-R axis II diagnoses following treatment of obsessive–compulsive disorder. *Am. J. Psychiatry*, **149**: 829–831.
2. Kozak M.J., Foa E.B. (1994) Obsessions, overvalued ideas, and delusions in obsessive–compulsive disorder. *Behav. Res. Ther.*, **32**: 343–353.
3. Salkovskis P.M. (1985) Obsessional-compulsive problems: a cognitive behavioural analysis. *Behav. Res. Ther.*, **23**: 571–583.
4. Black D.W., Noyes R. (1997) Obsessive–compulsive disorder and axis II. *Int. Rev. Psychiatry*, **9**: 111–118.
5. Lewis A. (1935) Problems of obsessional illness. *Proc. Roy. Soc. Med.*, **29**: 325–336.
6. Hollander E., Wong C.M. (1995) Obsessive–compulsive spectrum disorders. *J. Clin. Psychiatry*, **56** (Suppl. 4): 3–6.

6.15
Obsessive–Compulsive Personality Disorder: The African Dilemmas

Frank G. Njenga, Anna N. Nguithi and Rachel N. Kangethe[1]

For several reasons, obsessive–compulsive personality disorder (OCPD) is of great interest to the African psychiatrist. Firstly, it is a very difficult concept to get across in most African languages, and any attempt to describe it as a clinical entity is met with the questions: "What is so unusual about that? What is wrong with checking things many times?" Costa *et al.* capture more than a linguistic dilemma when they state that "whether OCPD is a valid disorder, one that reflects true psychopathology or better conceptualized as a maladaptive problem in living" is one among a number of questions we can raise that await future research and clinical consensus.

[1] *Kenya Institute of Stress Management, P.O. Box 73749, City Square, Nairobi 00200, Kenya*

The second and related problem concerns concepts such as affective constriction and the inability to express warm and tender emotions. In a practical sense, the African must have a "reason" for lacking such feelings for his relatives. If he does not, this is not a matter for doctors but rather a matter for the family to find a solution. Only bad people can fail to have protective and warm feelings for members of their clan and family. It is a concept that defies description, in particular if conceptualized within a medical model.

Culture has a definite bearing on the presentation of the clinical features of OCPD. In this regard, Okasha [1] states: "We find that the religious nature of upbringing and education has a key role in OCPD presentation behaviour". African culture has a great deal of magical belief and ritualistic behaviour. For example, before consuming alcohol, the Mugikuyu from Kenya must pour some to the ground for the consumption of the ancestors. It could be said that this is an act of compulsion, as its omission would cause much distress to the drinker who would fear loss of favour with his gods [2].

Personality traits are indicative of personality disorder if they lead to functional impairment or distress. In this respect, extreme orderliness and perfectionism may be a cause of interpersonal conflict. The often quoted African cultural difficulty to keep time becomes a source of conflict if one spouse is "normal" in not having much regard for time keeping while the other is obsessed with it. By its very nature, African culture dictates flexibility in many such social situations, allowing great elasticity to family visiting time, frequency of visits, number of visitors, number of hours or days they stay and the number of people expected for meals. In a sense, the very things that give order to the West (a measure of obsessionality, perfectionism) are looked down upon as manifestations of meanness. A spouse could find himself in serious problems from in-laws who interpret orderliness and time keeping as a sign of lack of respect for them. A lady who insists on checking and rechecking that she has all cups, spoons and other household items would have serious problems with in-laws and even neighbours, for not trusting them.

Evidence of OCPD sometimes comes to the clinician during the management of a spouse who develops features of depression as a result of keeping up with the demands for perfection and order. In a home frequented by many children from the extended family, the mother is forced to keep tidying up after the "tribe" if she expects peace in the home.

In a continent where malaria, tuberculosis, measles and AIDS are real killers, the psychiatrist talking about OCPD would be allowed to feel a little out of place. In countries where the majority live on less than a dollar a day, the situation becomes almost unbearable, when one considers the traditional modes of psychotherapy, which are very expensive. To further complicate life, these patients who are often rigid, inflexible and who seek absolute clarity in everything would find it hard going to a busy rural African health centre.

The African experience holds out opportunities for the elucidation of the nature of the condition. That the condition is uncommon, as is anorexia nervosa, creates the opportunity to research possible aetiological or protective factors. The virtual absence of treatment opportunities enables observation of the condition in its natural state, in particular with respect to its co-morbidity with Axis I disorders.

REFERENCES

1. Okasha A. (2000) Diagnosis of obsessive–compulsive disorder: a review. In *Obsessive–Compulsive Disorder* (Eds M. Maj, N. Sartorius, A. Okasha, J. Zohar), pp. 1–19. Wiley, Chichester.
2. Kenyatta J. (1938) *Facing Mount Kenya*. Martin Secker & Warburg, London.

Epilogue. The Renaissance of the Ancient Concept of Temperament (with a Focus on Affective Temperaments)

Hagop S. Akiskal[1,2] and Kareen Akiskal[1]

[1]International Mood Center, La Jolla, CA, USA
[2]University of California at San Diego, La Jolla, and Veterans Administration Hospital, 3350 La Jolla Village Drive, San Diego, CA 92161, USA

INTRODUCTION

This chapter is an epilogue on personality disorders. At the same time, it is a prologue on temperament, which, after a long neglect, is now gaining momentum in world psychiatry. Because temperament has not been formally studied in adults to the same extent as its clinical and officially sanctioned counterpart of personality disorders, this chapter provides a relatively brief account of current research within this perspective as well as its potential for a new understanding of the origin of mental disorders. Following a few remarks on the general construct of temperament, we expand on affective personalities.

Classically defined, temperament refers to emotional reactivity patterns in normal individuals. Individuals with each of the "sanguine", "melancholic" and "choleric" types are characterized by bias in their respective emotional reactivity towards mirth, sadness and anger. The phlegmatic lacks such reactivity and as a result is emotionally cold: such individuals do not "move" others. In more modern times, Kretschmer [1] described a schizothymic "temperament", which is in some respects reminiscent of the Graeco-Roman phlegmatic type. He contrasted the schizothymic to the cyclothymic temperament, which subsumes the other three classical temperaments. Through common language usage, as well as Eysenck's work [2] substituting "neuroticism" for the emotionality of the cyclothymic, temperament has come today to denote the affective personalities. Curiously, in the

Personality Disorders. Edited by Mario Maj, Hagop S. Akiskal, Juan E. Mezzich and Ahmed Okasha.
©2005 John Wiley & Sons Ltd: ISBN 0-470-09036-7

DSM-IV [3] and ICD-10 [4], they are classified on Axis I as "attenuated" mood disorders! As a result, there is inconsistency in these manuals: while the putative premorbid self of schizophrenic patients is described in homologous language (e.g. schizotypal), mood disorders do not have Axis II constructs homologous to them. Instead, a bipolar patient may be described as avoidant and obsessive (rather than depressive), as histrionic/borderline (rather than cyclothymic), or as narcissistic and psychopathic (rather than hyperthymic).

The present chapter can be viewed as a general commentary on the previous six chapters on personality disorders which, to a large extent, have omitted the emerging literature on affective temperaments. As such, it can also be viewed as a critique of the concept of personality disorders. The inadequacies of categorical personality diagnoses à la DSM-IV and ICD-10 include the following: (a) they are inordinately state-dependent; (b) mix symptoms, behaviours and traits; (c) in practice, rarely use significant others as informants; (d) involve substantial heterogeneity (e.g. borderline); (e) produce high rates of subjects with multiple diagnoses; (f) confound temporal consistency with inflexibility; (g) exclude those with subthreshold level of traits; (h) pay little respect for the adaptive role of personality.

The ancient concept of temperament (a "mixture" of traits) is particularly useful because it features adaptive traits useful in some environments, but vulnerable in other circumstances. Temperaments may have evolved to give adaptive resilience to human populations facing difficult social challenges. Although each temperament does not represent a perfect mixture of traits to face all challenges, the population at large consisting of different temperaments is "balanced", and poised to face adaptive challenges to the group or the species at large.

The ancient Greeks, Kraepelin [5] and Kretschmer [1] envisaged temperament to be in continuum with full-blown mood disorders. We recognize this perspective today in the concept of "spectrum" [6,7] from subthreshold to full-blown clinical illness. The subthreshold mood disorders are not only in continuum with more pathological mood states, but they also provide a bridge with normal affective conditions. In this context, temperament, as a construct encompassing affective personalities, is currently enjoying a renaissance as one of the possible substrates for the origin of mood disorders [8].

It is a curious fact that most subthreshold affective conditions—such as dysthymia, generalized anxiety disorder, and cyclothymia—though symptomatologically attenuated, tend to pursue a chronic course. This raises the question, partially addressed in this chapter, that these conditions in their trait expressions might serve some useful function, even as they burden the individual with cares and instability which could predispose to full-blown affective disease. By their very chronicity, these subaffective conditions pose difficult conceptual and clinical questions about their differentiation from personality disorders. Sceptics might argue that subthreshold affective conditions are nothing more than "neuroticism". Actually, a close examination of the Eysenck Personality Inventory [2], which ranges over a large terrain of depressiveness, anxiousness, emotionality, and mood lability among others, reveals low-grade intermittent affective symptomatology. And at least one genetic investigation has reported that neuroticism and major depression in women share substantial genetic underpinnings [9]. These data and considerations underscore the conceptual and practical difficulties of separating affective traits from subthreshold lifelong affective conditions.

To summarize, temperament classically refers to an adaptive mixture of traits which, in the extreme, can lead to illness or modify the expression of superimposed affective states. This is a conceptually and practically useful system for both scientists and clinicians. We will focus now on the three affective temperaments about which good data exist to address the issues raised above.

THE DEPRESSIVE (OR MELANCHOLIC) TYPE

History

This type is represented in official nosology (ICD-10, DSM-IV) in its subdepressive expression under the rubric of "dysthymia". The term "dysthymia" ("bad mood") originated in ancient Greece and is still in current use in that country with the same connotation [10]. In the Hippocratic school, it was considered as part of the broader concept of melancholia ("black bile"). A temperament predisposed to melancholia was also delineated, and referred to individuals who were lethargic, brooding and insecure.

Although Kraepelin [5] avoided using the term "temperament", he nonetheless delineated the "depressive disposition" as one of the constitutional foundations of affective episodes. The condition often began early in life, such that by adolescence many showed an increased sensitivity to life's sorrows and disappointments: they were tormented by guilt, had little confidence in their abilities, and suffered from low energy. As they grew into adulthood, they experienced "life with its activity [as] a burden which they habitually [bore] with dutiful self-denial without being compensated by the pleasures of existence: in some, these temperamental peculiarities were so marked that they could be considered morbid without the appearance of more severe, delimited attacks...". Subsequently, Kurt Schneider [11], in his opus Psychopathic Personalities, devoted considerable space to a depressive type whose entire existence was entrenched in suffering. Similar concepts have also appeared in the more contemporary German [12] and Japanese literature [13], with particular emphasis on self-critical attitudes, persistence in work habits, and devotion to others.

Proposed Diagnostic Criteria

Building on the foregoing rich phenomenological tradition, our research in Memphis [14] helped in operationalizing the core characteristics of such individuals encountered in contemporary practice: gloomy, sombre, and incapable of having fun; brooding, self-critical, and guilt-prone; lack of confidence, low self-esteem, preoccupation with failure; pessimistic, easily discouraged; easy to tire, sluggish, and bound to routine; non-assertive, self-denying, and devoted; shy and sensitive. Although two US [15,16] and one Italian study [17] have shown good psychometric properties for the depressive personality construct, a Japanese study [18] found that its work-oriented more adaptive facet (the melancholic type) could be distinct from an interpersonally vulnerable type prone to fatigue (the depressive type). Furthermore, German [19] and Turkish [20] work suggests that depressive traits as defined above overlap with the cognitive traits of generalized anxiety. More research is needed to further standardize the depressive type.

Prevalence

In two studies with good standardization of the depressive type, both among clinically well students, the rate was 3.7% in Italy [17] and 4.7% in Germany [21]. Females predominated in both. Those data accord with the rates of dysthymia in the community [22].

Description and Delimitation

The depressive type invests whatever energy he or she possesses into work, leaving none for leisure or social activities. According to Tellenbach [12], such dedication to work represents an overcompensation against depressive disorganization. Kretschmer [1] had earlier suggested that such persons were the backbone of society, devoting their lives to jobs that require dependability and great attention to detail. These features represent the obsessoid facet of the depressive type. Such individuals may seek outpatient counselling and psychotherapy for what some clinicians might consider "existential depression": individuals who complain that their life lacks lustre, joy, and meaning. Others present clinically because of an intensification of their gloom to the level of clinical depression.

The proverbial depressive personality will often complain of having been "depressed since birth" [23]. In the eloquent words of Kurt Schneider [11], "they view themselves as belonging to an 'aristocracy of suffering'". These hyperbolic descriptions of suffering in the absence of more objective signs of depression earn such individuals the label of "characterological depression". The fluctuating subdepressive picture, that merges imperceptibly with the patient's habitual self, leads to the customary clinical uncertainty as to whether such individuals belong to the affective or personality disorder domains. This confusion is best depicted in the DSM-IV decision to list it under dysthymia on Axis I and depressive personality as a proposed Axis II disorder.

Individuals with the depressive type [24] may consult their doctors for more fluctuating complaints consisting of gloominess, lethargy, self-doubt, and lack of joie de vivre; they typically work hard, but do not enjoy their work; if married, they are deadlocked in bitter and unhappy marriages which lead neither to reconciliation nor separation; for them, their entire existence is a burden: they are satisfied with nothing, complain of everything, and brood about the uselessness of existence. As a result, in the past those who could afford it were condemned to the couch—for what often proved to be interminable analysis—to delve into the origins of their "masochistic character structure".

To recapitulate, for nearly 2500 years physicians have described individuals with a low-grade lifelong depressive profile marked by gloominess, pessimism, low enjoyment of life, relatively low drive, yet endowed with self-critical attitudes and suffering for others. This constellation is as much a *virtue* as it is a disposition to melancholy, and many such individuals presenting clinically with dysthymia have various admixtures of major depression. This is compatible with a spectrum-concept of depressive illness [25] diagrammed in Figure E.1.

The depressive type can be complicated by both depressive episodes giving rise to the double depressive pattern [26], as well as by mania (giving rise to dysphoric mania [27]).

Ethological Considerations

Sensitivity to suffering, a cardinal feature of the depressive temperament, represents an important attribute in a species like ours, where caring for young and sick individuals is necessary for survival [28]. This temperament, historically the *anlage* of dysthymia, in the extreme often leads to clinical depression. These people tend to be self-denying and devote themselves to others: family, institutions, helping professions. They feel in greatest equilibrium when in harmony with others, conforming to social

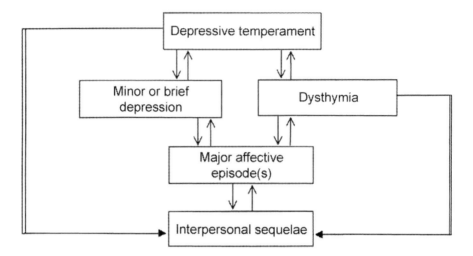

Figure E.1 Putative relationships within a broad depressive spectrum

norms and roles [29,30]. They develop clinical depression when unable to function in such roles, or when they lose them. A new study [31] sheds light on their assets and liabilities: the fact that the depressive type correlates positively with harm avoidance (+0.58) and negatively with novelty seeking (−0.10) suggests that their search for harmony and security in familiar, social and professional bonds is protective to a point; deficits in exploring the new would make their lives boring at best, and vulnerable to breakdown in situations of loss of the familiar. This type is predominant in females [17,21].

Therapeutic Aspects and Prognosis

Given the virtues of the depressive type documented above, Kurt Schneider [11] suggested that work was the best treatment for such individuals. Interpersonal psychotherapy [32] has also been proposed and, again, appears rational in light of the foregoing social-ethological formulation.

Extensive data [6] also support the contention idea that, when dysthymic, such individuals respond to the same type of psychopharmacotherapy as those with major depressive disorder.

Because depressive traits make their first appearance in juvenile years [33], identifying them at this early stage represents a special opportunity for prevention in child psychiatry and paediatrics.

THE CYCLOTHYMIC TYPE

History

Classical Greco-Roman psychological medicine did not include a cyclothymic type. Kraepelin [5] considered the cyclothymic disposition as one of the constitutional foundations from which manic-depressive illness arose. Kretschmer [1] went one step further and proposed that this constitution represented the core characteristic of the illness: some patients were more likely to oscillate in a sad direction, while others would more readily resonate with cheerful situations; these were merely viewed as variations in the cyclothymic oscillation between these two extremes. Kurt Schneider [11], who did not endorse the concept of "temperament", instead referred to "labile psychopaths" whose moods constantly moved in a dysphoric direction, and who bore no relationship to patients with manic-depressive psychosis. To confuse matters further, Schneider used the term "cyclothymia" as a synonym for manic-depressive illness. Today, "cyclothymia" is still sometimes used in this broader sense in Germanophone psychiatry. But in much of the rest of the world, cyclothymia (short for "cyclothymic disorder") is reserved for a form of extreme temperament related to bipolar disorder [34].

Cyclothymia, which in ICD-9 and DSM-II was subsumed under the affective personalities, was first introduced into DSM-III and DSM-IV and subsequently into ICD-10 as a form of attenuated chronic mood disorder. The diagnosis is not commonly made in clinical practice, because it is almost always seen when a patient presents with major depressive episodes, warranting the designation of "bipolar II" [14,28]. This usage conforms to Hecker's [35] historic description of cyclothymia.

Proposed Diagnostic Criteria

The criteria proposed by us [36] have been validated and standardized in the Pisa–San Diego study [37]. These are: lethargy alternating with eutonia; shaky self-esteem alternating between low self-confidence and overconfidence; decreased verbal output alternating with talkativeness; mental confusion alternating with sharpened and creative thinking; unexplained tearfulness alternating with excessive punning and jocularity; introverted self-absorption alternating with uninhibited people-seeking; hypersomnia alternating with decreased need for sleep; marked unevenness in quantity and quality of productivity-associated unusual working hours.

TABLE E.1   Prevalence of the cyclothymic temperament in different populations

Authors	Population (country)	Rates (%)
Akiskal *et al.* [34]	Mental health centre (USA)	10
Weissman and Myers [38]	Community (USA)	4
Depue *et al.* [39]	College students (USA)	6
Placidi *et al.* [17]	14–26-year-old students (Italy)	6
Erfurth *et al.* [21]	University students (Germany)	4.7

Prevalence

We found that 6.3% of a national cohort of 1010 mentally and physically healthy Italian students between the ages of 14 and 26 years of age [17] scored above two standard deviations for cyclothymia; this was more prevalent in females, with a ratio of 3:2. Such data testify to the fact that a cyclothymic disposition can be accurately measured and is prevalent. Table E.1 summarizes the rates of cyclothymia in different populations.

Description and Delimitation

By definition, individuals with cyclothymia report very short cycles of depression and hypomania that fail to meet the sustained duration criterion for these syndromes [14,34]. As such, they are distinct from rapid-cycling bipolar disorder. At various times, they exhibit the entire range of manifestations required for the diagnosis of depression and hypomania, but only for a few days at a time. These mini-cycles follow each other in an irregular fashion, often changing abruptly from one mood to another, with only rare interposition of "even" periods. The unpredictability of mood swings is a major source of distress for cyclothymes, as they do not know from moment to moment how they will feel. One subject described it as follows: "My moods swing like a pendulum, from one extreme to another". The rapid mood shifts, which undermine one's sense of self, may lead to the misleading diagnostic label of borderline personality. However, in the latter, mood swings are almost always dysphoric in nature. The mood swings of cyclothymes are biphasic and go beyond mere alternation between dysphoric and buoyant moods, involving eutonia alternating with anergic periods, people-seeking with self-absorption, sharpened thinking with mental paralysis, laconic speech with talkativeness; and low self-confidence with overconfidence.

The mood swings of cyclothymes can lead to major social maladjustments. At one time or another, labile angry or irritable moods are observed in virtually all [34]. However, these are not limited to the premenstrual phase in women. Unlike those with epilepsy, cyclothymes are aware of their "fits of anger", which lead to considerable personal and social embarrassment after they subside. They often feel "on edge, restless, and aimlessly driven"; family and friends report that during these periods patients seem inconsiderate and hostile toward people around them. The contribution of alcohol and sedative-hypnotic drugs to these moods cannot be denied, but the moods often occur in the absence of drugs.

The interpersonal costs of such unpredictable interpersonal explosiveness are often quite damaging. It is easy to understand how individuals with mercurial moods would charm others when in an expansive people-seeking mode, and rapidly alienate them when dysphoric. In effect, the life of many of these individuals is a tempestuous chain of intense but brief romantic liaisons [14], often with a series of unsuitable partners. These may alternate with sudden marriages, sometimes much above their social station (hypergamy). As expected, frequent marital separations, divorces, and sometimes remarriage to the same person occur. In the work arena, repeated and unpredictable shifts in work and study habits occur in most people with cyclothymia, giving rise to a dilettante biography [34]. Although some do better during their "high" periods, for others the occasional "even" periods are more conducive to meaningful work. It is sometimes unappreciated by clinicians inexperienced with bipolarity that "high periods" can be ones of disorganized and unpatterned busyness that could easily lead to a serious drop in *net* productivity. An alternating pattern of use of stimulants and sedatives further complicates the biographical instability of cyclothymes. Alternatively, the cyclothymic basis of mood swings in alcohol- or substance-abusing individuals can be documented by demonstrating mood swings before the onset of or well past the period of detoxification. In some cases, escalating mood instability makes its first appearance following abrupt drug or alcohol withdrawal.

Although cyclothymes are often confused with patients affected by adult attention-deficit/hyperactivity disorder (ADHD), their social warmth is a distinguishing characteristic. Furthermore, one-third of cyclothymes studied by us on a prospective basis [34] progressed to spontaneous affective episodes, predominantly evolving into hypomanias and clinical depression. Such switches were enhanced by antidepressants.

A larger National Institute of Mental Health study of patients with major depression who switched to bipolar II disorder during a prospective observation period of up to 11 years [40] found that a temperamental mix of "mood-labile", "energetic-active", and "daydreaming" traits (reminiscent of Kretschmer's concept of the cyclothymic temperament [1]) were the most specific predictors of such outcome.

Although cyclothymia can be sometimes complicated by full-blown manic-depressive illness, giving rise to mixed mania [27], it is more commonly associated with the bipolar II pattern (of recurrent major depression with self-limited hypomanias). In a French national study of patients with major depression [41], 88% of those with a cyclothymic disposition belonged to the bipolar II subtype.

The foregoing clinical and course characteristics suggest that a cyclothymic disposing to major depressive recurrences represents a distinct longitudinal pattern of "cyclothymic depression", which appears to capture the core features of bipolar II disorder in contemporary clinical practice [42]. Because hypomanic episodes cannot be easily ascertained by history, assessing cyclothymia in clinically depressed patients represents a more sensitive and specific approach to the diagnosis of bipolar II disorder [41].

Ethological Aspects

The flamboyant behaviour and the restless pursuit of romantic opportunities in cyclothymia suggest the hypothesis that its constituent traits may have evolved as a mechanism in sexual selection [28]. Even their creative bent in poetry, music, painting, or fashion design may have evolved to subserve such a mechanism.

Cyclothymic traits appear to lie on a polygenic continuum between excessive temperament and bipolar disorder. Indeed, clinically identified cyclothymes have patterns of familial affective illness, as one would expect for a *forme fruste* disorder [34].

Cyclothymia has also been observed in the juvenile offspring of bipolar probands [43]. Hypothetically, this temperament might represent one of the inherited trait diatheses for bipolar disorder. For instance, moody-temperamental individuals are over-represented in the "discordant" monozygotic co-twins of bipolar patients [44]. Alternatively, and in a more theoretical vein, bipolar illness might be the genetic reservoir for the desirable cyclothymic traits in the population at large [28]. These desirable traits, upheld in a recent study [31], correlated highly with novelty seeking (+0.49) and curiously positively with harm avoidance as well (+0.35). The latter might represent a "protective" break against dangerous levels of sensation seeking.

Therapeutic Considerations and Prognosis

Cyclothymes should be taught how to live with the extremes of their temperamental inclinations [45] and to seek professions where they determine the hours that they work. Marriage to a rich older spouse might sustain them for a while, but eventually interpersonal friction and sexual jealousy terminate such marriages. The artistically inclined among them should be encouraged to live in those parts of a city inhabited by artists and other intellectuals, where temperamental excesses are better tolerated. Ultimately, the decision to use mood stabilizers in such individuals should balance any benefits from decreased mood instability against the social and creative spurts that the cyclothymic disposition can bring to them.

Their clinical management represents a daunting task even for the psychiatrist who is willing to learn about the lifestyle of these individuals, not prejudging them by the more mundane norms of society. The psychiatrist should also be there to help them during the multiple crises of their lives. A low-dose atypical antipsychotic may temporarily help to diffuse such crises. It is only when a clinician has earned therapeutic alliance with a patient that the latter will permit limit-setting on his or her extravagant or outrageous behaviour. Parents might also benefit from some counselling, because the dilettante life of their children is often a source of great sorrow for them. Rarely, parents or spouses are rewarded by great artistic or intellectual achievement, which does not necessarily reduce the pain that the volatile cyclothymes bring to their loved ones. Kurt Schneider [11], writing about "labile psychopaths", admonished their kin "on their bad days... to keep out of their way as far as possible". Cyclothymes with some insight into their own temperament would give the same advice to their loved ones. A cautious trial of anticonvulsants [46,47] will often prove effective in those distressed enough by their behaviour to comply with such treatment.

The offspring of patients with bipolar disorder who exhibit a cyclothymic level of temperamental dysregulation represent a logical population for prevention studies. Molecular genetic testing will one day identify those moody individuals who carry the genes for bipolar disorder. At present, it would be useful to conservatively follow-up the cyclothymic offspring of people with bipolar disorders and provide them with psychoeducation about the necessity of avoiding stimulants and sleep deprivation. It may not be entirely possible to prohibit the use of moderate alcohol consumption, but benzodiazepines should be generally avoided. If they get depressed, it is important to protect them from the indiscriminate prescription of antidepressants, known to destabilize their moods further [14].

The topic of impulsive suicides in cyclothymes with superimposed major depression, well-documented by Rihmer et al. in Budapest [48], is beyond the limits of this chapter.

THE HYPERTHYMIC TYPE

History

Although well described by classical German psychiatrists (e.g. Schneider [11]), the hyperthymic type appears neither in DSM-IV nor in ICD-10. A lifelong disposition (hyperthymia) must be distinguished from short-lived hypomanic episodes. Indeed, it is best characterized as trait hypomania. It derives from the ancient Graeco-Roman "sanguine" temperament, believed to represent the optimal mixture of behavioural traits. They are full of zest, fun-loving, and prone to lechery: their habitual disposition is one of buoyant action orientation, extraverted people-seeking, overconfidence, and swift thinking.

They tend to drink alcohol, which can enhance their cheery disposition. Arataeus thought the combination could bring about mania [49].

The more adaptive, indeed "supernormal", attributes of individuals on the edge of mania have been given greater visibility in the modern psychiatric literature [14,50–53]. Typically short sleepers, hyperthymic individuals possess boundless energy to invest in sundry causes and projects, which often earn them leadership positions in the various professions and politics, yet their carefree attitudes and propensity for risk-taking can bring them to the brink of ruin; this is particularly true for their finances and sexual life, which can be marred by scandal. A hyperthymic lifestyle is so reinforcing that some of them resort to "augmenting" it with stimulants. In brief, while a hyperthymic temperament per se does not constitute affective pathology— indeed, it represents a constellation of adaptive traits—in excess it could lead to undesirable complications.

Proposed Diagnostic Criteria

Our most current diagnostic guidelines for a hyperthymic temperament, validated in the Pisa–San Diego [37] study, consist of the following traits on a habitual basis since at least early adulthood: cheerful, overoptimistic, or exuberant; extraverted and people-seeking, often to the point of being overinvolved or meddlesome; overtalkative, eloquent, and jocular; uninhibited, stimulus-seeking, and sexually-driven; vigorous, full of plans, improvident; overconfident, self-assured, and boastful attitudes that may reach grandiose proportions.

Prevalence

Extrapolating from studies on intermittent hypomania in the community [54]—i.e. strictly limited to subthreshold hypomania with early onset and persistent course—the prevalence of hyperthymic temperament has been estimated to be slightly under 1%. Eckblad and Chapman [55] reported a rate of 6% in a student population. The traits that constitute the hyperthymic profile are so desirable that normal individuals tend to endorse them. For instance, in a recent Pisa–San Diego collaborative study [17] involving 1010 students aged between 14 and 26 years, of whom 8.2% met the full criteria for hyperthymic temperament, all participants scored between the first and second positive standard deviation. Recent German work by Erfurth *et al.* [21] has succeeded in standardizing a self-report version, revealing a rate among university students of 2.1%. Thus, more work needs to be done on the psychometric standardization of this temperamental construct. On the other hand, all studies are consistent in showing marked male predominance.

Description and Delimitation

On the positive side, hyperthymic individuals are enterprising, ambitious and driven, often achieving considerable social and vocational prominence [51]. They are overrepresented among entertainers, business executives, self-made industrialists, politicians, high ranking military—indeed in all positions of leadership.

Abuse of stimulants is not so much an attempt to ward off depression and fatigue as an effort to enhance their already high-level drive and, sometimes, to further curtail their already reduced need for sleep. Hyperthymic individuals typically marry three or more times. Some, without entering into legally sanctioned matrimony, form three or more families in different cities; these men are capable of maintaining such relationships for long periods, testifying to their financial and personal resourcefulness, as well as their generosity towards their lovers and the offspring from such unions. Unlike the antisocial psychopath who is predatory on others and neglects or abuses his women and children, these men care for their loved ones [28]. But obviously such an "arrangement" involving women of different generations is complex, and a fertile soil for jealousy, drama, scandal, and tragedy. Nonetheless, it is not uncommon to see several women crying profusely and expressing their common grief at the funerals of these men!

Although individuals with hyperthymia optimally enjoy the advantage of their reduced need for sleep (giving more time and energy to invest in work and pleasure), some present clinically because of insomnia. Thus, in a predominantly male sample of executives presenting to a sleep centre [56], habitual sleep need was 4 to 5 hours; however, they had been intermittently bothered by "nervous energy" and difficulty falling asleep. Now, in late middle age, alcohol was no longer an effective hypnotic. Although they vigorously denied depressive and other mental symptoms (indeed, they had extremely low scores on self-rated depression), spouses or lovers provided collateral information about brief irritable-depressive dips, especially in the morning and, in some cases, more protracted "fatigue states" of days to weeks during which the subject would vegetate. Despite these depressive dips, these patients were distinguished from the constantly shifting moods of cyclothymic patients by the fact that the depressions arose from a baseline of trait hypomania of a more or less stable course.

A systematic retrospective review of the case records of people with manic-depressive illness whose course was dominated by manic episodes has been undertaken in Munich [29], yielding attributes overlapping with our proposed list: active, vivid, extraverted, verbally aggressive, self-assured, strong willed, engaged in self-employed professions, risk-taking, sensation-seeking, breaking social norms, spendthrift, and generous.

The hyperthymic temperament also emerged as the substrate for "classical" euphoric mania in the French Collaborative Study EPIMAN [27]. The fact that at least 10% of patients with major depression in an Italian study [57] could be characterized as premorbidly hyperthymic suggests that this temperament has relevance to both major affective poles. This is an important diagnostic consideration, because hyperthymia should be recognized as a genuine bipolar trait.

Ethological Aspects

Gardner's ethological analysis [52] of what constitutes "leadership" led to a description that overlaps with a hyperthymic profile: cheerfulness, joking, irrepressible infectious quality, unusual warmth, expansive, strong sense of confidence in one's abilities, scheming, robust, tireless, pushy, and meddlesome. Hypothetically, this temperament evolved in primates whose social life required leadership to better face challenges to the group, and its territory, from within and without.

Therapeutic Considerations and Prognosis

Little is known about the natural course of the hyperthymic temperament, except what can be reconstructed retrospectively from biographical and clinical studies [29]. Given their overoptimistic and self-assured style of thinking, these individuals feel perfectly fit in all areas of functioning and thus have no need to consult a psychiatrist. They do so only when forced by loved ones, e.g. when manic, depressed, or gravely addicted to alcohol or stimulant substances.

People with hyperthymia are action-oriented, and are not inclined to self-examination [28]. Furthermore, their hypertrophied sense of denial makes them poor candidates for psychotherapy. Alcohol consumption, which is common in these individuals, should not be abruptly interrupted because of the risk of the switch to a suicidal depression. If detoxification is necessary for health reasons, admission to a suitable inpatient facility should be arranged. The occasion might be profitably used for whatever counselling is deemed appropriate for life and health situations confronting them at the time.

It would appear that the hyperthymic's action-orientation without respite is deadly for the heart. They live intense but somewhat shorter lives. Their life can also be curtailed by physical risk-taking that may lead to accidents. Finally, they may kill themselves, during a depressive episode or on the threat of imminent scandal. It is likely that the mysterious suicides in many famous people, who seem to have everything, are due to such unrecognized factors.

The foregoing assets and liabilities of the hyperthymic type are best understood in light of a new study [31], where we found positive correlations between hyperthymia and novelty-seeking (0.34) and negative correlations between hyperthymia and harm-avoidance (-0.53). Thus, the action-oriented confident life style of the hyperthymic is vulnerable to lack of constraint from counterbalancing harm-avoidance.

PROPOSED LINKS BETWEEN THREE MAJOR SYSTEMS OF CLASSIFYING PERSONALITY AND ITS DISORDER

Table E.2 shows parallels between the system developed by Eysenck [2], DSM-IV [3] and Kurt Schneider [11]. Although Schneider did not use the term "temperament", his description of depressive and hyperthymic types coheres quite well with that of affective temperaments. While he did not include a cyclothymic type, his labile type significantly overlaps with the "irritable" [50] and dark [58] facet of cyclothymia. Such patients are often considered to be "borderline" [59,60]. We have defined an irritable type which has good psychometric properties [31], which will facilitate research in this complex interface. Interpersonal sensitivity [61,62] is another temperament dimension related to this affectively dysregulated realm [63]. At one level, they are subaffective disorders [64], but more complex in terms of psychic structure [65]. Further discussion of this topic is beyond the scope of this chapter.

DEVELOPMENT OF THE TEMPS-A

We have been using an interview-based diagnostic method for the affective personalities since 1975 [66]. During the last decade, interest in using our system was high among other clinicians and researchers. In particular, a self-

TABLE E.2 Comparison of Eysenck's concepts of temperament, DSM-IV Axis II and Schneider's system of classifying "psychopathic personalities"

Esyenck	DSM-IV	Schneider[a]
Extroversion	"Dramatic"	Explosive
	Antisocial	Affectionless
	Histrionic	Attention-seeking
	Narcissistic	Hyperthymic [?]
(+ neuroticism)	Borderline	Labile[b]
Psychoticism	"Eccentric"	
	Schizotypal	
	Paranoid	Fanatic
	Schizoid	
Neuroticism	"Anxious"	Asthenic
Introversion		
	Avoidant	Sensitive[c]
	Dependent	
	Compulsive	Insecure
	Depressive[d]	Depressive

[a]Although Schneider believed that his psychopathic personalities were unrelated to affective disorders, he provided excellent descriptions of what Kraepelin and Kretschmer considered as manic (hyperthymic) and depressive types.
[b] The labile psychopath is included in the Schedule for Affective Disorders and Schizophrenia as labile personality, which is in many ways similar to irritable cyclothymia in Kretschmer's system.
[c]The sensitive type in Schneider's schema does not have an equivalent on Axis II, but it is used under the concept of rejection sensitivity in the definition of atypical depression in DSM-IV. Actually Kretschmer used it as the personality of the self-referential "old-maid psychosis"; thus, it belongs to the psychoticism cluster. However, there is a great deal of data, beyond the scope of this chapter, to suggest that it is a transnosologic personality occurring in paranoid, obsessive–compulsive, social phobic, panic, bulimic, dysmorphophobic, and depressive disorders.
[d]Proposed for further study in the Appendix B of the DSM-IV.

rated version was needed to facilitate work by both groups of professionals. This led to the Semi-Structured Affective Temperament Interview (TEMPS-A) [31], whose short version is reproduced in Appendix 1, which has been translated into 10 languages: Italian, French, Portuguese, Greek, German, Danish, Hungarian, Turkish, Arabic and Japanese. We believe that this instrument will facilitate cross-talk between different systems of conceptualizing personality with the temperament perspective.

An unresolved issue in the classification of personality and temperament is the position of the cluster of anxious types [67,68]. The TEMPS-A measures only one of these, the anxious-worrying type [67]. Whether there exist distinct types of emotional reactivity along anxious and depressive lines is, according to Tyrer, to be answered in the negative [69]. Ultimately "neuroticism" may engulf most of the types described in this book, with the exception of the psychotic cluster and the affectionless antisocial. On the other hand, the Cloninger [70] and von Zerssen [71] systems are in their complexity unwieldy for practice but elegant in theory. The Five-Factor personality model [72], elegant too in theoretical and psychometric structure, presently appears more cogent for non-clinical populations. Kagan's work [73], though relevant to affective disorders, has curiously ignored the emerging literature on temperament reviewed in this chapter. Finally, terminological issues [74] as to what are "temperament", "character", "personality", and "personality disorder", continue to pose conceptual and methodological problems for the emerging field of personology [75].

In a more general vein, there may well not be one system that would meet all needs—e.g. practical diagnosis, definition of genetic endophenotypes, or utility in describing both normal and clinical subjects. The field of personology reflects the complexity of human nature. It is a fascinating emerging science, and the different perspectives described in this monograph reflect the different phenomenologic skills and measurement technologies required by this field.

REFERENCES

1. Kretschmer E. (1936) *Physique and Character*. Kegan Paul, Trench, Trubner, London.
2. Eysenck, H.E. (1987) The definition of personality disorders and the criteria appropriate for their description. *J. Person. Disord.*, **1**: 211–219.
3. American Psychiatric Association (1994) *Diagnostic and Statistical Manual of Mental Disorders*, 4th edn. American Psychiatric Association, Washington.
4. World Health Organization (1992) *The ICD-10 Classification of Mental and Behavioral Disorders*. World Health Organization, Geneva.
5. Kraepelin E. (1921) *Manic-depressive Insanity and Paranoia*. Livingstone, Edinburgh.
6. Akiskal H.S., Cassano G.B. (Eds) (1997) *Dysthymia and the Spectrum of Chronic Depressions*. Guilford, New York.
7. Akiskal H.S. (2002) The bipolar spectrum—the shaping of a new paradigm. *Curr. Psychiatry Rep.*, **4**: 1–3.
8. Akiskal H.S. (1996) The temperamental foundations of mood disorders. In *Interpersonal Factors in the Origin and Course of Affective Disorders* (Ed. C.H. Mundt), pp. 3–30. Gaskell, London.
9. Kendler K.S., Neale M.C., Kessler R.C., Heath A.C., Eaves L.J. (1993) A longitudinal twin study of personality and major depression in women. *Arch. Gen. Psychiatry*, **50**: 853–862.

10. Brieger P., Marneros A. (1997) Dysthymia and cyclothymia: historical origins and contemporary development. *J. Affect. Disord.*, **45**: 117–126.
11. Schneider K. (1958) *Psychopathic Personalities*. Thomas, Springfield.
12. Tellenbach H. (1980) *Melancholia*. Duquesne University Press, Pittsburgh.
13. Ueki H., Holzapfel C., Sakado K., Washino K., Inoue M., Ogawa N. (2004) Dimension of typus melancholicus on Kasahara's Inventory for the Melancholic Type Personality. *Psychopathology*, **37**: 53–58.
14. Akiskal H.S., Khani M.K., Scott-Strauss A. (1979) Cyclothymic temperamental disorders. *Psychiatr. Clin. North Am.*, **2**: 527–554.
15. Klein D.N. (1990) Depressive personality: reliability, validity, and relation to dysthymia. *J. Abnorm. Psychol.*, **99**: 412–421.
16. Gunderson J.G., Phillips K.A., Triebwasser J., Hirschfeld R.M. (1994) The Diagnostic Interview for Depressive Personality. *Am. J. Psychiatry*, **151**: 1300–1304.
17. Placidi G.F, Signoretta S., Liguori A., Gervasi R., Maremmani I., Akiskal H.S. (1998) The Semi-Structured Affective Temperament Interview (TEMPS-I): reliability and psychometric properties in 1010 14–26 year students. *J. Affect. Disord.*, **47**: 1–10.
18. Akiyama T., Tsuda H., Matsumoto S., Miyake Y., Kawamura Y., Akiskal K., Akiskal H.S. (in press) The proposed factor structure of temperament and personality in Japan: combining traits from TEMPS-A and MPT. *J. Affect. Disord.*
19. Erfurth A., Gerlach A.L., Hellweg I., Boenigk I., Michael N., Akiskal H.S. (in press) Studies on a German (Munster) version of the temperament autoquestionnaire TEMPS-A: construction and validation of the briefTEMPS-M. *J. Affect. Disord.*
20. Vahip S., Kesebir S., Alkan M., Yazic O., Akiskal K., Akiskal H. (in press) Affective temperaments in clinically-well subjects in Turkey: initial psychometric data on the TEMPS-A. *J. Affect. Disord.*
21. Erfurth A., Gerlach A.L., Michael N., Boenigh I., Hellweg I., Signoretta S., Akiskal K., Akiskal H.S. (in press) Distribution and gender effects of the subscales of a German version of the temperament autoquestionnaire brief-TEMPS-M in a university student population. *J. Affect. Disord.*
22. Weissman M.M., Leaf P.J., Bruce M.L., Florio L. (1988) The epidemiology of dysthymia in five communities: rates, risks, comorbidity, and treatment. *Am. J. Psychiatry*, **145**: 815–819.
23. Akiskal H.S. (1983) Dysthymic disorder: psychopathology of proposed chronic depressive subtypes. *Am. J. Psychiatry*, **140**: 11–20.
24. Akiskal H.S. (1996) Dysthymia as a temperamental variant of affective disorder. *Eur. Psychiatry*, **11** (Suppl. 3): 117s–122s.
25. Akiskal H.S. (1994) Dysthymia: clinical and external validity. *Acta Psychiatr. Scand.*, **89** (Suppl. 383): 19–23.
26. Keller M.B., Lavori P.W., Endicott J., Coryell W., Lerman G.L. (1983) Double depression: two-year follow-up. *Am. J. Psychiatry*, **140**: 689–694.
27. Akiskal H.S., Hantouche E.G., Bourgeois M.L., Azorin J.-M., Sechter D., Allilaire J.-F., Lancrenon S., Fraud J.-P., Châtenet-Duchêne L. (1998) Gender, temperament and the clinical picture in dysphoric mixed mania: findings from a French national study (EPIMAN). *J. Affect. Disord.*, **50**: 175–186.
28. Akiskal H.S. (2001) Dysthymia and cyclothymia in psychiatric practice a century after Kraepelin. *J. Affect. Disord.*, **62**: 17–31.
29. Possl J., von Zerssen D. (1990) A case history analysis of the "manic type" and the "melancholic type" of premorbid personality in affectively ill patients. *Eur. Arch. Psychiatry Neurol. Sci.*, **239**: 347–355.

30. Kraus A. (1996) Role performance, identity structure and psychosis in melancholic and manic-depressive patients. In *Interpersonal Factors in the Origin and Course of Affective Disorders* (Eds C. Mundt, M.J. Goldstein, K. Hahlweg, P. Fiedler), pp. 31–47. Royal College of Psychiatrists, London.

31. Akiskal H.S., Mendlowidz M.V., Girardin J.-L., Rapaport M.H., Kelsoe J.R., Gillin J.C., Smith T.L. (in press) TEMPS-A: validation of a short version of a self-rated instrument designed to measure variations in temperament. *J. Affect. Disord.*

32. Markowitz J.C. (1994) Psychotherapy of dysthymia. *Am. J. Psychiatry*, **151**: 1114–1121.

33. Kovacs M., Akiskal H.S., Gatsonis C., Parrone P.L. (1994) Childhood-onset dysthymic disorder: clinical features and prospective naturalistic outcome. *Arch. Gen. Psychiatry*, **51**: 365–374.

34. Akiskal H.S., Djenderedjian A.H., Rosenthal R.H., Khani M.K. (1977) Cyclothymic disorder: validating criteria for inclusion in the bipolar affective group. *Am. J. Psychiatry*, **134**: 1227–1233.

35. Koukopoulos A. (2003) Ewald Hecker's description of cyclothymia as a cyclical mood disorder: its relevance to the modern concept of bipolar II. *J. Affect. Disord.*, **73**: 199–205.

36. Akiskal H.S., Akiskal K. (1992) Cyclothymic, hyperthymic and depressive temperaments as subaffective variants of mood disorders. In *Annual Review of Psychiatry*, Vol. 11 (Eds A. Tasman, M.B. Riba), pp. 43–62. American Psychiatric Press, Washington.

37. Akiskal H.S., Placidi G.F., Signoretta S., Liguori A., Gervasi R., Maremmani I., Mallya G., Puzantian V.R. (1998) TEMPS-1. Delineating the most discriminant traits of cyclothymic, depressive, irritable and hyperthymic temperaments in a nonpatient population. *J. Affect. Disord.*, **51**: 7–19.

38. Weissman M.M., Myers J.K. (1978) Affective disorders in a US urban community, the use of research diagnostic criteria in an epidemiological survey. *Arch. Gen. Psychiatry*, **35**: 1304–1311.

39. Depue R.A., Slater J.F., Wolfstetter-Kausch H., Klein D., Goplerud E., Farr D. (1981) A behavioral paradigm for identifying persons at risk for bipolar depressive disorder: a conceptual framework and five validation studies. *J. Abnorm. Psychol.*, **90**: 381–437.

40. Akiskal H.S., Maser J.D., Zeller P., Endicott J., Coryell W., Keller M., Warshaw M., Clayton P., Goodwin F.K. (1995) Switching from "unipolar" to bipolar II: an 11-year prospective study of clinical and temperamental predictors in 559 patients. *Arch. Gen. Psychiatry*, **52**: 114–123.

41. Hantouche E.G., Akiskal H.S., Lancrenon S., Allilaire J.-F., Sechter D., Azorin J.-M., Bourgeois M., Fraud J.P., Chatenet-Duchene L. (1998) Systematic clinical methodology for validating bipolar-II disorder: data in midstream from a French national multisite study (EPIDEP). *J. Affect. Disord.*, **50**: 163–173.

42. Akiskal H.S. (1994) Dysthymic and cyclothymic depressions: Therapeutic considerations. *J. Clin. Psychiatry*, **55** (Suppl. 4): 46–52.

43. Akiskal H.S., Downs J., Jordan P., Watson S., Daugherty D., Pruitt D.B. (1985) Affective disorders in the referred children and younger siblings of manic-depressives: mode of onset and prospective course. *Arch. Gen. Psychiatry*, **42**: 996–1003.

44. Bertelsen A., Harvald B., Hauge M. (1977) A Danish twin study of manic-depressive disorders. *Br. J. Psychiatry*, **130**: 330–351.

45. Akiskal H.S. (2000) Dysthymia, cyclothymia and related chronic subthreshold mood disorders. In *New Oxford Textbook of Psychiatry* (Eds M. Gelder, J. Lopez-Ibor, N. Andreasen), pp. 736–749. Oxford University Press, London.

46. Deltito J. (1993) The effect of valproate on bipolar spectrum temperamental disorder. *J. Clin. Psychiatry*, **54**: 300–304.

47. Jacobsen P.M. (1993) Low-dose valproate: a new treatment for cyclothymia, mild rapid cycling disorders, and premenstrual syndrome. *J. Clin. Psychiatry*, **54**: 229–234.

48. Rihmer Z., Pestality P. (1999) Bipolar II disorder and suicidal behavior. *Psychiatr. Clin. North Am.*, **22**: 667–673.

49. Adams F. (Trans. and Ed.) (1856) *The Extant Works of Aretaeus, the Cappadocian.* Sydenham Society, London.

50. Akiskal H.S. (1992) Delineating irritable-choleric and hyperthymic temperaments as variants of cydothymia. *J. Person. Disord.*, **6**: 326–342.

51. Akiskal H.S., Akiskal K. (1988) Re-assessing the prevalence of bipolar disorders: clinical significance and artistic creativity. *Psychiatrie et Psychobiologie*, **3**: 29s–36s.

52. Gardner R. Jr (1982) Mechanisms in manic-depressive disorder: an evolutionary model. *Arch. Gen. Psychiatry*, **39**: 1436–1441.

53. Akhtar S. (1988) Hypomanic personality disorder. *Integr. Psychiatry*, **6**: 37–52.

54. Wicki W., Angst J. (1991) The Zurich study. X. Hypomania in a 28–30-year-old cohort. *Eur. Arch. Psychiatry Clin. Neurosci.*, **240**: 339–348.

55. Eckblad M., Chapman L.J. (1986) Development and validation of a scale for hypomanic personality. *J. Abnorm. Psychol.*, **95**: 214–222.

56. Akiskal H.S. (1984) Characterologic manifestations of affective disorders: Toward a new conceptualization. *Integr. Psychiatry*, **2**: 83–88.

57. Cassano G.B., Akiskal H.S., Savino M., Musetti L., Perugi G., Soriani A. (1992) Proposed subtypes of bipolar II and related disorders: with hypomanic episodes (or cyclothymia) and with hyperthymic temperament. *J. Affect. Disord.*, **26**: 127–140.

58. Akiskal H.S. Hantouche E.G., Allilaire J.-F. (2003) Bipolar II with and without cyclothymic temperament: "dark" and "sunny" expressions of soft bipolarity. *J. Affect. Disord.*, **73**: 49–57.

59. Stone M.H. (1980) *The Borderline Syndrome: Constitution, Personality and Adaptation.* McGraw-Hill, New York.

60. Coid J.W. (1993) An affective syndrome in psychopaths with borderline personality disorder? *Br. J. Psychiatry*, **162**: 641–650.

61. Boyce P., Parker G. (1989) Development of a scale to measure interpersonal sensitivity. *Aust. N. Zeal. J. Psychiatry*, **23**: 341–351.

62. Perugi G., Toni C., Travierso M.C., Akiskal H.S. (2003) The role of cyclothymia in atypical depression: toward a data-based reconceptualization of the borderline-bipolar II connection. *J. Affect. Disord.*, **73**: 87–98.

63. Akiskal H.S. (1981) Subaffective disorders: dysthymic, cyclothymic and bipolar II disorders in the 'borderline' realm. *Psychiatr. Clin. North Am.*, **4**: 25–46.

64. Herpertz S., Steinmeyer E.M., Sab H. (1998) On the conceptualisation of subaffective personality disorders. *Eur. Psychiatry*, **13**: 9–17.

65. Kernberg O.F. (1970) A psychoanalytic classification of character pathology. *J. Am. Psychoanal. Assoc.*, **18**: 800–822.

66. Akiskal H.S., Mallya G. (1987) Criteria for the "soft" bipolar spectrum: treatment implications. *Psychopharmacol. Bull.*, **23**: 68–73.

67. Akiskal H.S. (1998) Toward a definition of generalized anxiety disorder as an anxious temperament type. *Acta Psychiatr. Scand.*, **98** (Suppl. 393): 66–73.
68. Perugi G., Toni C., Benedetti A., Simonetti B., Musetti L., Akiskal H.S. (1998) Delineating a putative phobic-anxious temperament in 126 panic-agoraphobic patients: toward a rapprochement of European and US views. *J. Affect. Disord.*, **47**: 11–23.
69. Tyrer P. (1985) Neurosis divisible? *Lancet*, **1**: 685–688.
70. Cloninger C.R., Bayon C., Svrakic D.M. (1998) Measurement of temperament and character in mood disorders: a model of fundamental states as personality types. *J. Affect. Disord.*, **51**: 21–32.
71. Von Zerssen D. (2002) Development of an integrated model of personality, personality disorders and severe axis I disorders, with special reference to major affective disorders. *J. Affect. Disord.*, **68**: 143–158.
72. McCrae R.R., Costa P.T. Jr (2002) *Personality in Adulthood, Second Edition: A Five-Factor Theory Perspective.* Guilford, New York.
73. Kagan J., Snidman N., Arcus D., Reznick J.S. (1997) *Galen's Prophecy: Temperament in Human Nature.* Westview, Boulder.
74. von Zerssen D., Akiskal H.S. (1998) Personality factors in affective disorders: historical developments and current issues with special reference to the concepts of temperament and character. *J. Affect. Disord.*, **51**: 1–5.
75. Millon T. (1995) *Disorders of Personality: DSM-IV and Beyond*, 2nd edn. John Wiley & Sons, London.

APPENDIX 1. TEMPS-A SHORTENED VERSION [31][a]

We are interested in the kind of person you are. Please circle the following items only if they apply to you *for much of your life.*

1. My ability to think varies greatly from sharp to dull for no apparent reason.
2. I constantly switch between being lively and sluggish.
3. I get sudden shift in mood and energy.
4. The way I see things is sometimes vivid, but at other times lifeless.
5. My mood often changes for no reason.
6. I go back and forth between being outgoing and being withdrawn from others.
7. My moods and energy are either high or low, rarely in between.
8. I go back and forth between feeling overconfident and feeling unsure of myself.
9. My need for sleep varies a lot from just a few hours to more than 9 hours.

---

[a] Five factors: cyclothymic (1–12); depressive (13–20); irritable (21–28); hyperthymic (29–36); anxious-worrying (37–39).

10. I sometimes go to bed feeling great, and wake up in the morning feeling life is not worth living.
11. I can really like someone a lot, and then completely lose interest in them.
12. I am the kind of person who can be sad and happy at the same time.
13. People tell me I am unable to see the lighter side of things.
14. I'm the kind of person who doubts everything.
15. I am a very skeptical person.
16. I am by nature a dissatisfied person.
17. I'm a sad, unhappy person.
18. I think things often turn out for the worst.
19. I give up easily.
20. I complain a lot.
21. People tell me I blow up out of nowhere.
22. I can get so furious I could hurt someone.
23. I often get so mad that I will just trash everything.
24. When crossed, I could get into a fight.
25. When I disagree with someone, I can get into a heated argument.
26. When angry, I snap at people.
27. I am known to swear a lot.
28. I have been told that I become violent with just a few drinks.
29. I have a gift for speech, convincing and inspiring to others.
30. I often get many great ideas.
31. I love to tackle new projects, even if risky.
32. I like telling jokes, people tell me I'm humorous.
33. I have abilities and expertise in many fields.
34. I am totally comfortable even with people I hardly know.
35. I love to be with a lot of people.
36. I am the kind of person who likes to be the boss.
37. I am often fearful of someone in my family coming down with a serious disease.
38. I'm always thinking someone might break bad news to me about a family member.
39. When someone is late coming home, I fear they may have had an accident.

Index

Page numbers in *italic* indicate tables

Personality Disorders. Edited by Mario Maj, Hagop S. Akiskal, Juan E. Mezzich and Ahmed Okasha.
©2005 John Wiley & Sons Ltd: ISBN 0-470-09036-7

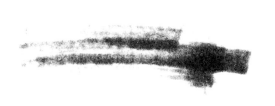